Hematology: Red Blood Cell Mechanisms and Clinical Implications

Hematology: Red Blood Cell Mechanisms and Clinical Implications

Editor: Chloe Thompson

AMERICAN
MEDICAL PUBLISHERS
www.americanmedicalpublishers.com

AMERICAN
MEDICAL PUBLISHERS
www.americanmedicalpublishers.com

Cataloging-in-Publication Data

Hematology : red blood cell mechanisms and clinical implications / edited by Chloe Thompson.
p. cm.
Includes bibliographical references and index.
ISBN 979-8-88740-176-8
1. Erythrocytes. 2. Blood cells. 3. Cells--Mechanical properties. 4. Blood--Diseases--Treatment.
5. Hematology. I. Thompson, Chloe.
RB45 .H46 2023
616.075 61--dc23

American Medical Publishers,
41 Flatbush Avenue,
1st Floor, New York,
NY 11217, USA

ISBN 979-8-88740-176-8 (Hardback)

Contents

Preface

Hematology is a branch of medical science concerned with the study of the blood and all components of blood. It also involves the diagnosis, treatment and prevention of diseases of blood, bone marrow, and immunologic and vascular systems. The red blood cells or erythrocytes are important cellular components of the blood. Their main function is to carry fresh oxygen from the lungs to the tissues. Carbon dioxide is removed from the body through the process of exhalation. The diseases related to red blood cells are caused due to a lack of iron or vitamins in the diet. Diseases of erythrocytes include several forms of anemia. It is a condition characterized by low count of healthy blood cells, which can transport adequate oxygen to different parts of the body. Major symptoms of anemia are tiredness, fast heart rate, pale skin, feeling cold, and in severe cases, heart failure. Some common forms of anemia are iron-deficiency anemia, sickle cell anemia, normocytic anemia, hemolytic anemia and fanconi anemia. This book unravels the recent studies in the field of hematology. It presents researches and studies on red blood cell mechanisms and clinical implications, performed by experts across the globe. Those in search of information to further their knowledge will be greatly assisted by this book.

All of the data presented henceforth, was collaborated in the wake of recent advancements in the field. The aim of this book is to present the diversified developments from across the globe in a comprehensible manner. The opinions expressed in each chapter belong solely to the contributing authors. Their interpretations of the topics are the integral part of this book, which I have carefully compiled for a better understanding of the readers.

At the end, I would like to thank all those who dedicated their time and efforts for the successful completion of this book. I also wish to convey my gratitude towards my friends and family who supported me at every step.

Editor

1

On the Mechanism of Human Red Blood Cell Longevity: Roles of Calcium, the Sodium Pump, PIEZO1 and Gardos Channels

Virgilio L. Lew and Teresa Tiffert**

Physiological Laboratory, Department of Physiology, Development and Neuroscience, University of Cambridge, Cambridge, United Kingdom

***Correspondence:**
Virgilio L. Lew
vll1@cam.ac.uk
Teresa Tiffert
jtt1000@cam.ac.uk

In a healthy adult, the transport of O_2 and CO_2 between lungs and tissues is performed by about $2 \cdot 10^{13}$ red blood cells, of which around $1.7 \cdot 10^{11}$ are renewed every day, a turnover resulting from an average circulatory lifespan of about 120 days. Cellular lifespan is the result of an evolutionary balance between the energy costs of maintaining cells in a fit functional state versus cell renewal. In this Review we examine how the set of passive and active membrane transporters of the mature red blood cells interact to maximize their circulatory longevity thus minimizing costs on expensive cell turnover. Red blood cell deformability is critical for optimal rheology and gas exchange functionality during capillary flow, best fulfilled when the volume of each human red blood cell is kept at a fraction of about 0.55–0.60 of the maximal spherical volume allowed by its membrane area, the optimal-volume-ratio range. The extent to which red blood cell volumes can be preserved within or near these narrow optimal-volume-ratio margins determines the potential for circulatory longevity. We show that the low cation permeability of red blood cells allows volume stability to be achieved with extraordinary cost-efficiency, favouring cell longevity over cell turnover. We suggest a mechanism by which the interplay of a declining sodium pump and two passive membrane transporters, the mechanosensitive PIEZO1 channel, a candidate mediator of P_{sickle} in sickle cells, and the Ca^{2+}-sensitive, K^+-selective Gardos channel, can implement red blood cell volume stability around the optimal-volume-ratio range, as required for extended circulatory longevity.

Keywords: human red blood cell, programmed senescence, calcium homeostasis, sodium pump, PIEZO1, Gardos channel, xerocytosis, erythrocyte longevity

INTRODUCTION

Human red blood cells (RBCs) have a prescribed lifespan of about 4 months before being cleared from the circulation. During this period, RBCs devoid of organelles and biosynthetic capacity experience irreversible age-related changes in metabolism, membrane transport, ionic composition, cortical cytoskeleton, and immune-reactivity, among others (Beutler, 1985b; Clark, 1988; Romero and Romero, 1999; Lew et al., 2007; Tiffert et al., 2007; Lutz, 2012; Franco et al., 2013; Lutz and Bogdanova, 2013). Nevertheless, under the microscope, the appearance of RBCs from healthy adults remains remarkably uniform, regardless of cell age. In narrow age-cohorts, the coefficient of variation in the haemoglobin concentration was found to be only about 3% (Lew et al., 1995). Such uniformity can only result from an erythroid production sequence that closely coordinates membrane area, volume, osmolyte, and haemoglobin contents in each cell, so that cells with larger areas also have larger volumes and haemoglobin contents, and vice versa. The mature RBC product is equipped with components capable of maintaining an extraordinary level of homogeneity in discoid appearance and haemoglobin concentration throughout a long circulatory lifespan (Svetina, 1982; Lew et al., 1995). That such manufacturing precision can be maintained by a bone marrow producing about $7 \cdot 10^9$ cells per hour in a normal adult is a truly remarkable feat of evolutionary bioautomation. And no less remarkable is the mechanism that enables the homeostatic stability of the RBCs throughout senescence. In this review we argue that maintenance of RBC longevity is driven primarily by the need to compensate for unavoidable reductions in sodium pump activity, which, if unchecked, would lead to cell swelling and early loss of the deformability required for normal capillary flow. We suggest that the need to maintain optimal circulatory performance has driven the evolution of a remarkably cost-efficient compensation strategy to preserve RBC volume and to extend RBC lifespan.

ON THE IMPORTANCE OF MAINTAINING RBC DISCOID SHAPE

Before considering *how* shape is maintained despite so much age-related change, let us try to answer *why*. Because selective pressures guide adaptive change to optimize function the answer must lie with the basic RBC function of mediating gas transfer between lungs and tissues. Gas exchange is a passive diffusional process that poses no direct metabolic demand, but requires a rheologically competent cell (Kaestner and Bogdanova, 2014). The discocyte shape allows RBCs to deform, fold, and squeeze against the endothelial walls of capillaries, exposing maximal surface area thus offering minimal diffusional distances for rapid O_2 and CO_2 exchanges across the capillary walls. Thus, maintenance of the discocyte shape is essential for preserving the optimal viability and functional capacity of the cells for an extended circulatory lifespan. In general, the basic requirement for optimal RBC rheology is maintenance of the cell volume substantially below the maximal spherical volume that can be accommodated by the membrane area of each cell. As stressed by Pivkin et al. (2016), the surface to volume ratio is by far the most important parameter of RBC deformability. In normal healthy human RBCs with favourable surface-volume ratios, rheology optimization is fulfilled by a discoid shape resulting from the biophysical properties of its membrane. In RBCs from other species the same optimization principles are fulfilled by a variety of other shapes, with different underlying cytoskeletal structures and biophysical properties (Cossins and Gibson, 1997).

RBC volumes are kept within 55–60% of their maximal spherical volumes. Let us call this the optimal volume ratio, or OVR. OVR is better known by its inverse, the critical haemolytic volume, which has values around 1.7 times the normal RBC volume (Ponder, 1948, 1950; Lew et al., 1995). With OVR values above 65% (swelling), and below 50% (dehydration), cell deformability and rheology become compromised, though by different mechanisms at each end (Secomb, 1987; Secomb and Hsu, 1995; Derganc et al., 2003; Fedosov et al., 2014a,b; Gompper and Fedosov, 2016; Lanotte et al., 2016). In this light, the discoid shape is simply the observable representation of OVR. Keeping RBC volumes within the physiological OVR range over such an extended circulatory longevity requires an extraordinary level of volume control, and this is where metabolic energy is invested.

KEY FEATURES OF VOLUME CONTROL IN HUMAN RBCS

Volume control in mature RBCs is entirely dependent on the combined function of a set of active and passive native membrane transporters (Garrahan and Glynn, 1967; Garrahan and Garay, 1974; Schatzmann, 1983; Rega and Garrahan, 1986; Carafoli, 1992). Maintenance of cellular homeostasis over extended periods of time, relying only on an assembly of native transporters unable to be repaired or replaced, represents an amazing evolutionary gamble. While ensuring cell stability under normal conditions, in inherited haematological disorders such as sickle cell disease (Lew and Bookchin, 2005), thalassaemia (Weatherall, 1997, 2004), or hereditary xerocytosis (Houston et al., 2011; Zarychanski et al., 2012; Andolfo et al., 2015; Alper, 2017; Fermo et al., 2017; Glogowska et al., 2017), altered membrane transport becomes a serious liability. In the following sections, the terms "permeability" and "leak" will be used to represent subsets of passive membrane transporters mediating the fluxes of the indicated substrates.

The volume stability of the highly water-permeable RBC depends on two key properties, a low permeability to cations, and a high permeability to neutral solutes such as glucose or urea. The low cation permeability severely rate-limits net salt and isoosmotic fluid transfer (Lew and Beaugé, 1979). The high neutral solute permeability allows rapid solute equilibration with minimal osmotic stress and volume displacement.

The most important evolutionary advantage associated with a low cation permeability is to allow volume control with negligible cost to RBC glycolytic metabolism and to the organism as a whole. The RBC ion leaks are balanced by two ATP-fuelled pumps, the sodium pump (ATP1) and the plasma membrane calcium pump (PMCA). The pump-leak turnover rate of Na^+ and K^+, of about 2–3 mmol/(L cells.h) in middle-age RBCs, representing mean population values, is sufficient to keep the Na^+ and K^+ concentration balance of the cells, and to offset the colloidosmotic swelling force of haemoglobin with minimal demand on glycolytic ATP production. The physiological pump-leak turnover rate of calcium in physiological conditions is about 20–50 μmol/(L cells.h; Lew et al., 1982), a rate three orders of magnitude below the Ca^{2+} extrusion capacity of a Ca^{2+}-saturated PMCA (Dagher and Lew, 1988; Lew et al., 2003). Thus, overall ATP turnover rates of about 1.0–2.0 mmol/(L cells.h) cover all the metabolic demands of normal, mature, middle-aged RBCs. In a healthy adult with a total red cell volume of ~2 L and a total body ATP turnover of ~5 mol/h, RBC ATP turnover contributes a negligible 0.04–0.06% to the total. This makes the low cation permeability of RBCs a most economical and efficient determinant of volume stability and preserved functional competence, enabling the evolution of a gas-carrier cell devoid of encumbering energy producing, and consuming structures and with a long circulatory lifespan. This is a general strategy, followed in many species, with substantial variations in the nature of the membrane transporters involved (Parker, 1973, 1978).

A FAILING SODIUM PUMP PRESENTS THE MAJOR CHALLENGE TO RBC LONGEVITY

An extended RBC lifespan is a major saver in expensive cell manufacture and turnover, and hence a powerful selective drive for cell preservation over replacement (Beutler, 1985a,b, 1986). In this light, the best recipe for extended RBC longevity would be maintenance of a constant volume and density within the OVR range. However, lack of biosynthetic capacity and protein renewal makes RBC volume stability vulnerable to cumulative damage of the enzymes and transporters involved in its control. Despite the robust antioxidant machinery of RBCs (Arese et al., 2005; Lutz, 2012; Lutz and Bogdanova, 2013), cumulative effects of non-enzymic oxidation, glycation, and of other processes, unavoidably alter protein structure and function (Beutler, 1985a,b, 1986; Gonzalez Flecha et al., 1999; Raftos et al., 2001; Keller et al., 2015; Piedrafita et al., 2015). Let us consider first the specific age-related changes relevant to volume control, and then the nature of the adaptive changes critical for extending the flow viability of aging RBCs.

Of the many documented changes observed in aging RBCs, those most threatening to volume stability are the gradual reduction in the activity of the sodium pump, and the progressive decline in glycolysis and ATP levels. From the vast body of experimental work in many different laboratories over the last six decades, the following essential facts emerge with uncontroversial consistency: (i) the number of sodium pumps per cell, estimated by ^{3}H-Ouabain binding, declines with RBC age by up to 70%; (ii) in aging RBCs the trans-membrane gradients of Na^+ and K^+ decline steadily, with increased Na^+ and decreased K^+ contents, all within relatively small variations in total $[Na^+] + [K^+]$; and (iii), ATP levels fall by up to 40% in aging RBCs (Cohen et al., 1976, 2008; Joiner and Lauf, 1978; Magnani et al., 1983; Cheng et al., 1984; Clark, 1988; Lew et al., 2007; Franco et al., 2013; Lutz and Bogdanova, 2013).

Dramatic changes were also documented in the activity of other transport-mediated processes, in particular the reductions in calcium pump and Gardos channels activity. However, Ca^{2+} extrusion and Gardos channel-mediated K^+ transport are hardly affected because of the huge native spare capacities of these transporters (Garcia-Sancho and Lew, 1988; Romero and Romero, 1997, 1999; Lew et al., 2003, 2007; Tiffert et al., 2007). Thus, the main focus for the need of volume control remains with the Na pump.

Decline in Na pump activity on its own would lead to a slow dissipation of the sodium and potassium gradients with a net gain of NaCl in excess of KCl loss, cell swelling and density decrease. The important issue to note here is that when RBCs start circulatory life, transiting from reticulocyte to mature RBC, their volume is at or just above the upper limit of the OVR (Rapoport, 1986). Therefore, any uncompensated decline in sodium pump activity, whatever its rate, would lead to increases in RBC volume, placing the volume ratio further above its optimal range and increasingly compromising rheology and gas exchange functionality with time, more so the higher the rate of pump inactivation. Thus, balancing the inevitable decline in sodium pump activity in order to keep the cells within safe OVR ranges would seem to offer the best conditions for RBC longevity to evolve.

THE AGE-DENSITY PATTERN

Instead of swelling, as predicted by uncompensated Na pump decline, mature RBCs shrink gradually with age. This was ascertained long ago by following the distribution of ^{59}Fe-labelled heme in layers of density-fractionated RBCs after a single intravenous injection of the isotope (Borun et al., 1957; Beutler, 1986; Clark, 1988). These experiments documented the senescence pattern of human RBCs, determined its duration, and established density separation as the method of choice to explore age-related changes in human RBC properties. However, a minor twist in this story has been systematically overlooked. When the ^{59}Fe activity ratios between top and bottom cell-density layers were monitored for up to 200 days following tracer injections, the ratios were seen to decline steadily, at variable rates in different subjects, up to day 70. But then, between days 70 and 120 the ratios changed direction suggesting a terminal density reversal (Borun et al., 1957). A minor part of this density reversal could be attributed to reutilization of diluted tracer, as discussed by Clark (1988), but most of it reflects a genuine and gradual reduction in the density of RBCs before their immune clearance from the circulation (Kay, 1975; Lutz et al., 1987; Lutz and Bogdanova, 2013), a view also supported by recent additional evidence (Bookchin et al., 2000; Franco et al., 2013; Lew and Tiffert, 2013). Explanation of this age-density pattern requires consideration of the transport processes involved in the control of RBC homeostasis.

MECHANISMS OF AGE-RELATED RBC DENSIFICATION AND TERMINAL REVERSAL

Two passive transporters of human RBCs deserve special attention: PIEZO1, a mechanosensitive ion channel (Zarychanski et al., 2012; Andolfo et al., 2013; Shmukler et al., 2014; Cinar et al., 2015; Kaestner, 2015; Alper, 2017; Glogowska et al., 2017), and the Ca^{2+}-sensitive, K^+-selective Gardos channel

(KCNN4) (Gardos, 1958; Lew and Ferreira, 1978; Ghanshani et al., 1998; Hoffman et al., 2003; Gottlieb et al., 2012; Gnanasambandam et al., 2015; Fermo et al., 2017; Rivera et al., 2017). PIEZO1 mutations were found to be responsible for marked RBC dehydration in hereditary xerocytosis (HX), a clinically heterogeneous family of congenital haemolytic anaemias. Detailed studies revealed that mutant channels exhibited a number of kinetic abnormalities relative to wild-type channels of which the most prominent was a marginally reduced inactivation kinetics following brief stretch-activation pulses (Bae et al., 2013). If a relatively small inactivation delay can lead to such a profound dehydration in RBCs from HX subjects (Glogowska et al., 2017), the wild-type channel may be expected to contribute to the progressive dehydration of normal RBCs over periods of weeks in the circulation. Moreover, in mice with specific deletion of PIEZO1 from the haematopietic system the RBCs were found to become over-hydrated just as expected from the removal of a transport pathway involved in a volume-balancing dehydration chain (Cahalan et al., 2015).

In addition, whole-cell patch-clamp recordings of normal human RBCs showed that brief suction pulses through the patch pipette elicited a Ca^{2+} influx sufficient to activate secondary currents through Gardos channels (Dyrda et al., 2010), well within the response expected from a brief and sharp increase in Ca^{2+} permeability through stretch-activated PIEZO1 channels in the microcirculation. This experimental condition is reminiscent of the one generated in sickled cells, where the same topology of membrane deformation is generated from inside the cells by protruding polymers of deoxy-haemoglobin S. In sickle cells, consecutive deoxygenation episodes triggered reversible increases in the calcium permeability of all the RBCs, but the dehydration response via Gardos channels proved to be a stochastic phenomenon in the RBC population (Lew et al., 1997). The deoxy-induced increase in permeability was named P_{sickle}. In cell-attached patch clamp recordings from sickle RBCs (Vandorpe et al., 2010), deoxygenation-induced P_{sickle} was found to be inhibited by GsMTx4, a specific inhibitor of mechanosensitive channels (Ostrow et al., 2003; Bae et al., 2011). In normal RBCs, the release of ATP under physiological levels of shear was shown to depend on the presence of external calcium and was also inhibited by GsMTx4, supporting the view that PIEZO1 mediates Ca^{2+} influx under normal circulatory shear stress (Larsen et al., 1981; Cinar et al., 2015).

Based on these considerations, PIEZO1 appears as a prime candidate for the mediation of RBC densification in normal RBC senescence, and also as the channel responsible for P_{sickle}, a key participant in the mechanism of sickle cell dehydration (Lew and Bookchin, 2005). It is the mechanical gating of this channel that makes PIEZO1 such a good candidate for translating stretch-induced circulatory RBC deformations into micro-dehydration events in normal senescence, and for polymer-induced membrane protrusions into P_{sickle} in sickle cells.

How would PIEZO1 lead to the dehydration of senescent RBCs? Because of its poor ion selectivity (Gnanasambandam et al., 2015), PIEZO1 activation would in principle contribute to general ion gradient dissipation. While minimal for Na^+, K^+, and Mg^{2+} with each brief PIEZO1 opening, the steep inward electrochemical gradient of Ca^{2+} would be expected to generate a transient peak of elevated $[Ca^{2+}]_i$. A significant proportion of such peaks may reach $[Ca^{2+}]_i$ levels activatory to Gardos channels, as with stochastic P_{sickle}, with cumulative downstream effects of selective KCl loss in excess of NaCl gains, leading to progressive and generalized cell dehydration and densification.

Participation of Gardos channels in the age-dependent densification of human RBCs has been suggested many times in the past. The required $[Ca^{2+}]_i$ elevations were attributed mostly to progressive PMCA weakness, aided by increases in Ca^{2+} permeability through undefined pathways. Given the large spare capacity of the PMCA it is difficult to estimate its real contribution. A weakening calcium pump may increase the frequency with which PIEZO1 generates Ca^{2+} peaks high enough to activate Gardos-channels, and also extend the duration of their active state by delayed Ca^{2+} extrusion (Dyrda et al., 2010).

ON THE MECHANISM OF PROGRAMMED SENESCENCE

The picture emerging from these considerations outlines a sequence of transport and homeostatic changes aimed at preserving the volume of aging RBCs within a narrow OVR range for as long as energy from fading metabolism, weakening sodium pumps, and enfeebled cation gradients can be sustained. An outline consistent with current knowledge suggests that the swelling tendency resulting from the declining activity of the sodium pump is opposed by net KCl and fluid losses resulting from periodic Gardos channel activation during capillary passages, elicited by brief surges in cell calcium via stretch-activated PIEZO1channels. The long-term cumulative effects of these opposing transport-mediated processes are a progressive dissipation of the sodium and potassium gradients, and a balanced volume control with a marginal, not functionally compromising increase in cell density for most of the lifespan of the cells. At some advanced stage, variable in RBCs from different subjects, sodium pump weakness and potassium gradient dissipation reach levels that can no longer prevent sustained net NaCl gains and RBC rehydration. This causes the densification trend to reverse and RBCs to swell, somehow signalling for terminal removal along the way (Kay, 1975; Beutler, 1986; Lutz and Bogdanova, 2013). In this light, terminal density reversal appears as a way of prolonging RBC longevity in a fit functional state within the OVR range, an opportunistic lifespan extension enabled by the preceding densification period. Thus, RBCs appear planned by evolution to last for as long as fit to function, not for obsolescence (Beutler, 1986).

This narrative outlines a hypothesis for the evolution and mechanism of the extended longevity of human RBCs consistent with current knowledge. At proof stage, a paper was published providing powerful new evidence in support of the mechanism hypothesized here. Kuchel and Shishmarev (2017) combined nuclear magnetic resonance spectroscopy measurements of ^{13}C signals of lactate production and of ^{133}Cs signals of K^+ congener fluxes with a most elegant experimental design in which RBCs embedded in gelatin gels of varied compositions could be exposed to reversible deformation protocols. Their results showed a clear calcium-dependent link between mechanical deformations, increased lactate production and increased Cs(K) fluxes. Additional experiments with the PIEZO1 activator yoda1 and PIEZO1 inhibitor GsMTx4 unambiguously identified PIEZO1 as the mediator of the deformation effects, starting with PIEZO1 activation allowing down-gradient Ca^{2+} influx. The ensuing $[Ca^{2+}]_i$ elevation stimulates PMCA activity with downstream lactate production, and activates Gardos channels increasing net Cs(K)-salt efflux and fluid loss. This is the same sequence suggested to participate in myriad micro-quantal deformation events in the capillary circulation as part of the hypothesized OVR control mechanism of RBC longevity.

AUTHOR CONTRIBUTIONS

All authors listed have made a substantial, direct and intellectual contribution to the work, and approved it for publication.

ACKNOWLEDGMENTS

We thank Daniel J. Lew for helpful discussions and insightful comments.

REFERENCES

Alper, S. L. (2017). Genetic diseases of PIEZO1 and PIEZO2 dysfunction. *Curr. Top. Membr.* 79, 97–134. doi: 10.1016/bs.ctm.2017.01.001

Andolfo, I., Alper, S. L., De Franceschi, L., Auriemma, C., Russo, R., De Falco, L., et al. (2013). Multiple clinical forms of dehydrated hereditary stomatocytosis arise from mutations in PIEZO1. *Blood* 121, 3925–3935, S1–S12. doi: 10.1182/blood-2013-02-482489

Andolfo, I., Russo, R., Manna, F., Shmukler, B. E., Gambale, A., Vitiello, G., et al. (2015). Novel Gardos channel mutations linked to dehydrated hereditary stomatocytosis (xerocytosis). *Am. J. Hematol.* 90, 921–926. doi: 10.1002/ajh.24117

Arese, P., Turrini, F., and Schwarzer, E. (2005). Band 3/complement-mediated recognition and removal of normally senescent and pathological human erythrocytes. *Cell. Physiol. Biochem.* 16, 133–146. doi: 10.1159/000089839

Bae, C., Gnanasambandam, R., Nicolai, C., Sachs, F., and Gottlieb, P. A. (2013). Xerocytosis is caused by mutations that alter the kinetics of the mechanosensitive channel PIEZO1. *Proc. Natl. Acad. Sci. U.S.A.* 110, E1162–E1168. doi: 10.1073/pnas.1219777110

Bae, C., Sachs, F., and Gottlieb, P. A. (2011). The mechanosensitive ion channel Piezo1 is inhibited by the peptide GsMTx4. *Biochemistry* 50, 6295–6300. doi: 10.1021/bi200770q

Beutler, E. (1985a). Biphasic loss of red cell enzyme activity during *in vivo* aging. *Prog. Clin. Biol. Res.* 195, 317–333.

Beutler, E. (1985b). How do red cell enzymes age? A new perspective. *Br. J. Haematol.* 61, 377–384. doi: 10.1111/j.1365-2141.1985.tb02841.x

Beutler, E. (1986). Planned obsolescence in humans and in other biosystems. *Perspect. Biol. Med.* 29, 175–179. doi: 10.1353/pbm.1986.0075

Bookchin, R. M., Etzion, Z., Sorette, M., Mohandas, N., Skepper, J. N., and Lew, V. L. (2000). Identification and characterization of a newly recognized population of high-Na^+, low-K^+, low-density sickle and normal red cells. *Proc. Natl. Acad. Sci. U.S.A.* 97, 8045–8050. doi: 10.1073/pnas.130198797

Borun, E. R., Figueroa, W. G., and Perry, S. M. (1957). The distribution of Fe^{59} tagged human erythrocytes in centrifuged specimens as a function of cell age. *J. Clin. Invest.* 36, 676–679. doi: 10.1172/JCI103468

Cahalan, S. M., Lukacs, V., Ranade, S. S., Chien, S., Bandell, M., and Patapoutian, A. (2015). Piezo1 links mechanical forces to red blood cell volume. *Elife* 4:e07370. doi: 10.7554/eLife.07370

Carafoli, E. (1992). The Ca^{2+} pump of the plasma membrane. *J. Biol. Chem.* 267, 2115–2118.

Cheng, J. T., Kahn, T., and Kaji, D. M. (1984). Mechanism of alteration of sodium potassium pump of erythrocytes from patients with chronic renal failure. *J. Clin. Invest.* 74, 1811–1820. doi: 10.1172/JCI111600

Cinar, E., Zhou, S., DeCourcey, J., Wang, Y., Waugh, R. E., and Wan, J. (2015). Piezo1 regulates mechanotransductive release of ATP from human RBCs. *Proc. Natl. Acad. Sci. U.S.A.* 112, 11783–11788. doi: 10.1073/pnas.1507309112

Clark, M. R. (1988). Senescence of red blood cells: progress and problems. *Physiol. Rev.* 68, 503–554.

Cohen, N. S., Ekholm, J. E., Luthra, M. G., and Hanahan, D. J. (1976). Biochemical characterization of density-separated human erythrocytes. *Biochim. Biophys. Acta* 419, 229–242. doi: 10.1016/0005-2736(76)90349-7

Cohen, R. M., Franco, R. S., Khera, P. K., Smith, E. P., Lindsell, C. J., Ciraolo, P. J., et al. (2008). Red cell life span heterogeneity in hematologically normal people is sufficient to alter HbA1c. *Blood* 112, 4284–4291. doi: 10.1182/blood-2008-04-154112

Cossins, A. R., and Gibson, J. S. (1997). Volume-sensitive transport systems and volume homeostasis in vertebrate red blood cells. *J. Exp. Biol.* 200(Pt 2), 343–352.

Dagher, G., and Lew, V. L. (1988). Maximal calcium extrusion capacity and stoichiometry of the human red cell calcium pump. *J. Physiol.* 407, 569–586. doi: 10.1113/jphysiol.1988.sp017432

Derganc, J., Bozic, B., Svetina, S., and Zeks, B. (2003). Equilibrium shapes of erythrocytes in rouleau formation. *Biophys. J.* 84, 1486–1492. doi: 10.1016/S0006-3495(03)74961-3

Dyrda, A., Cytlak, U., Ciuraszkiewicz, A., Lipinska, A., Cueff, A., Bouyer, G., et al. (2010). Local membrane deformations activate Ca^{2+}-dependent K^+ and anionic currents in intact human red blood cells. *PLoS ONE* 5:e9447. doi: 10.1371/journal.pone.0009447

Fedosov, D. A., Dao, M., Karniadakis, G. E., and Suresh, S. (2014a). Computational biorheology of human blood flow in health and disease. *Ann. Biomed. Eng.* 42, 368–387. doi: 10.1007/s10439-013-0922-3

Fedosov, D. A., Noguchi, H., and Gompper, G. (2014b). Multiscale modeling of blood flow: from single cells to blood rheology. *Biomech. Model. Mechanobiol.* 13, 239–258. doi: 10.1007/s10237-013-0497-9

Fermo, E., Bogdanova, A., Petkova-Kirova, P., Zaninoni, A., Marcello, A. P., Makhro, A., et al. (2017). 'Gardos Channelopathy': a variant of hereditary Stomatocytosis with complex molecular regulation. *Sci. Rep.* 7:1744. doi: 10.1038/s41598-017-01591-w

Franco, R. S., Puchulu-Campanella, M. E., Barber, L. A., Palascak, M. B., Joiner, C. H., Low, P. S., et al. (2013). Changes in the properties of normal human red blood cells during *in vivo* aging. *Am. J. Hematol.* 88, 44–51. doi: 10.1002/ajh.23344

Garcia-Sancho, J., and Lew, V. L. (1988). Heterogeneous calcium and adenosine triphosphate distribution in calcium-permeabilized human red cells. *J. Physiol.* 407, 523–539. doi: 10.1113/jphysiol.1988.sp017429

Gardos, G. (1958). The function of calcium in the potassium permeability of human erythrocytes. *Biochim. Biophys. Acta* 30, 653–654. doi: 10.1016/0006-3002(58)90124-0

Garrahan, P. J., and Garay, R. P. (1974). A kinetic study of the Na pump in red cells: its relevance to the mechanism of active transport. *Ann. N.Y. Acad. Sci.* 242, 445–458. doi: 10.1111/j.1749-6632.1974.tb19108.x

Garrahan, P. J., and Glynn, I. M. (1967). Facftors affecting the relative magnitudes of the sodium:potassium and sodium:sodium exchanges catalysed by the sodium pump. *J. Physiol.* 192, 189–216. doi: 10.1113/jphysiol.1967.sp008296

Ghanshani, S., Coleman, M., Gustavsson, P., Wu, A. C., Gargus, J. J., Gutman, G. A., et al. (1998). Human calcium-activated potassium channel gene *KCNN4* maps to chromosome 19q13.2 in the region deleted in diamond-blackfan anemia. *Genomics* 51, 160–161. doi: 10.1006/geno.1998.5333

Glogowska, E., Schneider, E. R., Maksimova, Y., Schulz, V. P., Lezon-Geyda, K., Wu, J., et al. (2017). Novel mechanisms of PIEZO1 dysfunction in hereditary xerocytosis. *Blood* 130, 1845–1856. doi: 10.1182/blood-2017-05-786004

Gnanasambandam, R., Bae, C., Gottlieb, P. A., and Sachs, F. (2015). Ionic selectivity and permeation properties of human PIEZO1 channels. *PLoS ONE* 10:e0125503. doi: 10.1371/journal.pone.0125503

Gompper, G., and Fedosov, D. A. (2016). Modeling microcirculatory blood flow: current state and future perspectives. *Wiley Interdiscip. Rev. Syst. Biol. Med.* 8, 157–168. doi: 10.1002/wsbm.1326

Gonzalez Flecha, F. L., Castello, P. R., Gagliardino, J. J., and Rossi, J. P. (1999). Molecular characterization of the glycated plasma membrane calcium pump. *J. Membr. Biol.* 171, 25–34. doi: 10.1007/s002329900555

Gottlieb, P. A., Bae, C., and Sachs, F. (2012). Gating the mechanical channel Piezo1: a comparison between whole-cell and patch recording. *Channels* 6, 282–289. doi: 10.4161/chan.21064

Hoffman, J. F., Joiner, W., Nehrke, K., Potapova, O., Foye, K., and Wickrema, A. (2003). The hSK4 (KCNN4) isoform is the Ca^{2+}-activated K^+ channel (Gardos channel) in human red blood cells. *Proc. Natl. Acad. Sci. U.S.A.* 100, 7366–7371. doi: 10.1073/pnas.1232342100

Houston, B. L., Zelinski, T., Israels, S. J., Coghlan, G., Chodirker, B. N., Gallagher, P. G., et al. (2011). Refinement of the hereditary xerocytosis locus on chromosome 16q in a large Canadian kindred. *Blood Cells Mol. Dis.* 47, 226–231. doi: 10.1016/j.bcmd.2011.08.001

Joiner, C. H., and Lauf, P. K. (1978). Ouabain binding and potassium transport in young and old populations of human red cells. *Membr. Biochem.* 1, 187–202. doi: 10.3109/09687687809063847

Kaestner, L. (2015). Channelizing the red blood cell: molecular biology competes with patch-clamp. *Front. Mol. Biosci.* 2:46. doi: 10.3389/fmolb.2015.00046

Kaestner, L., and Bogdanova, A. (2014). Regulation of red cell life-span, erythropoiesis, senescence, and clearance. *Front. Physiol.* 5:269. doi: 10.3389/fphys.2014.00269

Kay, M. M. (1975). Mechanism of removal of senescent cells by human macrophages in situ. *Proc. Natl. Acad. Sci. U.S.A.* 72, 3521–3525. doi: 10.1073/pnas.72.9.3521

Keller, M. A., Piedrafita, G., and Ralser, M. (2015). The widespread role of non-enzymatic reactions in cellular metabolism. *Curr. Opin. Biotechnol.* 34, 153–161. doi: 10.1016/j.copbio.2014.12.020

Kuchel, P. W., and Shishmarev, D. (2017). Accelerating metabolism and transmembrane cation flux by distorting red blood cells. *Sci. Adv.* 3:eaao1016. doi: 10.1126/sciadv.aao1016

Lanotte, L., Mauer, J., Mendez, S., Fedosov, D. A., Fromental, J. M., Claveria, V., et al. (2016). Red cells' dynamic morphologies govern blood shear thinning under microcirculatory flow conditions. *Proc. Natl. Acad. Sci. U.S.A.* 113, 13289–13294. doi: 10.1073/pnas.1608074113

Larsen, F. L., Katz, S., Roufogalis, B. D., and Brooks, D. E. (1981). Physiological shear stresses enhance the Ca^{2+} permeability of human erythrocytes. *Nature* 294, 667–668. doi: 10.1038/294667a0

Lew, V. L., and Beaugé, L. A. (1979). "Passive cation fluxes in red cell membranes," in *Transport Across Biological Membranes, Vol. II*, eds G. Giebisch, D. C. Tosteson, and H. H. Ussing (Berlin: Springer-Verlag), 85–115.

Lew, V. L., and Bookchin, R. M. (2005). Ion transport pathology in the mechanism of sickle cell dehydration. *Physiol. Rev.* 85, 179–200. doi: 10.1152/physrev.00052.2003

Lew, V. L., Daw, N., Etzion, Z., Tiffert, T., Muoma, A., Vanagas, L., et al. (2007). Effects of age-dependent membrane transport changes on the homeostasis of senescent human red blood cells. *Blood* 110, 1334–1342. doi: 10.1182/blood-2006-11-057232

Lew, V. L., Daw, N., Perdomo, D., Etzion, Z., Bookchin, R. M., and Tiffert, T. (2003). Distribution of plasma membrane Ca^{2+} pump activity in normal human red blood cells. *Blood* 102, 4206–4213. doi: 10.1182/blood-2003-06-1787

Lew, V. L., and Ferreira, H. G. (1978). "Calcium transport and the properties of a calcium-activated potassium channel in red cell membranes," in *Current Topics in Membranes and Transport, Vol. 10*, eds A. Kleinzeller and F. Bronner (New York, NY: Academic Press), 217–277.

Lew, V. L., Ortiz, O. E., and Bookchin, R. M. (1997). Stochastic nature and red cell population distribution of the sickling-induced Ca^{2+} permeability. *J. Clin. Invest.* 99, 2727–2735. doi: 10.1172/JCI119462

Lew, V. L., Raftos, J. E., Sorette, M. P., Bookchin, R. M., and Mohandas, N. (1995). Generation of normal human red cell volume, hemoglobin content and membrane area distributions, by "birth" or regulation? *Blood* 86, 334–341.

Lew, V. L., and Tiffert, T. (2013). The terminal density reversal phenomenon of aging human red blood cells. *Front. Physiol.* 4:171. doi: 10.3389/fphys.2013.00171

Lew, V. L., Tsien, R. Y., Miner, C., and Bookchin, R. M. (1982). Physiological $[Ca^{2+}]_i$ level and pump-leak turnover in intact red cells measured using an incorporated Ca chelator. *Nature* 298, 478–481. doi: 10.1038/298478a0

Lutz, H. U. (2012). Naturally occurring anti-band 3 antibodies in clearance of senescent and oxidatively stressed human red blood cells. *Transfus. Med. Hemother.* 39, 321–327. doi: 10.1159/000342171

Lutz, H. U., and Bogdanova, A. (2013). Mechanisms tagging senescent red blood cells for clearance in healthy humans. *Front. Physiol.* 4:387. doi: 10.3389/fphys.2013.00387

Lutz, H. U., Bussolino, F., Flepp, R., Fasler, S., Stammler, P., Kazatchkine, M. D., et al. (1987). Naturally occurring anti-band-3 antibodies and complement together mediate phagocytosis of oxidatively stressed human erythrocytes. *Proc. Natl. Acad. Sci. U.S.A* 84, 7368–7372. doi: 10.1073/pnas.84.21.7368

Magnani, M., Piatti, E., Serafini, N., Palma, F., Dacha, M., and Fornaini, G. (1983). The age-dependent metabolic decline of the red blood cell. *Mech. Ageing Dev.* 22, 295–308. doi: 10.1016/0047-6374(83)90084-2

Ostrow, K. L., Mammoser, A., Suchyna, T., Sachs, F., Oswald, R., Kubo, S., et al. (2003). cDNA sequence and *in vitro* folding of GsMTx4, a specific peptide inhibitor of mechanosensitive channels. *Toxicon* 42, 263–274. doi: 10.1016/S0041-0101(03)00141-7

Parker, J. C. (1973). Dog red blood cells. Adjustment of salt and water content *in vitro*. *J. Gen. Physiol.* 62, 147–156. doi: 10.1085/jgp.62.2.147

Parker, J. C. (1978). Sodium and calcium movements in dog red blood cells. *J. Gen. Physiol.* 71, 1–17. doi: 10.1085/jgp.71.1.1

Piedrafita, G., Keller, M. A., and Ralser, M. (2015). The impact of non-enzymatic reactions and enzyme promiscuity on cellular metabolism during (oxidative) stress conditions. *Biomolecules* 5, 2101–2122. doi: 10.3390/biom5032101

Pivkin, I. V., Peng, Z., Karniadakis, G. E., Buffet, P. A., Dao, M., and Suresh, S. (2016). Biomechanics of red blood cells in human spleen and consequences for physiology and disease. *Proc. Natl. Acad. Sci. U.S.A.* 113, 7804–7809. doi: 10.1073/pnas.1606751113

Ponder, E. (1948). *Hemolysis and Related Phenomena.* New York, NY: Grune & Stratton.

Ponder, E. (1950). Tonicity-volume relations in partially hemolyzed hypotonic systems. *J. Gen. Physiol.* 33, 177–193. doi: 10.1085/jgp.33.3.177

Raftos, J. E., Edgley, A., Bookchin, R. M., Etzion, Z., Lew, V. L., and Tiffert, T. (2001). Normal Ca^{2+} extrusion by the Ca^{2+} pump of intact red blood cells exposed to high glucose concentrations. *Am. J. Physiol. Cell Physiol.* 280, C1449–C1454. Available online at: http://ajpcell.physiology.org/content/280/6/C1449

Rapoport, S. M. (1986). *The Reticulocyte.* Boca Raton, FL: CRC Press.

Rega, A. F., and Garrahan, P. J. (1986). *The Ca^{2+} Pump of Plasma Membranes.* Boca Raton, FL: CRC Press.

Rivera, A., Vandorpe, D. H., Shmukler, B. E., Gallagher, D. R., Fikry, C. C., Kuypers, F. A., et al. (2017). Erythrocytes from hereditary xerocytosis patients heterozygous for KCNN4 V282M exhibit increased spontaneous Gardos channel-like activity inhibited by senicapoc. *Am. J. Hematol.* 92, E108–E110. doi: 10.1002/ajh.24716

Romero, P. J., and Romero, E. A. (1997). Differences in Ca^{2+} pumping activity between sub-populations of human red cells. *Cell Calcium* 21, 353–358. doi: 10.1016/S0143-4160(97)90028-2

Romero, P. J., and Romero, E. A. (1999). Effect of cell ageing on Ca^{2+} influx into human red cells. *Cell Calcium* 26, 131–137. doi: 10.1054/ceca.1999.0063

Schatzmann, H. J. (1983). The red cell calcium pump. *Annu. Rev. Physiol.* 45, 303–312. doi: 10.1146/annurev.ph.45.030183.001511

Secomb, T. W. (1987). Flow-dependent rheological properties of blood in capillaries. *Microvasc. Res.* 34, 46–58. doi: 10.1016/0026-2862(87)90078-1

Secomb, T. W., and Hsu, R. (1995). Red blood cell mechanics and functional capillary density. *Int. J. Microcirc. Clin. Exp.* 15, 250–254. doi: 10.1159/000179026

Shmukler, B. E., Vandorpe, D. H., Rivera, A., Auerbach, M., Brugnara, C., and Alper, S. L. (2014). Dehydrated stomatocytic anemia due to the heterozygous mutation R2456H in the mechanosensitive cation channel PIEZO1: a case report. *Blood Cells Mol. Dis.* 52, 53–54. doi: 10.1016/j.bcmd.2013.07.015

Svetina, S. (1982). Relations among variations in human red cell volume, density, membrane area, hemoglobin content and cation content. *J. Theor. Biol.* 95, 123–134. doi: 10.1016/0022-5193(82)90291-0

Tiffert, T., Daw, N., Etzion, Z., Bookchin, R. M., and Lew, V. L. (2007). Age decline in the activity of the Ca^{2+}-sensitive K^+ channel of human red blood cells. *J. Gen. Physiol.* 129, 429–436. doi: 10.1085/jgp.200709766

Vandorpe, D. H., Xu, C., Shmukler, B. E., Otterbein, L. E., Trudel, M., Sachs, F., et al. (2010). Hypoxia activates a Ca^{2+}-permeable cation conductance sensitive to carbon monoxide and to GsMTx-4 in human and mouse sickle erythrocytes. *PLoS ONE* 5:e8732. doi: 10.1371/journal.pone.0008732

Weatherall, D. J. (1997). The thalassaemias. *BMJ* 314, 1675–1678. doi: 10.1136/bmj.314.7095.1675

Weatherall, D. J. (2004). Thalassaemia: the long road from bedside to genome. *Nat. Rev. Genet.* 5, 625–631. doi: 10.1038/nrg1406

Zarychanski, R., Schulz, V. P., Houston, B. L., Maksimova, Y., Houston, D. S., Smith, B., et al. (2012). Mutations in the mechanotransduction protein PIEZO1 are associated with hereditary xerocytosis. *Blood* 120, 1908–1915. doi: 10.1182/blood-2012-04-422253

2

Is Increased Intracellular Calcium in Red Blood Cells a Common Component in the Molecular Mechanism Causing Anemia?

Laura Hertz[1†], *Rick Huisjes*[2†], *Esther Llaudet-Planas*[3], *Polina Petkova-Kirova*[1], *Asya Makhro*[4], *Jens G. Danielczok*[1], *Stephane Egee*[5,6,7], *Maria del Mar Mañú-Pereira*[3], *Richard van Wijk*[2], *Joan-Lluis Vives Corrons*[3], *Anna Bogdanova*[4] and *Lars Kaestner*[8,9]*

[1] Research Centre for Molecular Imaging and Screening, Medical School, Saarland University, Homburg, Germany, [2] Department of Clinical Chemistry and Haematology, University Medical Center Utrecht, Utrecht, Netherlands, [3] Red Blood Cell Defects and Hematopoietic Disorders Unit, Josep Carreras Leukaemia Research Institute, Barcelona, Spain, [4] Red Blood Cell Research Group, Institute of Veterinary Physiology, Vetsuisse Faculty and the Zurich Center for Integrative Human Physiology (ZIHP), University of Zurich, Zurich, Switzerland, [5] Centre National de la Recherche Scientifique, UMR 8227 Comparative Erythrocyte's Physiology, Roscoff, France, [6] Université Pierre et Marie Curie, Sorbonne Universités, Roscoff, France, [7] Laboratoire d'Excellence GR-Ex, Roscoff, France, [8] Theoretical Medicine and Biosciences, Saarland University, Homburg, Germany, [9] Experimental Physics, Saarland University, Saarbruecken, Germany

Correspondence:
Lars Kaestner
lars_kaestner@me.com

[†]These authors have contributed equally to this work.

For many hereditary disorders, although the underlying genetic mutation may be known, the molecular mechanism leading to hemolytic anemia is still unclear and needs further investigation. Previous studies revealed an increased intracellular Ca^{2+} in red blood cells (RBCs) from patients with sickle cell disease, thalassemia, or Gardos channelopathy. Therefore we analyzed RBCs' Ca^{2+} content from 35 patients with different types of anemia (16 patients with hereditary spherocytosis, 11 patients with hereditary xerocytosis, 5 patients with enzymopathies, and 3 patients with hemolytic anemia of unknown cause). Intracellular Ca^{2+} in RBCs was measured by fluorescence microscopy using the fluorescent Ca^{2+} indicator Fluo-4 and subsequent single cell analysis. We found that in RBCs from patients with hereditary spherocytosis and hereditary xerocytosis the intracellular Ca^{2+} levels were significantly increased compared to healthy control samples. For enzymopathies and hemolytic anemia of unknown cause the intracellular Ca^{2+} levels in RBCs were not significantly different. These results lead us to the hypothesis that increased Ca^{2+} levels in RBCs are a shared component in the mechanism causing an accelerated clearance of RBCs from the blood stream in channelopathies such as hereditary xerocytosis and in diseases involving defects of cytoskeletal components like hereditary spherocytosis. Future drug developments should benefit from targeting Ca^{2+} entry mediating molecular players leading to better therapies for patients.

Keywords: rare anemia, erythrocyte, calcium homeostasis, channelopathies, live cell imaging, spherocytosis, xerocytosis

INTRODUCTION

Anemia, defined as a hemoglobin concentration <11–13 g/dl, based on gender and age, affects 1.6 billion people worldwide (McLean et al., 2009). About 10% of these individuals are affected by rare anemias. This disease group includes ~90 different types of red blood cell (RBC) diseases, of which 80% are hereditary or congenital in nature. As the pathophysiology of most of these rare anemias is poorly understood, the appropriate treatment is often ineffective or even lacking.

Anemia in general has three major causes: blood loss, insufficient hematopoiesis, or facilitated removal of RBCs from the blood stream (Ossendorf, 2003). In hemolytic anemias the RBC premature clearance and shortened lifespan of RBCs are not compensated by enhanced RBC production giving rise to anemia (Dhaliwal et al., 2004). Many types of anemia can be assigned to mutations in a single protein. However, it is still unclear how these mutations transfer into an increased clearance of RBCs and what defines heterogeneity in disease severity. A prominent example is sickle cell disease. Described as a molecular disease as early as 1949 (Pauling et al., 1949), sickle cell disease is caused by a single point mutation in the ß-globin gene (Ingram, 1958). The mutated hemoglobin variant, HbS, is prone to polymerization and formation of HbS aggregates, that are even more likely to occur upon dehydration of RBCs (Layton and Nagel, 2010). Dehydration is largely mediated by high intracellular Ca^{2+}, subsequent activation of Gardos Channels and loss of K^{+} (Lew et al., 2002). Ca^{2+} uptake in sickle RBCs is abnormally high, and not always compensated by Ca^{2+} extrusion by the Ca^{2+} pumps resulting in an elevated intracellular Ca^{2+} content (Eaton et al., 1973; Tiffert et al., 2003). This increase in the Ca^{2+} content is attributed to highly abundant hyperactive NMDA receptors in membranes of patients' RBCs. Inhibition of Ca^{2+} uptake via these receptors could prevent dehydration and sickling of RBCs *in vitro* (Hänggi et al., 2014; Bogdanova et al., 2015). However, it remains elusive, how the mutation in the hemoglobin "causes" the increased Ca^{2+}-influx. The fact that vaso-occlusive crises in sickle cell disease patients occur sporadically (Rieber et al., 1977) points to a rather indirect connection. Increased intracellular Ca^{2+} levels were also found in RBCs from, e.g., beta thalassemia patients (Bookchin et al., 1988) or patients with Gardos channelopathy (Fermo et al., 2017). It is known that Ca^{2+} overload triggers several downstream events in RBCs (Bogdanova et al., 2013). One important effect is the impairment of the cytoskeletal stability, e.g., through activation of calpain and subsequent cleavage of membrane associated proteins (Inomata et al., 1993; Salamino et al., 1993). The activation of calmodulin and its interaction with the band 4.1R protein has been shown to decrease the affinity of 4.1R for its cytoskeletal interaction partners actin and spectrin and thereby loosening the cytoskeletal structure (Jarret and Kyte, 1979; Nunomura and Takakuwa, 2006). A decreased RBC volume is resulting from the Ca^{2+} dependent opening of the Gardos channel, which leads to loss of K^{+}, Cl^{-} and water (Gardos, 1958). Furthermore, increased Ca^{2+} levels lead to the disruption of the asymmetrical distribution of phospholipids in the plasma membrane. Phosphatidylserine, a lipid exclusively present in the inner leaflet of the membrane, becomes exposed on the outer membrane by activation of the scramblase and simultaneous inhibition of the flippase (Verkleij et al., 1973; Bitbol et al., 1987; Bassé et al., 1996; Woon et al., 1999). All these described changes in the cell physiology as well as the increased Ca^{2+} are signs of senescence (sometimes referred to as eryptosis) and prime the cells for clearance from the blood stream (Lutz and Bogdanova, 2013). A substantial increase in intracellular Ca^{2+} also increases the osmotic fragility with no strict correlation to cell volume and largely before cells reach spherocytic hemolysis volume (Cueff et al., 2010). This might be an additional mechanism of a decrease in RBC number associated to an elevated Ca^{2+}concentration. To what extent a Ca^{2+} induced increased vesiculation (Nguyen et al., 2011; Alaarg et al., 2013) may alter the RBC clearance is still unknown.

Here we aim to investigate if elevated intracellular Ca^{2+} levels are a general feature in the pathophysiology of hemolytic anemia and such provides a mechanistic link for an increased clearance of RBCs resulting in anemia of hemolytic patients.

MATERIALS AND METHODS

Participants

Patients diagnosed with different types of anemia were enrolled in the study after signed informed consent. Patient data were handled anonymously as outlined in the ethics applications. These applications were approved by the Medical Ethical Research Board (MERB) of the University Medical Center Utrecht, the Netherlands, (UMCU) under reference code 15/426M "Disturbed ion homeostasis in hereditary hemolytic anemia" and also by the Ethical Committee of Clinical Investigations of Hospital Clinic, Spain, (IDIBAPS) under the reference code 2013/8436. Exclusion criteria were erythrocyte transfusion in the past 90 days, age below 3 years and/or body weight lower than 18 kg. Blood from healthy control donors was anonymously obtained using the approved medical ethical protocol of 07/125 Mini Donor Dienst, also approved by the MERB of UMCU. The blood of the patient and the healthy donor anti-coagulated in lithium-heparin was shipped overnight from the University Medical Center Utrecht (Utrecht, The Netherlands) and from Institut d'Investigacions Biomèdiques August Pi i Sunyer/Hospital Clínic de Barcelona (Barcelona, Spain) to Saarland University (Homburg, Germany). All patients included in this study were genetically screened for mutations by next-generation sequencing and diagnosed with the following types of anemia: 16 patients included in this study were diagnosed with hereditary spherocytosis using golden standard techniques (EMA-binding, osmotic gradient ektacytometry and osmotic fragility test). Moreover, these 16 patients were screened for mutations by next-generation sequencing: 7 patients had mutations in *ANK1*, 4 patients had mutations in *SPTA1*, 3 patients in *SPTB*, and 2 patients showed mutations in *SLC4A1*). Eleven patients were diagnosed with hereditary xerocytosis (due to mutations in *PIEZO1*), 5 patients had enzymatic disorders (3 patients with glucose-6-phosphate dehydrogenase deficiency, 1 patient with glutamate-cysteine ligase deficiency, 1 patient with glutathione reductase deficiency) and 3 patients suffered from hemolytic anemia of unknown cause.

Calcium Imaging

Ca^{2+} imaging experiments were carried out with RBCs from 35 patient blood samples and 25 healthy transportation controls. Intracellular Ca^{2+} was measured from single cells as Fluo-4 (Thermo Fisher Scientific, Waltham, MA, USA) based fluorescence intensity as described before (Wang et al., 2014).

Data Analysis

Analysis of the fluorescence images was performed in ImageJ (Wayne Rasband, National Institutes of Health) and further processing of the data was done using Matlab (Mathworks, Natick, MA, USA) and GraphPad Prism (GraphPad Software Inc., La Jolla, CA, USA). For each patient and control at least 200 individual cells were analyzed. The mean fluorescence intensity values were plotted as box-and-whiskers. Boxes show median and 25th to 75th percentiles, whiskers are drawn down to 10th and up to 90th percentile. For cell-based analysis of single patients and controls, significance was checked using the Mann–Whitney test.

For patient-based analysis, patients were grouped in hereditary spherocytosis, hereditary xerocytosis, enzymopathies, and hemolytic anemia of unknown cause. As a statistical basis we used the median fluorescence intensity value from the single cell analysis for each patient and control sample. Intensity values from controls were normalized to their mean value, whereas patients were normalized to the corresponding shipping control. Significance was tested on not normalized raw data using the paired *t*-test when data showed a normal distribution (D'Agostino-Pearson normality test) otherwise with the Wilcoxon signed-rank test.

RESULTS

In this study, 35 patients with different types of hemolytic anemia were analyzed. Patients were grouped according to their disease into 4 subgroups: hereditary spherocytosis patients, hereditary xerocytosis patients, patients with enzymopathies and patients with unknown hemolytic anemia. For each subgroup, representative fluorescence images of Fluo-4 loaded RBCs from patients and corresponding transportation controls of healthy donors are depicted in **Figures 1A–D**.

Figures 1E–H show the cell-based statistical analysis for each patient and the corresponding control. Fluo-4 fluorescence intensity from single cells was measured and plotted. There was a huge variation in the intensity-correlated Ca^{2+} concentrations when comparing the samples taken altogether. However, when we compared samples within a particular shipment (identical transportation conditions), the Ca^{2+} concentrations were in a similar/comparable range. Therefore we always compared patients exclusively to their corresponding shipping controls.

In all 16 cases of hereditary spherocytosis we found that intracellular Ca^{2+} levels in RBCs were significantly elevated in patients compared to the corresponding healthy shipping control samples (**Figure 1E**). In hereditary xerocytosis 9 out of 11 patients showed increased Ca^{2+} levels, whereas for the other two patients no significant differences could be detected (**Figure 1H**, P50.1 and P51.2).

The group of unknown hemolytic anemia patients gave a more heterogeneous picture. The Ca^{2+} content in one patient was significantly increased, whereas the other two patients had significantly lower Ca^{2+} levels than the shipping control (**Figure 1F**, P30.1 vs. P31.1 and P32.1). The situation was similar for the enzymopathies: three patients (**Figure 1G**, P41.1, P42.1, P43.1) had an increased intracellular Ca^{2+} content, one was significantly lower and one patient showed no significant difference compared to its control (**Figure 1G**, P44.1 and P40.1, respectively).

The patient-based statistical analysis of the Ca^{2+} concentrations is depicted in **Figure 2A** and shows the paired and normalized analysis of all patients in comparison to all controls. Ca^{2+} levels in hemolytic anemia patients show a highly significant increase. **Figure 2B** shows the same analysis for subgroups of patients. The groups with hereditary spherocytosis and hereditary xerocytosis patients have significantly increased levels of intracellular Ca^{2+}, compared to the controls. Patients with enzymopathies depict an increase in the intracellular Ca^{2+} concentration but fail to reach significant changes. For patients with hemolytic anemia of unknown cause intracellular Ca^{2+} levels appear to be heterogeneous, because it is a non-systematic group composition.

DISCUSSION

Ca^{2+} Overload

In this study we monitored the intracellular Ca^{2+} levels in RBCs from patients with several types of hemolytic anemia. We found that in the analyzed cases of membranopathies, hereditary spherocytosis and hereditary xerocytosis, intracellular Ca^{2+} is significantly increased. **Figure 2C** depicts the proposed mechanism. Starting with the previously described sickle cell disease (compare Introduction) an increased number of NMDA receptors were identified to cause the abnormal uptake of Ca^{2+} (Hänggi et al., 2014). *In vitro*, this increase in Ca^{2+} can be reduced by NMDA blockers like Memantine and a pilot clinical trial investigating the effect of this drug on sickle cell disease patients is closed and the statistical analysis is currently on-going (Bogdanova et al., 2017). For other types of anemia the Ca^{2+} entry pathways are rather unclear. In the Gardos channelopathy it is suggested that Ca^{2+} enters via the mechanical activated Piezo1 channel (Fermo et al., 2017). We found several different mutations for the *PIEZO1* gene in the xerocytosis patients included in our study. A further characterization of how these mutations affect the physiology of the channel is still ongoing, but data in the literature show that six dehydrated hereditary stomatocytosis-causing mutations in the Piezo1 channel with five of them in the C-terminal 1/5 of the protein, result in a slowing of the inactivation kinetics of the channel and thus to a more active channel (Albuisson et al., 2013). However, independent of Ca^{2+} entry pathways also an impairment of Ca^{2+} extrusion (of residual Ca^{2+} influx) needs to be considered as an important factor for the Ca^{2+} homeostasis in RBCs. The plasma membrane Ca^{2+} ATPase (PMCA) is the only known active extrusion pathway for Ca^{2+} in RBCs and its transportation capacity is limited by the availability of ATP (Schatzmann, 1966; Pasini et al., 2006). It has been reported that Piezo1 can regulate the ATP release from human RBCs and that mutations in the channel can alter the released amount of ATP (Cinar et al., 2015). Therefore it

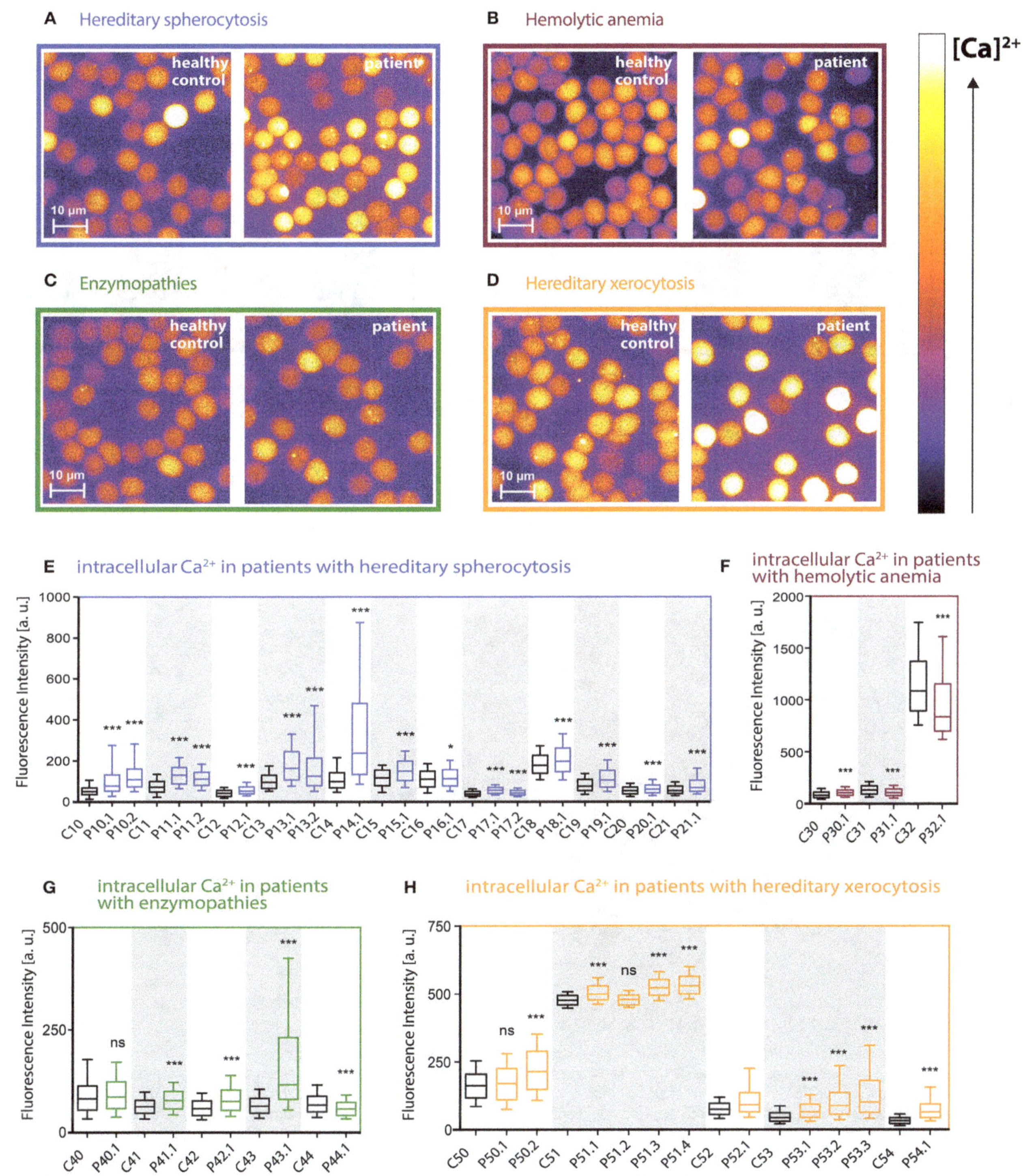

FIGURE 1 | Intracellular Ca^{2+} content in RBCs from patients with different types of hemolytic anemia. **(A–D)** Representative fluorescence images of Fluo-4 loaded RBCs from control and patient blood samples. Relative intracellular Ca^{2+} concentration is scaled from black (lowest) to white (highest). Patients were grouped according to their disease diagnosis: hereditary spherocytosis (blue), hemolytic anemia (purple), enzymopathies (green), hereditary xerocytosis (orange). **(E–H)** Statistical analysis of the mean Fluo-4 intensity values in arbitrary units from single cells for each group of patients and the corresponding control samples. Controls and patients that belong to the same shipment are highlighted with a white or gray background. Controls are displayed as black boxes, patients are colored in blue (hereditary spherocytosis), purple (unknown hemolytic anemia), green (enzymopathies), and orange (hereditary xerocytosis). Whiskers indicate the range between 10th and 90th percentiles. There is a huge variation in the intensity-correlated Ca^{2+} concentrations already within the control group of healthy donors. Significance was tested between each patient and the according shipping control sample (always the next control sample on left side) using the Mann–Whitney test (ns denotes $p > 0.5$, $^{*}p \leq 0.5$, $^{***}p \leq 0.01$).

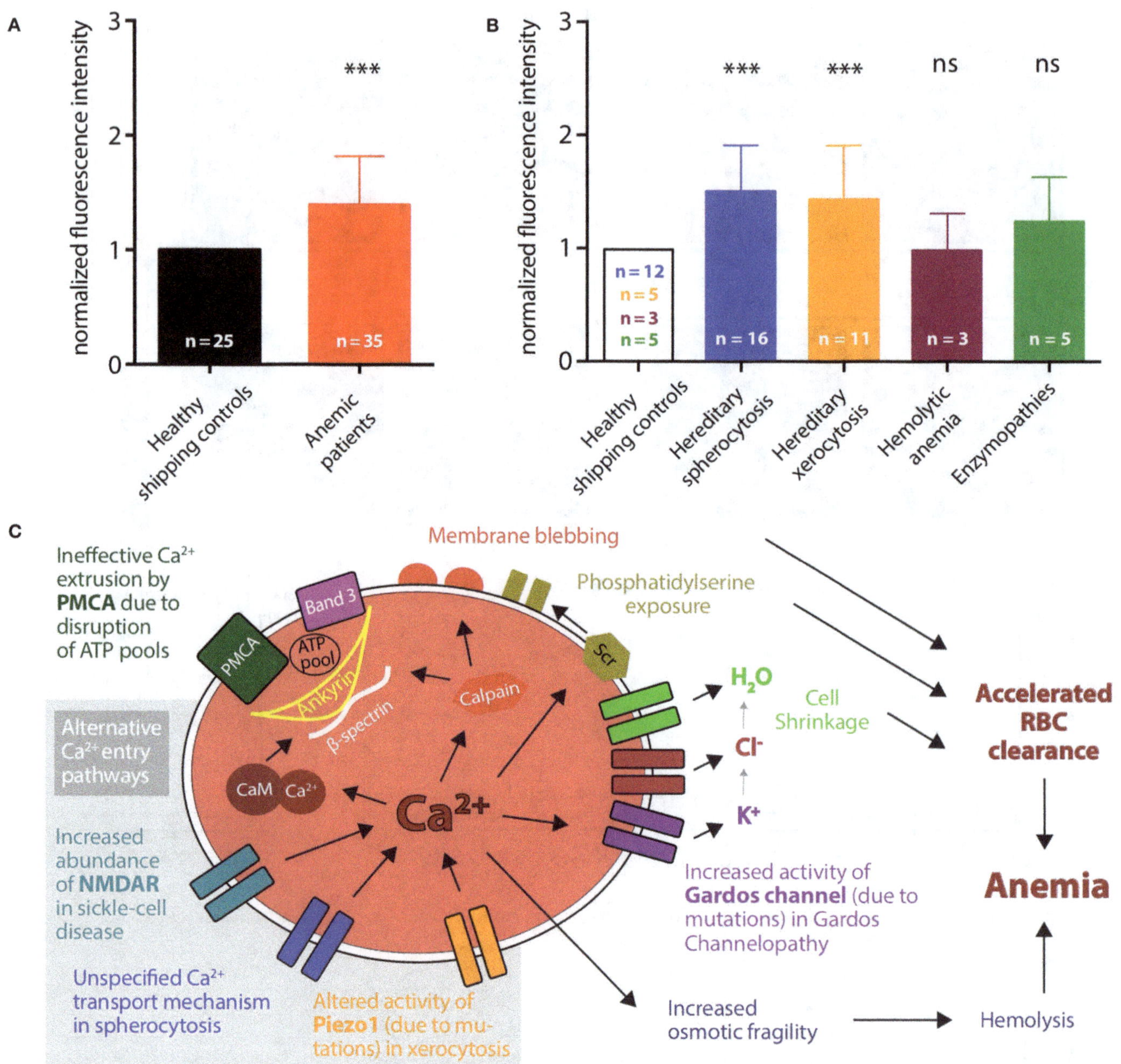

FIGURE 2 | Patient-based statistical analysis of intracellular Ca^{2+} levels and proposed mechanisms. **(A)** Statistical analysis of normalized median fluorescence intensity values for all 35 patients (red bar) and 25 healthy shipping controls (black bar). Significance was tested using the Wilcoxon signed-rank test (***$p \leq 0.01$). **(B)** Statistical analysis of normalized median fluorescence intensity values for controls and patients grouped by disease. Number of control samples differs for each disease group. Hereditary spherocytosis (blue): 16 patients and 12 controls, hereditary xerocytosis (orange): 12 patients and 5 controls, hemolytic anemia (purple): 3 patients and 3 controls, enzymopathies (green): 5 patients and 5 controls. Significance was tested using the paired *t*-test, when data showed a Gaussian distribution (D'Agostino-Pearson normality test), otherwise using the Wilcoxon signed-rank test (ns denotes $p > 0.5$, ***$p \leq 0.01$). **(C)** Proposed mechanisms leading to increased intracellular Ca^{2+} levels in diseased RBCs and accordingly to accelerated clearance of cells from the blood stream. Alternative or cumulating Ca^{2+} entry pathways are highlighted with gray background: increased abundance of NMDA-receptors (NMDAR), e.g., in sickle cell disease, altered activity of Piezo1, e.g., in hereditary xerocytosis, increased activity of Gardos Channel, e.g., in Gardos Channelopathy, or unspecified Ca^{2+} transport mechanisms. Additionally, ineffective extrusion of Ca^{2+} due to disruption of ATP pools fueling the plasma membrane Ca^{2+} ATPase (PMCA) can contribute. Several downstream processes follow Ca^{2+} overload in RBCs, e.g.: activation of calmodulin by formation of the Ca^{2+}-calmodulin complex (Ca-CaM) and activation of calpain, thereby loosening the cytoskeletal structure; activation of the scramblase (Scr) leading to exposure of phosphatidylserine on the outer leaflet of the membrane; activation of the Gardos channel followed by the efflux of K^+, Cl^- and H_2O and consecutive cell shrinkage.

is also possible that the detected Ca^{2+} overload in RBCs from xerocytosis patients is due to ATP depletion and ineffective Ca^{2+} extrusion. This would imply that glycolytic enzyme defects of the RBC, generally considered to lead to decreased ATP levels, would result in Ca^{2+} overload. The ATP needed to fuel the pump is trapped in membrane-associated complexes (ATP pools). Among others, identified components of these complexes are Band 3, ankyrin, and β-spectrin (Chu et al., 2012). Mutations in these proteins are found in the spherocytosis patients included in this study. If these mutations lead to a disruption of the complexes serving as ATP pools for the Ca^{2+} pump, the extrusion of Ca^{2+} will also be significantly reduced. Likewise, the general cytoskeleton stability is impaired in RBCs from spherocytosis patients. Changes in the mechanical stability of the cells may result in an activation of mechanosensitive channels, like Piezo1, again leading to an increase in intracellular Ca^{2+}. Both components (increased Ca^{2+} leak and decreased Ca^{2+} extrusion) could happen independent of each other or even mutually reinforce. We can exclude that the different values in fluorescence intensity are due to changes in cell volume: In a different study we tested volume changes, e.g., by osmotic swelling, and co-stained RBCs with Calcein Red-Orange, a dye insensitive to the Ca^{2+} concentration and intensity changes were negligible compared to intensity changes occurring in measurements probing the RBCs Ca^{2+} concentration (Danielczok et al., 2015). The delicate balance between Ca^{2+} entry and exit is likely to be influenced by mechanical stress. During their journey in the blood stream, RBCs experience hundreds squeezes when passing small capillaries and the spleen. To perform such experiments in artificial circulation systems *in vitro* became recently available based on microfluidic devices (Brust et al., 2014; Danielczok et al., 2015; Picot et al., 2015) and should be a future experimental focus.

The results we report do have a therapeutic impact: they illustrate that disease specific pharmacological targets should be upstream of the increase in intracellular Ca^{2+} to avoid all Ca^{2+} related effects that accumulate the processes facilitating RBC clearance as outlined in **Figure 2C**. In contrast pharmacological targets downstream of the action of intracellular Ca^{2+} may fail to address the major symptoms of the disease as it was shown for the Gardos channel inhibitor Senicapoc. In sickle cell disease patients it failed to improve acute vaso-occlusive crises (Ataga et al., 2011).

Blood Shipment

Having a critical look at our data from **Figures 1E–H** it is evident that the transportation process has a huge impact on the measured intracellular Ca^{2+} content in RBCs. Differences (within controls) are mainly not due to different transportation times (which were similar for all shipments) but to different transportation conditions, like temperature, vibration intensity and duration or other shipment related parameters that are out of our control. We choose Heparin as an anticoagulant because it does not interfere with the extracellular Ca^{2+}. Other standard anticoagulants like CPDA or EDTA bind the external Ca^{2+}, making internal Ca^{2+} measurements unreliable (Makhro et al., 2016). In the mentioned study transportation was simulated under laboratory conditions, which shows better results than the inconsistency of control samples within the present experiments (**Figures 1E–H**). In addition we do not know if intracellular Ca^{2+} levels during transportation are more severely influenced in patient RBCs compared to healthy controls, which presents an uncertainty of this study. Therefore future studies require investigations without cellular convolution by the shipment process, i.e., either a travel of the patient to specialized laboratories for single cell investigations or the establishment of such specialized mobile laboratories.

CONCLUSION

Considering our Ca^{2+} data and the results from studies on sickle cells and RBCs from patients with Gardos channelopathies, there is strong evidence that the Ca^{2+} overload in RBCs contributes to their accelerated clearance from the circulation and is a common part of the molecular mechanism in these types of anemia. The exact molecular regulation of the Ca^{2+} entry pathways requires further investigations. Future drug developments should benefit from targeting Ca^{2+} entry mediating molecular players, (as, e.g., Memantine for the treatment of sickle cell disease patients Bogdanova et al., 2017), leading to better therapies for patients.

AUTHOR CONTRIBUTIONS

LK, AB, RvW, JV defined the study and planed the experiments. LH, RH, EL, PP, JD, AM, MdM performed the acquisition and analysis. LH, SE, and LK interpreted the data. LH and LK drafted the manuscript. AB, RvW, JV, RH, SE, EL, PP, JD, AM, MdM critically revised the manuscript. All authors approved the final version of the manuscript.

ACKNOWLEDGMENTS

We would like to thank Prof. Peter Lipp (Institute for Molecular Cell Biology, Saarland University, Homburg/Saar, Germany) for letting us use the laboratory.

REFERENCES

Alaarg, A., Schiffelers, R. M., van Solinge, W. W., and van Wijk, R. (2013). Red blood cell vesiculation in hereditary hemolytic anemia. *Front. Physiol.* 4:365. doi: 10.3389/fphys.2013.00365

Albuisson, J., Murthy, S. E., Bandell, M., Coste, B., Louis-dit-Picard, H. L. N., Mathur, J., et al. (2013). Dehydrated hereditary stomatocytosis linked to gain-of-function mutations in mechanically activated PIEZO1 ion channels. *Nat. Commun.* 4, 165–119. doi: 10.1038/ncomms 2899

Ataga, K. I., Reid, M., Ballas, S. K., Yasin, Z., Bigelow, C., James, L. S., et al. (2011). Improvements in haemolysis and indicators of erythrocyte survival do not correlate with acute vaso-occlusive crises in patients with sickle cell disease: a phase III randomized, placebo-controlled, double-blind study of the Gardos channel blocker senicapoc (ICA-17043). *Br. J. Haematol.* 153, 92–104. doi: 10.1111/j.1365-2141.2010.08520.x

Bassé, F., Stout, J. G., Sims, P. J., and Wiedmer, T. (1996). Isolation of an erythrocyte membrane protein that mediates Ca^{2+}-dependent transbilayer movement of phospholipids. *J. Biol. Chem.* 271, 17205–17210. doi: 10.1074/jbc.271.29.17205

Bitbol, M., Fellmann, P., Zachowski, A., and Devaux, P. F. (1987). Ion regulation of phosphatidylserine and phosphatidylethanolamine outside-inside translocation in human erythrocytes. *Biochim. Biophys. Acta* 904, 268–282. doi: 10.1016/0005-2736(87)90376-2

Bogdanova, A., Makhro, A., and Kaestner, L. (2015). "Calcium handling in red blood cells of sickle cell disease patients," in *Sickle Cell Disease*, ed M. E. Lewis (Hauppauge, NY: Nova Science Publishers), 29–60.

Bogdanova, A., Makhro, A., Seiler, E., Gassmann, M., Hegemann, I., Muller, R., et al. (2017). "N-methyl D-glutamate receptor as a pharmacological target for treatment of sickle cell disease: effect of memantine on red cells of patients on a pilot clinical trial MemSID," in *21th Meeting of the European Red Cell Society* (Heidelberg). Abstract nr S03–02.

Bogdanova, A., Makhro, A., Wang, J., Lipp, P., and Kaestner, L. (2013). Calcium in red blood cells-a perilous balance. *Int. J. Mol. Sci.* 14, 9848–9872. doi: 10.3390/ijms14059848

Bookchin, R. M., Ortiz, O. E., Shalev, O., Tsurei, S., Rachmilewitz, E. A., Hockaday, A., et al. (1988). Calcium transport and ultrastructure of red cells in beta-thalassemia intermedia. *Blood* 72, 1602–1607.

Brust, M., Aouane, O., Thi baud, M., Flormann, D., Verdier, C., Kaestner, L., et al. (2014). The plasma protein fibrinogen stabilizes clusters of red blood cells in microcapillary flows. *Sci. Rep.* 4:4348. doi: 10.1038/srep04348

Chu, H., Puchulu-Campanella, E., Galan, J. A., Tao, W. A., Low, P. S., and Hoffman, J. F. (2012). Identification of cytoskeletal elements enclosing the ATP pools that fuel human red blood cell membrane cation pumps. *Proc. Natl. Acad. Sci. U.S.A.* 109, 12794–12799. doi: 10.1073/pnas.1209014109

Cinar, E., Zhou, S., DeCourcey, J., Wang, Y., Waugh, R. E., and Wan, J. (2015). Piezo1 regulates mechanotransductive release of ATP from human RBCs. *Proc. Natl. Acad. Sci. U.S.A.* 112, 11783–11788. doi: 10.1073/pnas.1507309112

Cueff, A., Seear, R., Dyrda, A., Bouyer, G., Eg e, S. P., Esposito, A., et al. (2010). Effects of elevated intracellular calcium on the osmotic fragility of human red blood cells. *Cell Calcium* 47, 29–36. doi: 10.1016/j.ceca.2009.11.002

Danielczok, J., Ruppenthal, S., Terriac, E., Lautenschläger, F., Lipp, P., and Kaestner, L. (2015). "Evidence for PIEZO1 involvment in pressure-dependent Ca^{2+}-increase in human red blood cells," in *20th Meeting of the European Red Cell Society* (Roscoff). Abstract nr 54.

Dhaliwal, G., Cornett, P., and Tierney, L. M. J. (2004). Hemolytic Anemia. *Am. Fam. Physician* 69, 2599–2606. Available online at: http://www.aafp.org/afp/2004/0601/p2599.html

Eaton, J. W., Jacob, H. S., Skelton, T. D., Swofford, H. S., and Kolpin, C. E. (1973). Elevated Erythrocyte Calcium in Sickle Cell Disease. *Nature* 246, 105–106. doi: 10.1038/246105a0

Fermo, E., Bogdanova, A., Petkova-Kirova, P., Zaninoni, A., Marcello, A. P., Makhro, A., et al. (2017). 'Gardos Channelopathy': a variant of hereditary Stomatocytosis with complex molecular regulation. *Sci. Rep.* 7:1744. doi: 10.1038/s41598-017-01591-w

Gardos, G. (1958). The function of calcium in the potassium permability of human erythrocytes. *Biochim. Biophys. Acta* 30, 653–654. doi: 10.1016/0006-3002(58)90124-0

Hänggi, P., Makhro, A., Gassmann, M., Schmugge, M., Goede, J. S., Speer, O., et al. (2014). Red blood cells of sickle cell disease patients exhibit abnormally high abundance of N-methyl D-aspartate receptors mediating excessive calcium uptake. *Br. J. Haematol.* 167, 252–264. doi: 10.1111/bjh.13028

Ingram, V. M. (1958). Abnormal human haemoglobins. I. The comparison of normal human and sickle-cell haemoglobins by fingerprinting. *Biochim. Biophys. Acta* 28, 539–545. doi: 10.1016/0006-3002(58)90516-X

Inomata, M., Nakamura, M., Imajoh-Ohmi, S., and Kawashima, S. (1993). A variety of calpain/calpastatin systems in mammalian erythrocytes. *Biochim. Biophys. Acta* 1178, 207–214. doi: 10.1016/0167-4889(93)90011-D

Jarret, H. W., and Kyte, J. (1979). Human erytrocyte calmodulin. *J. Biol. Chem.* 254, 8237–8244.

Layton, D. M., and Nagel, R. L. (2010). "Hemoglobinopathies due to structural mutations," in *Molecular Hematology*, eds D. Provan and J. G. Gribben (Chicester: Wiley-Blackwell), 179–195.

Lew, V. L., Etzion, Z., and Bookchin, R. M. (2002). Dehydration response of sickle cells to sickling-induced Ca. *Blood* 99, 2578–2585. doi: 10.1182/blood.V99.7.2578

Lutz, H. U., and Bogdanova, A. (2013). Mechanisms tagging senescent red blood cells for clearance in healthy humans. *Front. Physiol.* 4:387. doi: 10.3389/fphys.2013.00387

Makhro, A., Huisjes, R., Verhagen, L. P., Ma-ú-Pereira, M. D. M., Llaudet-Planas, E., Petkova-Kirova, P., et al. (2016). Red cell properties after different modes of blood transportation. *Front. Physiol.* 7:288. doi: 10.3389/fphys.2016.00288

McLean, E. E., Cogswell, M. M., Egli, I. I., Wojdyla, D. D., and de Benoist, B. B. (2009). Worldwide prevalence of anaemia, WHO vitamin and mineral nutrition information system, 1993-2005. *Public Health Nutr.* 12, 444–454. doi: 10.1017/S1368980008002401

Nguyen, D. B., Wagner-Britz, L., Maia, S., Steffen, P., Wagner, C., Kaestner, L., et al. (2011). Regulation of phosphatidylserine exposure in red blood cells. *Cell. Physiol. Biochem.* 28, 847–856. doi: 10.1159/000335798

Nunomura, W., and Takakuwa, Y. (2006). Regulation of protein 4.1R interactions with membrane proteins by Ca^{2+} and calmodulin. *Front. Biosci.* 11, 1522–1539. doi: 10.2741/1901

Ossendorf, M. (2003). "Erythrozyten," in *Integrative Klinische Chemie und Laboratoriumsmedizin Pathophysiologie, Pathobiochemie, Hämatologie*, ed H. Renz (Berlin; New York, NY: de Gruyter), 157–184.

Pasini, E. M., Kirkegaard, M., Mortensen, P., Lutz, H. U., Thomas, A. W., and Mann, M. (2006). In-depth analysis of the membrane and cytosolic proteome of red blood cells. *Blood* 108, 791–801. doi: 10.1182/blood-2005-11-007799

Pauling, L., Itano, H. A., Singer, S. J., and Wells, I. C. (1949). Sickle cell anemia a molecular disease. *Science* 110, 543–548. doi: 10.1126/science.110.2865.543

Picot, J., Ndour, P. A., Lefevre, S. D., El Nemer, W., and Tawfik, H., Galimand, J., et al. (2015). A biomimetic microfluidic chip to study the circulation and mechanical retention of red blood cells in the spleen. *Am. J. Hematol.* 90, 339–345. doi: 10.1002/ajh.23941

Rieber, E. E., Veliz, G., and Pollack, S. (1977). Red cells in sickle cell crisis: observations on the pathophysiology of crisis. *Blood* 49, 967–979.

Salamino, F., De Tullio, R., Mengotti, P., Viotti, P. L., Melloni, E., and Pontremoli, S. (1993). Site-directed activation of calpain is promoted by a membrane-associated natural activator protein. *Biochem. J.* 290, 191–197. doi: 10.1042/bj2900191

Schatzmann, H. J. (1966). ATP-dependent Ca^{++}-extrusion from human red cells. *Experientia* 22, 364–365. doi: 10.1007/BF01901136

Tiffert, T., Bookchin, R. M., and Lew, V. L. (2003). "Calcium homeostasis in normal and abnormal human red cells," in *Red Cell Membrane Transport in Health and Disease*, eds I. Bernhardt and J. C. Ellory (Berlin; Heidelberg: Springer), 373–405.

Verkleij, A. J., Zwaal, R. F., Roelofsen, B., Comfurius, P., Kastelijn, D., and van Deenen, L. L. (1973). The asymmetric distribution of phospholipids in the human red cell membrane. A combined study using phospholipases and freeze-etch electron microscopy. *Biochim. Biophys. Acta* 323, 178–193. doi: 10.1016/0005-2736(73)90143-0

Wang, J., van Bentum, K., Sester, U., and Kaestner, L. (2014). Calcium homeostasis in red blood cells of dialysis patients in dependence of erythropoietin treatment. *Front. Physiol.* 5:16. doi: 10.3389/fphys.2014.00016

Woon, L. A., Holland, J. W., Kable, E. P. W., and Roufogalis, B. D. (1999). Ca^{2+} sensitivity of phospholipid scrambling in human red cell ghosts. *Cell Calcium* 25, 313–320. doi: 10.1054/ceca.1999.0029

3

Red Blood Cell Passage of Small Capillaries Is Associated with Transient Ca^{2+}-Mediated Adaptations

Jens G. Danielczok[1], Emmanuel Terriac[2,3], Laura Hertz[1], Polina Petkova-Kirova[1], Franziska Lautenschläger[2,3], Matthias W. Laschke[4] and Lars Kaestner[2,5]*

[1] *Institute for Molecular Cell Biology, Saarland University, Homburg, Germany,* [2] *Experimental Physics, Saarland University, Saarbrücken, Germany,* [3] *Leibniz Institute for New Materials, Saarbrücken, Germany,* [4] *Institute for Clinical and Experimental Surgery, Saarland University, Homburg, Germany,* [5] *Theoretical Medicine and Biosciences, Saarland University, Homburg, Germany*

Correspondence:
Lars Kaestner
lars_kaestner@me.com

When red blood cells (RBCs) pass constrictions or small capillaries they need to pass apertures falling well below their own cross section size. We used different means of mechanical stimulations (hypoosmotic swelling, local mechanical stimulation, passing through microfluidic constrictions) to observe cellular responses of human RBCs in terms of intracellular Ca^{2+}-signaling by confocal microscopy of Fluo-4 loaded RBCs. We were able to confirm our *in vitro* results in a mouse dorsal skinfold chamber model showing a transiently increased intracellular Ca^{2+} when RBCs were passing through small capillaries *in vivo*. Furthermore, we performed the above-mentioned *in vitro* experiments as well as measurements of RBCs filterability under various pharmacological manipulations (GsMTx-4, TRAM-34) to explore the molecular mechanism of the Ca^{2+}-signaling. Based on these experiments we conclude that mechanical stimulation of RBCs activates mechano-sensitive channels most likely Piezo1. This channel activity allows Ca^{2+} to enter the cell, leading to a transient activation of the Gardos-channel associated with K^+, Cl^-, and water loss, i.e., with a transient volume adaptation facilitating the passage of the RBCs through the constriction.

Keywords: RBC deformation, Piezo1, hSK4 (KCNN4), Ca^{2+} imaging, microfluidics, dorsal skinfold chamber

INTRODUCTION

The physiological function of the Gardos-channel, a Ca^{2+}-activated K^+-channel (Gardos, 1958) in the red blood cell (RBC), that was later identified as the hSK4 (KCNN4) channel (Hoffman et al., 2003), was obscure for decades. It was regarded as a RBC suicidal mechanism (Andrews and Low, 1999; Kaestner and Bernhardt, 2002; Lang and Qadri, 2012) including the process of dehydration associated with Gardos-channel activity (Begenisich et al., 2004; Lew et al., 2005). Such a concept was mainly consequent to the observation that an increase in the intracellular RBC Ca^{2+}-concentration was associated with numerous processes leading in their synergistic effects to cell death (Bogdanova et al., 2013). The Gardos-channel fits well into this concept as it requires Ca^{2+} to be activated and its activation results in K^+-loss associated with loss in Cl^- and water and hence in cell shrinkage. In addition within the recent years hereditary anemic disorders have been associated with mutations in the Gardos-channel (Glogowska et al., 2015; Fermo et al., 2017).

Furthermore, several sources of Ca^{2+}-entry have been identified in RBCs, like a non-selective voltage-activated cation channel (Kaestner et al., 2000), $Ca_V2.1$ (Andrews et al., 2002), TRPC6 (Foller et al., 2008), VDAC (Bouyer et al., 2011), or NMDA-receptors (Makhro et al., 2013). Complementary, an increased activity of these channels has been associated with pathophysiological conditions such as prostaglandin E_2 and lysophosphatidic acid release from activated platelets (Li et al., 1996; Yang et al., 2000; Kaestner et al., 2004, 2012), malaria infection (Bouyer et al., 2011) and anemias like sickle cell disease or rare anemia (Hänggi et al., 2014; Hertz et al., 2017).

During the past years a new player was discovered, Piezo1, a mechano-sensitive non-selective cation channel (Coste et al., 2010; Gottlieb and Sachs, 2012; Gottlieb et al., 2012) that is also abundant in RBCs (Zarychanski et al., 2012; Albuisson et al., 2013; Kaestner, 2015). This discovery initiated studies to link mechanical stress associated Piezo1 activity with RBC volume regulation by Gardos-channel activity (Gallagher, 2013; Faucherre et al., 2014; Cahalan et al., 2015). However, these studies have either been performed in animal models (Faucherre et al., 2014; Cahalan et al., 2015) or in relation to pathophysiological conditions (Glogowska and Gallagher, 2015). Here, we investigate healthy human RBCs subjected to different forms of mechanical stimulation using intracellular Ca^{2+} changes as a read-out parameter and compare their behavior when Piezo1 is inhibited by the toxin GsMTx-4 (Bae et al., 2011).

MATERIALS AND METHODS

Human RBCs

Blood sampling from humans was approved by the ethical committee (Ärztekammer des Saarlandes, approval number 132/08) upon informed consent. Blood was collected in 9 mL heparin tubes (Vacuette, Becton, Dickinson and Co., Franklin Lakes, NJ, USA) and immediately used for measurements as recommended (Makhro et al., 2016). All treatments and measurements of RBCs were performed in a laboratory of biological safety level S2. Blood was washed three times in Tyrode solution containing in mM: 135 NaCl, 5.4 KCl, 10 Glucose, 10 HEPES, 1.8 $CaCl_2$, 1 $MgCl_2$, pH 7.35 adjusted with NaOH, 300 mOsmol/kg H_2O. The washing procedure was based on 3 min centrifugation with 1,000 × g, supernatant and buffy coat were removed by aspiration. All experiments were performed at least three times with RBCs from three different donors.

Cell Staining and Pharmacological Interventions

During the staining procedure and the experiments, RBCs were kept in Tyrode solution and incubated with Fluo-4, AM or Calcein Red-Orange, AM (both ThermoFisher Scientific, Waltham, MA, USA) at a concentration of 5 μM (from a 1 mM stock solution in dimethyl sulfoxide (DMSO) containing 20% Pluronic F-127) for 1 h. After the staining, cells were washed three times by 3 min centrifugation with 1,000 × g. Then RBCs were plated on coverslips and 20 min were allowed for sedimentation and deesterification of the Fluo-4. Mechano-sensitive channels and the Gardos-channel were inhibited by GsMTx-4 and TRAM-34, respectively. GsMTx-4 was purchased from Alomone Labs (Jerusalem, Israel) and TRAM-34 from Sigma-Aldrich (St. Louis, MO, USA). For both substances, stock solutions were prepared at 1 mM in aqua dest. Further applications were performed at concentrations indicated in the experimental description.

Confocal Imaging

Confocal imaging was performed with a 2D-array kilobeam scanner (Infinity-4, VisiTech Int., Sunderland, UK) as previously described (Danielczok et al., 2017). In short, excitation was performed with a 491 nm DPSS laser (Calypso, Cobolt, Solna, Sweden). The confocal scanner was attached to an inverted microscope (TE2000-U, Nikon, Tokyo, Japan) utilizing a 60x objective (NA 1.4) and using a confocal aperture of 64 μm. Image acquisition was done with an EM-CCD camera (iXon887, Andor, Belfast, UK) cooled down to −50°C and used in frame transfer mode. Exposure time was 2,000 ms for the measurements at stasis and 500 ms for the microfluidic experiments at a 1 × 1 binning and a pixel read-out of 10 MHz. A pre-amplification of 2.4 and an EM-gain of 180 was applied. The entire measurement process was software controlled (VoxCellScan, VisiTech Int., Sunderland, UK). The data analysis concept was previously described (Wang et al., 2013) and image analysis is detailed below. Further data analysis and determination of the maximal cellular response was processed in Igor Pro 6.2 (WaveMetrics, Portland, Oregon, USA) with custom made macros.

Mechanical Stimulation

Mechanical stimulation was done either by application of a hypoosmotic solution or by touching the RBC with a micropipette. For the hypoosmotic solution Tyrode solution (see section Human RBCs above) was diluted by aqua dest. until an osmolarity of 200 mosml was reached. Osmolarity was measured using a vapor pressure osmometer (Vapro, Wescor, South Logan, UT, USA). Solution was applied by a local gravity driven perfusion system where the continuous flow of Tyrode solution was switched to the hypoosmotic solution. For pipette stimulation pipettes were made in the same manner as for patch-clamping RBCs (Thomas et al., 2001), in detail glas pipettes were pulled from glas capillaries (GB150-8P, Science Products, Berlin, Germany) on a DMZ Universal Puller (Seitz, Munich, Germany). Pipettes were prefilled with Tyrode solution and to avoid capillary effects the back end of the pipette was closed with a putty plug. Pipettes were fixed in a patch-clamp pipette holder (HEKA, Lambrecht, Germany). For navigating the pipette a hydraulic micromanipulator WR-6 (Narishige, Tokyo, Japan) was utilized.

Microfluidic Chips

The channels used for the experiments of cells flowing through narrow constrictions are similar to those used in a previous study (Thiam et al., 2016). The custom-made mold used in the study, bearing many combinations of channels and constriction sizes (length and width), was replicated with epoxy resist (Soloplast R123) (Heuzé et al., 2011). PDMS RTV 615 (Momentive) and its curing agent were mixed to a ratio 10:1 (w/w), cast in the mold and cured for 2 h at 70°C. The hardened PDMS was then cut and drilled in the inlets with an 18 G needle and was then bound, after plasma activation (Harrick PDC, 30 s treatment), to a glass-bottom dish (FD35, World Precision Instrument). From the available sizes, the set of channels used in this study were 5 μm high and 8 μm wide, with constrictions of 3 μm wide and 10 μm long. Cells were pushed through the channel by a programmable syringe pump (NE-1000, New Era Pump Systems, Farmingdale, NY, USA) such that RBCs reached a flow speed in the range of 3–5 μm/s.

Preparation of Dorsal Skinfold Chamber and *in Vivo* Imaging

Animals

The *in vivo* experiments were performed in 12- to 14-week old male C57BL/6 mice with a body weight of 24–26 g. The animals were bred and housed in open cages in the conventional animal husbandry of the Institute for Clinical & Experimental Surgery (Saarland University, Germany) in a temperature-controlled environment under a 12 h/12 h light-dark cycle and had free access to drinking water and standard pellet food (Altromin, Lage, Germany). All experiments were approved by the local governmental animal care committee (approval Number 06/2015) and were conducted in accordance with the German legislation on protection of animals and the NIH Guidelines for the Care and Use of Laboratory Animals (Institute of Laboratory Animal Resources, National Research Council, Washington, USA).

Dorsal Skinfold Chamber Model

Red blood cell passage of small capillaries was analyzed in the dorsal skinfold chamber model, which provides continuous microscopic access to the microcirculation of the striated skin muscle and the underlying subcutaneous tissue (Laschke and Menger, 2016). For the implantation of the chamber, the mice were anesthetized by i.p. injection of ketamine (75 mg/kg body weight; Ursotamin®; Serumwerke Bernburg, Bernburg, Germany) and xylazine (15 mg/kg body weight; Rompun®; Bayer, Leverkusen, Germany). Subsequently, two symmetrical titanium frames (Irola Industriekomponenten GmbH & Co. KG, Schonach, Germany) were implanted on the extended dorsal skinfold of the animals in a stepwise procedure, as described previously in detail (Laschke et al., 2011). Within the area of the observation window, one layer of skin was completely removed in a circular area of ~15 mm in diameter. The remaining layers (striated skin muscle, subcutaneous tissue and skin) were finally covered with a removable cover glass. To exclude alterations of the microcirculation due to the surgical intervention, the mice were allowed to recover for 48 h.

In Vivo Microscopy

In vivo microscopic analyses were performed as previously described (Brust et al., 2014). In detail, the mice were anesthetized and a fine polyethylene catheter (PE10, 0.28 mm internal diameter) was inserted into the A. carotis for application of labeled RBCs. Then, the animals were put in lateral decubital position on a plexiglas pad and the dorsal skinfold chamber was attached to the microscopic stage of an upright microscope (E600; Nikon, Tokyo, Japan) equipped with a 40x, NA 0.8, water immersion objective and a halogen lamp attached to a fluorescein isothiocyanate (FITC) filterset (excitation 465–495 nm, emission 515–555 nm). For labeling RBCs blood samples were taken from siblings and *ex vivo* stained with Fluo-4, AM as described above. Up to 0.5 mL of stained RBCs were transfused directly prior to the imaging experiments. The microscopic images were recorded using a charge-coupled device video camera (iXon Ultra; Andor, Belfast, UK) connected to a PC system at an acquisition speed of 212 images per second (4.5 ms exposure time, 2 × 2 binning, shift speed 0.3 μs, readout rate 17 MHz). For image processing, the black and white pictures were changed into a "fire" look-up table for better visualization.

Measuring Fiterability

Blood samples were centrifuged at 1,000 × g for 20 min. Plasma was aspirated and mixed with phosphate buffered saline (PBS) (1:10). Erythrocytes were mixed with Tyrode solution (1:1) and washed three times (1,000 × g, 5 min). Filterability was tested by a modified method originally developed for the depletion of leukocytes (Beutler et al., 1976; Minetti et al., 2013). Filter paper (Whatman No. 4, GE Healthcare, UK) was pressed in a 3 mL syringe (Omnifix Solo Lure, Braun, Germany) and 200 mg Sigma- and 100 mg Alpha-Cellulose was added. The syringe was filled further with 2 mL Tyrode solution and shaked to allow the cellulose to mix. After the Tyrode drained, the syringe was primed with 2 mL of the diluted plasma. Subsequently, 500 μL of the RBC/Tyrode mixture was added at stopped flow conditions. Another 2 mL of Tyrode solution was carefully added. The flow through the syringe was started and the filtrate collected for exactly 1 min. The amount of RBCs was related to the amount of hemoglobin, which was determined photometrically. To standardize the measurements different forms of hemoglobin were converted to hemiglobincyanid as previously described (Meyer-Wilmes and Remmer, 1956). Absorption was measured at 546 nm (Lambda Bio+, Perkin Elmer, Waltham, MA, USA).

Image Analysis

All image analysis was performed in ImageJ (Wayne Rasband, National Institute of Health, USA). For the images displayed in the figures a look-up table named "fire" was applied. To extract data from the images raw data were used. First a background subtraction was performed (subtraction of an image just without the cells). Then regions of interest (ROI) were defined for each cell or for each position of the cell when analyzing cells in flow. To create graphs of cellular responses we presented the fluorescence intensity as self ratios F/F_0, i.e., the entire fluorescence trace was divided by the fluorescence value at the beginning of the recording to normalize the starting conditions and to compensate for cellular differences in dye loading or hemoglobin concentration (Kaestner et al., 2006).

Statistics

For all statistical analysis the Gaussian distribution of the dataset was checked by the D'Agostino and Pearson omnibus normality test. For data with Gaussian distribution the mean value ± the standard error of mean (SEM) was plotted as column graphs. Testing for significant differences was performed with a paired

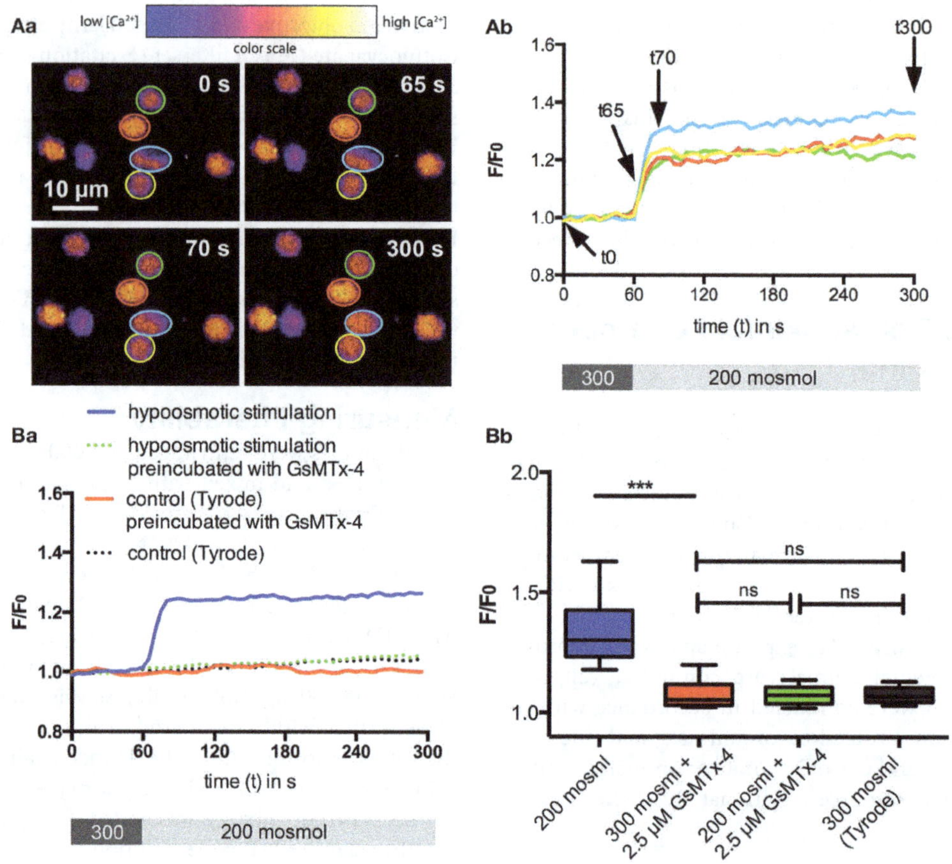

FIGURE 1 | Ca^{2+}-signaling of RBCs after hypoosmotic treatment. RBCs in Tyrode solution were exposed to 200 mosmol solution. **(A)** depicts confocal example images at four time points **(Aa)** and example traces **(Ab)** indicating the time points displayed in **(Aa)** with arrows. The cellular Ca^{2+}-response as fluorescence intensity (F/F_0) of the Ca^{2+}-fluorophor Fluo-4 is plotted over time. The color-coded regions of interest in **(Aa)** correspond to the colors of the traces in **(Ab)**. Below the graph in **(Ab)** the protocol of the solution application (60 s, 300 mosmol followed by 240 s 200 mosml) is provided. **(B)** shows the statistical analysis. For each condition between 160 and 210 cells from three different donors were analyzed. The median fluorescence trace (F/F_0) over time of all cells is depicted in **(Ba)**. Below the graph the protocol of the solution application (60 s, 300 mosmol followed by 240 s 200 mosml) is provided. The analysis of the cellular maximal response (F/F_0) is depicted in **(Bb)**. The response under hypoosmotic conditions in the absence of GsMTx-4 is significantly different relative to all other conditions measured ($p < 0.001$; ***).

t-test, wheras $p < 0.0001$ was denoted with four stars (****) and non-significant differences abbreviated with "ns."

Datasets with a non-Gaussian distribution were visualized as box-plots representing the median and the 25–75th percentile and whiskers representing the 5–95th percentile. Significance was tested with Mann-Whitney test and significance levels were indicated with three stars (***) for $p < 0.001$, with one star (*) for $p < 0.05$ and "ns" for not significant.

All graph presentations and statistical tests were performed in GraphPad Prism (GraphPad Software, La Jolla, CA, USA).

RESULTS

RBC Ca^{2+}-Response after Mechanical Stimulation in Stasis

In an initial experiment we aimed to check if basic mechanical stimulation by osmotic swelling leads to an activity of mechano-sensitive channels in RBCs. We challenged the cells with a 200 mosmol solution and used the change in intracellular free Ca^{2+} as a read-out parameter. The results of the microscopic measurements using the Ca^{2+}-fluorophore Fluo-4 are summarized in **Figure 1**. In contrast to hormonal-like stimulations (Wang et al., 2013), RBCs showed qualitatively a very homogeneous response, i.e., all cells responded immediately with an increase in intracellular Ca^{2+}, just the extent of the increase varied between the cells. This Ca^{2+}-increase could be completely blocked by preincubation of the RBCs with 2.5 µM GsMTx-4 (**Figure 1Bb**, green box), a widely used inhibitor of Piezo1 (Bae et al., 2011), whereas GsMTx-4 itself had no effect on cells in isosmotic solution (**Figure 1Bb**, red box).

Next we tested if local mechanical stimulation by poking an individual RBC with a micropipette would also lead to an increase in intracellular Ca^{2+}. The results of these experiments are presented in **Figure 2**. Touching the cell with the micropipette resulted in an immediate increase in intracellular Ca^{2+}, which could be inhibited by preincubation with 2.5 µM GsMTx-4 (**Figures 2A,B**). Furthermore, we could even identify the spot where the micropipette was touching the cell as the source

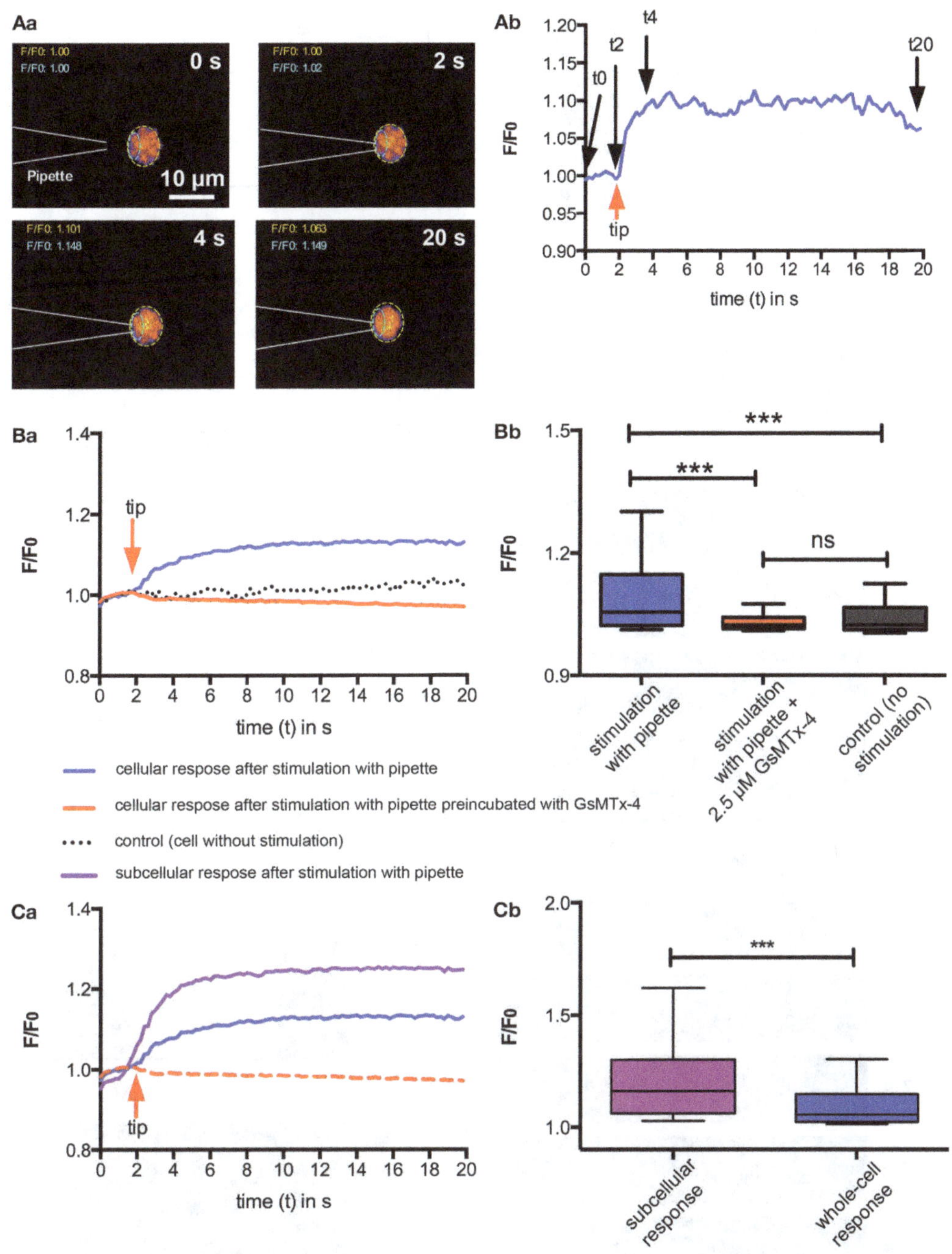

FIGURE 2 | Ca^{2+}-signaling of RBC after local mechanical stimulation. Individual RBCs were mechanically stimulated using a micropipette. **(A)** exemplifies a typical experiment. Fluorescent confocal images of a Fluo-4 loaded cell when touched by a micropipette at four time points are shown in **(Aa)**. The color scale is the same as in **Figure 1Aa**. Since the pipette is not visible in the fluorescent image, its position is drawn in the images by dashed white lines. The fluorescence intensity (F/F_0) of the region of interest (ROI) indicated by the dashed yellow line in **(Aa)** is plotted in **(Ab)** indicating the time point when the pipette touches the cell (red arrow) and the time points of the images displayed in **(Aa)** (black arrows). **(B)** depicts the statistical analysis comparing pipette stimulation in the absence and presence of GsMTx-4 with unstimulated RBCs. For each condition between 74 and 76 cells from three different donors were analyzed. The median fluorescence trace (F/F_0) over time of all cells is depicted in **(Ba)**. The red arrow indicates the time point when the pipette was touching the RBC. The analysis of the cellular maximal response (F/F_0) is depicted in **(Bb)**. The response of the mechanical stimulation in the absence of GsMTx-4 is significantly different relative to all other conditions measured ($p < 0.001$; ***). **(C)** Compares the cellular response of 76 RBCs as depicted in **(B)** with the local (subcellular) fluorescence intensity at the spot where the micropipette is touching the cell as indicated by the ROI outlined with cyan dashed lines in **(Aa)**. The median fluorescence trace (F/F_0) over time of all cells is depicted in **(Ca)**. The red arrow indicates the time point when the pipette was touching the RBC. For a better comparison the blue and the red lines are replotted from **(Ba)**. The comparison of the local (subcellular) and cellular (whole-cell) maximum response (F/F_0) is depicted in **(Cb)**. The local response is significantly higher than the whole-cell response ($p < 0.001$; ***).

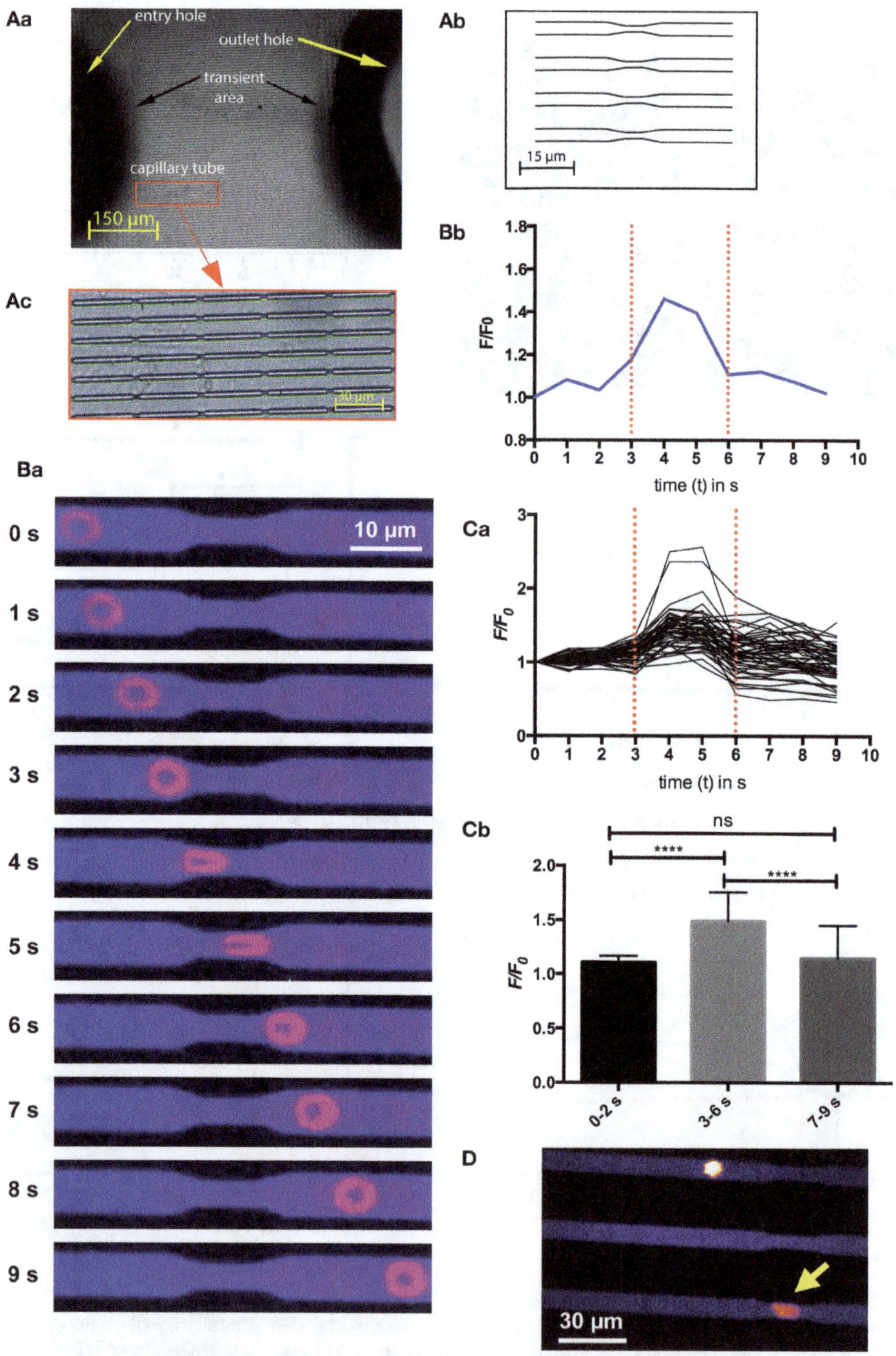

FIGURE 3 | Ca^{2+}-signaling of a RBC passing through constrictions in a microfluidic chip. **(A)** depicts the design of the microfluidic chip used. A photographic overview with labeled parts of the chip is given in **(Aa)**, whereas a schematic overview of parallel channels with constrictions to simulate capillaries is drawn in **(Ab)**. In contrast, the real appearance of the channels with repetitive constrictions is displayed in **(Ac)**. **(B)** exemplifies a typical experiment. Fluorescent confocal images of a Fluo-4 loaded cell when passing through the microfluidic channel at 10 time points are shown in **(Ba)**. The color scale is the same as in **Figure 1Aa**. The fluorescence intensity (F/F_0) of the RBC at the 10 time points shown in **(Ba)** is plotted in **(Bb)** indicating the start and the end of the constriction by red dotted lines. A video of this experiment is available in the supplemental material (Supplemental Video 1). **(C)** depicts the analysis of 52 cells measured while passing through the constriction. The fluorescence intensity (F/F_0) traces of all measured RBCs are plotted in **(Ca)**. The statistical analysis of the maximal fluorescence intensity (F/F_0) at time points before the constriction (0–2 s), when passing through the constriction (3–6 s) and after passing through the constriction (7–9 s) is depicted in **(Cb)**. The increase in Ca^{2+}, while passing through the constriction is highly significant ($p < 0.0001$; ****). **(D)** Shows an image of RBCs treated with 1 µM GsMTx-4 getting stuck in the microfluidic channels. The yellow arrow points to a cell sticking in a constriction. To better judge the resting state of the cell please refer to Supplemental Video 2.

of the Ca^{2+}-entry, because maximal intensity values in the vicinity of this spot (**Figure 2Aa**, cyan region of interest) reached higher than the values considering the full cellular confocal cross section (**Figure 2C**). To exclude the increase in fluorescence intensity was caused by an artifact (e.g., cellular compression and putative increase in Fluo-4 concentration) we performed control experiments with a simultaneous Calcein Red-Orange staining, a dye that is insensitive to Ca^{2+} and other ions but still has a cytoplasmic localisation. The Calcein Red-Orange fluorescence was constant during the entire measurement indicating (i) that the cell membrane was not damaged and (ii) lack of volume related artifacts in the fluorescence intensity.

RBC Ca^{2+}-Response While Passing through Constrictions in Microfluidic Channels

Since RBCs experience a mechanical stimulation when small capillaries or interendothelial slits in the spleen, we designed a microfluidic chip that would mimic such a constriction (**Figure 3A**). The measurement procedure as well as the statistical analysis are depicted in **Figures 3B,C** as well as in Supplemental Video 1. The cells indeed showed a transient increase in intracellular Ca^{2+} when passing through the constriction. In similarity to the previous experiments (**Figures 1**, **2**) all cells reacted with such a Ca^{2+} increase just to a different degree. The hypothesis that we are facing a mechanism of adaptive volume regulation initiated by mechano-sensitive channels is supported by attempts to perform the same experiments as presented in **Figure 3B** with RBCs preincubated with GsMTx-4. Under these conditions the channels of the microfluidic chip were clogged immediately preventing any cellular analysis (**Figure 3D** and Supplemental Video 2). This was confirmed for GsMTx-4 concentrations in the range of 2.5 – 0.1 μM.

In Vivo RBC Ca^{2+}-Response While Passing through Capillaries

To answer the question if the results from the microfluidic channels are of physiological relevance, we aimed for *in vivo* measurements and chose the mouse model utilizing

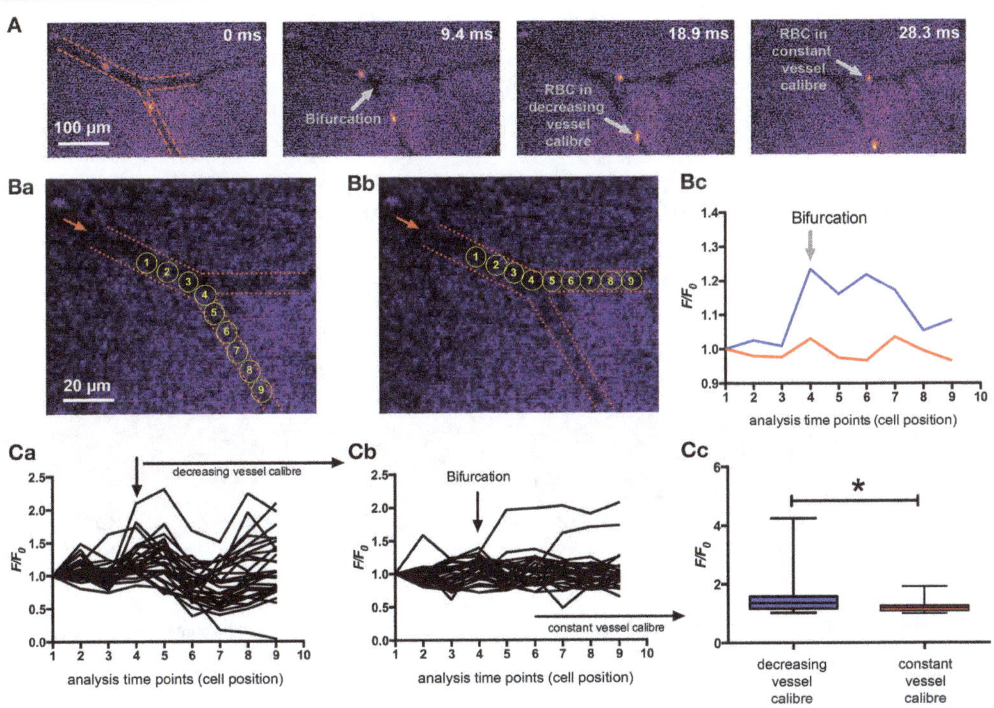

FIGURE 4 | *In vivo* Ca^{2+}-signaling of mouse RBCs when passing through capillaries. Mouse RBCs were *ex vivo* stained with Fluo-4 and then re-injected into the mouse circulation. Fluorescence imaging of capillaries was performed in the dorsal skinfold chamber. **(A)** Shows representative snapshots of RBCs passing a bifurcation. For the 30 ms sequence only every second recorded image is presented. For a better orientation the vessel walls are indicated by red dashed lines in the leftmost image and further annotations (gray) are added in the other images. **(B)** depicts the positions where fluorescence intensity (F/F_0) was analyzed for a decreasing vessel caliber **(Ba)** and for a constant vessel caliber **(Bb)** of the same example section as in **(A)**. The dashed red lines mark the vessel walls, the red arrow indicates the blood flow direction and the yellow circles depict the analysis positions which are plotted in the following diagrams. Example fluorescence traces of the two cells analyzed as pointed out in **(Ba,Bb)** are shown in **(Bc)**. Videos of these two example cells are available in the supplemental material (Supplemental Videos 3, 4, respectively). **(C)** depicts the analysis of 30 cells passing through a capillary with decreasing vessel caliber and 28 cells passing through a capillary with constant vessel caliber. Analysis was performed at three vessel-bifurcations in two mice. The fluorescence intensity (F/F_0) traces of all measured RBCs passing through a capillary with decreasing vessel caliber is plotted in **(Ca)**, while the traces of all measured RBCs passing a capillary with constant vessel caliber is plotted in **(Cb)**. The statistical analysis of the maximal fluorescence intensity (F/F_0) of RBCs from both groups is depicted in **(Cc)**. The increase in Ca^{2+}, while passing through a vessel with decreasing caliber is significant ($p = 0.014$; *).

a dorsal skinfold chamber for the optical imaging. Mouse RBCs were stained with Fluo-4 *ex vivo* and then reinjected into the circulation. The fast movement of the RBCs in the capillaries required high speed fluorescence imaging at a frame rate exceeding the 200 Hz. We chose imaging positions of capillary bifurcations, where one vessel showed a decreasing caliber while the other one remained fairly constant in order to have constrictions and a control condition in the same image sequence. Representative recordings are depicted in Supplemental Videos 3 and 4. **Figure 4** summarizes the analysis of RBCs in three of such bifurcations (from 2 mice). We could identify a significantly higher Ca^{2+} in the RBCs passing through the vessel with the decreased caliber compared to control conditions (**Figure 4C**).

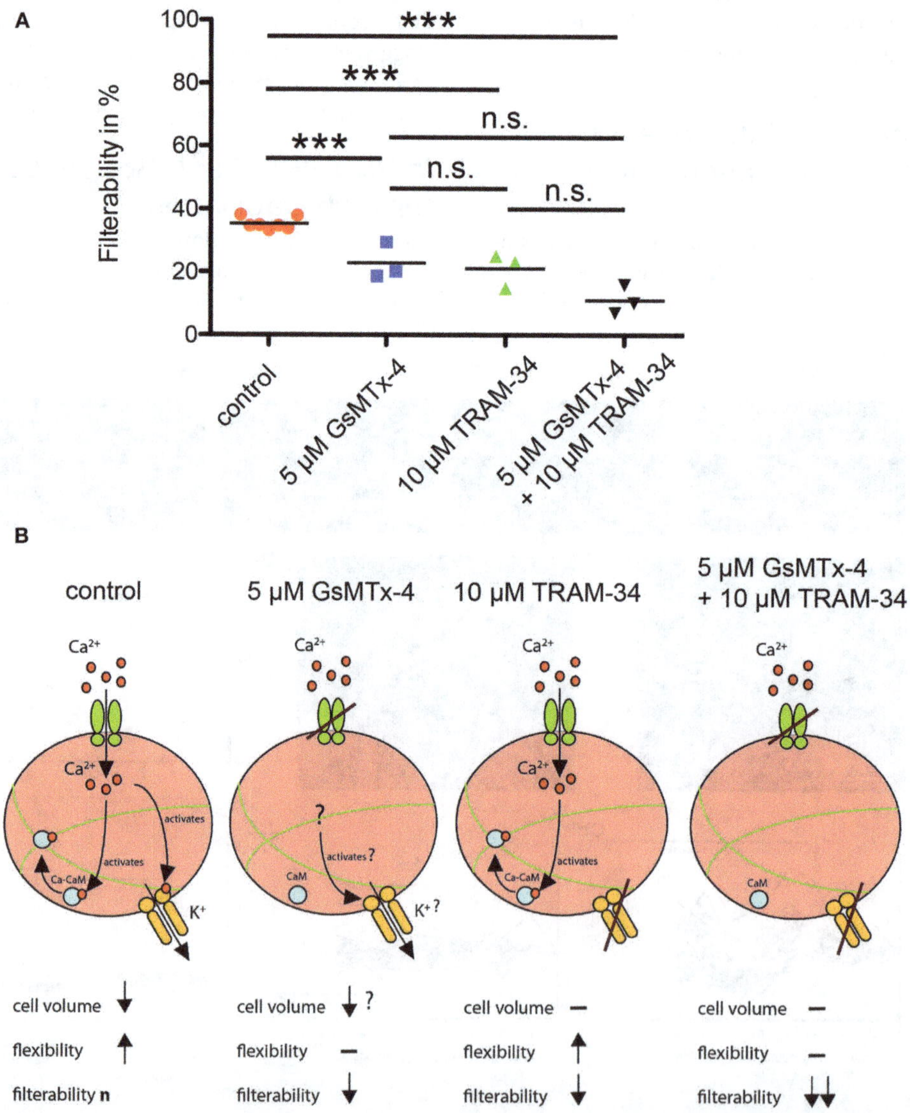

FIGURE 5 | RBC filterability and putative mechanisms. **(A)** shows measurements of the filterability of RBCs under control conditions (red circles) and in the presence of GsMTx-4, a blocker of the Piezo1 ion channel (blue squares), in the presence of TRAM-34, an inhibitor of the Gardos-channel (green triangles) and in the presence of both drugs (black triangles; ***$p < 0.001$). A summary of these data was already published in a different context (Fermo et al., 2017). **(B)** visualizes the putative mechanism for all four experimental conditions depicted in **(A)**. Under control conditions interaction of the RBC with the cellulose activates mechanosensitive channels such as Piezo1 (green channel symbol), Ca^{2+} (red circles) can enter the cell. Ca^{2+} activates the Gardos-channel (orange channel symbol) and by formation of the calcium-calmodulin complex (Ca-CaM; associated blue and red circles) loosens the cross-linked spectrin tetramers (green lines). For a more detailed description of this process see Discussion. These processes will reduce the cell volume and increase the flexibility of the cell resulting in the "normal" filterability n. If GsMTx-4 blocks the Piezo1, the Ca^{2+}-entry pathway is impaired and the above-described process is diminished. However, it is not clear if Ca^{2+}-permeable channels other than Piezo1 are involved, and hence a slight adaptation in cell volume occurs. If TRAM-34 blocks the Gardos-channel, Ca^{2+} may still enter the cell through Piezo1, which should still allow the modification of the spectrin network but not the volume adaptation resulting in decreased filterability. If both Piezo1 and Gardos-channel are inhibited all mechanisms described above are blocked with the expected consequence for the RBCs' filterability.

Measurements of RBCs Filterability

In order to test if our microscopic results have a macroscopic implication, we measured the filterability of human blood samples and compared it with samples preincubated with 5 μM GsMTx-4 or 10 μM TRAM-34, a Gardos-channel inhibitor, or with both substances simultaneously (**Figure 5A**). Any of the applied pharmacological interventions, i.e., any impairment of the proposed mechano-sensitive volume regulation (**Figure 5B**), significantly reduced the RBC filterability.

DISCUSSION

We investigated RBCs after various modes of mechanical stimulation: osmotic swelling (**Figure 1**), poking individual cells with a micropipette (**Figure 2**) and squeezing cells through a constriction in a microfluidic channel (**Figure 3**). To transfer this scenario to *in vivo* conditions we used a mouse model (**Figure 4**) and finally we performed macroscopic measurements on cell populations (**Figure 5**). All these measurements gave consistent data supporting our hypothesis outlined in **Figure 6**. When RBCs are passing through a capillary with a diameter smaller than the cross-section of a RBC or interendothelial slits in the spleen, they need to be super-deformable and undergo a transient volume decrease. We could show that all kinds of mechanical stimulation resulted in an intracellular increase in Ca^{2+}. We did not demonstrate the molecular identity mediating the Ca^{2+}-entry but based on the knowledge of mechano-sensitive channels in the human RBC (Cinar et al., 2015; Kaestner, 2015), the sensitivity of our measurements for GsMTx-4 (Bae et al., 2011 and **Figures 1B**, **2B**, **5**) and the comparison of our results with knock-out animals (Faucherre et al., 2014; Cahalan et al., 2015) it is very likely that Piezo1 is the mechano-sensitive "Ca^{2+}-source." However, involvement of other mechano-sensitive transport cannot be excluded. NMDA-receptors which are also present in the RBC-population (Makhro et al., 2013) show a mechano-sensitivity but it is not sensitive to GsMTx-4 (Maneshi et al., 2017).

Considering the long lasting Ca^{2+}-signals in **Figures 1**, **2**, we have to admit that in both cases the mechanical stimulation (osmotic pressure and pipette touching the cell) lasted during the entire experiment, Piezo1 activation would suggest a transient Ca^{2+}-entry. If Ca^{2+} entry would have been carried exclusively through the Piezo1 channel, due to the inactivation kinetics of the channel, such an entry would suddenly stop. Indeed the Ca^{2+}-level remains constant after the initial increase pointing to an equilibrium between Ca^{2+}-extrusion by the Ca^{2+}-pump and Ca^{2+} entry. A special case for such an equilibrium could be Piezo1 inactivation and the failure of the Ca^{2+}-pump, e.g., by Ca^{2+}-mediated destruction of the pump fuelling ATP-pools (Chu et al., 2012). For a transient mechanical stimulation, e.g., when passing through a constriction, (**Figures 3**, **4**) the associated Ca^{2+} signal as expected was also transient.

Once Ca^{2+} enters the RBCs it initiates a plethora of processes in a concentration dependent manner (Bogdanova et al., 2013). One of them (responsible for the dehydration—compare Introduction) is the Gardos-channel, which was also challenged by application of TRAM-34 in the measurements of

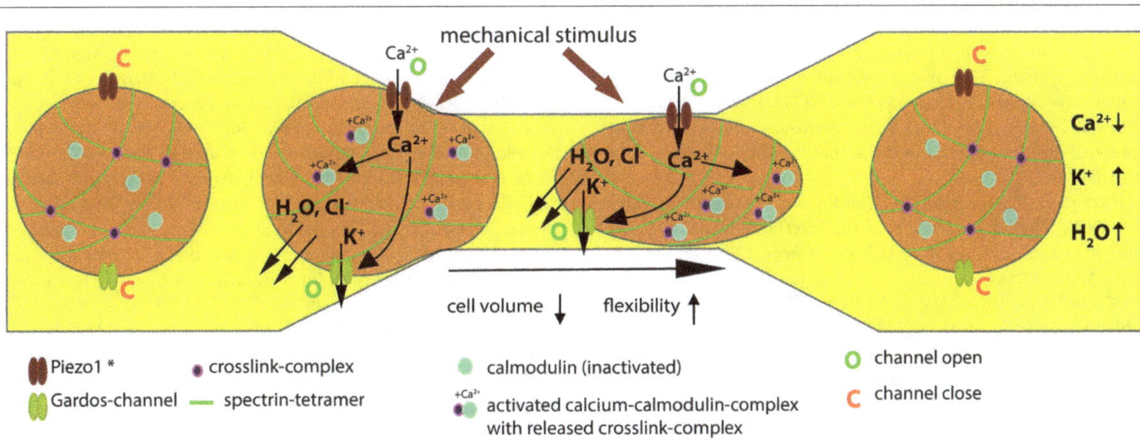

FIGURE 6 | Evidence based hypothesis of the Ca^{2+}-signaling mechanism when RBCs pass capillaries. The description of a RBC passing through a constriction is described from left to right. Under laminar flow of RBCs in the vessel, for both Piezo1 and the Gardos-channel the open probability is very low and they can be regarded as being in a closed state (denoted by a "C" next to the channel symbols). *In this scheme Piezo1 denotes the most probably involved molecular player but could also be a different mechanosensitive mechanism. As the RBC enters a constriction and the cell comes in mechanical contact with the vessel wall, this mechanical stimulus activates Piezo1 (denoted by a "O" next to the channel symbol). Since Piezo1 is a non-selective cation-channel (Gottlieb and Sachs, 2012) and in view of the tremendous gradient for Ca^{2+} across the membrane (Tiffert et al., 2003), Ca^{2+} will enter the cell. This will activate the Gardos-channel (denoted by a "O" next to the channel symbol) and the calcium-calmodulin complex (Ca-CaM) will be formed (associated blue and pink circles). Activation of the Gardos-channel will result in loss of K^+, Cl^- and water, i.e., in cell shrinkage. The Ca-CaM destabilizes the actin—addusin—Band 4.1 complex and the cross-linked spectrin network becomes more flexible (interrupted green lines). For a more detailed description of this process see Discussion. Both processes facilitate the passage of the RBC trough the constriction. Both, Piezo1 and Gardos-channels are likely to inactivate and close (denoted by a "C" next to the channel symbols). Na^+/K^+-pump and Ca^{2+}-pump (not shown in scheme) will restore the original ion concentrations and such the RBC volume will return to its original size. Likewise the Ca-CaM will inactivate resulting in the dissociation of the calmodolin (blue circles) and thus the cross-linking of the spectrin tetramers (pink circles at cross-section of green lines).

the filterability (**Figure 5**). In addition to the Gardos-channel mediated dehydration, in **Figure 6** we render a further Ca^{2+}-dependent process, the Ca^{2+} binding to calmodulin, forming the Ca^{2+}-calmodulin complex (Ca-CaM). Protein Band 4.1 and adducin interact with Ca-CaM. Adducin binds to actin blocking elongation of the fast-growing (barbing) ends of actin filaments within the junctional complexes. Interaction with Ca-CaM down-regulates capping activity of adducin regulating thereby actin filament assembly (Kuhlman et al., 1996). Furthermore, adducin tetramers participate in docking of carbonic anhydrase II to band 3 tetramers. When interacting with the band 3 dimers anchoring the spectrin network to the membrane, the junctional complex becomes a part of bigger multi-protein complexes known as 4.1R-complexes. Interaction of the 4.1R-complex with Ca-CaM triggers the reduction of the affinity of this protein to all interacting partners. As a result, spectrin network interaction with the integral proteins becomes loose and finally the RBC show an increased flexibility (Bogdanova et al., 2013).

Our data allow a transfer of knowledge originally achieved with knock-out approaches of Piezo1 in zebrafish (Faucherre et al., 2014) and mice (Cahalan et al., 2015) to human RBCs as outlined above. Furthermore, comparing our micropipette poking experiments with very similar patch-clamp experiments with human RBCs (Dyrda et al., 2010), showing a mechanical stimulation followed by the activation of the Gardos-channel is in support of the Piezo1—Gardos-channel interplay for transient volume adaptation.

AUTHOR CONTRIBUTIONS

LK defined the study, JD, FL, ML, and LK planned the experiments. JD, ET, LH, PP-K, ML, and LK performed the acquisition and analysis. JD, PP-K, and LK interpreted the data. JD drafted the figures and LK drafted the manuscript. ET, LH, PP-K, FL, and ML critically revised the manuscript. All authors approved the final version of the manuscript.

ACKNOWLEDGMENTS

The authors like to thank Prof. P. Lipp for providing the laboratory for the Ca^{2+} measurements.

REFERENCES

Albuisson, J., Murthy, S. E., Bandell, M., Coste, B., Louis-Dit-Picard, H., Mathur, J., et al. (2013). Dehydrated hereditary stomatocytosis linked to gain-of-function mutations in mechanically activated PIEZO1 ion channels. *Nat. Commun.* 4:1884. doi: 10.1038/ncomms2899

Andrews, D. A., and Low, P. S. (1999). Role of red blood cells in thrombosis. *Curr. Opin. Hematol.* 6, 76–82. doi: 10.1097/00062752-199903000-00004

Andrews, D. A., Yang, L., and Low, P. S. (2002). Phorbol ester stimulates a protein kinase C-mediated agatoxin-TK-sensitive calcium permeability pathway in human red blood cells. *Blood* 100, 3392–3399. doi: 10.1182/blood.V100.9.3392

Bae, C., Sachs, F., and Gottlieb, P. A. (2011). The mechanosensitive ion channel Piezo1 is inhibited by the peptide GsMTx4. *Biochemistry* 50, 6295–6300. doi: 10.1021/bi200770q

Begenisich, T., Nakamoto, T., Ovitt, C. E., Nehrke, K., Brugnara, C., Alper, S. L., et al. (2004). Physiological roles of the intermediate conductance, Ca^{2+}-activated potassium channel Kcnn4. *J. Biol. Chem.* 279, 47681–47687. doi: 10.1074/jbc.M409627200

Beutler, E., West, C., and Blume, K. G. (1976). Removal of leukocytes and platelets from whole-blood. *J. Lab. Clin. Med.* 88, 328–333.

Bogdanova, A., Makhro, A., Wang, J., Lipp, P., and Kaestner, L. (2013). Calcium in red blood cells-a perilous balance. *Int. J. Mol. Sci.* 14, 9848–9872. doi: 10.3390/ijms14059848

Bouyer, G., Cueff, A., Egée, S., Kmiecik, J., Maksimova, Y., Glogowska, E., et al. (2011). Erythrocyte peripheral type benzodiazepine receptor/voltage-dependent anion channels are upregulated by *Plasmodium falciparum*. *Blood* 118, 2305–2312. doi: 10.1182/blood-2011-01-329300

Brust, M., Aouane, O., Thiébaud, M., Flormann, D., Verdier, C., Kaestner, L., et al. (2014). The plasma protein fibrinogen stabilizes clusters of red blood cells in microcapillary flows. *Sci. Rep.* 4:4348. doi: 10.1038/srep04348

Cahalan, S. M., Lukacs, V., Ranade, S. S., Chien, S., Bandell, M., and Patapoutian, A. (2015). Piezo1 links mechanical forces to red blood cell volume. *Elife* 4:e07370. doi: 10.7554/eLife.07370

Chu, H., Puchulu-Campanella, E., Galan, J. A., Tao, W. A., Low, P. S., and Hoffman, J. F. (2012). Identification of cytoskeletal elements enclosing the ATP pools that fuel human red blood cell membrane cation pumps. *Proc. Natl. Acad. Sci. U.S.A.* 109, 12794–12799. doi: 10.1073/pnas.1209014109

Cinar, E., Zhou, S., DeCourcey, J., Wang, Y., Waugh, R. E., and Wan, J. (2015). Piezo1 regulates mechanotransductive release of ATP from human RBCs. *Proc. Natl. Acad. Sci. U.S.A.* 112, 11783–11788. doi: 10.1073/pnas.1507309112

Coste, B., Mathur, J., Schmidt, M., Earley, T. J., Ranade, S., Petrus, M. J., et al. (2010). Piezo1 and Piezo2 are essential components of distinct mechanically activated cation channels. *Science* 330, 55–60. doi: 10.1126/science.1193270

Danielczok, J., Hertz, L., Ruppenthal, S., Kaiser, E., Petkova-Kirova, P., Bogdanova, A., et al. (2017). Does erythropoietin regulate TRPC channels in red blood cells? *Cell. Physiol. Biochem.* 41, 1219–1228. doi: 10.1159/000464384

Dyrda, A., Cytlak, U., Ciuraszkiewicz, A., Lipinska, A., Cueff, A., Bouyer, G., et al. (2010). Local membrane deformations activate Ca^{2+}-dependent K+ and anionic currents in intact human red blood cells. *PLoS ONE* 5:e9447. doi: 10.1371/journal.pone.0009447

Faucherre, A., Kissa, K., Nargeot, J., Mangoni, M. E., and Jopling, C. (2014). Piezo1 plays a role in erythrocyte volume homeostasis. *Haematologica* 99, 70–75. doi: 10.3324/haematol.2013.086090

Fermo, E., Bogdanova, A., Petkova-Kirova, P., Zaninoni, A., Marcello, A. P., Makhro, A., et al. (2017). "Gardos Channelopathy": a variant of hereditary Stomatocytosis with complex molecular regulation. *Sci. Rep.* 7:1744. doi: 10.1038/s41598-017-01591-w

Foller, M., Kasinathan, R. S., Koka, S., Lang, C., Shumilina, E. V., Birnbaumer, L., et al. (2008). TRPC6 contributes to the Ca(2+) leak of human erythrocytes. *Cell. Physiol. Biochem.* 21, 183–192. doi: 10.1159/000113760

Gallagher, P. G. (2013). Disorders of red cell volume regulation. *Curr. Opin. Hematol.* 20, 201–207. doi: 10.1097/MOH.0b013e32835f6870

Gardos, G. (1958). The function of calcium in the potassium permeability of human erythrocytes. *Biochim. Biophys. Acta* 30, 653–654. doi: 10.1016/0006-3002(58)90124-0

Glogowska, E., and Gallagher, P. G. (2015). Disorders of erythrocyte volume homeostasis. *Int. J. Lab. Hematol.* 37(Suppl. 1), 85–91. doi: 10.1111/ijlh.12357

Glogowska, E., Lezon-Geyda, K., Maksimova, Y., Schulz, V. P., and Gallagher, P. G. (2015). Mutations in the Gardos channel (KCNN4) are associated with hereditary xerocytosis. *Blood* 126, 1281–1284. doi: 10.1182/blood-2015-07-657957

Gottlieb, P. A., Bae, C., and Sachs, F. (2012). Gating the mechanical channel Piezo1: a comparison between whole-cell and patch recording. *Channels* 6, 282–289. doi: 10.4161/chan.21064

Gottlieb, P. A., and Sachs, F. (2012). Piezo1: properties of a cation selective mechanical channel. *Channels* 6, 214–219. doi: 10.4161/chan.21050

Hänggi, P., Makhro, A., Gassmann, M., Schmugge, M., Goede, J. S., Speer, O., et al. (2014). Red blood cells of sickle cell disease patients exhibit abnormally high abundance of N-methyl D-aspartate receptors mediating excessive calcium uptake. *Br. J. Haematol.* 167, 252–264. doi: 10.1111/bjh.13028

Hertz, L., Huisjes, R., Llaudet-Planas, E., Petkova-Kirova, P., Makhro, A., Danielczok, J. G., et al. (2017). Is increased intracellular calcium in red blood cells a common component in the molecular mechanism causing anemia? *Front. Physiol.* 8:673. doi: 10.3389/fphys.2017.00673

Heuzé, M. L., Collin, O., Terriac, E., Lennon-Duménil, A.-M., and Piel, M. (2011). Cell migration in confinement: a micro-channel-based assay. *Methods Mol. Biol.* 769, 415–434. doi: 10.1007/978-1-61779-207-6_28

Hoffman, J. F., Joiner, W., Nehrke, K., Potapova, O., Foye, K., and Wickrema, A. (2003). The hSK4 (KCNN4) isoform is the Ca^{2+}-activated K^+ channel (Gardos channel) in human red blood cells. *Proc. Natl. Acad. Sci. U.S.A.* 100, 7366–7371. doi: 10.1073/pnas.1232342100

Kaestner, L. (2015). Channelizing the red blood cell: molecular biology competes with patch-clamp. *Front. Mol. Biosci.* 2:46. doi: 10.3389/fmolb.2015.00046

Kaestner, L., and Bernhardt, I. (2002). Ion channels in the human red blood cell membrane: their further investigation and physiological relevance. *Bioelectrochemistry* 55, 71–74. doi: 10.1016/S1567-5394(01)00164-5

Kaestner, L., Christophersen, P., Bernhardt, I., and Bennekou, P. (2000). The non-selective voltage-activated cation channel in the human red blood cell membrane: reconciliation between two conflicting reports and further characterisation. *Bioelectrochemistry* 52, 117–125. doi: 10.1016/S0302-4598(00)00110-0

Kaestner, L., Steffen, P., Nguyen, D. B., Wang, J., Wagner-Britz, L., Jung, A., et al. (2012). Lysophosphatidic acid induced red blood cell aggregation *in vitro*. *Bioelectrochemistry* 87, 89–95. doi: 10.1016/j.bioelechem.2011.08.004

Kaestner, L., Tabellion, W., Lipp, P., and Bernhardt, I. (2004). Prostaglandin E_2 activates channel-mediated calcium entry in human erythrocytes: an indication for a blood clot formation supporting process. *Thromb. Haemost.* 92, 1269–1272. doi: 10.1160/TH04-06-0338

Kaestner, L., Tabellion, W., Weiss, E., Bernhardt, I., and Lipp, P. (2006). Calcium imaging of individual erythrocytes: problems and approaches. *Cell Calcium* 39, 13–19. doi: 10.1016/j.ceca.2005.09.004

Kuhlman, P. A., Hughes, C. A., Bennett, V., and Fowler, V. M. (1996). A new function for adducin. Calcium/calmodulin-regulated capping of the barbed ends of actin filaments. *J. Biol. Chem.* 271, 7986–7991. doi: 10.1074/jbc.271.14.7986

Lang, F., and Qadri, S. M. (2012). Mechanisms and significance of eryptosis, the suicidal death of erythrocytes. *Blood Purif.* 33, 125–130. doi: 10.1159/000334163

Laschke, M. W., and Menger, M. D. (2016). The dorsal skinfold chamber: a versatile tool for preclinical research in tissue engineering and regenerative medicine. *Eur. Cell Mater.* 32, 202–215. doi: 10.22203/eCM.v032a13

Laschke, M. W., Vollmar, B., and Menger, M. D. (2011). The dorsal skinfold chamber: window into the dynamic interaction of biomaterials with their surrounding host tissue. *Eur. Cell. Mater.* 22, 147–164. discussion: 164–167. doi: 10.22203/eCM.v022a12

Lew, V. L., Tiffert, T., Etzion, Z., Perdomo, D., Daw, N., Macdonald, L., et al. (2005). Distribution of dehydration rates generated by maximal Gardos-channel activation in normal and sickle red blood cells. *Blood* 105, 361–367. doi: 10.1182/blood-2004-01-0125

Li, Q., Jungmann, V., Kiyatkin, A., and Low, P. S. (1996). Prostaglandin E_2 stimulates a Ca^{2+}-dependent K^+ channel in human erythrocytes and alters cell volume and filterability. *J. Biol. Chem* 271, 18651–18656. doi: 10.1074/jbc.271.31.18651

Makhro, A., Hanggi, P., Goede, J. S., Wang, J., Brüggemann, A., Gassmann, M., et al. (2013). N-methyl D-aspartate (NMDA) receptors in human erythroid precursor cells and in circulating red blood cells contribute to the intracellular calcium regulation. *Am. J. Physiol.Cell Physiol.* 305, C1123–C1138. doi: 10.1152/ajpcell.00031.2013

Makhro, A., Huisjes, R., Verhagen, L. P., Mañú Pereira, M. D. M., Llaudet-Planas, E., Petkova-Kirova, P., et al. (2016). Red cell properties after different modes of blood transportation. *Front. Physiol.* 7:288. doi: 10.3389/fphys.2016.00288

Maneshi, M. M., Maki, B., Gnanasambandam, R., Belin, S., Popescu, G. K., Sachs, F., et al. (2017). Mechanical stress activates NMDA receptors in the absence of agonists. *Sci. Rep.* 7:39610. doi: 10.1038/srep39610

Meyer-Wilmes, J., and Remmer, H. (1956). Die standardisierung des roten blutfarbstoffes durch Hämiglobincyanid. *Naunyn Schmiedebergs Arch.* 229, 441–449. doi: 10.1007/BF00247016

Minetti, G., Egée, S., Mörsdorf, D., Steffen, P., Makhro, A., Achilli, C., et al. (2013). Red cell investigations: art and artefacts. *Blood Rev.* 27, 91–101. doi: 10.1016/j.blre.2013.02.002

Thiam, H.-R., Vargas, P., Carpi, N., Crespo, C. L., Raab, M., Terriac, E., et al. (2016). Perinuclear Arp2/3-driven actin polymerization enables nuclear deformation to facilitate cell migration through complex environments. *Nat. Commun.* 7:10997. doi: 10.1038/ncomms10997

Thomas, S. L., Egée, S., Lapaix, F., Kaestner, L., Staines, H. M., and Ellory, J. C. (2001). Malaria parasite *Plasmodium gallinaceum* up-regulates host red blood cell channels. *FEBS Lett.* 500, 45–51. doi: 10.1016/S0014-5793(01)02579-0

Tiffert, T., Bookchin, R. M., and Lew, V. L. (2003). "Calcium Homeostasis in normal and abnormal human red cells," in *Red Cell Membrane Transport in Health and Disease*, eds I. Bernhardt and C. Ellory (Berlin; Heidelberg: Springer Verlag), 373–405.

Wang, J., Wagner-Britz, L., Bogdanova, A., Ruppenthal, S., Wiesen, K., Kaiser, E., et al. (2013). Morphologically homogeneous red blood cells present a heterogeneous response to hormonal stimulation. *PLoS ONE* 8:e67697. doi: 10.1371/journal.pone.0067697

Yang, L., Andrews, D. A., and Low, P. S. (2000). Lysophosphatidic acid opens a Ca^{++} channel in human erythrocytes. *Blood* 95, 2420–2425.

Zarychanski, R., Schulz, V. P., Houston, B. L., Maksimova, Y., Houston, D. S., Smith, B., et al. (2012). Mutations in the mechanotransduction protein PIEZO1 are associated with hereditary xerocytosis. *Blood* 120, 1908–1915. doi: 10.1182/blood-2012-04-422253

4

The Molecular Basis for Altered Cation Permeability in Hereditary Stomatocytic Human Red Blood Cells

*Joanna F. Flatt and Lesley J. Bruce**

Bristol Institute for Transfusion Sciences, NHS Blood and Transplant, Bristol, United Kingdom

Correspondence:
Lesley J. Bruce
lesley.bruce@nhsbt.nhs.uk

Normal human RBCs have a very low basal permeability (leak) to cations, which is continuously corrected by the Na,K-ATPase. The leak is temperature-dependent, and this temperature dependence has been evaluated in the presence of inhibitors to exclude the activity of the Na,K-ATPase and NaK2Cl transporter. The severity of the RBC cation leak is altered in various conditions, most notably the hereditary stomatocytosis group of conditions. Pedigrees within this group have been classified into distinct phenotypes according to various factors, including the severity and temperature-dependence of the cation leak. As recent breakthroughs have provided more information regarding the molecular basis of hereditary stomatocytosis, it has become clear that these phenotypes elegantly segregate with distinct genetic backgrounds. The cryohydrocytosis phenotype, including South-east Asian Ovalocytosis, results from mutations in *SLC4A1*, and the very rare condition, stomatin-deficient cryohydrocytosis, is caused by mutations in *SLC2A1*. Mutations in *RHAG* cause the very leaky condition over-hydrated stomatocytosis, and mutations in *ABCB6* result in familial pseudohyperkalemia. All of the above are large multi-spanning membrane proteins and the mutations may either modify the structure of these proteins, resulting in formation of a cation pore, or otherwise disrupt the membrane to allow unregulated cation movement across the membrane. More recently mutations have been found in two RBC cation channels, *PIEZO1* and *KCNN4*, which result in dehydrated stomatocytosis. These mutations alter the activation and deactivation kinetics of these channels, leading to increased opening and allowing greater cation fluxes than in wild type.

Keywords: hereditary stomatocytosis, familial pseudohyperkalemia, SLC4A1, SLC2A1, RhAG, ABCB6, PIEZO1, KCNN4

INTRODUCTION

At first glance, mature human red blood cells (RBCs) appear to be simply membranes packed full of hemoglobin, carrying the respiratory gases oxygen and carbon dioxide around the body. They lack all cellular organelles, even the seemingly indispensible nucleus and mitochondria, enabling the maximum volume of the cells to be occupied by hemoglobin. Consequently, RBCs contain extremely high concentrations of hemoglobin (30–35 g/dL) and other impermeant solutes, creating an osmotic imbalance between the intracellular space and the surrounding plasma. Upon closer inspection, the RBC membrane has a greater role to play in RBC function than solely to contain the large amounts of hemoglobin required for oxygen transport. Interactions between RBC membrane proteins and the underlying cytoskeleton maintain the RBC's unique biconcave discoid shape that enables the 6 μm cell to deform and pass through 3 μm capillaries and splenic slits. Some of the most abundant RBC membrane proteins are fundamental to the rapid and efficient transport gases, for example Rh-associated glycoprotein (RhAG) and aquaporin 1 (AQP1) transport neutral gases such as carbon dioxide (Endeward et al., 2006) and maybe oxygen and/or nitric oxide (Burton and Anstee, 2008). The glucose transporter 1 (GLUT1) transports essential metabolites such as glucose (for energy) and dehydroascorbic acid (DHA; for redox homeostasis). The most abundant RBC membrane protein, band 3, exchanges bicarbonate to the plasma in exchange for chloride, a process that is crucial for the efficient transport of carbon dioxide in the blood. This high membrane permeability to anions is in contrast to its very low permeability to cations. In human RBCs it is thought that the cell utilizes its low cation permeability to counteract the osmotic effect of the high solute concentration within the RBCs. Cation gradients across the membrane are actively maintained by pumps keeping intracellular sodium low and intracellular potassium high. This mechanism is tightly regulated to ensure that there is no uncontrolled movement of water into or out of the RBC and is fundamental to cellular volume control (reviewed in Gallagher, 2017).

CATION PUMPS, TRANSPORTERS AND CHANNELS IN THE RBC MEMBRANE

Human RBC membranes contain a number of different cation pumps, transporters and channels (Gallagher, 2017). The major protein responsible for maintaining the high potassium, low sodium intracellular state is the Na,K-ATPase, which is an ATP-dependent pump that exchanges 3 sodium ions outwards for 2 potassium ions inwards. Its activity can be specifically inhibited with ouabain. A second major physiologically-active transporter is the NaK2Cl cotransporter (NKCC1), which usually moves 1 Na^+, 1 K^+, and 2 Cl^- into the cell from the extracellular space, although transport can occur in both directions across the membrane. The NaK2Cl cotransporter is inhibited by the drugs bumetanide and furosemide, cell swelling and urea (Lim et al., 1995), and is expressed in numerous cell types. Another ion transporter present in the RBC membrane is the potassium chloride cotransporter (KCC3), which is stimulated by cell swelling and urea. This protein cotransports both potassium and chloride out of the cell, which are accompanied by water and leads to a decrease in cell volume (Lauf and Adragna, 2000). The Na-H exchanger (NHE1) is present in RBCs and many other cell types, and is involved in cell volume and pH control. It can be inhibited with the drug amiloride. The cytoplasmic domain of NHE1 interacts with the cytoskeletal protein 4.1, which may play a part in its regulation (Nunomura et al., 2012). It is activated by cell shrinking, which is associated with phosphorylation of a number of residues of NHE1 (Rigor et al., 2011). The non-selective, voltage-dependent cation (NSVDC) channel (Bennekou and Christopherson, 2003) and the K(Na)/H exchanger (Bernhardt and Weiss, 2003) are both activated in low ionic strength conditions and may play a role in cation loss in low chloride media, but probably have little role in cation homeostasis at physiological pH and tonicity.

Many of these transporters are regulated by changes in cell volume (swelling and/or shrinkage). The mechanisms underlying this are likely to involve protein-protein interactions, transporter phosphorylation, and cell chloride concentrations (Flatman, 2002). Other cation transporting proteins are not thought to play a major role within homeostatic physiological conditions. These include the calcium-activated potassium channel, KCNN4, known as KCa3.1 or the Gardos channel (Hoffman et al., 2003). Elevation of intracellular calcium levels activates the Gardos channel to its open conformation, allowing potassium efflux and consequent rapid cellular dehydration. However, this channel usually exists in its dormant closed state, as intracellular calcium is extruded by the Ca^{2+}-ATPase. Although the RBC membrane has been very well studied, new insights continue to be made concerning the proteins present and their role in RBC function. There is some evidence from studies in mice that the Kell/XK complex is involved in the regulation of cation homeostasis, as the absence of XK leads to elevated intracellular calcium levels and Gardos channel activation (Rivera et al., 2013a).

Fairly recently it was discovered that the RBC membrane contains a mechanosensitive cation channel, PIEZO1 (Zarychanski et al., 2012). PIEZO1 is encoded by the gene *FAM38A* and can be inhibited by the stretch-activated channel inhibitor, tarantula toxin GsMTx4 (Bae et al., 2011). A synthetic small molecule called Yoda1 has been shown to act as a specific PIEZO1 agonist, and may prove to be an important tool for full investigation of the biophysical properties of the channel (Syeda et al., 2015). PIEZO1 has been knocked down in zebrafish and mouse, resulting in swelling and lysis of RBCs, suggesting that it is important for cell volume control (Faucherre et al., 2014; Cahalan et al., 2015), and it has been shown to be important for vascular development (Ranade et al., 2014). Evidence from a recent study by Cahalan et al. suggests that PIEZO1-mediated calcium influx activates the Gardos channel and triggers cellular dehydration. This mechanism has been hypothesized to aid the RBC's passage through the microvasculature by allowing it to reduce its volume in response to mechanical stimulation or shear stress (Cahalan et al., 2015). It will be interesting to discover whether PIEZO1 is directly involved in regulating other RBC membrane cation transporters that are variously stimulated or inhibited by cell swelling, raising the exciting possibility that PIEZO1 is the master regulator of RBC volume control.

NORMAL MEMBRANE ION DISTRIBUTION AND FLUXES

In normal human RBCs there is a very low basal permeability to cations. At body temperature, this "leak" is corrected by the Na,K-ATPase, which is present in RBCs at a low copy number, but is sufficient to maintain the sodium/potassium electrochemical gradients. This basal cation permeability can be measured in the presence of the inhibitors ouabain and bumetanide, in order the exclude the activity of the Na,K-ATPase and NaK2Cl transporter, respectively. The temperature-dependence of the potassium leak has been evaluated, and it exhibits an unusual pattern. From 37°C downwards the leak decreases with temperature in a monotonic manner. The minimum of the leak occurs at around 8°C, but below 10°C the leak actually increases with decreasing temperature, resulting in a U-shaped graph (**Figure 1**) (Stewart et al., 1980; Coles and Stewart, 1999). The explanation for this pattern is not known, and comparisons with other species' RBCs revealed that human RBCs appear to be unique in this feature (Hall and Willis, 1986).

COMPARISON OF HUMAN WITH OTHER SPECIES' RBCS

Intriguingly, this use of cation gradients for regulation of cell volume in human RBCs does not appear to be a common feature of other mammals' RBCs. Dogs, sheep and cows are all species in which individuals' RBC phenotype may be categorized as either "high K" or "low K" (Chan et al., 1964; Gibson, 2003). In dogs the "low K" phenotype is most common, and this is inherited in an autosomal dominant manner. Despite the fact that the potassium levels of "high K" dog RBCs are most similar to the normal state of human RBCs, they exhibit signs of overhydration, including increased osmotic fragility, increased cell size, reduced cell hemoglobin concentration and reduced RBC lifespan. Studies of dog RBCs suggest that they employ a different mechanism for regulating their volume, predominantly involving the Na/H exchanger and KCl cotransporter (Parker et al., 1990). "High K" dog RBCs have higher levels of the Na,K-ATPase, which is thought to be responsible for the unusual cation gradients, and in this species its expression appears to be detrimental. It has been shown that both "low K" and "high K" dog reticulocytes express Na,K-ATPase and produce exosomes containing the protein, but "high K" erythroid progenitor cells express higher levels (Komatsu et al., 2010). The genetic basis of the "high K" vs. "low K" phenotype has not yet been established, but may provide a clue concerning the regulation of Na,K-ATPase expression.

Studies using duck RBCs have shown that their volume regulation involves coordinated transport by NaK2Cl cotransporter and KCl cotransporter proteins (Lytle and McManus, 2002), highlighting that there are many ways to control RBC volume, utilizing different transporters to achieve this goal.

Mice are often used as a model for the human system, however evaluation of a number of different mouse strains has revealed that their cation content and transporter activity are different depending on the strain and gender of the mouse (Rivera et al., 2013b). These observations may be useful in the investigation of genetic determinants of ion transport.

CONDITIONS INVOLVING DISTURBANCES IN ION FLUXES

It has become apparent that a number of factors can affect the cation permeability of the human RBC membrane. These include the use of certain drugs and oxidation of membranes. A recent study using aquaporin-9 knock-out mouse RBCs showed that oxidative modification of aquaporin-9 increases the cation permeability of the RBC membrane (Kucherenko et al., 2012). The presence of certain disease states results in aberrant membrane ion flux. Increased cation permeability has been recorded in thalassemia and chronic dyserythropoietic anemia (CDA), where the bone marrow is under continual stress (Wiley, 1981). Cation fluxes are also disturbed in a group of inherited disorders collectively known as the hereditary stomatocytoses. Although a common theme running throughout these disorders is that cation permeability of the RBC membrane is perturbed, these disorders show wide heterogeneity in the severity and characteristics of their cation leaks and also accompanying symptoms (**Table 1**). These are an extensively-studied group whose molecular bases remained unknown for a long time, but for the vast majority these have now been elucidated and form the basis of this review.

HEREDITARY STOMATOCYTOSES

Despite the lack of information concerning the molecular cause(s) of the hereditary stomatocytoses (HSt), great efforts were made to thoroughly characterize the cation leaks exhibited by the known pedigrees. These analyses further underlined the wide heterogeneity of the disorders. Prof. G. Stewart classified the pedigrees into distinct types according to various factors, including the severity and temperature-dependence of the cation leak (Stewart, 2004) (**Table 1**, **Figure 1**). As recent breakthroughs have provided more information regarding the molecular basis of HSt, it has become clear that these phenotypes elegantly segregate with distinct genetic backgrounds.

HST MUTATIONS IN LARGE MULTI-SPANNING MEMBRANE PROTEINS

Band 3 Mutations

Cryohydrocytosis

Cryohydrocytosis (CHC) is so named because of the temperature-dependence of the cation leak. Although CHC cells have increased basal cation permeability at physiological temperatures, this leak becomes much more pronounced when the cells are cooled to below 10°C (**Figure 1B**). Cryohydrocytosis was the first of the hereditary stomatocytoses in which the genetic basis was established. Heterozygous single amino acid substitutions in the band 3 protein (SLC4A1) were identified in 11 stomatocytosis pedigrees (Bruce et al., 2005). Band 3 is responsible for anion exchange across the plasma membrane, however in each of these pedigrees the mutant band 3 proteins were unable to transport anions even when expressed in the RBC membrane. Instead, expression of the mutant protein resulted in the temperature-sensitive increase in the permeability of the RBC membrane to cations.

All of the band 3 HSt mutations identified so far occur within the transmembrane domain between spans 8 and 12, the region that forms the transport channel of band 3 (**Figure 2**;

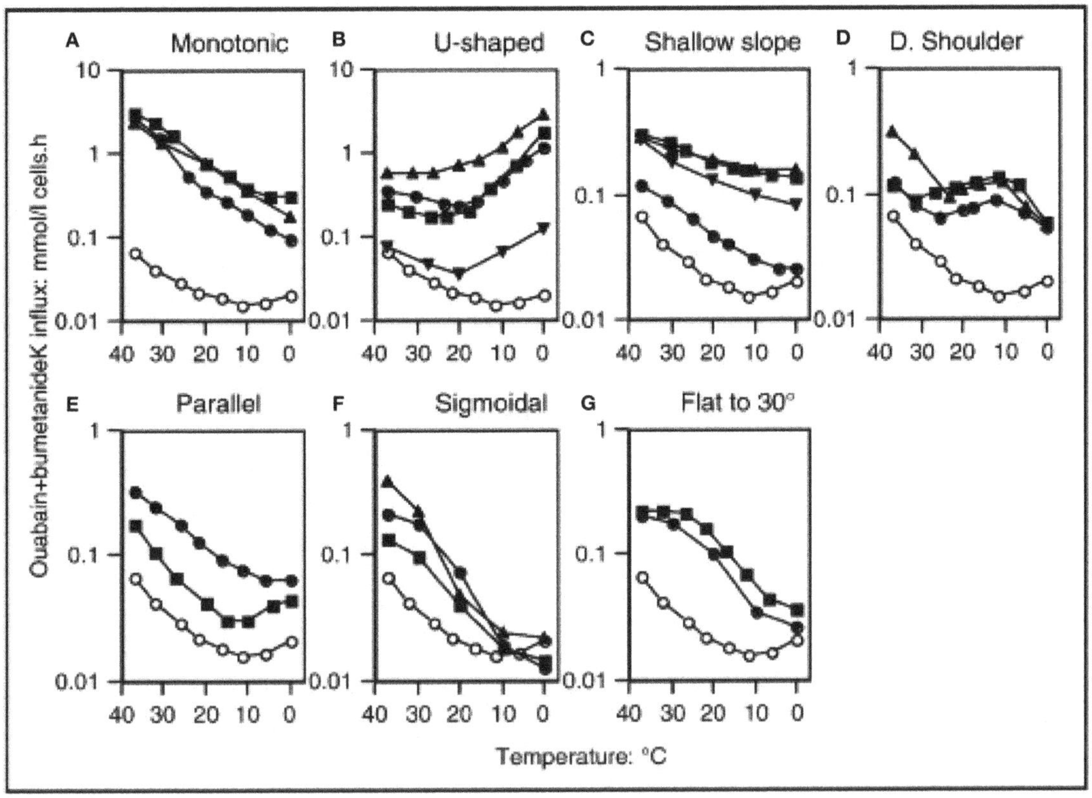

Panel	Symbol (all closed)	Pedigree	Type of HSt	Gene	Mutation
A	Circle	Brighton	OHSt-1	RHAG	Phe65Ser
	Square	Harrow	OHSt-2	RHAG	Ile61Arg
	Triangle	Albequerque	OHSt-1	RHAG	Phe65Ser
B	Circle	Hemel	CHC	SLC4A1	Ser731Pro
	Square	Hurstpierpoint	CHC	SLC4A1	His734Gln
	Triangle	Montpellier	sdCHC	SLC2A1	Gly286Asp
	Inverted triangle	Cardiff	FP (Cardiff)	ABCB6	Arg723Gln
C	Circle	Edinburgh	FP*	PIEZO1	Thr2127Met
	Square	Blackburn	"Blackburn"	SLC4A1	Leu687Pro
	Triangle	Darlington	"Blackburn"	SLC4A1	Leu687Pro
	Inverted triangle	Bergen	"Blackburn"	Unknown	Bergheim, 2003
D	Circle	Chiswick	FP (Chiswick)	ABCB6	Arg375Gln
	Square	Bow	FP (Chiswick)	ABCB6	Arg375Trp
	Triangle	Falkirk	FP (Chiswick)	ABCB6	Arg375Trp
E	Circle	Woking	DHSt (Woking)	unknown	Jarvis 2001
	Square	Omagh	DHSt	ABCB6	Arg276Trp
F	Circle	Bury St Edmunds	DHSt+ascites	unknown	(unpublished)
	Square	Sunderland	DHSt+ascites	unknown	Basu et al. (2003)
	Triangle	West London		unknown	(unpublished)
G	Circle	Birmingham	DHSt/FP (M'brough)	Ala492Thr	Gore 2004
	Square	Middlesbrough	DHSt/FP (M'brough)	unknown	Gore 2004

*FP: As measured at RT 20°C not 4°C.

FIGURE 1 | Temperature dependence of "leak" potassium flux in different leaky membrane variants among the hereditary stomatocytosis conditions. Open symbols denote normal red cells. Closed symbols denote patients, detailed below and in the Table. Potassium influx was measured using ^{86}Rb as a tracer. The medium contained (mM): Na^+, 145: K^+, 5; Cl^-, 150, MOPS, 15 (pH 7.4 at 20°C); glucose, 5; ouabain, 0.1; bumetanide, 0.1. Reproduced with permission from Stewart (2004).

Arakawa et al., 2015; Reithmeier et al., 2016). The mutant proteins were shown to be expressed in the CHC patients' RBCs and they induced a cation leak when expressed heterologously in *Xenopus levis* oocytes. The ouabain and bumetanide insensitive cation leak could be inhibited with a range of specific band 3 inhibitors, supporting the hypothesis that the cation leak is

TABLE 1 | Hereditary stomatocytosis pedigrees and other cation-leaky membrane disorders.

Clinical/hematology								Genetics/biochemistry		
Phenotype	**Pedigree**	**RBC morphology**	**Thromb.**	**Lipid**	**Leak rate**	**Temp dependence**	**References**	**Gene**	**Genotype**	**References**
OHSt 1	Stockport	Stomatocytes	+	Normal	× 40	Monotonic	Lock et al., 1961	*RHAG*	Phe65Ser	Bruce et al., 2009
OHSt 1	Albuquerque	Stomatocytes	No splen.	Normal	× 40	Monotonic	Fricke et al., 2004	*RHAG*	Phe65Ser	Bruce et al., 2009
OHSt 1	Brighton	Stomatocytes (30–40%)	+		× 40	Monotonic	Meadow, 1967	*RHAG*	Phe65Ser	Bruce et al., 2009
OHSt 1	Toulouse	Stomatocytes	No splen.		× 40	Monotonic	Fricke et al., 2004	*RHAG*	Phe65Ser	Bruce et al., 2009
OHSt 1	Grenoble	Stomatocytes (15–20%)	No splen.		× 40	Monotonic	Morlé et al., 1989	*RHAG*	Phe65Ser	Bruce et al., 2009
OHSt 1	Nancy	Stomatocytes (10–20%)	Unknown		× 40	Monotonic	Bruce et al., 2009	*RHAG*	Phe65Ser	Bruce et al., 2009
OHSt 2	Harrow	Stomatocytes	No splen.		× 40	Monotonic	Fricke et al., 2004	*RHAG*	Ile61Arg	Bruce et al., 2009
sdCHC + neuro.	Montpellier	Stomatocytes	No splen.		× 10	U-shaped	Fricke et al., 2004	*SLC2A1*	Gly286Asp	Flatt et al., 2011
sdCHC + neuro.	San Francisco	Unknown	No splen.		× 10	U-shaped	Fricke et al., 2004	*SLC2A1*	ΔIle435/436	Flatt et al., 2011
sdCHC + neuro.	n/a	Echinocytes, stomatocytes	No splen.			n.t.	Bawazir et al., 2012	*SLC2A1*	ΔIle435/436	Bawazir et al., 2012
PED + cation leak	n/a	Echinocytes (14–40%)	No splen.			n.t.	Weber et al., 2008	*SLC2A1*	Δ282–285	Weber et al., 2008
CHC	Hemel	Stomatocytes (30%)	–	+ ether	× 4	U-shaped	Coles et al., 1999a	*SLC4A1*	Ser731Pro	Bruce et al., 2005
CHC	Watford	Stomatocytes	–	+ ether	× 4	U-shaped	Coles et al., 1999a	*SLC4A1*	Ser731Pro	Bruce et al., 2005
CHC	Bushey	Stomatocytes	–	+ ether	× 4	U-shaped	Haines et al., 2001a	*SLC4A1*	Ser731Pro	Bruce et al., 2005
CHC	Milton Keynes		No splen.		× 4	U-shaped	Stewart, 2004	*SLC4A1*	Ser731Pro	Bruce et al., 2005
CHC	Hurstpierpoint	Stomatocytes (15–20%)	–	Normal	× 4	U-shaped	Haines et al., 2001a	*SLC4A1*	His734Arg	Bruce et al., 2005
CHC	Zurich		No splen.		× 4	U-shaped	Stewart, 2004	*SLC4A1*	His734Arg	Bruce et al., 2005
CHC	Islington					n.t.	Stewart, 2004	n.t.		
CHC	n/a	Stomatocytes, spherocytes			× 3	U-shaped	Guizouarn et al., 2011	*SLC4A1*	Ser762Arg	Guizouarn et al., 2011
SAO	n/a	Stomatocytic ovalocytes			× 2	U-shaped	Guizouarn et al., 2011	*SLC4A1*	Δ400–408	Tanner et al., 1991
HS-LTL	Cricklewood	Spherocytes	No splen.				Bruce et al., 2005	*SLC4A1*	Arg760Gln	Bruce et al., 2005
HS-LTL	Dagenham	Spherocytes	No splen.				Bruce et al., 2005	*SLC4A1*	Arg760Gln	Bruce et al., 2005
HS-LTL	Eastbourne	Spherocytes	+				Gore et al., 2002a	*SLC4A1*	Asp705Tyr	Bruce et al., 2005
HSt Blackburn	Blackburn	Stomatocytes	+	Normal	× 4	Shallow slope	Coles et al., 1999b	*SLC4A1*	Leu687Pro	Bruce et al., 2005
HSt Blackburn	Darlington	Stomatocytes (5–10%)	+		× 3	Shallow slope	Gore et al., 2004	*SLC4A1*	Leu687Pro	Bruce et al., 2005
HSt Blackburn	Bergen		+		× 4	Shallow slope	Stewart, 2004	n.t.		
HSt Blackburn	St. Etienne		+		× 4	Shallow slope	Stewart, 2004	n.t.		
Band 3 New Haven	Patient 1	Rare stomatocytes					Stewart et al., 2010	*SLC4A1*	Glu758Lys	Stewart et al., 2010
Band 3 New Haven	Patient 2	Mild anisocytosis					Stewart et al., 2010	*SLC4A1*	Glu758Lys	Stewart et al., 2010
HSt variant	Stanford	Normal, rare stomatocytes	Unknown		× 6		Stewart et al., 2011	*SLC4A1*	Arg730Cys	Stewart et al., 2011
Band 3 Ceinge + dyseryth.	Ceinge	Anisopoikilocytosis					Iolascon et al., 2009	*SLC4A1*	Gly796Arg	Iolascon et al., 2009
FP	Cardiff	Normal	No splen.	+ ether	× 1	U-shaped	Gore et al., 2002b	*ABCB6*	Arg723Gln	Bawazir et al., 2014
FP	Cumbria	Normal			× 1	U-shaped	Bawazir et al., 2014	*ABCB6*	Arg723Gln	Bawazir et al., 2014
FP	Harrow	Normal			× 1	U-shaped	Bawazir et al., 2014	*ABCB6*	Arg723Gln	Bawazir et al., 2014
FP	Cardiff-2						Andolfo et al., 2016	*ABCB6*	Arg723Gln /Arg276Trp	Andolfo et al., 2016
FP	Bolivian						Andolfo et al., 2016	*ABCB6*	Val454Ala	Andolfo et al., 2016
FP	Lille						Dagher et al., 1989	*ABCB6*	Arg375Gln	Andolfo et al., 2013a
FP	Chiswick	Normal	No splen.	Normal	× 1.5	Shoulder	Haines et al., 2001b	*ABCB6*	Arg375Gln	Bawazir et al., 2014
FP	White City						Bawazir et al., 2014	*ABCB6*	Arg375Gln	Bawazir et al., 2014
FP	Falkirk		No splen.	Normal	× 1.5	Shoulder	Haines et al., 2001a	*ABCB6*	Arg375Trp	Andolfo et al., 2013a
FP	Bow	Normal, rare stomatocytes	No splen.	Normal	× 1.5	Shoulder	Gore et al., 2004	*ABCB6*	Arg375Trp	Andolfo et al., 2013a
FP/DHSt	Irish		+				Stewart et al., 1996	*ABCB6*	Arg276Trp	Andolfo et al., 2016
DHSt M'brough	Middlesbrough	Target cells, rare stomatocytes			× 4	Flat to 30	Gore et al., 2004			
DHSt M'brough	Birmingham	Target cells			× 2	Flat to 30	Gore et al., 2004			
HSt variant	Woking	Stomatocytes (5–10%)	No splen.		× 4	Parallel	Jarvis et al., 2001			
DHSt + ascites	Bury St. Edmunds				× 2	Sigmoidal	Stewart, 2004			

(Continued)

TABLE 1 | Continued

Clinical/hematology								Genetics/biochemistry		
Phenotype	**Pedigree**	**RBC morphology**	**Thromb.**	**Lipid**	**Leak rate**	**Temp dependence**	**References**	**Gene**	**Genotype**	**References**
DHSt + ascites	Sunderland	Anisocytosis, target cells	No splen.		× 2	Sigmoidal	Basu et al., 2003			
DHSt	Kyoto	Rare stomatocytes		+ PC			Imashuku et al., 2016	*FAM38A*	Glu2496GluLeuGlu	Imashuku et al., 2016
DHSt	Case 1						Albuisson et al., 2013	*FAM38A*	Glu2496GluLeuGlu	Albuisson et al., 2013
DHSt	Case 2						Albuisson et al., 2013	*FAM38A*	Glu2496GluLeuGlu	Albuisson et al., 2013
DHSt	Case 3						Albuisson et al., 2013	*FAM38A*	Glu2496GluLeuGlu	Albuisson et al., 2013
DHSt	Case 5						Albuisson et al., 2013	*FAM38A*	Glu2496GluLeuGlu	Albuisson et al., 2013
DHSt	Case 6						Albuisson et al., 2013	*FAM38A*	Glu2496GluLeuGlu	Albuisson et al., 2013
DHSt	Case 7						Albuisson et al., 2013	*FAM38A*	Glu2496GluLeuGlu	Albuisson et al., 2013
DHSt + ascites	Vesoul		+		× 2		Grootenboer et al., 2000	*FAM38A*	Glu2496GluLeuGlu	Albuisson et al., 2013
DHSt + FP	Family 3		+	+PC			Carli et al., 2007	*FAM38A*	Glu2496GluLeuGlu	Albuisson et al., 2013
DHSt + ascites	Patient 6		No splen				Glogowska et al., 2017	*FAM38A*	Glu2496GluLeuGlu	Glogowska et al., 2017
DHSt	Patient 7		No splen				Glogowska et al., 2017	*FAM38A*	Glu2496GluLeuGlu	Glogowska et al., 2017
DHSt + ascites	Patient 8		+				Glogowska et al., 2017	*FAM38A*	Glu2496GluLeuGlu	Glogowska et al., 2017
DHSt	Patient 9		+				Glogowska et al., 2017	*FAM38A*	Glu2496GluLeuGlu	Glogowska et al., 2017
DHSt	Family A (UK)	Schistocytes, rare stomatocytes					Andolfo et al., 2018a	*FAM38A*	Glu2496GluLeuGlu	Andolfo et al., 2018a
DHSt	Family B (Italy)	Schistocytes, rare stomatocytes					Andolfo et al., 2018a	*FAM38A*	Glu2496GluLeuGlu/ Arg1864His	Andolfo et al., 2018a
DHSt + FP	Arras		+				Grootenboer et al., 2000	*FAM38A*	Arg2488Gln /Gly718Ser	Andolfo et al., 2013b
DHSt	Boston	Target cells					Platt et al., 1981	*FAM38A*	Arg2488Gln	Archer et al., 2014
DHSt + ascites	Patient 3		No splen				Glogowska et al., 2017	*FAM38A*	Arg2488Gln	Glogowska et al., 2017
DHSt	Canada	Target cells, schistocytes					Houston et al., 2011	*FAM38A*	Arg2456His	Zarychanski et al., 2012 Bae et al., 2013
DHSt	San Francisco						Grootenboer et al., 2000	*FAM38A*	Arg2456His	Andolfo et al., 2013b; Bae et al., 2013
DHSt	Rosedale	Macrocytes, stomatocytes					Shmukler et al., 2014	*FAM38A*	Arg2456His	Shmukler et al., 2014
DHSt	Denmark	Normal					Sandberg et al., 2014	*FAM38A*	Arg2456His	Sandberg et al., 2014
DHSt + ascites	Nantes family 1	Target cells, rare stomatocytes					Beneteau et al., 2014	*FAM38A*	Arg2456His	Beneteau et al., 2014
DHSt + ascites	Nantes family 2	Target cells, rare stomatocytes					Beneteau et al., 2014	*FAM38A*	Arg2456His	Beneteau et al., 2014
DHSt	Burnley		No splen.	+ PC	× 2	Parallel	Stewart, 2004	*FAM38A*	Arg2456His	Unpublished, LJ Bruce 2018
DHSt	Nuneaton		+	+ PC	× 2	Parallel	Stewart, 2004	*FAM38A*	Arg2456His	Unpublished, LJ Bruce 2018
DHSt	Patient 4		No splen				Glogowska et al., 2017	*FAM38A*	Arg2302His	Glogowska et al., 2017
DHSt	New York	Stomatocytes (up to 35% hom)		Normal			Miller et al., 1971	*FAM38A*	Met2225Arg	Zarychanski et al., 2012; Bae et al., 2013
DHSt	Dax						Grootenboer et al., 2000	*FAM38A*	2166-2169delLys	Andolfo et al., 2013b
DHSt + FP	Edinburgh	Target cells	No splen.	Normal	× 1.1	Shallow slope	Stewart and Ellory, 1985	*FAM38A*	Thr2127Met	Andolfo et al., 2013b
DHSt	Case 8						Albuisson et al., 2013	*FAM38A*	Thr2127Met	Albuisson et al., 2013
DHSt	Patient 2		No splen				Glogowska et al., 2017	*FAM38A*	Arg2088Gly	Glogowska et al., 2017
DHSt + FP	Vanves	Rare stomatocytes			× 1.5		Grootenboer et al., 2000	*FAM38A*	Ala2020Thr	Albuisson et al., 2013
DHSt	Essex						Carella et al., 1998	*FAM38A*	Ala2020Val/Ser1117Leu	Andolfo et al., 2013b
DHSt		Stomatocytes					Paessler and Hartung, 2015	*FAM38A*	c.6239_6256dup18	Paessler and Hartung, 2015
DHSt	Troyes		+				Grootenboer et al., 2000	*FAM38A*	Ala2003Asp	Andolfo et al., 2013b
DHSt	Patient 1		No splen				Glogowska et al., 2017	*FAM38A*	Arg1943Gln	Glogowska et al., 2017
DHSt	Case 4	Rare stomatocytes					Syfuss et al., 2006	*FAM38A*	Arg1358Pro	Albuisson et al., 2013
DHSt + FP + ascites	Bicetre						Grootenboer et al., 2000	*FAM38A*	Arg808Gln/Gly782Ser	Andolfo et al., 2013b
DHSt	Italy	Stomatocytes	+				Fermo et al., 2017	*KCNN4*	Arg352His	Rapetti-Mauss et al., 2015
DHSt	France	Anisocytosis					Rapetti-Mauss et al., 2015	*KCNN4*	Arg352His	Rapetti-Mauss et al., 2015
DHSt	Poland	Anisocytosis					Rapetti-Mauss et al., 2015	*KCNN4*	Arg352His	Andolfo et al., 2015
DHSt	Naples	Anisopoikilocytosis, stomatocytes					Andolfo et al., 2015	*KCNN4*	Arg352His	Andolfo et al., 2015; Glogowska et al., 2015
DHSt	Worcester				× 3		Grootenboer et al., 2000	*KCNN4*	Val282Met	Glogowska et al., 2015
DHSt	French/Irish	Target cells, acanthocytes					Glader et al., 1974	*KCNN4*	Val282Glu	Fermo et al., 2017

mediated directly through the transport channel of band 3 (Bruce et al., 2005). There is variability in the phenotype depending on the mutation. Two mutations were initially identified as corresponding to the classic CHC phenotype: Ser731Pro and His734Gln (Bruce et al., 2005), both occurring very close to each other in transmembrane domain 10 of band 3 (Arakawa et al., 2015). His734 is an essential residue for anion transport and Ser731 lie close to the transport site (Arakawa et al., 2015). Further CHC mutations have since been reported in the same region of the protein, including Ser762Arg (Guizouarn et al., 2011) in span 11 of band 3. This residue interacts with His734 in TM10 (Arakawa et al., 2015; Reithmeier et al., 2016).

One subtype within the cryohydrocytosis group referred to as HS-LTL (hereditary spherocytosis with low temperature leak) results from the mutation Asp705Tyr or Arg760Gln (Bruce et al., 2005) and shows some overlap with the hereditary spherocytosis (HS) group of disorders. In those disorders the vertical link between the RBC cytoskeleton and the membrane is disrupted because of defects in the structurally important proteins band 3, protein 4.2 or ankyrin. In typical HS (without a cation leak) the mutant band 3 may be too misfolded to reach the membrane at all, or the mutant mRNA is unstable and is degraded. The remaining wild type allele produces functional band 3, but not in sufficient quantity to fully compensate for the lost structural interactions. The weakening of the link between the membrane and the underlying cytoskeleton results in the loss of membrane, producing small and dense spherocytic cells. In HS-LTL there is a deficiency in the vertical interactions between the cytoskeleton and band 3 in the membrane, resulting in the same spherocytic morphology, but the difference is that some of the mutant band 3 is successfully trafficked to the membrane, despite being misfolded. Once expressed at the plasma membrane the mutant protein causes a RBC cation leak.

Southeast Asian Ovalocytosis

Southeast Asian Ovalocytosis (SAO) cells are morphologically abnormal, showing large oval cells often with double slits on blood films. The mutation in SAO band 3 is a 9 amino acid deletion at residues 400–408 (Tanner et al., 1991) (**Figure 2**). This region is situated close to the boundary of the large cytoplasmic N-terminal domain and the transmembrane domain and it is known to affect the normal folding of band 3 (Kuma et al., 2002). Like CHC band 3, the SAO band 3 is expressed in the RBC membrane but is misfolded and cannot transport anions. Early *in vitro* studies of SAO RBCs indicated that these cells were resistant to invasion by the malaria parasite, *Plasmodium falciparum* (Hadley et al., 1983). However, further experimental study showed that a significant part of this effect is caused by depletion in the cellular levels of ATP upon storage of these cells (Dluzewski et al., 1992). This is an effect resulting from a cold-induced cation leak (Bruce et al., 1999), which is almost indistinguishable from that observed in CHC (Guizouarn et al., 2011). However, the SAO mutation has been shown to confer protection from cerebral malaria—a serious complication that can arise from *P. falciparum* infection (Allen et al., 1999), and this could explain the prevalence of SAO in low-lying parts of Papua New Guinea and South East Asia.

Other HSt Caused by Band 3 Mutations

HSt Blackburn is another distinct type of cation leak with a characteristic temperature-dependence. This has previously been described as the "shallow slope" type, where cells exhibit a cation leak 4–5 times greater than normal cells at 37°C, but as the temperature lowers only a small decrease in this leak is observed (**Figure 1C**; Coles and Stewart, 1999). This phenotype is associated with a band 3 point mutation, Leu687Pro, which prevents normal anion exchange function and produces a cation leak when expressed in *X. levis* oocytes (Bruce et al., 2005). Leu687 is at the C-terminus of TM8, which packs against TM3 and TM10 (**Figure 2**). TM8 is at the interface of the core and gate domains of band 3 (Arakawa et al., 2015) and therefore key to the normal functioning of band 3.

Band 3 New Haven (Glu758Lys) has been reported in 2 patients (Stewart et al., 2010). Expressing this mutant band 3 in oocytes produced anion exchange activity only when GPA was co-expressed, but the cation leak associated with its expression was GPA-independent. These characteristics are in contrast to other HSt band 3 mutations, where anion exchange was completely abolished. The same group also reported a further band 3 mutation in HSt (Arg730Cys) (Stewart et al., 2011). The temperature-dependence of the leaks caused by these two mutations were not characterized.

Band 3 Ceinge (Gly796Arg) is an interesting HSt variant, as this pedigree exhibited signs of dyserythropoiesis and no mutations were found in *CDAN1*, the gene associated with chronic dyserythropoietic anemia (CDA) type 1. Analysis of the membranes also revealed increased tyrosine phosphorylation of band 3 and other membrane proteins (Iolascon et al., 2009).

RhAG Mutations

Overhydrated Hereditary Stomatocytosis

The most severe cation leak in the hereditary stomatocytoses can be found in a condition known as overhydrated hereditary stomatocytosis (OHSt). At 37°C the cation leak can be as high as 40 times greater than normal; the temperature dependence profile shows a simple pattern of increasing leak with increasing temperature (**Figure 1A**; Coles and Stewart, 1999). Heterozygous mutations in *RHAG* are associated with this disorder—Phe65Ser and Ile61Arg—and again these fall within a transmembrane span (Bruce et al., 2009). This gene encodes the Rh-associated glycoprotein (RhAG), which is distantly related to ammonia transporters in bacteria and yeast (Marini et al., 1997). Molecular modeling of the mutant RhAG suggests that the Phe65Ser mutation causes a significant widening of the central transport channel, converting it into a non-selective cation pore (Bruce et al., 2009). Ile61Arg is also predicted to widen the central channel, but not to the same extent. It was noted that larger structural changes may occur, which would allow passage of cations. In addition, there is experimental evidence that the OHSt mutation Phe65Ser prevents the transport of ammonia, which is thought to be the normal substrate of RhAG (Genetet et al., 2012).

A metabolomics study of four individuals with OHSt has provided an insight into the downstream effects of this RhAG mutation (Darghouth et al., 2011). The authors found that the glycolytic pathway is overactive in OHSt RBCs, with a build-up

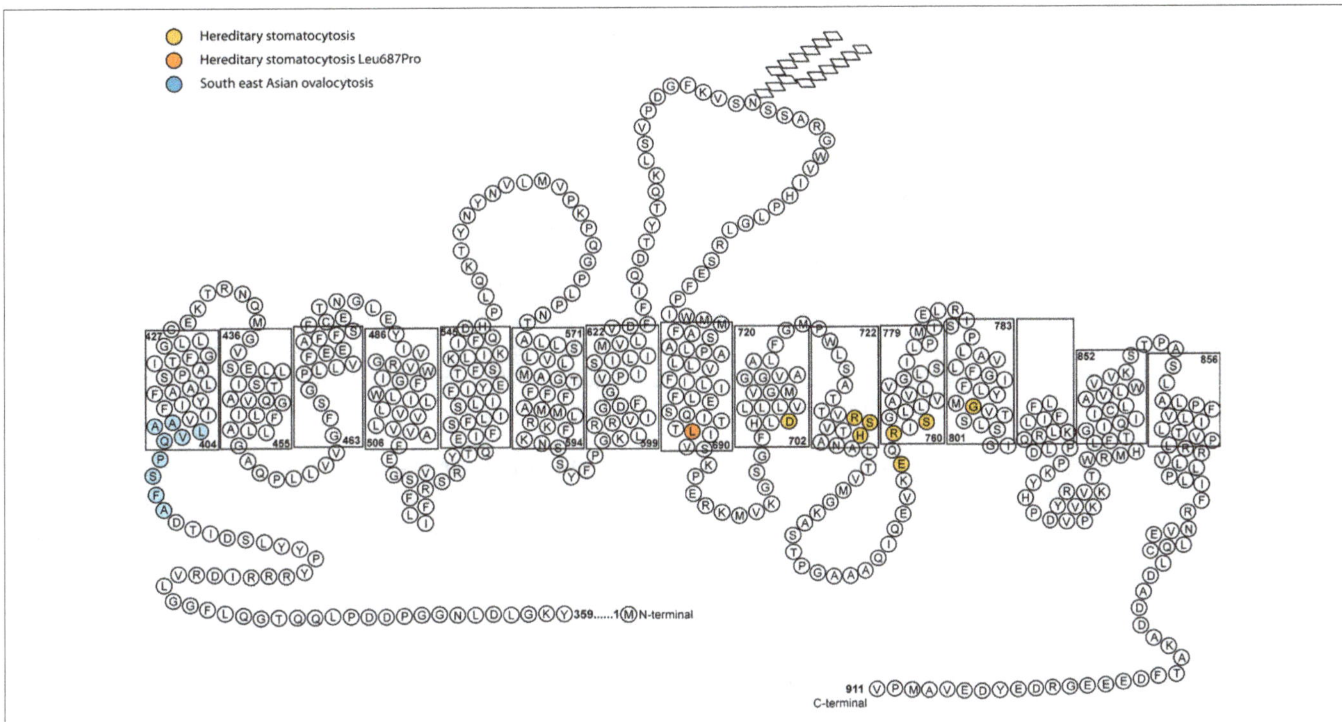

FIGURE 2 | Diagram of the membrane domain of band 3 showing the membrane spans and HSt mutations. The length of the membrane spans mimics that determined from the crystal structure by Arakawa et al. (2015). In the final structure the half transmembrane span 3 and half transmembrane span 10 form a full transmembrane domain (TM) jointly (Arakawa et al., 2015). The nine amino acid residues deleted in SAO band 3 are shown in blue. The amino acid residues associated with HSt are shown in orange. The Asp705Tyr (TM9), Arg730Cys (TM10), Ser731Pro (TM10), His734Arg (TM10) Glu758Lys (TM11), Arg760Gln (TM11), and Ser762Arg (TM11) mutations all occur close to the anion binding site of band 3. The Gly796Arg mutation is in TM12 and may affect helix-helix packing. The Leu687Pro mutation is near the C-terminus of TM8 which is at the interface of the core and gate domains. Movement between these two domains is required for anion transport and substitution of Leu687 with a proline residue may restrict this movement (Arakawa et al., 2015).

of glycolysis end products. This is consistent with an increased energy demand in OHSt cells, possibly resulting from elevated activity of the Na,K-ATPase attempting to maintain normal cation gradients. An unexpected finding in the metabolomics study was an alteration in levels of certain members of oxidation pathways, raising the possibility that OHSt RBCs may also suffer from previously unrecognized oxidative stress (Darghouth et al., 2011).

Stomatin

Stomatin first attracted attention when it was observed to be deficient in the membranes of overhydrated stomatocytosis RBCs, and was named after the disease (Lande et al., 1982; Stewart et al., 1992). Initially it appeared that the disease must be caused by the absence of this protein, however further investigation revealed that stomatin deficiency was a secondary effect of the disorder (Fricke et al., 2003). It is now known that the primary defect is mutation in RhAG. Since then, a second type of hereditary stomatocytosis has been observed to be deficient in stomatin (sdCHC, see below).

Interestingly, the levels of stomatin are also significantly higher in dog RBCs of the "high K" phenotype and its expression can be used as a marker for the phenotype (Komatsu et al., 2010).

The precise role of stomatin in the RBC has become a long-running debate, although potential roles have been plentiful. Studies using a wide variety of organisms have provided evidence that stomatin is involved in cholesterol binding, actin binding, vesiculation and regulation of ion channels. In species unable to synthesize vitamin C *de novo*, stomatin converts GLUT1 into a transporter of oxidized vitamin C (dehydroascorbic acid; DHA), which is crucial for its recycling (Montel-Hagen et al., 2008).

Cross-linking experiments also implicate stomatin in RBC protein complexes with GLUT1, band 3, aquaporin-1 and other membrane transporters and proteins (Rungaldier et al., 2013). Stomatin is able to form higher order homo-oligomeric complexes in the RBC membrane and probably acts as a scaffolding protein (Salzer and Prohaska, 2001).

Rh$_{null}$

The molecular basis of Rh$_{null}$ (regulator type) is mutation in both alleles of *RHAG*, resulting in the absence of RhAG and its closely associated partner proteins from the RBC membrane. Rh$_{null}$ (amorph type) occurs when an RhD-negative individual also has mutations in both alleles of *RHCE*, in which case RhAG is only weakly expressed (Cartron, 1999). This deficiency of the Rh protein complex is associated with a number of as yet unexplained features including altered membrane phospholipid asymmetry, occasional stomato-spherocytic morphology and a mild cation leak (reviewed by Cartron, 1999). Patients usually experience chronic mild to moderate hemolytic anemia.

Analysis of morphologically normal Rh_{null} RBCs revealed normal cation and water content but an increase in the basal membrane permeability to potassium and the ouabain and bumetanide sensitive potassium permeability. Consistent with the observed increase in active potassium transport, the number of Na,K-ATPase molecules in the Rh_{null} RBCs was greater than normal by 35–45% (Lauf and Joiner, 1976). The temperature-dependence of the leak has not been established.

There is evidence that protein-lipid interactions are altered in Rh_{null} RBCs (Dorn-Zachertz and Zimmer, 1981). Band 3 has been shown to interact strongly with RhAG, so its absence is likely to disrupt the correct formation of the band 3 macrocomplex (Bruce et al., 2003). More work is needed to elucidate the mechanism behind the increased cation permeability previously observed in 2 cases of Rh_{null}. However, the lack of availability of this extremely rare blood type is restrictive for comprehensive studies.

GLUT1 Mutations

Stomatin-deficient cryohydrocytosis (sdCHC) is a very rare type of HSt, and has only been reported in 3 patients to date (Bawazir et al., 2012). Alongside a RBC cation leak that is 10 times greater than normal at 37°C (**Figure 1B**) these patients also suffer from numerous non-hematological symptoms that do not occur in any of the other types of hereditary stomatocytosis. These include cataracts and a debilitating neurological phenotype comprising seizures and severe learning difficulties. The gene responsible has been identified as *SLC2A1*, encoding glucose transporter isoform 1 (GLUT1). GLUT1 is the major glucose transporter expressed in RBCs and at the blood-brain barrier. Two distinct mutations in *SLC2A1* have been found in sdCHC patients (Flatt et al., 2011). In the Montpellier pedigree a single amino acid substitution mutation was found (Gly286Asp), whilst the San Francisco pedigree exhibited a single amino acid deletion (Ile435 or Ile436). In an analogous situation to the RhAG mutants in OHSt and some of the band 3 mutants in CHC, the GLUT1 mutants lost their ability to transport their usual substrate, and instead induced a cation leak when expressed heterologously in *X. levis* oocytes.

GLUT1 mutations have also been shown to result in a RBC cation leak in one pedigree suffering from another condition called paroxysmal exertion-induced dyskinesia (PED) (Weber et al., 2008). In PED involuntary movements are brought on by exercise, and it is not normally associated with a RBC cation leak. In this case the mutation in GLUT1 was identified as a deletion of residues 282–285, which is immediately adjacent to the substitution mutation identified in sdCHC. This mutation occurs within transmembrane span 7, which has been shown to be crucial for transport function. Modeling of the mutant protein suggested that the central pore is widened. Unlike in sdCHC, these RBCs exhibited spiky protrusions (echinocytosis), which are often associated with cellular dehydration. The permeability of the RBCs to sodium, potassium and calcium was increased, raising the possibility that calcium influx might be sufficient to activate the Gardos channel and trigger rapid potassium efflux and cellular dehydration, explaining the echinocytosis (Weber et al., 2008).

Mutations in GLUT1 are also associated with GLUT1-deficiency syndrome (GLUT1-DS). This disorder shows some heterogeneity in its severity and symptoms (Brockmann, 2009). However, there does appear to be a correlation between the effect on glucose transport and clinical severity (Rotstein et al., 2010). Inactivating mutations in one allele result in ~50% reduction in glucose transport, and these are the most common form of GLUT1-DS. Other missense mutations appear to impact glucose transport in a minor way, resulting in an asymptomatic or mild phenotype. Compound heterozygosity or homozygosity for a "mild" mutation could therefore result in a severe phenotype where glucose transport is reduced by more than 50%. A reduction of 75% or more is likely to be embryonic lethal (Rotstein et al., 2010).

ABCB6 Mutations

The condition, familial pseudohyperkalemia (FP), is a very mild form of HSt that can often be asymptomatic. The condition was first reported in 1979 (Stewart et al., 1979), although FP in this cohort was later shown to map to the 16q23-ter locus (Iolascon et al., 1999) and result from a mutation in PIEZO1 (Andolfo et al., 2013b). A detailed analysis of the temperature sensitivity of the potassium flux was described in 1985 (Meenaghan et al., 1985). At the physiological temperature of 37°C the cation leak is practically indistinguishable from normal, being only 1.1–1.5 times the normal rate (Stewart, 2004). The close to normal cation permeability at 37°C means that samples of FP blood when tested immediately after venesection show normal hematological parameters. However, after cooling to room temperature and/or refrigeration the cation leak is "activated" and a rise in plasma potassium occurs after a period of cool or room temperature storage. Although all FP cases share this feature, the heterogeneity in the temperature-dependence of their cation leaks means that the degree of potassium efflux varies between the different subtypes at different temperatures.

The temperature dependences of the cation leaks in the FP pedigrees are shown in **Figure 1**, and include U-shaped (**Figure 1B**), shallow slope (**Figure 1C**) and shoulder types (**Figure 1D**). All show a cation leak very similar to the control at 37°C which increases as the temperature decreases. The molecular bases of a number of FP pedigrees have been determined recently, with mutations in the ATP-binding cassette family member B6 (ABCB6) identified as responsible (Andolfo et al., 2013a, 2016; Bawazir et al., 2014). The ABCB6 protein is a porphyrin transporter that is considered to be a mitochondrial protein, but has also been detected in lysosomes and the RBC plasma membrane (Kiss et al., 2012). Indeed, it has also been discovered that ABCB6 carries the antigens of the Langereis blood group system (Helias et al., 2012).

Two of the *ABCB6* mutations affect the same residue in the protein (R375Q and R375W) and both of these changes result in the same temperature-dependence profile in their cation leak (shoulder type with a peak at 10°C, (**Figure 1D**). A different mutation in ABCB6 is associated with the Cardiff pedigree (R723Q), whose cation leak shows a U-shaped temperature-dependence (**Figure 1B**). Hence, the cation leak in this type of FP only becomes apparent at temperatures lower than 20°C and further increases as the temperature decreases. Although the vast majority of FP mutations seem to be very rare, the SNP database suggests that the R723Q mutation has a frequency of 1 in 500 (Bawazir et al., 2014). The temperature-dependent activation of these leaks during the processing and storage of RBC concentrates for use in transfusion medicine should be a concern when selecting units for transfusion of high-risk patients such as neonates (Bawazir et al., 2014).

Three further mutations in ABCB6 have been reported in FP families. The Arg276Trp mutation has been found alone, and in trans to the Arg723Gln mutation, in two separate families (Andolfo et al., 2016), and the Val454Ala mutation has been found in a Bolivian family (Andolfo et al., 2016). Andolfo et al. present data to show that the Arg276Trp and Val454Ala mutations increase cation permeability of HEK293 cells over-expressing these mutant ABCB6 proteins, and show evidence of a slight increase in cation permeability in FP RBCs with the Arg276Trp mutation. Interestingly the family with the Arg276Trp mutation is the Irish family from Omagh that were initially classified as DHSt with FP (**Table 1**; Stewart et al., 1996). The temperature profile was assigned as parallel (**Figure 1E**) but may fit better in the U-shaped classification (**Figure 1B**) as the temperature profile is similar to the FP-Cardiff profile although milder (note the different Y-axis scales on **Figures 1B,D**). It would not be expected that the Arg276Trp mutation would cause a large difference in cation permeability because it is classified as "benign" in the Single Nucleotide Polymorphism database: https://www.ncbi.nlm.nih.gov/projects/SNP/snp_ref.cgi?rs=57467915 and this mutant has a fairly high population frequency in the European population. This would therefore be expected to have caused more problems with blood storage and transfusion than have been reported. The high population frequency of this mutation underlines the fact that FP is an under-diagnosed condition (Andolfo et al., 2018a,b).

Unresolved—HSt Woking

An unusual case of hereditary stomatocytosis has been reported in which there is a significant cation leak (5 times greater than normal, but with a normal temperature dependence pattern), yet there was minimal hemolysis observed and nearly normal osmotic fragility (Jarvis et al., 2001). The affected offspring of the propositus experienced an even milder phenotype. The authors speculated that the discrepancy between the grossly abnormal cation content and mild phenotype was because the sodium and potassium abnormalities were relatively balanced (Jarvis et al., 2001). The genetic basis for this variant is unknown and has not been mapped.

HST MUTATIONS IN AFFECTING THE REGULATION OF CATION CHANNELS

PIEZO1 Mutations

Dehydrated hereditary stomatocytosis (DHSt; also known as hereditary xerocytosis) is a condition, similar to FP that falls at the milder end of the cation leaky spectrum. DHSt RBCs exhibit an elevation in their passive cation leak at 37°C of around twice normal, and the temperature-dependence profiles of the leak (shown in **Figure 1, Table 1**) have been reported as shallow slope (**Figure 1C**), parallel (**Figure 1D**), sigmoidal (**Figure 1E**) or flat to 30°C (**Figure 1G**). This can mean that the relative increase in cation permeability of DHSt cells is augmented at lower temperatures. Indeed, all four panels show an increased cation leak relative to the control at 20°C, most markedly in the parallel and flat to 30°C profiles, however only the parallel profile shows an increased cation leak at 4°C (**Figure 1**). It should be noted that most of the profiles shown in the shallow slope graph (**Figure 1C**) are the HSt Blackburn type caused by mutations in *SLC4A1*. With hind sight, it may be that the Edinburgh profile would fit better as a mild form of the parallel profile. This tendency for DHSt RBCs to have a very minor difference in cation permeability at 37°C but maintain an increased cation leak, relative to the control, at lower temperature explains why DHSt is so often associated with pseudohyperkalemia.

The nature of the cation leak in DHSt cells is imbalanced, in that there is a greater loss of potassium from the cells than the increase in sodium, which leads to dehydration of the RBC. The dehydrated cells are accordingly more osmotically resistant than controls, and also have an unexplained increased susceptibility to oxidants (Harm et al., 1979). Individuals with DHSt exhibit mild hemolytic anemia with increased reticulocytes and macrocytosis. Unlike in other hemolytic anemias, splenectomy is not recommended for patients with DHSt because it often results in thrombo-embolic events (Stewart et al., 1996).

After a long search for the molecular basis of DHSt a breakthrough was finally made, where mutations in the gene encoding PIEZO1, *FAM38A*, were discovered to be associated with the disorder (Zarychanski et al., 2012). The PIEZO1 protein forms part of a mechanosensitive transduction channel (Coste et al., 2010). PIEZO1 is a very large protein, predicted to cross the membrane 36–39 times and has been identified in RBC membranes using mass spectrometry and Western blotting methods (Zarychanski et al., 2012; Andolfo et al., 2013b). It has been shown to induce cationic fluxes in response to mechanical stimulation in eukaryotic cells (Coste et al., 2010). Expression of wild type PIEZO1 in *X. levis* oocytes resulted in mechano-stimulated currents that were not observed in uninjected oocytes. These currents were also observed in PIEZO1-expressing oocytes subjected to hypotonic and hypertonic induced swelling and shrinkage, respectively (Andolfo et al., 2013b). Comparison of the conductances of normal and DHSt (with mutation R2456H) RBCs using cell-attached recording showed that DHSt cells exhibited a conductance that could be inhibited with tarantula toxin, GsMTx-4, supporting the hypothesis that the cation leak is mediated by PIEZO1 (Andolfo et al., 2013b). Expression of DHSt mutant PIEZO1 proteins in HEK293T cells revealed that all six of the tested mutations result in slower inactivation of the current (Albuisson et al., 2013). This gain-of-function pattern would be consistent with the observed dehydrated phenotype. Conversely knockdown of PIEZO1 in zebrafish or mouse results in swollen cells (Faucherre et al., 2014; Cahalan et al., 2015).

It therefore seems probable that different mutations in the two genes known to be associated with DHSt and FP can result in highly similar phenotypes. Equally, different mutations within the same gene can result in distinct phenotypes, as has also been seen in the other stomatocytosis variants. For example, some mutations affect the transport ability of the proteins while others do not, and the two *RHAG* mutations resulting in OHSt give rise to subtly different phenotypes (**Table 1**). Although the ability of PIEZO1 or ABCB6 to transport their usual substrates has not been fully characterized in DHSt and FP RBCs, it is possible that inhibited transport may affect the resulting phenotype. This is particularly interesting in the case of PIEZO1, which has been shown to act as a stretch sensor in RBCs and to play a key role in RBC volume regulation (Zarychanski et al., 2012). Recent studies have shown that the DHSt mutations in PIEZO1 cause a partial gain-of-function phenotype (Albuisson et al., 2013; Andolfo et al., 2013b). Generation of mechanically activated currents inactivate more slowly than wild type. However in addition to delayed channel inactivation, additional alterations have been found in mutant PIEZO1 channel kinetics, differences in response to osmotic stress, and altered membrane protein trafficking, predicting variant alleles that worsen or ameliorate erythrocyte hydration (Glogowska et al., 2017).

DHSt is occasionally associated with perinatal ascites (buildup of fluid in the baby's abdominal cavity) and/or nuchal translucency (buildup of fluid at the back of the baby's head observed during ultrasound scans) (Entezami et al., 1996; Ami et al., 2009). Andolfo et al. (2013b) investigated the tissue expression pattern of PIEZO1 and found that it was expressed in the peritoneal lymphatic vessels in fetal, but not adult, samples. This expression pattern is consistent with the observed phenotype of edema that spontaneously self-corrects just after birth (Andolfo et al., 2013b). It is of interest that the mutations detected in DHSt with associated ascites have also been found in DHSt cases where ascites has not been reported. It is possible that this is an under-reported condition, and that some cases have not been detected or diagnosed, especially when the edema resolves prenatally (personal communication from Prof Jean Delaunay, 2013). The severity of the edema appears to vary between cases, even those with the same mutation in PIEZO1, and may suggest the presence of a modifying gene. In recent years, numerous PIEZO1 mutations have been reported associated with DHSt alone, DHSt with pseudohyperkalemia and /or with edema (see **Table 1**).

Gardos Channel Mutations

After the breakthrough discovery that mutations in PIEZO1 cause various forms of DHSt, several groups have recently published studies showing that mutations in the Gardos channel (heterozygous substitutions Val282Glu, Val282Met, Arg352His), encoded by the gene *KCNN4*, are associated with DHSt (Andolfo et al., 2015; Glogowska et al., 2015; Rapetti-Mauss et al., 2015). Functional analysis of the R352H mutant suggested that it was 10-fold more sensitive to activation by calcium and also remained in the open conformation longer than the wild type protein (Rapetti-Mauss et al., 2015).

These findings have led to the hypothesis that DHSt result from a malfunction in the regulation of the joint activity of the Gardos channel and PIEZO1. In wild-type RBC, passage through constricted splenic slits or small capillary beds is associated with transient calcium-mediated adaptions (Danielczok et al., 2017). It is proposed that this transient increase in intracellular calcium is mediated by the opening of the PIEZO1 channel, which opens in response to the shear stress of the constricted space. The rise in intracellular calcium then causes the Gardos channel to open with the loss of potassium, followed by chloride ions and water, thus dehydrating the cell. This would make the Gardos channel the essential determinant of RBC dehydration in HSt (Rapetti-Mauss et al., 2017), regardless of whether the mutation was in PIEZO1 causing a prolonged influx of calcium or in KCNN4 making the Gardos channel more sensitive to intracellular calcium.

Despite the discovery of the genes responsible for DHSt, it is still not clear why many individuals with DHSt have been reported to exhibit a propensity to iron overload (Syfuss et al., 2006). It has been suggested that dyserythropoiesis in these conditions may play a role but this is yet to be confirmed (Andolfo et al., 2015).

ORIGIN OF THE CATION LEAK IN THE HEREDITARY STOMATOCYTOSES

Once it was discovered that band 3 mutations result in a cation leak, the mechanism of the leak was debated. In the initial report it was suggested that cation movements were conducted directly though the mutant band 3, and further investigation of the band 3 CHC mutations supported this proposal (Bruce et al., 2005; Guizouarn et al., 2007). However, Bogdanova et al. reported increased cation transport via the K(Na)/H exchanger and the K,Cl cotransporter in CHC RBCs leading to the proposal of an alternative mechanism whereby the mutant band 3 activates other endogenous transporters in the membrane, causing the cation imbalance (Bogdanova et al., 2010; Stewart et al., 2010). It is interesting to note that cation-leaky band 3 point mutations are mainly clustered around the same region in the protein, between transmembrane span 8 and span 12, the region of the protein intimately involved in anion transport (Arakawa et al., 2015) (**Figure 2**). The exception to this is the Leu687Pro mutation which is in TM 8 at the interface of the core and gate domains. This mutation may obstruct the movement between these two domains and thereby affect anion exchange and the correct packing of the protein (**Figure 2**).

Modeling RhAG based on the structure of *Nitrosomonas europea* Rh50 protein predicted that the OHSt mutations resulted in widening of the central channel and its conversion into a cation pore (Bruce et al., 2009). The leak in OHSt increases with temperature in a linear pattern, consistent with the hypothesis of the conversion of RhAG into a constitutively open cation channel. The more complex temperature-dependence of the other HSt leaks might suggest a less clear cut mechanism of cation leak. In the cryohydrocytosis types, the leak is even enhanced at lower temperatures. The GLUT1 mutations responsible for sdCHC have been modeled, with Gly286Asp predicted to result in a more rigid protein structure and Ile435DEL predicted to result in longer range conformational changes that are hard to model accurately (Flatt et al., 2011). This distinct temperature dependence and lack of structural evidence for the formation of a pore suggest that the cation leak may not be conducted directly through the transport channel of GLUT1. Instead, the leak may be mediated via altered protein-protein or protein-lipid interactions. Both band 3 and GLUT1 have been shown to participate in larger protein complexes (Bruce et al., 2003; Khan et al., 2008), so it is conceivable that small alterations in their structures, and resultant macro-structures, could provide gaps through which the leak could occur. Alternatively, small alterations in protein-lipid interactions could provide a pathway for cations across the membrane. It is becoming more evident that the surfaces of proteins contain specific lipid binding sites that are important for the proper expression and function of the protein in the membrane (reviewed by Palsdottir and Hunte, 2004). Perturbation of these interactions could be thought of as a weakening of the lipid "seal" around the protein. At lower temperatures membranes become more rigid, which could exacerbate the poor fit of lipids around mutant proteins and their multi-protein complexes and provide an explanation for how and why the leaks worsen at low temperatures.

Given that mutations in 4 different large multi-spanning membrane proteins have now been associated with these cation leaky conditions it seems unlikely that a distinct cation transporter pathway is being activated and causing the cation imbalance. Rather, it appears to be the general rule that mutation in any large multi-spanning membrane protein can provoke a cation leak if it is expressed at the RBC plasma membrane.

More recently the discovery and characterization of mutations in PIEZO1 and the Gardos channel in DHSt have been made. This has revealed a second, alternative mechanism behind HSt, in which an over-active mutant cation channel is responsible for the observed increase in membrane permeability to cations.

OTHER INCIDENCES OF STOMATOCYTIC MORPHOLOGY

The presence of stomatocytes in the blood is not exclusive to the cation-leaky disorders. Phytosterolemia is a recessively-inherited condition in which cholesterols and plant-derived sterols are absorbed from the gut in a deregulated manner. The excess of phytosterols in the blood can result in stomatocytosis and large platelets (Rees et al., 2005). It is thought that the phytosterols are able to partition into the membranes of circulating RBCs and selectively expand the inner leaflet of the bilayer, inducing an inward curve in the membrane that leads to the adoption of stomatocytic morphology. Indeed, the quantity of stomatocytic cells can vary widely, and they are often not overtly predominant in blood smears from hereditary stomatocytosis pedigrees. Blood smears commonly appear normal in familial pseudohyperkalemia and in DHSt abnormal cells are principally target cells, not stomatocytes.

SUMMARY

At present the evidence strongly suggests that there are two distinct mechanisms underlying the pathological increase in cation permeability of the RBC membrane in hereditary stomatocytosis. Modifications in a variety of multi-spanning membrane proteins including band 3, RhAG, GLUT1 and ABCB6 can result in formation of a cation pore or otherwise disrupt the membrane to allow unregulated cation movement across the membrane. Alternatively, modifications to existing cation channels such as PIEZO1 and the Gardos channel can alter their activation and deactivation kinetics, leading to increased opening and allowing greater cation fluxes than in wild type. The degree and character of the "leakiness" in these conditions can vary greatly, illustrated by the diverse phenotypes found in HSt.

AUTHOR CONTRIBUTIONS

Both authors conceived and developed the ideas in this review. JF wrote the paper and LB edited and updated it.

REFERENCES

Albuisson, J., Murthy, S. E., Bandell, M., Coste, B., Louis-Dit-Picard, H., Mathur, J., et al. (2013). Dehydrated hereditary stomatocytosis linked to gain-of-function mutations in mechanically activated PIEZO1 ion channels. *Nat. Commun.* 4:1884. doi: doi: 10.1038/ncomms2899

Allen, S. J., O'Donnell, A., Alexander, N. D., Mgone, C. S., Peto, T. E., Clegg, J. B., et al. (1999). Prevention of cerebral malaria in children in Papua New Guinea by southeast Asian ovalocytosis band 3. *Am. J. Trop. Med. Hyg.* 60, 1056–1060. doi: 10.4269/ajtmh.1999.60.1056

Ami, O., Picone, O., Garçon, L., Castel, C., Guitton, C., Delaunay, J., et al. (2009). First-trimester nuchal abnormalities secondary to dehydrated hereditary stomatocytosis. *Prenat. Diagn.* 29, 1071–1074. doi: 10.1002/pd.2342

Andolfo, I., Alper, S. L., De Franceschi, L., Auriemma, C., Russo, R., De Falco, L., et al. (2013b). Multiple clinical forms of dehydrated hereditary stomatocytosis arise from mutations in PIEZO1. *Blood* 121, 3925–3935. doi: 10.1182/blood-2013-02-482489

Andolfo, I., Alper, S. L., Delaunay, J., Auriemma, C., Russo, R., Asci, R., et al. (2013a). Missense mutations in the ABCB6 transporter cause dominant familial pseudohyperkalemia. *Am. J. Hematol.* 88, 66–72. doi: 10.1002/ajh.23357

Andolfo, I., Manna, F., De Rosa, G., Rosato, B. E., Gambale, A., Tomaiuolo, G., et al. (2018a). PIEZO1-R1864H rare variant accounts for a genetic phenotype-modifier role in dehydrated hereditary stomatocytosis. *Haematologica* 103, e94–e97. doi: 10.3324/haematol.2017.180687

Andolfo, I., Russo, R., Gambale, A., and Iolascon, A. (2018b). Hereditary stomatocytosis: an underdiagnosed condition. *Am. J. Hematol.* 93, 107–121. doi: 10.1002/ajh.24929

Andolfo, I., Russo, R., Manna, F., De Rosa, G., Gambale, A., Zouwail, S., et al. (2016). Functional characterization of novel ABCB6 mutations and their clinical implications in familial pseudohyperkalemia. *Haematologica* 101, 909–917. doi: 10.3324/haematol.2016.142372

Andolfo, I., Russo, R., Manna, F., Shmukler, B. E., Gambale, A., Vitiello, G., et al. (2015). Novel Gardos channel mutations linked to dehydrated hereditary stomatocytosis (Xerocytosis). *Am. J. Hematol.* 90, 921–926. doi: 10.1002/ajh.24117

Arakawa, T., Kobayashi-Yurugi, T., Alguel, Y., Iwanari, H., Hatae, H., Iwata, M., et al. (2015). Crystal structure of the anion exchanger domain of human erythrocyte band 3. *Science* 350, 680–684. doi: 10.1126/science.aaa4335

Archer, N. M., Shmukler, B. E., Andolfo, I., Vandorpe, D. H., Gnanasambandam, R., Higgins, J. M., et al. (2014). Hereditary xerocytosis revisited. *Am. J. Hematol.* 89, 1142–1146. doi: 10.1002/ajh.23799

Bae, C., Gnanasambandam, R., Nicolai, C., Sachs, F., and Gottlieb, P. A. (2013). Xerocytosis is caused by mutations that alter the kinetics of the mechanosensitive channel PIEZO1. *Proc. Natl. Acad. Sci. U.S.A.* 110, E1162–E1168. doi: 10.1073/pnas.1219777110

Bae, C., Sachs, F., and Gottlieb, P. A. (2011). The mechanosensitive ion channel Piezo1 is inhibited by the peptide GsMTx4. *Biochemistry* 50, 6295–6300. doi: 10.1021/bi200770q

Basu, A. P., Carey, P., Cynober, T., Chetty, M., Delaunay, J., Stewart, G. W., et al. (2003). Dehydrated hereditary stomatocytosis with transient perinatal ascites. *Arch. Dis. Child. Fetal Neonatal Ed.* 88, F438–F439. doi: 10.1136/fn.88.5.F438

Bawazir, W. M., Flatt, J. F., Wallis, J. P., Rendon, A., Cardigan, R. A., New, H. V., et al. (2014). Familial pseudohyperkalemia in blood donors: a novel mutation with implications for transfusion practice. *Transfusion* 54, 3043–3050. doi: 10.1111/trf.12757

Bawazir, W. M., Gevers, E. F., Flatt, J. F., Ang, A. L., Jacobs, B., Oren, C., et al. (2012). An infant with pseudohyperkalemia, hemolysis, and seizures: cation-leaky GLUT1-deficiency syndrome due to a SLC2A1 mutation. *J. Clin. Endocrinol. Metab.* 97, E987–E993. doi: 10.1210/jc.2012-1399

Beneteau, C., Thierry, G., Blesson, S., Le Vaillant, C., Picard, V., Béné, M., et al. (2014). Recurrent mutation in the PIEZO1 gene in two families of hereditary xerocytosis with fetal hydrops. *Clin. Genet.* 85, 293–295. doi: 10.1111/cge.12147

Bennekou, P., and Christopherson, P. (2003). "Ion channels" in *Red Cell Membrane Transport*, eds I. Bernhardt and J. C. Ellory (Berlin; Heidelberg: Springer-Verlag), 139–152.

Bernhardt, I., and Weiss, E. (2003). "Passive membrane permeability for ions and the membrane potential" in *Red Cell Membrane Transport*, eds I. Bernhardt and J. C. Ellory (Berlin; Heidelberg: Springer-Verlag), 83–109.

Bogdanova, A., Goede, J. S., Weiss, E., Bogdanov, N., Bennekou, P., Bernhardt, I., et al. (2010). Cryohydrocytosis: increased activity of cation carriers in red cells from a patient with a band 3 mutation. *Haematologica* 95, 189–198. doi: 10.3324/haematol.2009.010215

Brockmann, K. (2009). The expanding phenotype of GLUT1-deficiency syndrome. *Brain Dev.* 31, 545–552. doi: 10.1016/j.braindev.2009.02.008

Bruce, L. J., Beckmann, R., Ribeiro, M. L., Peters, L. L., Chasis, J. A., Delaunay, J., et al. (2003). A band 3-based macrocomplex of integral and peripheral proteins in the RBC membrane. *Blood* 101, 4180–4188. doi: 10.1182/blood-2002-09-2824

Bruce, L. J., Guizouarn, H., Burton, N. M., Gabillat, N., Poole, J., Flatt, J. F., et al. (2009). The monovalent cation leak in overhydrated stomatocytic red blood cells results from amino acid substitutions in the Rh-associated glycoprotein. *Blood* 113, 1350–1357. doi: 10.1182/blood-2008-07-171140

Bruce, L. J., Ring, S. M., Ridgwell, K., Reardon, D. M., Seymour, C. A., Van Dort, H. M., et al. (1999). South-east asian ovalocytic (SAO) erythrocytes have a cold sensitive cation leak: implications for *in vitro* studies on stored SAO red cells. *Biochim. Biophys. Acta* 1416, 258–270. doi: 10.1016/S0005-2736(98)00231-4

Bruce, L. J., Robinson, H. C., Guizouarn, H., Borgese, F., Harrison, P., King, M. J., et al. (2005). Monovalent cation leaks in human red cells caused by single amino-acid substitutions in the transport domain of the band 3 chloride-bicarbonate exchanger, AE1. *Nat. Genet.* 37, 1258–1263. doi: 10.1038/ng1656

Burton, N. M., and Anstee, D. J. (2008). Structure, function and significance of Rh proteins in red cells. *Curr. Opin. Hematol.* 15, 625–630. doi: 10.1097/MOH.0b013e328311f422

Cahalan, S. M., Lukacs, V., Ranade, S. S., Chien, S., Bandell, M., and Patapoutian, A. (2015). Piezo1 links mechanical forces to red blood cell volume. *Elife.* 4. doi: 10.7554/eLife.07370

Carella, M., Stewart, G., Ajetunmobi, J. F., Perrotta, S., Grootenboer, S., Tchernia, G., et al. (1998). Genomewide search for dehydrated hereditary stomatocytosis (hereditary xerocytosis): mapping of locus to chromosome 16 (16q23-qter). *Am. J. Hum. Genet.* 63, 810–816. doi: 10.1086/302024

Carli, P., Graffin, B., Gisserot, O., Landais, C., and De Jaureguiberry, J. P. (2007). Recurrence of thromboembolic disease after splenectomy for hereditary xerocytosis. *Rev. Med. Interne.* 28, 879–881. doi: 10.1016/j.revmed.2007.05.012

Cartron, J. P. (1999). RH blood group system and molecular basis of Rh-deficiency. *Baillieres. Best Pract. Res. Clin. Haematol.* 12, 655–689. doi: 10.1053/beha.1999.0047

Chan, P. C., Calabrese, V., and Theil, L. S. (1964). Species differences in the effect of sodium and potassium ions on the ATPase of erythrocyte membranes. *Biochim. Biophys. Acta* 79, 424–426. doi: 10.1016/0926-6577(64)90028-2

Coles, S. E., Chetty, M. C., Ho, M. M., Nicolaou, A., Kearney, J. W., Wright, S. D., et al. (1999a). Two British families with variants of the "cryohydrocytosis" form of hereditary stomatocytosis. *Br. J. Haematol.* 105, 1055–1065.

Coles, S. E., Ho, M. M., Chetty, M. C., Nicolaou, A., and Stewart, G. W. (1999b). A variant of hereditary stomatocytosis with marked pseudohyperkalaemia. *Br. J. Haematol.* 104, 275–283.

Coles, S. E., and Stewart, G. W. (1999). Temperature effects on cation transport in hereditary stomatocytosis and allied disorders. *Int. J. Exp. Pathol.* 80, 251–258. doi: 10.1046/j.1365-2613.1999.00120.x

Coste, B., Mathur, J., Schmidt, M., Earley, T. J., Ranade, S., Petrus, M. J., et al. (2010). Piezo1 and Piezo2 are essential components of distinct mechanically activated cation channels. *Science* 330, 55–60. doi: 10.1126/science.1193270

Dagher, G., Vantyghem, M. C., Doise, B., Lallau, G., Racadot, A., and Lefebvre, J. (1989). Altered erythrocyte cation permeability in familial pseudohyperkalaemia. *Clin. Sci.* 77, 213–216. doi: 10.1042/cs0770213

Danielczok, J. G., Terriac, E., Hertz, L., Petkova-Kirova, P., Lautenschläger, F., Laschke, M. W., et al. (2017). Red blood cell passage of small capillaries is associated with transient $Ca2^{+}$-mediated adaptations. *Front. Physiol.* 8:979. doi: 10.3389/fphys.2017.00979

Darghouth, D., Koehl, B., Heilier, J. F., Madalinski, G., Bovee, P., Bosman, G., et al. (2011). Alterations of red blood cell metabolome in overhydrated hereditary stomatocytosis. *Haematologica* 96, 1861–1865. doi: 10.3324/haematol.2011.045179

Dluzewski, A. R., Nash, G. B., Wilson, R. J., Reardon, D. M., and Gratzer, W. B. (1992). Invasion of hereditary ovalocytes by *Plasmodium falciparum in vitro* and its relation to intracellular ATP concentration. *Mol. Biochem. Parasitol.* 55, 1–7. doi: 10.1016/0166-6851(92)90121-Y

Dorn-Zachertz, D., and Zimmer, G. (1981). Different protein-lipid interaction in human red blood cell membrane of Rh positive and Rh negative blood compared with Rhnull. *Z Naturforsch. C* 36, 988–996.

Endeward, V., Cartron, J. P., Ripoche, P., and Gros, G. (2006). Red cell membrane CO2 permeability in normal human blood and in blood deficient in various blood groups, and effect of DIDS. *Transfus. Clin. Biol.* 13, 123–127. doi: 10.1016/j.tracli.2006.02.007

Entezami, M., Becker, R., Menssen, H. D., Marcinkowski, M., and Versmold, H. T. (1996). Xerocytosis with concomitant intrauterine ascites: first description and therapeutic approach. *Blood* 87, 5392–5393.

Faucherre, A., Kissa, K., Nargeot, J., Mangoni, M., and Jopling, C. (2014). Piezo1 plays a role in erythrocyte volume homeostasis. *Haematologica* 99, 70–75. doi: 10.3324/haematol.2013.086090

Fermo, E., Bogdanova, A., Petkova-Kirova, P., Zaninoni, A., Marcello, A. P., Makhro, A., et al. (2017). "Gardos Channelopathy:" a variant of hereditary Stomatocytosis with complex molecular regulation. *Sci. Rep.* 7:1744. doi: 10.1038/s41598-017-01591-w

Flatman, P. W. (2002). Regulation of Na-K-2Cl cotransport by phosphorylation and protein-protein interactions. *Biochim. Biophys. Acta* 1566, 140–151. doi: 10.1016/S0005-2736(02)00586-2

Flatt, J. F., Guizouarn, H., Burton, N. M., Borgese, F., Tomlinson, R. J., Forsyth, R. J., et al. (2011). Stomatin-deficient cryohydrocytosis results from mutations in SLC2A1: a novel form of GLUT1 deficiency syndrome. *Blood* 118, 5267–5277. doi: 10.1182/blood-2010-12-326645

Fricke, B., Argent, A. C., Chetty, M. C., Pizzey, A. R., Turner, E. J., Ho, M. M., et al. (2003). The "stomatin" gene and protein in overhydrated hereditary stomatocytosis. *Blood*. 102, 2268–2277. doi: 10.1182/blood-2002-06-1705

Fricke, B., Jarvis, H. G., Reid, C. D., Aguilar-Martinez, P., Robert, A., Quittet, P., et al. (2004). Four new cases of stomatin-deficient hereditary stomatocytosis syndrome: association of the stomatin-deficient cryohydrocytosis variant with neurological dysfunction. *Br. J. Haematol.* 125, 796–803. doi: 10.1111/j.1365-2141.2004.04965.x

Gallagher, P. G. (2017). Disorders of erythrocyte hydration. *Blood* 130, 2699–2708. doi: 10.1182/blood-2017-04-590810

Genetet, S., Ripoche, P., Picot, J., Bigot, S., Delaunay, J., Armari-Alla, C., et al. (2012). Human RhAG ammonia channel is impaired by the Phe65Ser mutation in overhydrated stomatocytic red cells. *Am. J. Physiol. Cell Physiol.* 302, C419–C428. doi: 10.1152/ajpcell.00092.2011

Gibson, J. S. (2003). "Comparative physiology of red cell membrane transport," in *Red Cell Membrane Transport*, eds I. Bernhardt and J. C. Ellory (Berlin; Heidelberg: Springer-Verlag), 721–734.

Glader, B. E., Fortier, N., Albala, M. M., and Nathan, D. G. (1974). Congenital hemolytic anemia associated with dehydrated erythrocytes and increased potassium loss. *N. Engl. J. Med.* 291, 491–496. doi: 10.1056/NEJM197409052911003

Glogowska, E., Lezon-Geyda, K., Maksimova, Y., Schulz, V. P., and Gallagher, P. G. (2015). Mutations in the Gardos channel (KCNN4) are associated with hereditary xerocytosis. *Blood* 126, 1281–1284. doi: 10.1182/blood-2015-07-657957

Glogowska, E., Schneider, E. R., Maksimova, Y., Schulz, V. P., Lezon-Geyda, K., Wu, J., et al. (2017). Novel mechanisms of PIEZO1 dysfunction in hereditary xerocytosis. *Blood* 130, 1845–1856. doi: 10.1182/blood-2017-05-786004

Gore, D. M., Chetty, M. C., Coles, S. C., Gover, P. M., and Stewart, G. W. (2002a). Hereditary spherocytosis with a low temperature Na/K leak and thrombosis. *Br. J. Haematol.* 117(Suppl. 1), 9–10.

Gore, D. M., Chetty, M. C., Fisher, J., Nicolaou, A., and Stewart, G. W. (2002b). Familial pseudohyperkalaemia Cardiff: a mild version of cryohydrocytosis. *Br. J. Haematol.* 117, 212–214.

Gore, D. M., Layton, M., Sinha, A. K., Williamson, P. J., Vaidya, B., Connolly, V., et al. (2004). Four pedigrees of the cation-leaky hereditary stomatocytosis class presenting with pseudohyperkalaemia. *Novel profile of temperature dependence of* Na^+*-*K^+ *leak in a xerocytic form. Br. J. Haematol.* 125, 521–527. doi: 10.1111/j.1365-2141.2004.04944.x

Grootenboer, S., Schischmanoff, P. O., Laurendeau, I., Cynober, T., Tchernia, G., Dommergues, J. P., et al. (2000). Pleiotropic syndrome of dehydrated hereditary stomatocytosis, pseudohyperkalemia, and perinatal edema maps to 16q23-q24. *Blood* 96, 2599–2605.

Guizouarn, H., Borgese, F., Gabillat, N., Harrison, P., Goede, J. S., McMahon, C., et al. (2011). South-east Asian ovalocytosis and the cryohydrocytosis form of hereditary stomatocytosis show virtually indistinguishable cation permeability defects. *Br. J. Haematol.* 152, 655–664. doi: 10.1111/j.1365-2141.2010.08454.x

Guizouarn, H., Martial, S., Gabillat, N., and Borgese, F. (2007). Point mutations involved in red cell stomatocytosis convert the electroneutral anion exchanger 1 to a nonselective cation conductance. *Blood* 110, 2158–2165. doi: 10.1182/blood-2006-12-063420

Hadley, T., Saul, A., Lamont, G., Hudson, D. E., Miller, L. H., and Kidson, C. (1983). Resistance of Melanesian elliptocytes (ovalocytes) to invasion by Plasmodium knowlesi and *Plasmodium falciparum* malaria parasites *in vitro*. *J. Clin. Invest.* 71, 780–782. doi: 10.1172/JCI110827

Haines, P. G., Crawley, C., Chetty, M. C., Jarvis, H., Coles, S. E., Fisher, J., et al. (2001b). Familial pseudohyperkalaemia Chiswick: a novel congenital thermotropic variant of K and Na transport across the human red cell membrane. *Br. J. Haematol.* 112, 469–474.

Haines, P. G., Jarvis, H. G., King, S., Noormohamed, F. H., Chetty, M. C., Fisher, J., et al. (2001a). Two further British families with the "cryohydrocytosis" form of hereditary stomatocytosis. *Br. J. Haematol.* 113, 932–937.

Hall, A. C., and Willis, J. S. (1986). The temperature dependence of passive potassium permeability in mammalian erythrocytes. *Cryobiology* 23, 395–405. doi: 10.1016/0011-2240(86)90024-6

Harm, W., Fortier, N. L., Lutz, H. U., Fairbanks, G., and Snyder, L. M. (1979). Increased erythrocyte lipid peroxidation in hereditary xerocytosis. *Clin. Chim. Acta* 99, 121–128. doi: 10.1016/0009-8981(79)90034-2

Helias, V., Saison, C., Ballif, B. A., Peyrard, T., Takahashi, J., Takahashi, H., et al. (2012). ABCB6 is dispensable for erythropoiesis and specifies the new blood group system Langereis. *Nat. Genet.* 44, 170–173. doi: 10.1038/ng.1069

Hoffman, J. F., Joiner, W., Nehrke, K., Potapova, O., Foye, K., and Wickrema, A. (2003). The hSK4 (KCNN4) isoform is the Ca2+-activated K+ channel (Gardos channel) in human red blood cells. *Proc. Natl. Acad. Sci. U.S.A.* 100, 7366–7371. doi: 10.1073/pnas.1232342100

Houston, B. L., Zelinski, T., Israels, S. J., Coghlan, G., Chodirker, B. N., Gallagher, P. G., et al. (2011). Refinement of the hereditary xerocytosis locus on chromosome 16q in a large Canadian kindred. *Blood Cells Mol. Dis.* 47, 226–231. doi: 10.1016/j.bcmd.2011.08.001

Imashuku, S., Muramatsu, H., Sugihara, T., Okuno, Y., Wang, X., Yoshida, K., et al. (2016). PIEZO1 gene mutation in a Japanese family with hereditary high phosphatidylcholine hemolytic anemia and hemochromatosis-induced diabetes mellitus. *Int. J. Hematol.* 104, 125–129. doi: 10.1007/s12185-016-1970-x

Iolascon, A., De Falco, L., Borgese, F., Esposito, M. R., Avvisati, R. A., Izzo, P., et al. (2009). A novel erythroid anion exchange variant (Gly796Arg) of hereditary stomatocytosis associated with dyserythropoiesis. *Haematologica* 94, 1049–1059. doi: 10.3324/haematol.2008.002873

Iolascon, A., Stewart, G. W., Ajetunmobi, J. F., Perrotta, S., Delaunay, J., Carella, M., et al. (1999). Familial pseudohyperkalemia maps to the same locus as dehydrated hereditary stomatocytosis (hereditary xerocytosis). *Blood* 93, 3120–3123.

Jarvis, H. G., Chetty, M. C., Nicolaou, A., Fisher, J., Miller, A., and Stewart, G. W. (2001). A novel stomatocytosis variant showing marked abnormalities in intracellular [Na] and [K] with minimal haemolysis. *Eur. J. Haematol.* 66, 412–414. doi: 10.1034/j.1600-0609.2001.066006412.x

Khan, A. A., Hanada, T., Mohseni, M., Jeong, J. J., Zeng, L., Gaetani, M., et al. (2008). Dematin and adducin provide a novel link between the spectrin cytoskeleton and human erythrocyte membrane by directly interacting with glucose transporter-1. *J. Biol. Chem.* 283, 14600–14609. doi: 10.1074/jbc.M707818200

Kiss, K., Brozik, A., Kucsma, N., Toth, A., Gera, M., Berry, L., et al. (2012). Shifting the paradigm: the putative mitochondrial protein ABCB6 resides in the lysosomes of cells and in the plasma membrane of erythrocytes. *PLoS ONE* 7:e37378. doi: 10.1371/journal.pone.0037378

Komatsu, T., Sato, K., Otsuka, Y., Arashiki, N., Tanaka, K., Tamahara, S., et al. (2010). Parallel reductions in stomatin and Na,K-ATPase through the exosomal pathway during reticulocyte maturation in dogs: stomatin as a genotypic and phenotypic marker of high K^+ and low K^+ red cells. *J. Vet. Med. Sci.* 72, 893–901. doi: 10.1292/jvms.10-0030

Kucherenko, Y. V., Huber, S. M., Nielsen, S., and Lang, F. (2012). Decreased redox-sensitive erythrocyte cation channel activity in aquaporin 9-deficient mice. *J. Membr. Biol.* 245, 797–805. doi: 10.1007/s00232-012-9482-y

Kuma, H., Abe, Y., Askin, D., Bruce, L. J., Hamasaki, T., Tanner, M. J., et al. (2002). Molecular basis and functional consequences of the dominant effects of the mutant band 3 on the structure of normal band 3 in Southeast Asian ovalocytosis. *Biochemistry* 41, 3311–3320. doi: 10.1021/bi011678

Lande, W. M., Thiemann, P. V., and Mentzer, W. C. Jr. (1982). Missing band 7 membrane protein in two patients with high Na, low K erythrocytes. *J. Clin. Invest.* 70, 1273–1280. doi: 10.1172/JCI110726

Lauf, P. K., and Adragna, N. C. (2000). K-Cl cotransport: properties and molecular mechanism. *Cell. Physiol. Biochem.* 10, 341–354. doi: 10.1159/000016357

Lauf, P. K., and Joiner, C. H. (1976). Increased potassium transport and ouabain binding in human Rhnull red blood cells. *Blood* 48, 457–468.

Lim, J., Gasson, C., and Kaji, D. M. (1995). Urea inhibits NaK2Cl cotransport in human erythrocytes. *J. Clin. Invest.* 96, 2126–2132. doi: 10.1172/JCI118266

Lock, S. P., Smith, R. S., and Hardisty, R. M. (1961). Stomatocytosis: a hereditary red cell anomally associated with haemolytic anaemia. *Br. J. Haematol.* 7, 303–314. doi: 10.1111/j.1365-2141.1961.tb00341.x

Lytle, C., and McManus, T. (2002). Coordinate modulation of Na-K-2Cl cotransport and K-Cl cotransport by cell volume and chloride. *Am. J. Physiol. Cell Physiol.* 283, C1422–C1431. doi: 10.1152/ajpcell.00130.2002

Marini, A. M., Urrestarazu, A., Beauwens, R., and André, B. (1997). The Rh (rhesus) blood group polypeptides are related to $NH4^+$ transporters. *Trends Biochem. Sci.* 22, 460–461. doi: 10.1016/S0968-0004(97)01132-8

Meadow, S. R. (1967). Stomatocytosis. *Proc. R. Soc. Med.* 60, 13–15.

Meenaghan, M., Follett, G. F., and Brophy, P. J. (1985). Temperature sensitivity of potassium flux into red blood cells in the familial pseudohyperkalaemia syndrome. *Biochim. Biophys. Acta* 821, 72–78. doi: 10.1016/0005-2736(85)90155-5

Miller, D. R., Rickles, F. R., Lichtman, M. A., La Celle, P. L., Bates, J., and Weed, R. I. (1971). A new variant of hereditary hemolytic anemia with stomatocytosis and erythrocyte cation abnormality. *Blood* 38, 184–204.

Montel-Hagen, A., Kinet, S., Manel, N., Mongellaz, C., Prohaska, R., Battini, J. L., et al. (2008). Erythrocyte Glut1 triggers dehydroascorbic acid uptake in mammals unable to synthesize vitamin C. *Cell* 132, 1039–1048. doi: 10.1016/j.cell.2008.01.042

Morlé, L., Pothier, B., Alloisio, N., Féo, C., Garay, R., Bost, M., et al. (1989). Reduction of membrane band 7 and activation of volume stimulated (K+, Cl-)-cotransport in a case of congenital stomatocytosis. *Br. J. Haematol.* 71, 141–146. doi: 10.1111/j.1365-2141.1989.tb06288.x

Nunomura, W., Denker, S. P., Barber, D. L., Takakuwa, Y., and Gascard, P. (2012). Characterization of cytoskeletal protein 4.1R interaction with NHE1 (Na(+)/H(+) exchanger isoform 1). *Biochem. J.* 446, 427–435. doi: 10.1042/BJ20120535

Paessler, M., and Hartung, H. (2015). Dehydrated hereditary stomatocytosis masquerading as MDS. *Blood* 125:1841.

Palsdottir, H., and Hunte, C. (2004). Lipids in membrane protein structures. *Biochim. Biophys. Acta* 1666, 2–18. doi: 10.1016/j.bbamem.2004.06.012

Parker, J. C., McManus, T. J., Starke, L. C., and Gitelman, H. J. (1990). Coordinated regulation of Na/H exchange and [K-Cl] cotransport in dog red cells. *J. Gen. Physiol.* 96, 1141–1152. doi: 10.1085/jgp.96.6.1141

Platt, O. S., Lux, S. E., and Nathan, D. G. (1981). Exercise-induced hemolysis in xerocytosis. Erythrocyte dehydration and shear sensitivity. *J. Clin. Invest.* 68, 631–638. doi: 10.1172/JCI110297

Ranade, S. S., Qiu, Z., Woo, S. H., Hur, S. S., Murthy, S. E., Cahalan, S. M., et al. (2014). Piezo1, a mechanically activated ion channel, is required for vascular development in mice. *Proc. Natl. Acad. Sci. U.S.A.* 111, 10347–10352. doi: 10.1073/pnas.1409233111

Rapetti-Mauss, R., Lacoste, C., Picard, V., Guitton, C., Pontou-Lombard, E., Loosveld, M., et al. (2015). A mutation in the Gardos channel is associated with hereditary xerocytosis. *Blood* 126, 1273–1280. doi: 10.1182/blood-2015-04-642496

Rapetti-Mauss, R., Picard, V., Guitton, C., Ghazal, K., Proulle, V., Badens, C., et al. (2017). Red blood cell Gardos channel (KCNN4): the essential determinant of erythrocyte dehydration in hereditary xerocytosis. *Haematologica* 102, e415–e418. doi: 10.3324/haematol.2017.171389

Rees, D. C., Iolascon, A., Carella, M., O'marcaigh, A. S., Kendra, J. R., Jowitt, S. N., et al. (2005). Stomatocytic haemolysis and macrothrombocytopenia (Mediterranean stomatocytosis/macrothrombocytopenia) is the haematological presentation of phytosterolaemia. *Br. J. Haematol.* 130, 297–309. doi: 10.1111/j.1365-2141.2005.05599.x

Reithmeier, R. A., Casey, J. R., Kalli, A. C., Sansom, M. S., Alguel, Y., and Iwata, S. (2016). Band 3, the human red cell chloride/bicarbonate anion exchanger (AE1, SLC4A1), in a structural context. *Biochim. Biophys. Acta* 1858(7 Pt A):1507–1532. doi: 10.1016/j.bbamem.2016.03.030

Rigor, R. R., Damoc, C., Phinney, B. S., and Cala, P. M. (2011). Phosphorylation and activation of the plasma membrane Na+/H+ exchanger (NHE1) during osmotic cell shrinkage. *PLoS ONE* 6:e29210. doi: 10.1371/journal.pone.0029210

Rivera, A., Kam, S. Y., Ho, M., Romero, J. R., and Lee, S. (2013a). Ablation of the Kell/Xk complex alters erythrocyte divalent cation homeostasis. *Blood Cells Mol. Dis.* 50, 80–85. doi: 10.1016/j.bcmd.2012.10.002

Rivera, A., Zee, R. Y., Alper, S. L., Peters, L. L., and Brugnara, C. (2013b). Strain-specific variations in cation content and transport in mouse erythrocytes. *Physiol. Genomics* 45, 343–350. doi: 10.1152/physiolgenomics.00143.2012

Rotstein, M., Engelstad, K., Yang, H., Wang, D., Levy, B., Chung, W. K., et al. (2010). Glut1 deficiency: inheritance pattern determined by haploinsufficiency. *Ann. Neurol.* 68, 955–958. doi: 10.1002/ana.22088

Rungaldier, S., Oberwagner, W., Salzer, U., Csaszar, E., and Prohaska, R. (2013). Stomatin interacts with GLUT1/SLC2A1, band 3/SLC4A1, and aquaporin-1 in human erythrocyte membrane domains. *Biochim. Biophys. Acta* 1828, 956–966. doi: 10.1016/j.bbamem.2012.11.030

Salzer, U., and Prohaska, R. (2001). Stomatin, flotillin-1, and flotillin-2 are major integral proteins of erythrocyte lipid rafts. *Blood* 97, 1141–1143. doi: 10.1182/blood.V97.4.1141

Sandberg, M. B., Nybo, M., Birgens, H., and Frederiksen, H. (2014). Hereditary xerocytosis and familial haemolysis due to mutation in the PIEZO1 gene: a simple diagnostic approach. *Int. J. Lab. Hematol.* 36, e62–e65. doi: 10.1111/ijlh.12172

Shmukler, B. E., Vandorpe, D. H., Rivera, A., Auerbach, M., Brugnara, C., and Alper, S. L. (2014). Dehydrated stomatocytic anemia due to the heterozygous mutation R2456H in the mechanosensitive cation channel PIEZO1: a case report. *Blood Cells Mol. Dis.* 52, 53–54. doi: 10.1016/j.bcmd.2013.07.015

Stewart, A. K., Kedar, P. S., Shmukler, B. E., Vandorpe, D. H., Hsu, A., Glader, B., et al. (2011). Functional characterization and modified rescue of novel AE1 mutation R730C associated with overhydrated cation leak stomatocytosis. *Am. J. Physiol. Cell Physiol.* 300, C1034–C1046. doi: 10.1152/ajpcell.00447.2010

Stewart, A. K., Vandorpe, D. H., Heneghan, J. F., Chebib, F., Stolpe, K., Akhavein, A., et al. (2010). The GPA-dependent, spherostomatocytosis mutant AE1 E758K induces GPA-independent, endogenous cation transport in amphibian oocytes. *Am. J. Physiol. Cell Physiol.* 298, C283–C297. doi: 10.1152/ajpcell.00444.2009

Stewart, G. W. (2004). Hemolytic disease due to membrane ion channel disorders. *Curr. Opin. Hematol.* 11, 244–250. doi: 10.1097/01.moh.0000132240.20671.33

Stewart, G. W., Amess, J. A., Eber, S. W., Kingswood, C., Lane, P. A., Smith, B. D., et al. (1996). Thrombo-embolic disease after splenectomy for hereditary stomatocytosis. *Br. J. Haematol.* 93, 303–310. doi: 10.1046/j.1365-2141.1996.4881033.x

Stewart, G. W., Corrall, R. J., Fyffe, J. A., Stockdill, G., and Strong, J. A. (1979). Familial pseudohyperkalaemia. A new syndrome. *Lancet* 2, 175–177.

Stewart, G. W., and Ellory, J. C. (1985). A family with mild hereditary xerocytosis showing high membrane cation permeability at low temperatures. *Clin. Sci.* 69, 309–319. doi: 10.1042/cs0690309

Stewart, G. W., Ellory, J. C., and Klein, R. A. (1980). Increased human red cell cation passive permeability below 12 degrees C. *Nature* 286, 403–404. doi: 10.1038/286403a0

Stewart, G. W., Hepworth-Jones, B. E., Keen, J. N., Dash, B. C., Argent, A. C., and Casimir, C. M. (1992). Isolation of cDNA coding for an ubiquitous membrane protein deficient in high Na+, low K+ stomatocytic erythrocytes. *Blood* 79, 1593–1601.

Syeda, R., Xu, J., Dubin, A. E., Coste, B., Mathur, J., Huynh, T., et al. (2015). Chemical activation of the mechanotransduction channel Piezo1. *Elife* 4. doi: 10.7554/eLife.07369

Syfuss, P. Y., Ciupea, A., Brahimi, S., Cynober, T., Stewart, G. W., Grandchamp, B., et al. (2006). Mild dehydrated hereditary stomatocytosis revealed by marked hepatosiderosis. *Clin. Lab. Haematol.* 28, 270–274. doi: 10.1111/j.1365-2257.2006.00774.x

Tanner, M. J., Bruce, L., Martin, P. G., Rearden, D. M., and Jones, G. L. (1991). Melanesian hereditary ovalocytes have a deletion in red cell band 3. *Blood* 78, 2785–2786.

Weber, Y. G., Storch, A., Wuttke, T. V., Brockmann, K., Kempfle, J., Maljevic, S., et al. (2008). GLUT1 mutations are a cause of paroxysmal exertion-induced dyskinesias and induce hemolytic anemia by a cation leak. *J. Clin. Invest.* 118, 2157–2168. doi: 10.1172/JCI34438

Wiley, J. S. (1981). Increased erythrocyte cation permeability in thalassemia and conditions of marrow stress. *J. Clin. Invest.* 67, 917–922. doi: 10.1172/JCI110140

Zarychanski, R., Schulz, V. P., Houston, B. L., Maksimova, Y., Houston, D. S., Smith, B., et al. (2012). Mutations in the mechanotransduction protein PIEZO1 are associated with hereditary xerocytosis. *Blood* 120, 1908–1915. doi: 10.1182/blood-2012-04-422253

5

Influence of Standard Laboratory Procedures on Measures of Erythrocyte Damage

*Lena Wiegmann[1], Diane A. de Zélicourt[1,2], Oliver Speer[3], Alissa Muller[4], Jeroen S. Goede[5,6], Burkhardt Seifert[7] and Vartan Kurtcuoglu[1,2,6,8]**

[1] *The Interface Group, Institute of Physiology, University of Zurich, Zurich, Switzerland,* [2] *National Center of Competence in Research, Kidney.CH, Zurich, Switzerland,* [3] *Division of Haematology, University Children's Hospital Zurich, Zurich, Switzerland,* [4] *Department of Health Sciences and Technology, ETH Zurich, Zurich, Switzerland,* [5] *Department of Haematology, Kantonsspital Winterthur, Winterthur, Switzerland,* [6] *Zurich Center for Integrative Human Physiology, University of Zurich, Zurich, Switzerland,* [7] *Department of Biostatistics, Epidemiology, Biostatistics and Prevention Institute, University of Zurich, Zurich, Switzerland,* [8] *Neuroscience Center Zurich, University of Zurich, Zurich, Switzerland*

***Correspondence:**
Vartan Kurtcuoglu
vartan.kurtcuoglu@uzh.ch

The ability to characterize the mechanical properties of erythrocytes is important in clinical and research contexts: to diagnose and monitor hematologic disorders, as well as to optimize the design of cardiovascular implants and blood circulating devices with respect to blood damage. However, investigation of red blood cell (RBC) properties generally involves preparatory and processing steps. Even though these impose mechanical stresses on cells, little is known about their impact on the final measurement results. In this study, we investigated the effect of centrifuging, vortexing, pipetting, and high pressures on several markers of mechanical blood damage and RBC membrane properties. Using human venous blood, we analyzed erythrocyte damage by measuring free hemoglobin, phosphatidylserine exposure by flow cytometry, RBC deformability by ektacytometry and the parameters of a complete blood count. We observed increased levels of free hemoglobin for all tested procedures. The release of hemoglobin into plasma depended significantly on the level of stress. Elevated pressures and centrifuging also altered mean cell volume (MCV) and mean corpuscular hemoglobin (MCH), suggesting changes in erythrocyte population, and membrane properties. Our results show that the effects of blood handling can significantly influence erythrocyte damage metrics. Careful quantification of this influence as well as other unwanted secondary effects should thus be included in experimental protocols and accounted for in clinical laboratories.

Keywords: red blood cells, erythrocytes, centrifugation, vortexing, pipetting, free hemoglobin, ektacytometry

INTRODUCTION

Erythrocytes, or red blood cells (RBCs), constitute the majority of blood cellular components and are responsible for the vital transport of oxygen and carbon dioxide throughout the body. The mechanical properties and physical integrity of the erythrocyte plasma membrane are central to this function, allowing RBCs to undergo considerable deformations and travel through the smallest capillaries. In converse, impaired RBC membrane properties and deformability yield severe pathological phenotypes, including sickle cell anemia, spherocytosis, stomatocytosis, and elliptocytosis. Beyond hereditary diseases, blood damage is also often an acquired condition due to cardiovascular implants such as artificial heart valves or ventricular assist devices

(Shapira et al., 2009; Kirklin et al., 2015). The ability to characterize RBC mechanical properties is therefore important in both clinical and research contexts: firstly, to diagnose and monitor hematological disorders and, secondly, to understand hemolysis pathways and optimize the design of implantable or extracorporeal devices in order to minimize the induced blood damage.

Mechanical forces acting on RBCs range from those found physiologically in the cardiovascular system to pathophysiological stresses present in implants or during (inappropriate) handling. The range of the cells' reaction naturally also varies from deformation to changes in volume to cell rupture. The essential role in volume homeostasis of Piezo1, a mechanically activated cation channel in the RBC membrane, was recently shown (Cahalan et al., 2015). Activation of Piezo1 due to mechanical loading leads to Ca^{2+} influx, which in turn triggers the dehydration of the cells. This mechanism of volume reduction in response to stress could improve the RBCs' ability to travel through the smallest capillaries (Cahalan et al., 2015) and was also hypothesized to promote oxygen/CO_2 exchange in the periphery, which was observed following mechanical stimulation of RBCs (Rao et al., 2009). If the stresses acting on the cell exceed its loading capacity, pore formation (Zhao et al., 2006) or complete membrane rupture (Rand, 1964) occurs, and all cytosolic content including hemoglobin is released into the plasma.

In clinical laboratories, several parameters are carefully and specifically analyzed to judge a patient's hematological status. Standardized operating procedures, careful selection of controls and participation in round robin tests ensure a high quality and reproducibility of the results (Gunter et al., 1996; Lippi et al., 2006; Plebani, 2007). At the same time, protocols involve several preparation and intermediate steps, such as pipetting, mixing, and centrifuging, which impose mechanical stresses on the cells. Little is known about their influence on the final laboratory results.

This similarly holds true for *in vitro* experiments for research purposes and the systematic investigation of shear stress effects on cell integrity (Zhao et al., 2006; Quinn et al., 2011). To reproduce mechanical stresses in artificial organs such as ventricular assist devices or across artificial heart valves, researchers often rely on *in vitro* systems such as viscometers or microchannels (Leverett et al., 1972; Sutton et al., 1997; Paul et al., 2003; Korin et al., 2007). Yet, irrespective of proper control of the shear stress levels within the actual experimental apparatus, these experiments again include handling steps for the preparation of cells, for their placement in the apparatus and for preparation of samples for subsequent analysis. Secondary experimental effects, inherent to the geometric configuration and setup of the apparatus, may also influence the measurement end-points. One such example is the occurrence of high pressures required to drive blood through microchannels. A thorough understanding of the contribution of these different forces to the measurement endpoints is therefore of critical importance for the interpretation of the results and optimization of the laboratory procedures. Still, to date, little literature is available addressing this.

Damage due to centrifugal forces has been demonstrated on different cell lines, but not on erythrocytes (Katkov and Mazur, 1998; Ferraro et al., 2011). Similarly, the effect of pipetting and elevated pressures was studied on other cell types (Kay et al., 2004; Heng et al., 2007). Various mixing methods were compared (Bai et al., 2012), identifying vortexing as the most stress intensive method. However, the induced cell damage was not quantified. For RBCs, the influence of standard laboratory procedures on hemolysis has mostly been studied in the context of transfusion medicine. Delay between collection and separation, large variation in centrifuging speeds, rapid anticoagulation, as well as shaking and mixing were found to yield increased levels of hemolysis in blood bags (Sowemimo-Coker, 2002). Along the lines of testing handling artifacts on RBCs, the effect of different modes of transportation, reflected in variations in anticoagulation and temperature in simulated shipment conditions, was investigated in Makhro et al. (2016).

While these studies clearly indicate that potentially any handling associated with large forces may be detrimental to cells, it remains unclear to what extent and in what fashion RBCs will incur damage. Next to hemolysis, mechanical stress-induced changes to the plasma membrane deserve attention. Here we address this knowledge gap by investigating the effect of centrifuging, vortexing, pipetting, and high pressures on several markers of mechanical blood damage and erythrocyte membrane properties.

MATERIALS AND METHODS

Subjects

We used venous whole blood of 22 healthy volunteers. Blood was collected with a syringe from a venous catheter (20G) in an antecubital vein. It was anticoagulated either with lithium heparin or ethylenediaminetetraacetic acid (EDTA) depending on the subsequent analysis. The study was approved by the Ethics Commission of the Canton of Zurich, and conformed to the Declaration of Helsinki. Subjects gave written informed consent to participation. The collected samples were randomly assigned to experimental setups and analyses and each donor's blood was used for multiple experiments. Experiments were started immediately after drawing blood and performed at room temperature. The experimental order was randomized and the last experiment was always completed within a maximum of 2 h of blood draw. Blood awaiting experimental testing was kept at 4°C to minimize changes in hemorheological properties (Baskurt et al., 2009). The analysis procedures as described in section Analyses were initiated right after the end of the experiments and completed within a maximum of 6 h. The experimental and analysis workflows are explained in the next sections.

Experimental Setups

Figure 1 provides an overview of the experimental setups presented in this study. We investigated the effect of pressure, centrifuging, vortexing, and pipetting, and for each one of these four methods tested a range of setup parameters such as stressor magnitude or exposure time. Centrifuging

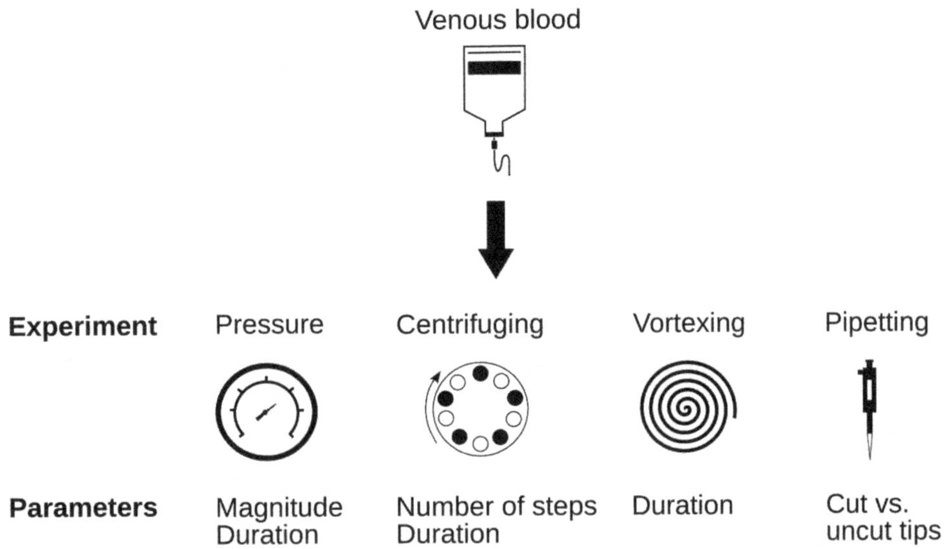

FIGURE 1 | Overview over the experimental setups presented in this study.

and pipetting are routinely used both in hematology and research laboratories. Although, vortexing is usually avoided in RBC handling, it was nevertheless included here to explore the upper bound of applied stresses in a laboratory context. Finally, repeated exposure to pressure plateaus was motivated by the conditions typically experienced by RBCs in experimental microchannel setups. Detailed descriptions of the different experimental conditions are provided in the following subsections.

High Pressure

In-vitro microchannel setups typically involve repeated cell exposure to high pressures, required to drive the cell suspension through channels and constrictions. To assess the effect of these repeated pressure exposures independently of other forces, notably independently of shear stresses, the samples were exposed to pressure sequences in custom-built pressure chambers driven by compressed nitrogen. A pressure sequence consisted of square pressure waveforms including 10 repeated cycles of high and low pressures. High pressure plateaus (P_{high}) were maintained for a duration T_{high}, where P_{high} was set to either 3, 5, or 7 bars and T_{high} to 1 or 30 s for short or long exposures, respectively. T_{high} and P_{high} remained constant within a given experimental sequence. In all sequences, samples were allowed to recover for 30 s at low (ambient) pressure between two consecutive high pressure plateaus. Pressure relative to the atmosphere was monitored with a pressure sensor (PBT-RB010SG1SSNAMA0Z, Sick AG, Waldkirch, Germany). The number of tested samples is indicated in the respective figure caption in the Results section. Controls for this experiment were kept at room temperature in petri dishes (Fisher Scientific, Waltham MA, USA) as used in the pressure chambers for 5 min (short exposure experiment) respectively 10 min (long exposure experiment).

Centrifugation

All centrifugation experiments were performed in the same benchtop centrifuge (Eppendorf Centrifuge 5415D, Eppendorf AG, Hamburg, Germany) at 900 g, a centrifuging speed that was chosen according to a diagnostic standard operation procedure at the erythrocyte laboratory, University Children's Hospital, Zurich. Samples were centrifuged for 5 or 10 consecutive minutes; 1, 2, or 4 times in a row. Energic mixing is required to resuspend the pellet before analysis or the next centrifugation cycle. In these experiments, the samples were vortexed for 2 s after each centrifugation. Controls were kept at room temperature in Eppendorf tubes as used in the experiments and vortexed for 2 s before analysis. The number of tested samples is indicated in the figure caption in the Results section. Per design, comparison of the controls vs. single centrifugation elucidates damage induced by centrifugation only, while comparison against samples centrifuged two to four times, demonstrates the damage induced by repeated centrifuging and mixing/vortexing cycles (see also section Discussion for in depth discussion).

Vortexing

Vortexing was included as representative of extreme stressors on RBCs. Samples were placed into 1.5 ml Eppendorf tubes and vortexed once for 20 or 40 s in a standard laboratory vortexer (Genie, VWR International, Rednor, USA). The number of tested samples is indicated in the figure caption in the Results section. Controls were kept at room temperature in the same Eppendorf tubes without vortexing.

Pipetting

To test whether cutting the front end of pipet tips makes pipetting less harmful for RBCs, we compared samples that were pipetted in and out 10 times in a row with and without cut tip to controls.

The repeated exposure was carried out to amplify possible effects on the cells. Pipet tips used were standard 1,000 μl tips (Tip One, Starlab, Milton Keynes, United Kingdom). Cut tips were cut 7 mm above the tip end. The number of tested samples is indicated in the figure caption in the Results section. Controls were kept at room temperature in the same Eppendorf tubes as used in the experiments.

Naturally, all experiments involved one pipetting step before and after the experiment. It was pursued as gently as possible to keep forces on the cells as low as possible. As a reference, the pipetting rate used in the pipetting experiments was 639 μl/s (51.1 ± 1.1 s for 10 consecutive cycles of pipetting 1,000 μl), compared to a rate of 392 μl/s for the gentle pipetting. Since these gentle pipetting steps are also applied on every control sample, the measured differences are not affected.

Analyses

Figure 2 provides an overview of the analyses conducted in this study. We analyzed multiple parameters indicative for mechanical blood damage and RBC membrane properties.

Free Hemoglobin

The samples were anticoagulated using lithium heparin. To avoid additional mechanical stresses, plasma separation was not achieved via centrifuging but via sedimentation for 180 min. The sedimentation period was started immediately after finishing the experiments. After separation, the plasma was pipetted gently and frozen at −20°C for later analysis.

Free hemoglobin (Hb) in plasma was measured using photospectrometry at 415, 450, and 700 nm and the final Hb concentration was calculated according to (Fairbanks et al., 1992):

$$C_{Hb}[\text{mg/ml}] = 1.55 \cdot A_{415} - 1.3 \cdot A_{450} - 1.24 \cdot A_{700}$$

The first term represents the known absorption coefficient of hemoglobin, while the second and third term correct for absorption by bilirubin and turbidity. Note that this formulation can yield negative values, which clinically are cut-off and represented by a concentration of 0 mg/ml free hemoglobin. In this study, we kept the original values (whether positive or negative) in order to maintain a valid distribution for subsequent statistical analysis. Triplets of each sample were measured. The reported value corresponds to the arithmetic mean of the three measurements.

Ektacytometry

Ektacytometry is currently the most widely used technique for the measurement of RBC deformability (Baskurt et al., 2009). Clinically, it is applied for the diagnosis of several erythrocyte membranopathies, such as hereditary spherocytosis, stomatocytosis, and ellipsocytosis. Here, we used this method to detect changes in the general deformation behavior of the cells. In an ektacytometry measurement, EDTA anticoagulated whole blood is mixed with viscous solutions of different osmolalities, and the elongation index (EI) of the RBCs under constant shear is measured using laser diffraction. The minimal osmolality with measurable EI (Omin) corresponds to the osmotic fragility measured in other applications. All measurements were performed in a Lorrca Maxsis Osmoscan (RR Mechatronics, Hoorn, The Netherlands). Blood samples were analyzed according to the standard protocol for this machine, which involves mixing of the sample in iso-osmolar polyvinylpyrrolidone solution (RR mechatronics) before analysis.

Phosphatidylserine Expression

Phosphatidylserine is a membrane phospholipid and its externalization a marker for macrophage clearance (Boas et al., 1998). Therefore, it is also interpreted as a marker of RBC damage (Lutz and Bogdanova, 2013). We measured its expression levels using flow cytometry using a protocol similar to the one described in Kuypers et al. (1996).

Normal sample preparation

Blood was anticoagulated using lithium heparin. Erythrocytes were labeled using allophycocyanin (APC) anti-human CD235ab antibody staining and PS expression was measured using fluorescein isothiocyanate (FITC) labeled annexin V. All reagents were ordered from BioLegend Europe (London, United Kingdom). Cells were incubated for 20 min in complete darkness after mixing 5 μl of APC-CD235ab and FITC-annexin V with 95 μl of annexin binding buffer and 5 μl of whole blood. Four hundred microliters of buffer where then added and everything was mixed using the vortex before the solution was transferred to Falcon polystyrene tubes (Fisher Scientific, Waltham MA, USA), which were prefilled with 500 μl of the same buffer.

Controls

We used the following controls: an unstained tube, an APC negative control, a FITC negative control, the two Fluorescence Minus One (FMO) controls and a fully stained control with a 50/50 mixture of normal and PS-positive blood. For the APC negative control, we used a peripheral blood mononuclear cell (PBMC) solution. The unstained control was intended to detect the level of background fluorescence of the system. The FITC negative control contained phosphate buffered saline (PBS) buffer instead of annexin V binding buffer. In the FMOs and the all-in control, we used blood that was prepared to contain an increased amount of PS-positive cells. Details of these protocols are described hereafter.

Preparation of PS-positive blood

Blood was treated with *N*-Ethylmaleimide (NEM; Sigma-Aldrich, St. Louis, Missouri, USA), which inhibits the aminophospholipid translocase, and afterwards mixed with calcium ionophore A23817 (Sigma-Aldrich), to induce membrane lipid scrambling (Kuypers et al., 1996). After washing the cells once with PBS, 10 mM NEM buffer solution was added to resuspend the cell pellet. The solution was then incubated for 30 min, and afterwards centrifuged for 5 min at 835 g to remove the supernatant. After another washing step, the cell pellet was resuspended in 2 mM calcium buffer solution and incubated during 3 min at 37°C. Six microliters of 1 mM calcium ionophore solution (in DMSO) were then added and incubated during 1 h at room temperature. Thereafter, the solution was centrifuged for 5 min at 835 g to remove the supernatant. The cells were washed once with 2.5 mM EDTA buffer solution and three times with

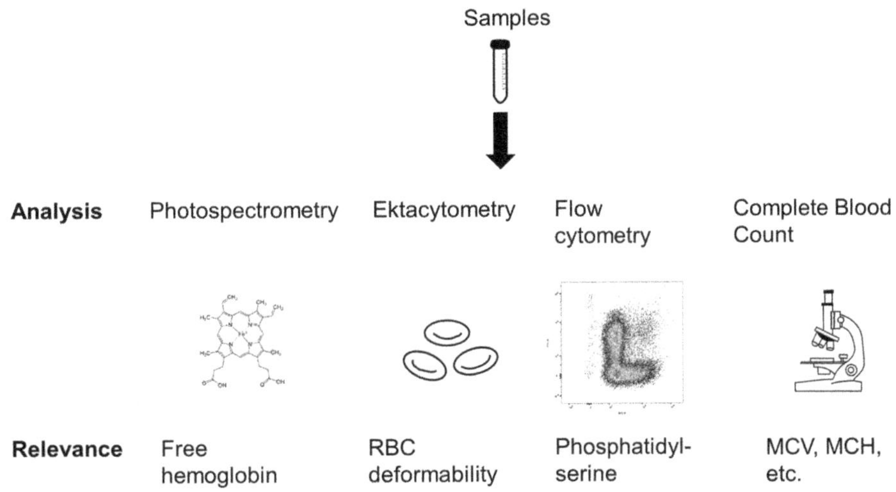

FIGURE 2 | Overview of the analyses performed in this study. MCV, Mean cell volume; MCH, Mean corpuscular hemoglobin. Sources: Tube: https://pixabay.com/en/tube-conical-test-measured-305147/; Heme: https://commons.wikimedia.org/wiki/File:Heme_b.svg; Microscope: https://pixabay.com/en/microscope-lab-chemistry-science-2223268/.

cell staining buffer (BioLegend Europe). The cell pellet was then resuspended in 0.3 ml PBS and used as what is described here as "PS-positive blood."

Preparation of PBMCs

A solution of PBMCs was produced using Ficoll-Paque separation. Whole blood was diluted in 2–4x 2 mM EDTA buffer (pH 7.2). For the density gradient centrifugation, 5 ml of Ficoll (GE Healthcare, Little Chalfont, United Kingdom) were filled into a 15 ml tube, afterwards 7 ml of the diluted blood was added. After centrifugation at 800 g for 20 min, PBMCs were gently pipetted off, washed with PBS and the cell pellet resuspended in PBS.

Flow cytometry

The flow cytometric analysis was performed in a BD FACS Canto II (BD Biosciences, Franklin Lakes, New Jersey, USA). In our gating strategy, we initially gated for singlets using forward scatter height vs. width. Afterwards, we selected APC-positive cells (erythrocytes) and, finally, compared the number of FITC-positive cells across samples.

Complete Blood Count (CBC)

A routine CBC was conducted using an Advia 2120i system (Siemens Healthcare, Erlangen, Germany) in all samples that also underwent ektacytometry testing.

Statistics

Numerical values are reported as either absolute or normalized by their respective control to account for inter-subject variability. Statistical analyses were conducted using the IBM SPSS Statistics 23 software (IBM Corporation, Armonk, USA). We performed a linear mixed model analysis with the subject as random effect. *Post-hoc* analysis was according to Tukey-HSD (Tukey, 1977). *P*-values below 0.05 are considered significant and are indicated in the respective figures.

RESULTS

Pressure

We exposed the samples to a series of high pressure peaks, lasting 1 or 30 s each. Exposure to high pressures significantly increased plasma free hemoglobin (**Figures 3A,B**). The higher the pressure level, the more hemoglobin was released from the RBCs. While the magnitude of the pressure had a significant effect on free Hb levels, there was no difference between the two exposure times suggesting that the duration of the exposure did not play a major role. Increasing pressures were also associated with a significant decrease in mean cell volume (MCV, **Figure 3C**). The mean corpuscular hemoglobin (MCH, **Figure 3D**) decreased with increasing pressure, but this decrease was not statistically significant, while the MCH concentration (MCHC, Figure S1) stayed constant. Neither the ektacytometric measurement nor the phosphatidylserine expression showed any differences for samples exposed to elevated levels of pressure compared to controls (Figures S4, S8A).

Centrifugation

In these experiments, we centrifuged samples at 900 g for either 5 or 10 min. Sample centrifugation increased the plasma free hemoglobin from a mean baseline value of 61 mg/l up to 79 mg/l (**Figure 4A**). This behavior was observed for samples centrifuged for 5 min as well as for those centrifuged for 10 min. Overall, we observed higher absolute free Hb values for samples centrifuged for 5 min.

The MCV increased slightly with centrifugation (**Figure 4B**), while MCH (**Figure 4C**) and MCHC (**Figure 4D**) did not change significantly, though showing a trend to increase. Neither phosphatidylserine expression nor parameters measured in ektacytometry were influenced by centrifugation (Figures S5, S8B).

To assess the influence of more than one centrifugation step, the samples had to be resuspended in between centrifugations by

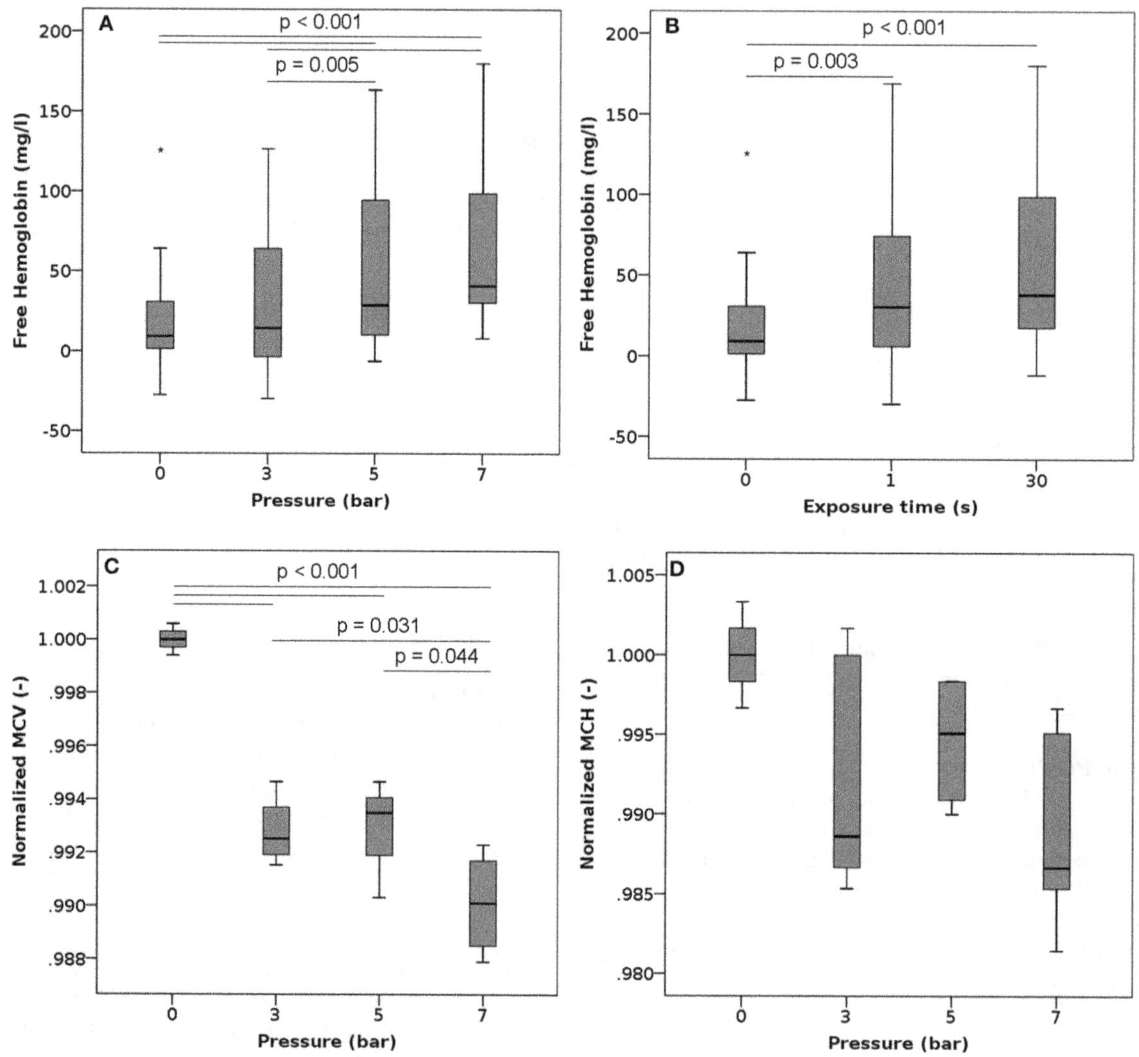

FIGURE 3 | Free hemoglobin, MCV and MCH after exposure to high pressure. Blood samples were exposed to high pressures (varying between 3 and 7 bars) 10 times (single exposure duration of 1 or 30 s) with a 30 s recovery period between two consecutive exposures. **(A)** Free hemoglobin as a function of the pressure level (irrespective of the exposure time) $n = 18$, 22, 20, and 21 for high pressures of 0, 3, 5, and 7 bar, respectively. **(B)** Free hemoglobin as a function of the exposure duration (irrespective of the pressure level) $n = 18$, 33, and 30 for exposures of 0, 1, and 30 s, respectively. **(C)** Normalized mean cell volume as a function of the pressure level (exposure time 1 s). Reported values have been normalized by the mean of the corresponding control measurements. $n = 4$, 4, 3, and 4 for high pressures of 0, 3, 5, and 7 bar, respectively. **(D)** Normalized mean corpuscular hemoglobin as a function of the pressure level (exposure time 1 s). Reported values have been normalized by the mean of the corresponding control measurements. $n = 4$, 4, 3, and 4 for high pressures of 0, 3, 5, and 7 bar, respectively.

a short vortexing step. Consequently, we measured a combined effect of centrifuging and vortexing for these samples. Free Hb increased with an increasing number of centrifugation and resuspension steps (Figure S9A), while maximum deformability as measured by ektacytometry, EI_{max}, slightly decreased (Figure S9D).

Vortexing

In these experiments, blood samples were vortexed for either 20 or 40 s. Such vortexing led to significant increase in plasma free hemoglobin (**Figure 5**), resulting in the highest levels of free hemoglobin in plasma observed within this study. This increase in released Hb was strongly dependent on the duration of vortexing. None of the characteristics measured within the complete blood count, ektacytometry, and measurement of PS-expression showed any significant changes after vortexing (Figures S2, S6, S8B).

Pipetting

To test the effects of pipetting and strategies proposed to potentially moderate them, we pipetted the samples 10 times in a row using either normal or cut pipet tips. Pipetting induced a statistically significant increase in free hemoglobin compared to controls irrespective of the tip used (**Figure 6**), and there

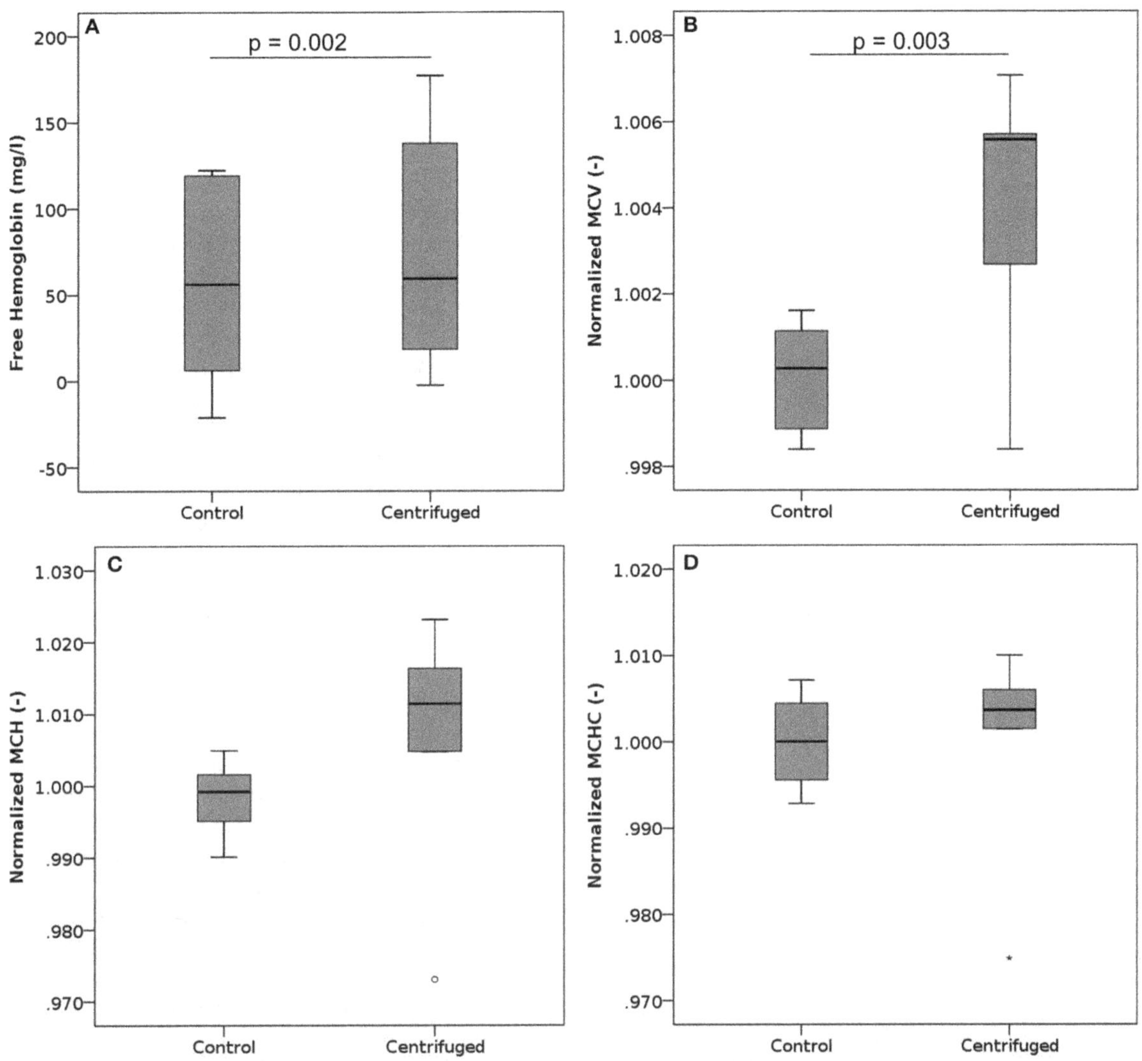

FIGURE 4 | Free hemoglobin, MCV, MCH, and MCHC after centrifugation. Blood samples where centrifuged at 900 g. **(A)** Free hemoglobin after centrifugation for 5 or 10 min. The black line indicates the median, while the mean values are 61 mg/l and 79 mg/l for controls and centrifuged samples, respectively. *n* per group = 12. **(B)** Normalized mean cell volume after centrifugation for 5 min. Reported values have been normalized by the mean of the corresponding control measurements. *n* per group = 6. **(C)** Normalized mean corpuscular hemoglobin after centrifugation for 5 min. Reported values have been normalized by the mean of the corresponding control measurements. *n* per group = 6. **(D)** Normalized mean corpuscular hemoglobin concentration after centrifugation for 5 min. Reported values have been normalized by the mean of the corresponding control measurements. *n* per group = 6.

was no difference between samples that were pipetted with normal or cut tips. No changes were noted in the ektacytometry curves, phosphatidylserine expression or in any of the parameters measured within the CBC (Figures S3, S7, S8C).

DISCUSSION

While the connection between mechanical forces and hemolysis is well-acknowledged, it has mostly been considered in research applications, for example to investigate shear stress-induced hemolysis in cardiovascular implants. However, RBC exposure to supra-physiological forces does not only occur in implants, but also during blood handling. Here we have investigated hemolytic and other stress-induced changes to RBC caused by exposure to high pressures, centrifuging, vortexing, and pipetting, thereby surveying the main mechanical stressors in laboratories and experimental blood handling.

Our results show that high pressures, centrifuging, vortexing, and pipetting all yield increased levels of free hemoglobin, implying that the forces associated with these methods already translate into hemolytic damage. Among these methods, vortexing whole blood samples led to the highest increase in plasma free hemoglobin, with values reaching a mean of 260 and 400 mg/l after vortexing for 20 and 40 s, respectively. Similar findings have been made in orbital shakers, wherein lysis occurred after some time, possibly due to prolonged fatigue

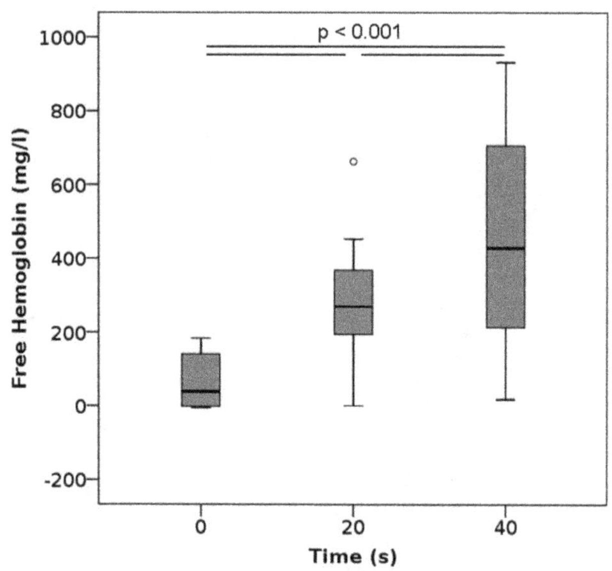

FIGURE 5 | Free hemoglobin after vortexing as a function of the vortexing time. *n* per group = 12.

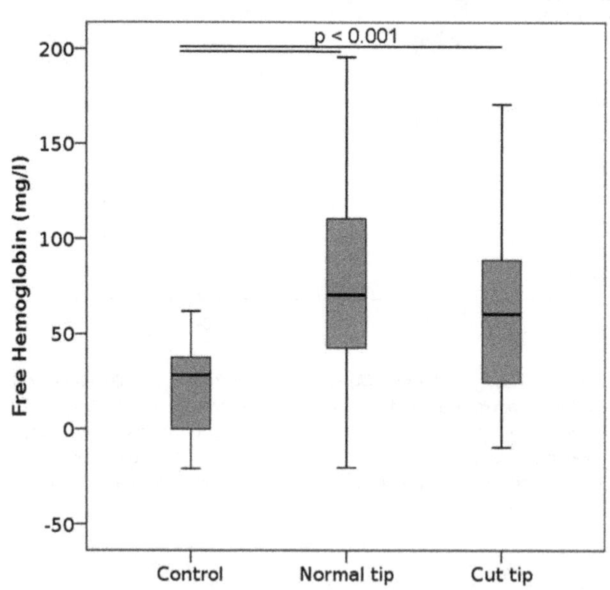

FIGURE 6 | Free hemoglobin after pipetting. Blood samples were primed and relieved from the pipet 10 consecutive times. The pipet tip was either normal or cut 7 mm away from the leading edge. *n* per group = 12.

(Zhang et al., 1995). Vortexing as well as shaking impose shear stresses on the cells, which RBCs are generally vulnerable to Leverett et al. (1972). Numerical simulations of the flow fields induced by rotators, orbital shakers, magnetic stirrers, and vortex mixers identified vortexing as the method that induced the largest shear stresses within the samples (Bai et al., 2012). While vortexing RBCs is generally avoided in hematology laboratories, we investigated it here as a representative of extreme stresses on the cells. As evidenced by our results, these stresses are clearly detrimental. Since we did not observe an effect on MCV or MCH, the release of hemoglobin induced by vortexing seems to be governed by complete lysis of the cells, irrespective of their size. Even though vortexing durations of 20 or 40 s are long in an experimental context, these results clearly show that vortexing *per se* is harmful to RBCs and should be avoided not only in clinical laboratories, but also in research applications.

Pipetting also induces shear forces on the cells, the magnitude of which increases as the pipette tip diameter decreases. Using large pipettes and cutting the foremost edge of the pipette tip to increase the tip diameter had thus been suggested as a means to reduce the stress on cells and mechanical damage (Exadactylos et al., 2003; Miao and Jiang, 2007). Investigating the effect of repetitive pipetting with standard or cut tips, our results confirmed that pipetting increases free hemoglobin compared to controls, but did not reveal any significant differences between the types of pipette tip used. The suction area of the cut tips was a factor of 14 larger than that of the regular tips, which may not have had a strong enough effect to be detected with our sample size. Alternatively, it is also possible that even though the shear stresses were significantly reduced in the cut pipet tips, the effect on erythrocyte lysis was counterbalanced by the creation of sharper edges. The latter option would point toward the need to round the edges after cutting. However, we do not have enough evidence to favor one interpretation over the other. We thus conclude that pipette tip sectioning does not appear to be effective in reducing pipetting induced hemolysis and may therefore not be a useful addition to the analysis workflow.

In the pressure experiments, plasma hemoglobin increased with higher pressure plateaus, but not with longer exposure times. The recovery pressure and time over which the pressure was varied were constant throughout the experimental conditions. Accordingly, the pressure gradient increased with increasing high pressure levels. Independence from the exposure time may thereby point to the temporal pressure gradients, more than to the absolute pressure values, as the predominant factor for the observed increase in plasma hemoglobin. This hypothesis is in accordance with previous findings in other cell lines. Pressure gradient, and not exposure duration, has been put forth as a primary determinant of epithelial cell damage (Kay et al., 2004). The fact that RBCs might be sensitive to pressure gradients thus warrants particular attention in research settings: For example, if high pressures are required to drive blood through a microchannel, then the rate of pressure changes along the channel should be considered in addition to the shear stresses experienced by the cells in the test section.

Our experiments revealed lysis and changes of mechanical properties after centrifuging RBCs, even though the applied centrifugal force (900 g) was at the lower end of the spectrum of commonly used forces in laboratories. This is especially noteworthy given that centrifugation is very commonly performed both in laboratory practice as well as in research experiments in preparatory steps. Between two consecutive centrifuging steps, cells were resuspended with a short vortex period, which is likely to have increased blood damage.

Consequently, the results for multiple centrifugation steps reflect a combined effect of centrifuging and resuspension (Figure S9). However, since we already observed a statistically significant increase in free hemoglobin between controls and one centrifugation step (mean values of 61 mg/l vs. 79 mg/l, $p = 0.002$), with both control and experiment including one vortexing event, it is reasonable to state that centrifugation is by itself a process that induces blood damage. It is difficult to estimate the level of damage induced by experiments published in literature a posteriori, as these often only report the centrifugation speed (rpm) instead of the relative centrifugal forces (rcf), which, without knowledge of the rotor diameter, do not reveal the applied forces (Sutton et al., 1997; Zhao et al., 2006; Quinn et al., 2011). The need to consider such "processing lesions" in addition to the well-known storage lesions was already pointed out by Urbina et al. who noted that the centrifuging performed to extract erythrocyte concentrate from whole blood donations changed RBC shape and MCH (Urbina et al., 2016).

We also observed overall higher values of free hemoglobin for samples centrifuged for 5 min compared to those centrifuged for 10 min. This may be due to an unintended bias toward male subjects in these samples (100% male subjects in samples selected for the 5 min centrifuging steps vs. 25% of male subjects for the samples selected for 10 min). It is known that females have 80% more young RBCs and 85% fewer old RBCs than males (Kameneva et al., 1999), and that old RBCs have a significantly increased mechanical fragility and rigidity compared to young ones (Sutera et al., 1985). Older RBCs are thus more susceptible to damage, which may explain the higher values of plasma free Hb noted in the 5 min, males-only, group. We also observed an increased amount of PS-positive cells in this subject group, which supports this interpretation. The results shown for the other experimental procedures (pressure, pipetting, vortexing) were not affected by this sex bias, since the study used a paired design wherein the blood from each donor was exposed to all tested conditions, including control.

Vortexing and pipetting did not yield any notable changes in the ektacytometry curves, phosphatidylserine expression, or in any of the parameters measured within the CBC (Figures S2, S3, S6, S8). For pipetting, this absence of notable changes may be explained by the relatively low overall damage level that was measured. However, this does not hold true for vortexing, which induced significantly elevated levels of plasma hemoglobin. This may suggest that the noted cell damage resulted from complete cell lysis affecting RBCs uniformly, irrespective of their size and age.

In contrast to the above, centrifuging and elevated pressures were also associated with changes in RBC properties (**Figures 3, 4**). Centrifuging induced a subtle increase in mean cellular volume, pointing at a destruction of older and smaller RBCs. Also, the maximum deformability decreased with an increasing number of combined resuspension and centrifuging steps (Figure S9D), a behavior that was not observed in the experiments solely involving vortexing (Figure S6D). While the magnitude of the noted changes in mean cellular volume and maximum deformability remained small, these two observations combined are of relevance for both clinical laboratories and researchers: they suggest that even if the remaining cells maintain sufficient membrane integrity not to release significant amounts of intracellular hemoglobin, their mechanical properties may still be altered by repeated centrifugation and resuspension. This finding is also supported by Urbina et al. who observed significant morphological changes, including the appearance of abnormal shapes (echinocytes), after centrifugation (Urbina et al., 2016).

Elevated pressures, on the other hand, led to a decrease of mean RBC volume, a trend toward decreasing MCH and constant MCHC compared to controls. One possible interpretation of the decrease in volume may be the destruction of larger cells. This would be in contrast to previous reports that suggested that mechanical stresses, albeit mostly shear stresses, would affect smaller, older cells first and thus lead to increased MCV (Sakota et al., 2008). Alternatively, this observed cell shrinkage could also point toward a channel-mediated loss of cytosolic content due to the mechanical load (Cahalan et al., 2015). Since we also observed increased levels of plasma free Hb, it could be hypothesized that the weaker cells suffer from complete lysis, while the remainder of the RBC population reacts with cell shrinkage following Ca^{2+} influx (Bogdanova et al., 2013). Otherwise, high pressures have been noted to alter the permeability of the bilayer cell membrane (MacDonald, 1984), such that cytosolic content, including hemoglobin, could be released into the plasma without full cell lysis. Compared to the conditions explored here, those experiments were conducted at extreme pressure levels (250–1,500 bar). Yet, the simultaneous reduction in corpuscular volume and increase in free Hb observed in our pressure experiments could hint at a similar mechanism.

From a clinical perspective, one limitation of this study is the sole investigation of hematologically healthy patients. It might be of interest to characterize whether RBCs with known membrane alterations, such as in patients with sickle cell disease or hereditary spherocytosis, react differently to the same levels of centrifuging, vortexing, and pipetting. Determining whether or not different RBC properties are associated with different reactions to standard procedures would be of relevance for the diagnosis workup, as this could interfere with correct interpretation of results and introduce a bias in the comparison of a given patient's hematological characteristics against standard healthy values. From an experimental perspective, a limitation of this study is the limited applicability of quantitative results to other experimental protocols or setups. This study should thus primarily raise awareness that both preparatory steps as well as secondary factors inherent to an experimental setup should be systematically checked for their influence on the selected study endpoints. Finally, given the small magnitude of the noted changes in CBC parameters, one should also carefully consider potential artifacts introduced by the measurement method. The Advia hematology system uses optical scattering as working principle. We confirmed the trends of increasing MCV after centrifuging and decreasing MCV after exposure to high pressures also in an impedance-based system (Sysmex NX-100, Sysmex K. K., Kobe, Japan), indicating that the noted differences in MCV, although arguably small, were not artefactual. However, manual analysis may be needed for a conclusive answer.

CONCLUSION

Within a standard laboratory workflow, there are multiple steps that expose cells to mechanical stress. Here, we investigated the effect of centrifuging, vortexing, pipetting, and pressure on human RBCs. All procedures significantly increased the free hemoglobin in plasma, the measured hemolysis increasing with the vortexing time or the applied pressure. Elevated pressures and centrifugation also altered MCV and MCH. Careful quantification of the influence of these steps as well as of other unwanted secondary effects should be included in experimental protocols and should be checked for in clinical laboratories.

AUTHOR CONTRIBUTIONS

LW conducted the experiments and performed the data analysis. DdZ supervised the experimental study design and interpretation. OS enabled the measurements of free hemoglobin. AM and JG contributed to the ektacytometry measurements. OS and JG guided the clinical interpretation. BS did the statistical analyses. VK conceived the study and directed the research. All authors wrote the manuscript.

ACKNOWLEDGMENTS

We would like to thank Kristina Koch for her work on the flow cytometry protocols. The authors gratefully acknowledge the financial support provided by the Swiss National Science Foundation through grant 200021_147193 CINDY, Marie Heim-Vögtlin fellowship PMPDP2_151255, NCCR Kidney.CH and the Stavros Niarchos Foundation. This work is part of the Zurich Heart Project of Hochschulmedizin Zurich.

REFERENCES

Bai, G., Bee, J. S., Biddlecombe, J. G., Chen, Q., and Leach, W. T. (2012). Computational fluid dynamics (CFD) insights into agitation stress methods in biopharmaceutical development. *Int. J. Pharm.* 423, 264–280. doi: 10.1016/j.ijpharm.2011.11.044

Baskurt, O., Boynard, M., Cokelet, G., Connes, P., Cooke, B. M., Forconi, S., et al. (2009). New guidelines for hemorheological laboratory techniques. *Clin. Hemorheol. Microcirc.* 42, 75–97. doi: 10.3233/CH-2009-1202

Boas, F. E., Forman, L., and Beutler, E. (1998). Phosphatidylserine exposure and red cell viability in red cell aging and in hemolytic anemia. *Proc. Natl. Acad. Sci. U.S.A.* 95, 3077–3081. doi: 10.1073/pnas.95.6.3077

Bogdanova, A., Makhro, A., Wang, J., Lipp, P., and Kaestner, L. (2013). Calcium in red blood cells-a perilous balance. *Int. J. Mol. Sci.* 14, 9848–9872. doi: 10.3390/ijms14059848

Cahalan, S. M., Lukacs, V., Ranade, S. S., Chien, S., Bandell, M., and Patapoutian, A. (2015). Piezo1 links mechanical forces to red blood cell volume. *Elife* 4, 1–12. doi: 10.7554/eLife.07370

Exadactylos, A., Geffen, A. J., and Panagiotaki, P. (2003). Population structure of Dover sole *Solea solea*: RAPD and allozyme data indicate divergence in European stocks. *Mar. Ecol. Prog. Ser.* 246, 253–264. doi: 10.3354/meps246253

Fairbanks, V. F., Ziesmer, S. C., and O'Brien, P. C. (1992). Methods for measuring plasma hemoglobin in micromolar concentration compared. *Clin. Chem.* 38, 132–140.

Ferraro, G. A., De Francesco, F., Tirino, V., Cataldo, C., Rossano, F., Nicoletti, G., et al. (2011). Effects of a new centrifugation method on adipose cell viability for autologous fat grafting. *Aesthetic Plast. Surg.* 35, 341–348. doi: 10.1007/s00266-010-9613-8

Gunter, E. W., Bowman, B. A., Caudill, S. P., Twite, D. B., Adams, M. J., and Sampson, E. J. (1996). Results of an international round robin for serum and whole-blood folate. *Clin. Chem.* 42, 1689–1694.

Heng, B. C., Liu, H., Ge, Z., and Cao, T. (2007). Mechanical dissociation of human embryonic stem cell colonies by manual scraping after collagenase treatment is much more detrimental to cellular viability than is trypsinization with gentle pipetting. *Biotechnol. Appl. Biochem.* 47, 33–37. doi: 10.1042/BA20060151

Kameneva, M. V., Watach, M. J., and Borovetz, H. S. (1999). Gender difference in rheologic properties of blood and risk of cardiovascular diseases. *Clin. Hemorheol. Microcirc.* 21, 357–363.

Katkov, I. I., and Mazur, P. (1998). Influence of centrifugation regimes on motility, yield and cell assications of mouse spermatozoa. *J. Androl.* 19, 232–241. doi: 10.1002/j.1939-4640.1998.tb01993.x

Kay, S. S., Bilek, A. M., Dee, K. C., and Gaver, D. P. (2004). Pressure gradient, not exposure duration, determines the extent of epithelial cell damage in a model of pulmonary airway reopening. *J. Appl. Physiol.* 97, 269–276. doi: 10.1152/japplphysiol.01288.2003

Kirklin, J. K., Naftel, D. C., Pagani, F. D., Kormos, R. L., Stevenson, L. W., Blume, E. D., et al. (2015). Seventh INTERMACS annual report: 15,000 patients and counting. *J. Hear. Lung Transplant.* 34, 1495–1504. doi: 10.1016/j.healun.2015.10.003

Korin, N., Bransky, A., and Dinnar, U. (2007). Theoretical model and experimental study of red blood cell (RBC) deformation in microchannels. *J. Biomech.* 40, 2088–2095. doi: 10.1016/j.jbiomech.2006.10.004

Kuypers, F. A., Lewis, R. A., Hua, M., Schott, M. A., Discher, D., Ernst, J. D., et al. (1996). Detection of altered membrane phospholipid asymmetry in subpopulations of human red blood cells using fluorescently labeled annexin V. *Blood* 87, 1179–1187.

Leverett, L., Hellums, J., Alfrey, C., and Lynch, E. C. (1972). Red blood cell damage by shear stress. *Biophys. J.* 12, 257–273. doi: 10.1016/S0006-3495(72)86085-5

Lippi, G., Guidi, G. C., Mattiuzzi, C., and Plebani, M. (2006). Preanalytical variability: the dark side of the moon in laboratory testing. *Clin. Chem. Lab. Med.* 44, 358–365. doi: 10.1515/CCLM.2006.073

Lutz, H. U., and Bogdanova, A. (2013). Mechanisms tagging senescent red blood cells for clearance in healthy humans. *Front. Physiol.* 4:387. doi: 10.3389/fphys.2013.00387

MacDonald, A. G. (1984). The effects of pressure on the molecular structure and physiological functions of cell membranes. *Philos. Trans. R. Soc. L.* 304, 47–68. doi: 10.1098/rstb.1984.0008

Makhro, A., Huisjes, R., Verhagen, L. P., del Manu-Pereira, M., Llaudet-Planas, E., Petkova-Kirova, P., et al. (2016). Red cell properties after different modes of blood transportation. *Front. Physiol.* 7:288. doi: 10.3389/fphys.2016.00288

Miao, Y., and Jiang, L. (2007). Transient expression of fluorescent fusion proteins in protoplasts of suspension cultured cells. *Nat. Protoc.* 2, 2348–2353. doi: 10.1038/nprot.2007.360

Paul, R., Apel, J., Klaus, S., Schügner, F., Schwindke, P., and Reul, H. (2003). Shear stress related blood damage in laminar Couette flow. *Artif. Organs* 27, 517–529. doi: 10.1046/j.1525-1594.2003.07103.x

Plebani, M. (2007). Errors in laboratory medicine and patient safety: the road ahead. *Clin. Chem. Lab. Med.* 45, 700–707. doi: 10.1515/CCLM.2007.170

Quinn, D. J., Pivkin, I., Wong, S. Y., Chiam, K.-H., Dao, M., Karniadakis, G. E., et al. (2011). Combined simulation and experimental study of large deformation of red blood cells in microfluidic systems. *Ann. Biomed. Eng.* 39, 1041–1050. doi: 10.1007/s10439-010-0232-y

Rand, R. P. (1964). Mechanical properties of the red cell membrane: II. Viscoelastic breakdown of the membrane. *Biophys. J.* 4, 303–316. doi: 10.1016/S0006-3495(64)86784-9

Rao, S., Bálint, S., Cossins, B., Guallar, V., and Petrov, D. (2009). Raman study of mechanically induced oxygenation state transition of red blood cells using optical tweezers. *Biophys. J.* 96, 209–216. doi: 10.1529/biophysj.108.139097

Sakota, D., Sakamoto, R., Sobajima, H., Yokoyama, N., Waguri, S., Ohuchi, K., et al. (2008). Mechanical damage of red blood cells by rotary blood pumps: selective destruction of aged red blood cells and subhemolytic trauma. *Artif. Organs* 32, 785–791. doi: 10.1111/j.1525-1594.2008.00631.x

Shapira, Y., Vaturi, M., and Sagie, A. (2009). Hemolysis associated with prosthetic heart valves: a review. *Cardiol. Rev.* 17, 121–124. doi: 10.1097/CRD.0b013e31819f1a83

Sowemimo-Coker, S. O. (2002). Red blood cell hemolysis during processing. *Transfus. Med. Rev.* 16, 46–60. doi: 10.1053/tmrv.2002.29404

Sutera, S. P., Gardner, R. A., Boyland, C. W., Carroll, G. L., Chang, K. C., Marvel, J. S., et al. (1985). Age-related changes in deformability of human erythrocytes. *Blood* 65, 275–282.

Sutton, N., Tracey, M. C., Johnston, I. D., Greenaway, R. S., and Rampling, M. W. (1997). A novel instrument for studying the flow behaviour of erythrocytes through microchannels simulating human blood capillaries. *Microvasc. Res.* 53, 272–281. doi: 10.1006/mvre.1997.2014

Tukey, J. W. (1977). "Exploratory data analysis," in *Addison-Wesley Series in Behavioral Science. Quantitative Methods* (Massachusetts: Addison-Wesley Educational Publishers Inc.), 5–23.

Urbina, A., Godoy-Silva, R., Hoyos, M., and Camacho, M. (2016). Acute hydrodynamic damage induced by SPLITT fractionation and centrifugation in red blood cells. *J. Chromatogr. B Anal. Technol. Biomed. Life Sci.* 1020, 53–61. doi: 10.1016/j.jchromb.2016.03.025

Zhang, Z., Chisti, Y., and Moo-young, M. (1995). Effects of the hydrodynamic environment and shear protectants on survival of erythrocytes in suspension. *J. Biotechnol.* 43, 33–40. doi: 10.1016/0168-1656(95)00111-8

Zhao, R., Antaki, J. F., Naik, T., Bachman, T. N., Kameneva, M. V., and Wu, Z. J. (2006). Microscopic investigation of erythrocyte deformation dynamics. *Biorheology* 43, 747–765.

6

Increased Reactive Oxygen Species and Cell Cycle Defects Contribute to Anemia in the RASA3 Mutant Mouse Model *scat*

Emily S. Hartman[1†], Elena C. Brindley[1,2†], Julien Papoin[1], Steven L. Ciciotte[3], Yue Zhao[3], Luanne L. Peters[3‡] and Lionel Blanc[1,4*‡]

[1] Laboratory of Developmental Erythropoiesis, Center for Autoimmune, Musculoskeletal and Hematopoietic Diseases, The Feinstein Institute for Medical Research, Manhasset, NY, United States, [2] Donald and Barbara Zucker School of Medicine at Hofstra/Northwell, Hempstead, NY, United States, [3] The Jackson Laboratory, Bar Harbor, ME, United States, [4] Department of Molecular Medicine and Pediatrics, Donald and Barbara Zucker School of Medicine at Hofstra/Northwell, Hempstead, NY, United States

***Correspondence:**
Lionel Blanc
LBlanc@northwell.edu

† These authors have contributed equally to this work.

‡ Co-senior authors

RASA3 is a Ras GTPase activating protein that plays a critical role in blood formation. The autosomal recessive mouse model *scat* (severe combined anemia and thrombocytopenia) carries a missense mutation in *Rasa3*. Homozygotes present with a phenotype characteristic of bone marrow failure that is accompanied by alternating episodes of crisis and remission. The mechanism leading to impaired erythropoiesis and peripheral cell destruction as evidenced by membrane fragmentation in *scat* is unclear, although we previously reported that the mislocalization of RASA3 to the cytosol of reticulocytes and mature red cells plays a role in the disease. In this study, we further characterized the bone marrow failure in *scat* and found that RASA3 plays a central role in cell cycle progression and maintenance of reactive oxygen species (ROS) levels during terminal erythroid differentiation, without inducing apoptosis of the precursors. In *scat* mice undergoing crises, there is a consistent pattern of an increased proportion of cells in the G_0/G_1 phase at the basophilic and polychromatophilic stages of erythroid differentiation, suggesting that RASA3 is involved in the G_1 checkpoint. However, this increase in G_1 is transient, and either resolves or becomes indiscernible by the orthochromatic stage. In addition, while ROS levels are normal early in erythropoiesis, there is accumulation of superoxide levels at the reticulocyte stage (DHE increased 40% in *scat;* $p = 0.02$) even though mitochondria, a potential source for ROS, are eliminated normally. Surprisingly, apoptosis is significantly decreased in the *scat* bone marrow at the proerythroblastic (15.3%; $p = 0.004$), polychromatophilic (8.5%; $p = 0.01$), and orthochromatic (4.2%; $p = 0.02$) stages. Together, these data indicate that ROS accumulation at the reticulocyte stage, without apoptosis, contributes to the membrane fragmentation observed in *scat*. Finally, the cell cycle defect and increased levels of ROS suggest that *scat* is a model of bone marrow failure with characteristics of aplastic anemia.

Keywords: erythropoiesis, mouse models, anemia, aplastic, bone marrow failure syndromes, reactive oxygen species (ROS), cell cycle, apoptosis

INTRODUCTION

Every day, a healthy individual's bone marrow produces 200 billion erythrocytes in the process of erythropoiesis. Bone marrow failure syndromes (BMFS) are a diverse group of inherited or acquired disorders characterized by varying degrees of hematopoietic failure and a predisposition to hematologic malignancies (Shimamura and Alter, 2010). While targetable molecular markers associated with the various subclasses of BMFS have recently been identified, the full molecular pathogeneses of these diseases are likely a complex interaction between genetic changes at the hematopoietic stem cell level and alterations in the hematopoietic niche of the bone marrow itself, and these mechanisms have yet to be fully elucidated (Rankin et al., 2015). Aplastic anemia (AA) is one of the most commonly diagnosed BMFS, with over 2,500 new cases each year in North America and in Europe alone, and is characterized by a hypocellular bone marrow and ineffective hematopoiesis of the erythroid, megakaryocyte, and granulocyte/monocyte lineages (Guinan, 2011; Bodine and Berliner, 2014). At the molecular level, AA is characterized by increased levels of reactive oxygen species (ROS) and defective DNA repair mechanisms (Khincha and Savage, 2013; Richardson et al., 2015).

Like most BMFS, AA can either be acquired or inherited. Acquired AA appears to be an immune-mediated suppression of the bone marrow and is thus responsive, in most cases, to immunosuppressive therapy (Miano and Dufour, 2015). Inherited AA, however, has a complex variety of pathogeneses. Although many of the patients with BMFS have identifiable causes, 30–40% of cases still have unknown etiologies, including cases of inherited AA (Peters et al., 2013). Spontaneous and engineered models of bone marrow failure have allowed focused study of these uncharacterized molecular mechanisms. One such spontaneous model is the autosomal recessive *scat* (severe combined anemia and thrombocytopenia) mouse model; *scat* carries a missense mutation in the protein-coding *Rasa3* gene (Blanc et al., 2012).

RASA3, a Ras-GTPase Activating Protein (GAP), has previously been found to play a key role in normal blood formation. This protein acts to negatively regulate the small GTPase Ras, and its localization to the membrane is required for normal function (Fukuda and Mikoshiba, 1996). The specific *Rasa3* mutation in the *scat* mouse results in the mislocalization of RASA3 to the cytosol and thus loss of RASA3 function, which leads to increased levels of active GTP-bound Ras (Blanc et al., 2012). *scat* mice interestingly cycle between hematologic crisis and remission, regardless of the cytosolic localization of RASA3, suggesting that a secreted factor may mediate the crisis-remission transition. The first crisis begins *in utero* and lasts until ~P9. Mice that survive the first crisis will progress to remission, during which there is a striking normalization of hematologic parameters and physical appearance. Some mice then enter a second crisis, during which there is over 90% mortality by 4 weeks of age, likely due to bone marrow failure and the resulting peripheral pancytopenia (Blanc et al., 2012). Overall, the mechanism of the cyclic phenotype in *scat* mouse is unknown and offers unique opportunities to study the onset and resolution of bone marrow failure.

In this study, we further characterized the bone marrow failure in *scat* and found that RASA3 plays a central role in cell cycle progression and maintenance of ROS levels during terminal erythroid differentiation. We observed that in mice undergoing crisis episodes, the G_0/G_1 phase is transiently increased at the basophilic and polychromatophilic stages, suggesting that RASA3 is involved in regulating the G_1 checkpoint. In addition, while ROS levels are normal early in erythropoiesis, we observed an accumulation of ROS at the reticulocyte stage in *scat* mice. However, mitochondria, a potential source of ROS, are eliminated normally at the reticulocyte stage, suggesting that mitochondrial metabolism and ROS production may be altered prior to removal. Surprisingly, apoptosis is not increased, but rather significantly decreased at several stages of erythroid differentiation in *scat* during crisis events. Together, these data suggest that *scat* is a model of bone marrow failure with some of the molecular characteristics of AA. To begin testing the hypothesis that a secreted factor may be mediating the cyclic phenotype, we also characterized the differences in the plasma cytokine profile of *scat* mice during crisis compared to wild type. We observed that galectin-1 is significantly decreased in *scat* mice in crisis compared to wild type.

MATERIALS AND METHODS

Animals

All experimental mice were 14–21 days old, which corresponds to the second crisis event of the *scat* mice. All protocols were performed according to NIH animal care guidelines, as approved and enforced by the Institutional Animal Care and Use Committees at Northwell Health and The Jackson Laboratory.

Erythroblast, Red Cell, and Plasma/Serum Collection

Bone marrow was flushed and dissociated with cold PBS containing 0.5% (weight/volume) bovine serum albumin (BSA) and 2 mM Ethylenediaminetetraacetic acid (EDTA), pH 8.0 (Invitrogen). Spleens were dissociated in cold PBS with 0.5% BSA only. Cells were filtered using a 70 μm cell strainer and CD45 depleted using anti-mouse CD45-conjugated microbeads and magnetic columns as per manufacturer instructions (Miltenyi). Circulating red cells, containing both reticulocytes and erythrocytes, were obtained by cardiac puncture. To obtain plasma or serum, whole blood with or without EDTA was centrifuged at 600 *g* for 5 min and the plasma/serum removed.

Erythroid Surface Markers Used for Flow Cytometry

Terminal erythropoiesis was monitored using CD44, Ter119, and FSC (Forward Scatter) as markers of differentiation. While Ter119 is increased during differentiation, CD44 is lost as the erythroblasts differentiate.

Depending on the experimental purpose, reticulocyte maturation was monitored using whether CD71 and Ter119 (ROS content); or MitoTracker Red (MTR) and thiazole orange (TO, mitochondria analysis). All of these markers except for Ter119 are lost during reticulocyte maturation.

Reactive Oxygen Species Detection by Flow Cytometry

Samples were blocked with rat anti-mouse CD16/32 (2.5 μg/10^6 cells) for 5 min at room temperature (RT) followed by staining with a cell surface marker cocktail for 15 min at RT protected from light. Spleen and bone marrow samples were stained with rat anti-mouse CD44 APC-conjugated (0.5 μg/10^6 cells), rat anti-mouse CD45R/CDllb/Ly6G APC-Cy7-conjugated (0.3 μg/10^6 cells), and rat anti-mouse Ter119 V450-conjugated (0.5 μg/10^6 cells) for CM-H2DCFDA (DCF, Invitrogen) or rat anti-mouse Ter119 FITC-conjugated (1 μg/10^6 cells) for Dihydroethidium (DHE, Invitrogen). Peripheral blood samples were stained with rat anti-mouse Ter119 V450-conjugated (0.5 μg/10^6 cells) and either rat anti-mouse CD71 PE-conjugated (0.2 μg/10^6 cells) for DCF or rat anti-mouse CD71 FITC-conjugated (0.625 μg/10^6 cells) for DHE. Samples were washed twice in PBS and stained with either DHE or DCF. DHE diluted in warm IMDM/1% FBS was added to spleen and bone marrow samples at a 0.4 μM final concentration, and to RBC at a 4 μM final concentration. DCF diluted in warm 1x PBS was added at a 25 μM final concentration for all samples. DHE and DCF were added to the samples and incubated for 30 min at 37°C protected from light. All samples were washed and resuspended for flow analysis. Data was collected using the BD LSRFortessa cytometer and subsequently analyzed with FlowJo software. All cell surface marker antibodies were from BD Biosciences.

Cell Cycle Analysis by Flow Cytometry

Bone marrow cells were isolated and CD45-depleted as above, blocked with rat anti-mouse CD16/32 (2.5 μg/10^6 cells) for 5 min at RT, and stained with an antibody cocktail of rat anti-mouse Ter119 FITC-conjugated (1 μg/10^6 cells), CD44 APC-conjugated (0.5 μg/10^6 cells), and CD45R/CDllb/Ly6G APC-Cy7-conjugated (0.3 μg/10^6 cells) for 15 min at RT in the dark (Liu et al., 2013). Samples were washed in PBS/0.5% BSA, resuspended in 10 μg/mL Hoechst 33342 (Invitrogen) in warm IMDM/1%FBS (1 mL/10^6 cells), and incubated at 37°C for 30 min in the dark. Samples were resuspended in 500 μL of 1× PBS with the addition of 0.25 μg of 7AAD (BD Biosciences) to identify dead cells. Data was collected using the BD LSRFortessa cytometer and analyzed using FlowJo software.

Cytokine Array

Plasma was separated from circulating red cells as described above and then frozen at −80°C until future use. Cytokine levels were semi-quantitated using the Abcam 97-target Mouse Cytokine Antibody Array according to the manufacturer's protocol (ab169820). Briefly, plasma samples were diluted 1:20 in the 1× blocking buffer provided. Membranes were imaged with the Bio-Rad ChemiDoc™ MP. Quantification was performed using Gilles Carpentier's *Dot Blot Analyzer for ImageJ* from the ImageJ website macros/toolsets folder, according to documentation at image.bio.methods.free.fr/dotblot.html.

ELISA Analysis of Galectin-1 Levels in Mouse Plasma and Serum

Plasma samples were obtained as mentioned above, and serum samples were obtained in the same manner but without the use of EDTA. Both plasma and serum samples were used to demonstrate consistency across collection methods (de Jager et al., 2009). Prior to loading, all samples were diluted 1:10 in dilution buffer provided with Abcam's Mouse Galectin 1 ELISA Kit (ab119595), and the kit was run according to manufacturer's protocol. The plate was read on a spectrophotometer at 450 nm at RT. Galectin-1 concentrations of each sample were extrapolated using the standard curve created on Microsoft Excel and analyzed by comparing *scat* and wild type measures by unpaired *t*-test using GraphPad Prism software.

Apoptosis Analysis by Flow Cytometry

Apoptosis was assessed using Annexin V as per manufacturer (BD Biosciences). All samples were stained with the cell surface marker antibodies as discussed in the cell cycle methods section, followed by staining with Annexin V and 7AAD. The protocol was modified by using 1 μg of Annexin V and 0.25 μg of 7AAD for 1 × 10^6 cells. Apoptosis data was collected using the BD LSRFortessa cytometer and analyzed using FlowJo software.

Mitochondria Analysis

Mitophagy was assessed using MitoTracker Red CMXRos (MTR; Molecular Probes) and TO (BD Biosciences) as described (Zhang et al., 2009). Doubly stained reticulocytes were obtained by sequential staining with MTR, then TO. MTR fluorescence emission between 600 and 620 nm was collected after 562 nm laser excitation using a BD LSR II flow cytometry analyzer (BD Biosciences).

Transmission Electron Microscopy

For analysis by transmission electron microscopy, peripheral blood reticulocytes and red cells were fixed in 4% paraformaldehyde, 0.1% glutaraldehyde, and 1% sucrose in 0.1 M cacodylate buffer for 1 h at 4°C, then washed in 0.1 M buffer at pH 7.4; remaining aldehydes were quenched with 50 mM ammonium chloride. The fixed cells were then dehydrated and embedded in LR-White Resin, sectioned to 50–70 nm thickness, and examined in a Philips-410 electron microscope.

Statistics

Statistical evaluations between different experimental groups were performed using GraphPad Prism 7 (unpaired *t*-test) and $p < 0.05$ was considered to indicate statistical significance.

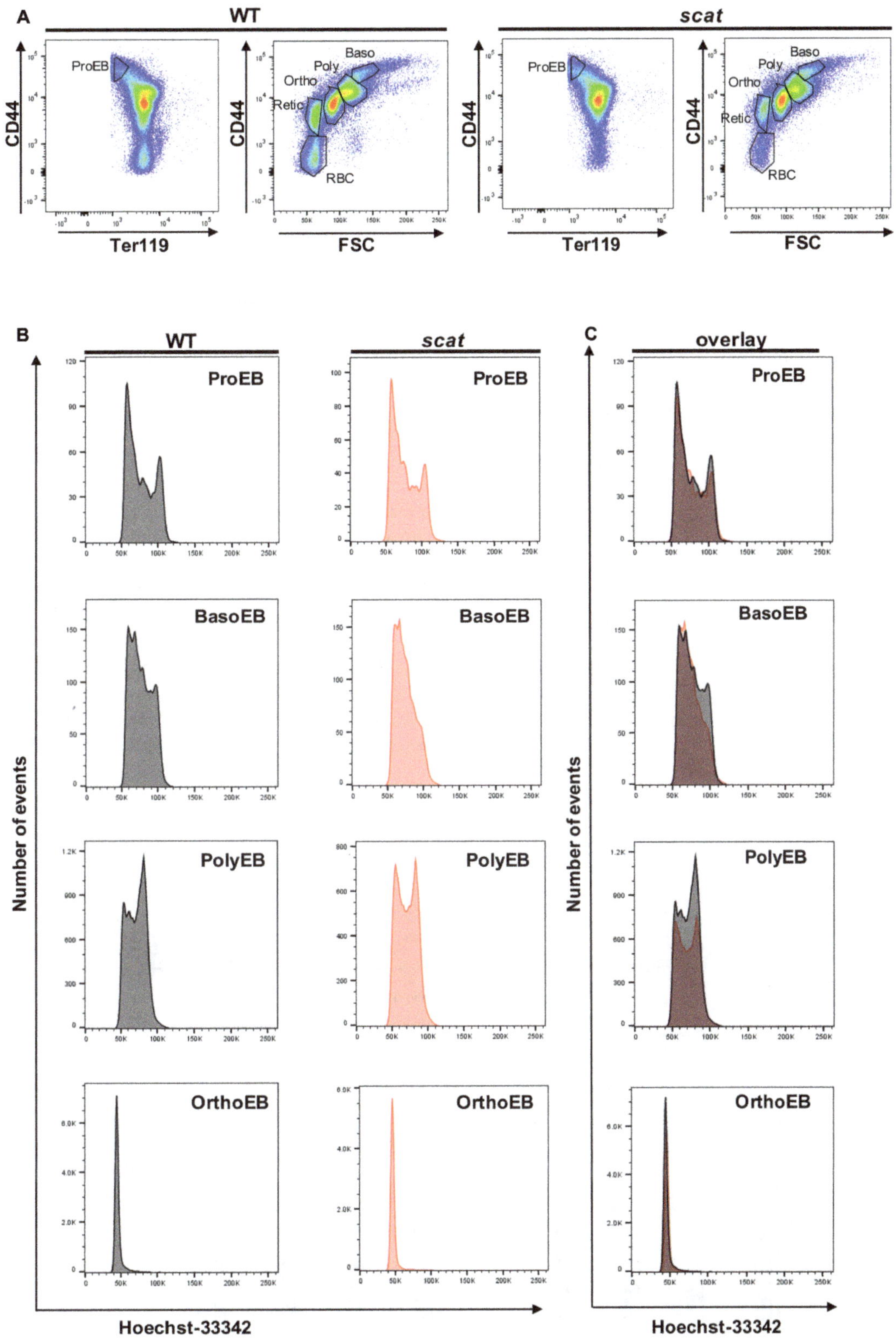

FIGURE 1 | Hoechst staining reveals altered cell cycling in the basophilic and polychromatophilic stages of erythropoiesis in *scat* mice. **(A)** Gating of CD45-depleted, Ter119 positive bone marrow cells based on CD44 surface expression in wild type and *scat*. **(B)** Wild type and *scat* cells were stained with Hoechst dye (10 μg/mL) and analyzed as individual erythropoietic populations by flow cytometry. **(C)** Representative cell cycle patterns are suggestive of an accumulation of cells in the G_0/G_1 phase during erythropoiesis in *scat* mice. Representative pattern from five independent experiments.

RESULTS

scat Presents With Cell Cycle Defects at the Basophilic and Polychromatophilic Stages

We previously reported an accumulation of erythroid precursors at the polychromatophilic and orthochromatic stages in the *scat* mouse model (Blanc et al., 2012), suggesting potential cell cycle defects. Therefore, we isolated the bone marrow from wild type and *scat* mice and measured the cell cycle progression at each of the erythroid differentiation stages using the DNA-binding dye Hoechst-33342 along with the erythroid cell surface markers CD44, Ter119, and FSC. Throughout differentiation, erythroid cells lose the adhesion molecule CD44, gain the membrane glycoprotein associated-Ter119, and decrease in size, allowing analysis of distinct developing populations (Liu et al., 2013; **Figure 1A**). While the pattern was similar between wild type and *scat* within the proerythroblast population, we observed different patterns of DNA content at the basophilic and polychromatophilic stages that demonstrate a failure to progress out of G_0/G_1 into S or G_2 in *scat,* indicating a defect at the G_1 checkpoint. However, we observed that the pattern either normalizes or becomes indiscernible by the orthochromatic stage, as orthochromatic erythroblasts in both *scat* and wild type mice are almost entirely in the G_0/G_1 phase, consistent with previously published studies (Pop et al., 2010; **Figures 1B,C**). Thus, we conclude that *Rasa3* plays a critical role in the G_1 checkpoint at the basophilic and polychromatophilic stages of erythroid differentiation.

Reactive Oxygen Species (ROS) Accumulate at the Proerythroblastic and Reticulocyte Stages in *scat*

Having shown that the cell cycle is altered specifically at the basophilic and polychromatophilic stages, we then hypothesized that increased levels of ROS could be involved in the mechanism leading to crisis in *scat.* To evaluate cytosolic peroxide and superoxide generation in wild type and *scat,* we used DCF and DHE, respectively, as previously described by George et al. (2013). We assessed ROS production in the spleen, bone marrow, and peripheral blood of the mice. A qualitative overlay of the superoxide and general oxidative stress signals in the spleens of wild type and *scat* indicate a relatively similar level of ROS levels (**Figure 2A**). However, when we quantified these ROS levels, we observed a significant increase in the peroxide levels at the proerythroblastic stage of *scat* spleen (**Figure 2B**; $P < 0.05$). We also noticed a trend toward increased levels of ROS throughout erythroid differentiation (**Figure 2B**, left panel). The same trend is observed in the bone marrow (Supplementary Figure 1). This increase in ROS does not seem to be due to an increase in cytosolic superoxide, as DHE levels remain unchanged in *scat* throughout differentiation, and comparable to those observed in WT (**Figure 2B**, right panel and Supplementary Figure 1).

Reactive oxygen species play a role in the regulation of the red cell lifespan (Friedman et al., 2004). Therefore, we evaluated these ROS levels in the peripheral blood of the mice. By using CD71 and Ter119 as markers, one can discriminate between reticulocytes and erythrocytes (**Figure 3A**). Due to the young age of the mice (less than 3 weeks old), there is a noticeable

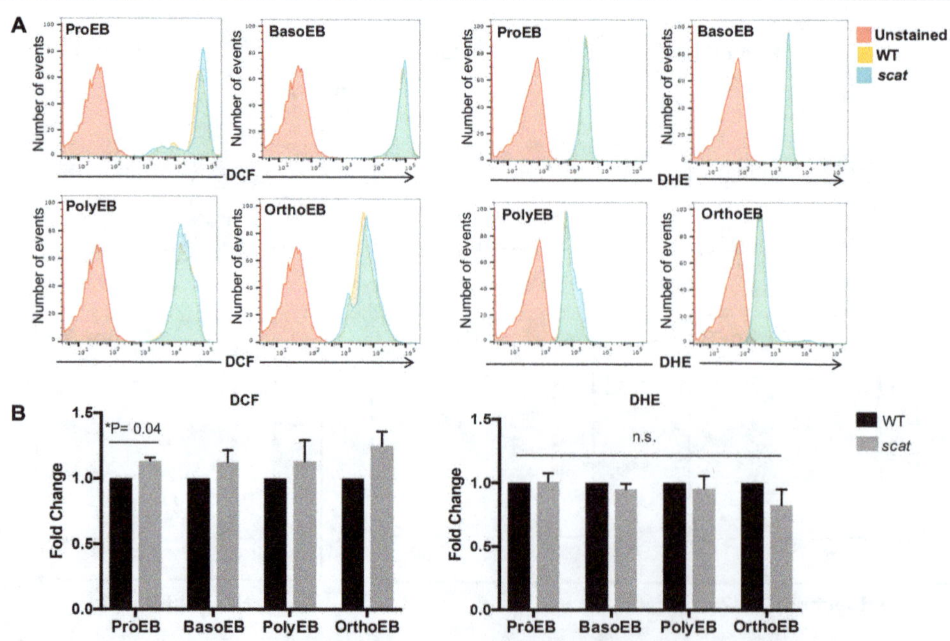

FIGURE 2 | There is an increase in peroxide levels at the proerythroblastic stage of erythropoiesis in the spleen of *scat* mice. **(A)** Representative histograms showing the levels of DCF (four left panels) and DHE (four right panels) in the spleen measured as fluorescence intensity. **(B)** Quantification of DCF and DHE levels by population in the spleen of wild type and *scat* mice. Measured as fold change normalized to wild type ($n = 6$ for DCF and $n = 14$ for DHE).

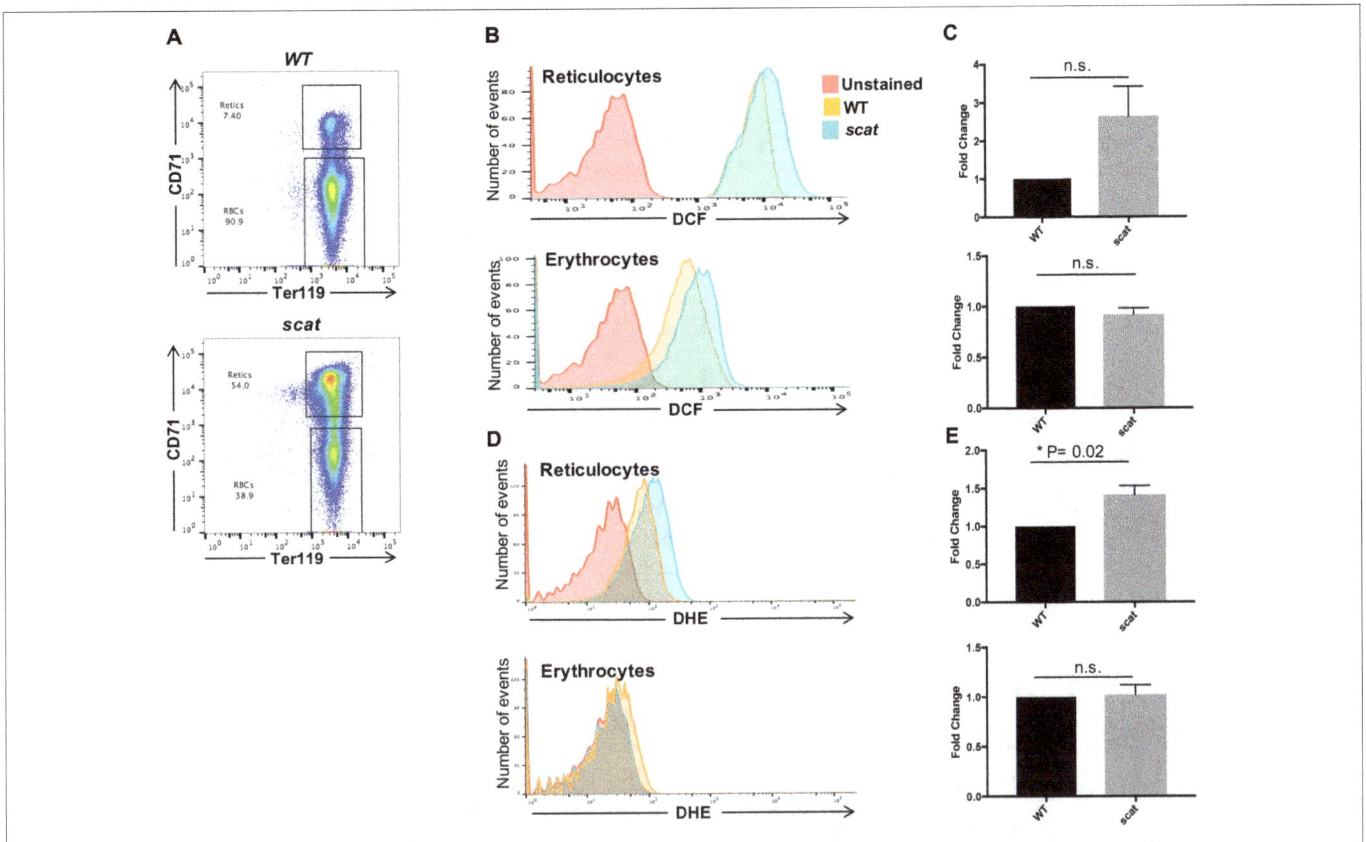

FIGURE 3 | Increased ROS in *scat* crisis reticulocytes. **(A)** Representative gating of reticulocytes and erythrocytes based on levels of CD71 in wild type and *scat* peripheral blood. **(B)** Representative histograms showing the levels of DCF measured as fluorescence intensity in reticulocytes and erythrocytes. **(C)** Quantification of DCF levels in reticulocytes and erythrocytes based on fold change. **(D)** Representative histograms showing the levels of DHE measured as fluorescence intensity in reticulocytes and erythrocytes. **(E)** Quantification of DHE levels in reticulocytes and erythrocytes based on fold change (n = 11 for DCF and n = 9 for DHE).

amount of reticulocytes in the bloodstream of WT animals. We observed that the trend toward increased DCF levels seen in the spleen (**Figure 2B**) is also present in *scat* reticulocytes (**Figures 3B,C**, upper panels). However, the increased levels of ROS normalize during reticulocyte maturation, as erythrocytes do not show an increase in DCF (**Figures 3B,C**, lower panels). Surprisingly, and unlike what we observed in the spleen, DHE levels are increased 1.4 times in *scat* reticulocytes compared to WT (**Figures 3D,E**, upper panels; P = 0.02). Nevertheless, this increase is transient, and the DHE levels normalize at the erythrocyte stage (**Figures 3D,E**, lower panels). Taken together, these results suggest that there is a transient increase in ROS, both early and late in erythroid differentiation in *scat*.

Mitochondria Are Eliminated Normally at the Reticulocyte Stage in the *scat* Mice

Mitochondria are an important source of ROS and are among the last organelles to be eliminated at the reticulocyte stage (Ney, 2011). Therefore, we assessed mitochondrial clearance during reticulocyte maturation in both WT and *scat* using MTR and TO as markers for mitochondria and reticulocyte maturation by RNA content, respectively. As shown in **Figure 4A**, no evidence of abnormal mitochondrial retention is seen in *scat*. While there is an increased overall number of reticulocytes in *scat* compared to WT due to the compensatory reticulocytosis, there are no $TO^-/MitR^+$ events, indicating no mature reticulocytes (TO^-) with mitochondria present. In addition, electron microscopy performed on the peripheral blood of WT and *scat* animals demonstrates that no aberrant mitochondria are observed in the *scat* reticulocytes (**Figure 4B**). Thus, we conclude that the increased ROS levels observed at the reticulocyte stage are not a byproduct of improper mitochondria elimination.

Apoptosis Is Decreased in *scat* During Erythropoiesis

Given the increased ROS in the reticulocytes and the overall cellular stress associated with the bone marrow failure observed in *scat*, we elected to investigate apoptosis at each stage of erythroid differentiation in the bone marrow and spleen. To do so, we used the markers Annexin V and 7AAD in addition to CD44, Ter119, and FSC as described previously (Liu et al., 2013). No significant increase in the overall percentage of early apoptotic (Annexin V^+ $7AAD^-$), late apoptotic (Annexin V^+ $7AAD^+$), or necrotic (Annexin V^- $7AAD^+$) cells in *scat* were seen compared to their littermate controls. However, we observed a significant decrease in

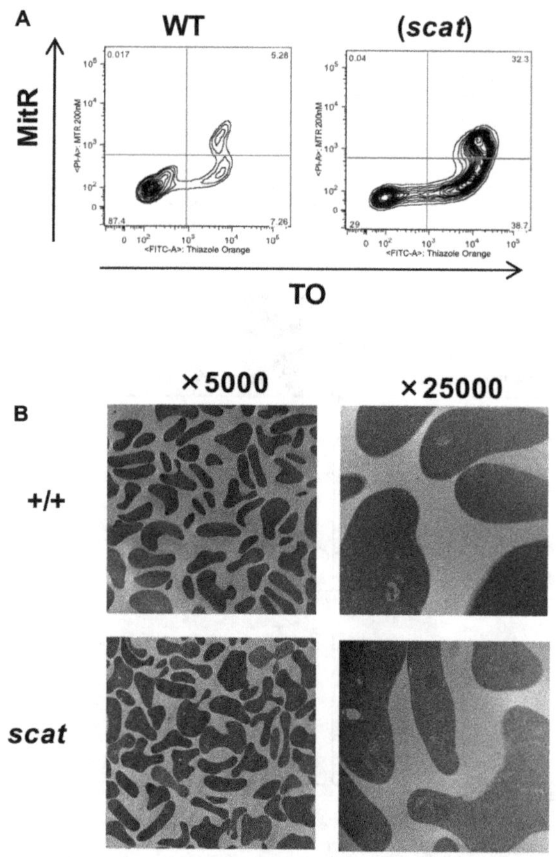

FIGURE 4 | Mitochondria are removed normally during erythropoiesis in *scat* mice. **(A)** Analysis of wild type and *scat* peripheral blood by flow cytometry using markers for mitochondria (MitR) and RNA content of reticulocytes (TO). Early reticulocytes are ribosome-positive, mitochondria-positive (upper right quadrant), late reticulocytes ribosome-positive, mitochondria-negative (lower right quadrant), and retained mitochondria ribosome-negative, mitochondria-positive (upper left quadrant). No evidence for increased mitochondrial retention is seen. Representative pattern from five independent experiments. **(B)** Electron microscopy of RBCs in wild type and *scat* mice shows no evidence of mitochondria retention.

the percentage of late apoptotic cells in the bone marrow (Supplementary Figure 2; $P < 0.05$). Additionally, when we quantified early apoptosis based on each individual erythroid population, we noticed a significant decrease in apoptosis in both scat bone marrow and spleen proerythroblastic, polychromatic, and orthochromatic stages (**Figures 5A,B**; $P < 0.05$). Together, these data suggest that loss of function in *Rasa3* leads to decreased apoptosis.

scat Mice Demonstrate Decreased Plasma and Serum Levels of Galectin-1

One of the most striking aspects of the *scat* phenotype is the cyclic remission that includes normalization or near normalization of hematologic parameters and external physical manifestations of anemia and thrombocytopenia. The fact that remission occurs without a correction to RASA3's aberrant location in the cytosol led to the hypothesis that a secreted factor may be mediating its onset. To test this hypothesis, we analyzed plasma cytokine profiles by cytokine array and identified several targets of interest, including galectin-1 (**Figure 6A**). Galectin-1 is a known mediator of stromal cell-to-stem cell interactions and transduction of intracellular signaling in the bone marrow hematopoietic niche (Liu and Rabinovich, 2010; Rabinovich and Vidal, 2011), and its levels were significantly decreased in *scat* mice during crisis compared to wild type (**Figure 6B**, 23326.5 ± 21439.72 vs. 31019.63897 ± 20110.65161; $P < 0.05$), making it our initial focus. Interestingly, well-known inflammatory mediators such as IL-1β and IL-6, were not significantly different between wild type and *scat*. To verify these results, we performed an ELISA on serum and plasma samples from *scat* and littermate wild type mice and indeed found significantly decreased levels of galectin-1 in samples from *scat* mice (**Figure 6C**, 2487.917 ± 606.1 pg/mL vs. 5562.417 ± 652.4 pg/mL; $P < 0.05$). Together, these results suggest that galectin-1 may play a role in the cyclic phenotype or serve as a biomarker of the crisis-remission transition observed in *scat*.

DISCUSSION

In this study, we elucidate mechanisms contributing to anemia in *scat* mice during crisis events and propose a model in which loss of RASA3 function during erythropoiesis leads to dysregulation of several key cellular processes with the final result of anemia (**Figure 7**). In the bone marrow and spleen, impaired cell cycle progression and increased ROS inhibit proper proliferation and terminal differentiation, leading to eventual decreased red cell output, despite decreased apoptosis. In the periphery, increased ROS further contribute to anemia and secreted factors such as galectin-1 have a yet to be elucidated role in modulating erythropoiesis. The *scat* model is very unique in the context of existing mouse models of inherited bone marrow failures. Most current models focus on the immune-mediated pathogenesis of acquired AA (Scheinberg and Chen, 2013), and models of congenital AA have focused on mutations in DNA-repair pathways, such as the $Fanc^{-/-}$ models and more recent $Brca^{-/-}$ model (Parmar et al., 2009; Vasanthakumar et al., 2016). Therefore, *scat* and its loss of function mutation in *Rasa3* implicate a unique signaling axis in congenital AA. Further, though these other models of congenital AA have similar hematopoietic defects and possibly convergent molecular mechanisms, *scat* is the only existing model with a cyclic phenotype that offers key opportunities to study both the onset and remission of some aspects of bone marrow failure.

Cell cycle progression and erythropoiesis are intricately co-regulated. Proper alignment of cell cycle status with phases of erythroid maturation is crucial for regulating the transition from proliferative progenitors to increasingly differentiated precursors, allowing production of a sufficient number of fully mature red cells. Known cell cycle regulators have been shown to play key cell-intrinsic roles in promoting

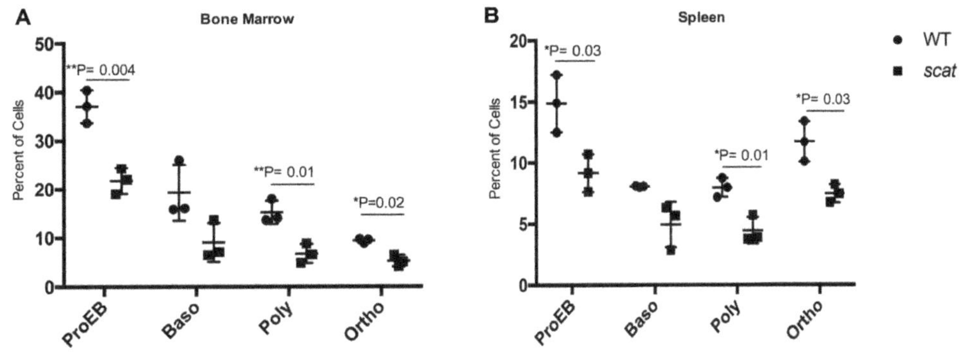

FIGURE 5 | Early apoptosis is significantly decreased in *scat* mice at three distinct erythroid populations. **(A)** Quantification of early apoptosis in the bone marrow of wild type and *scat* mice at the proerythroblastic, basophilic, polychromatophilic, and orthochromatic erythroid differentiation stages. **(B)** Quantification of early apoptosis in the spleen of wild type and *scat* mice at the proerythroblastic, basophilic, polychromatophilic, and orthochromatic erythroid differentiation stages (n = 3).

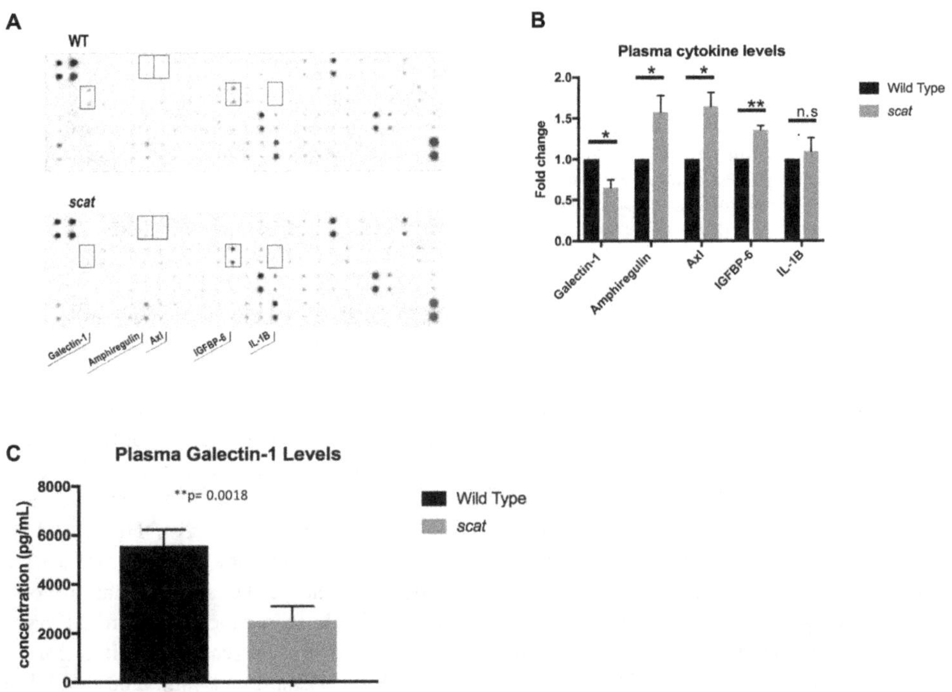

FIGURE 6 | Levels of specific cytokines, including galectin-1, are altered in *scat* plasma and serum. **(A)** Analysis of plasma samples from *scat* and littermate WT mice by cytokine array reveals significant differences in four cytokines: galectin-1, amphiregulin, Axl, IGFBP-6, and no significant difference in levels of IL-1B (n = 3). **(B)** Quantification of the fold change of the cytokines specified in **A**; galectin-1: p = 0.0154, amphiregulin: p = 0.0366, Axl: p = 0.0135, IGFBP-6: p = 0.0011, IL-1B: p = 0.5825. **(C)** ELISA analysis of plasma and serum samples diluted 1:10 verifies significantly decreased levels of galectin-1 in *scat* samples compared to littermate WT (n = 15; p = 0.0018). *p < 0.05 and **p < 0.01.

terminal erythroid differentiation (Sankaran et al., 2008). Further, Ras/Raf/MEK/ERK and Ras/PI3K/Akt pathways are known to control the transcription or regulation of key cell cycle regulators (Lee et al., 2008). Therefore, we examined the cell cycle status of individual erythroid differentiation populations in wild type and *scat* bone marrow. Our results demonstrate a pattern of accumulation in the G_0/G_1 phase in *scat*, suggestive of a defect at the G_1 checkpoint that normalizes or becomes indiscernible by the orthochromatic stage. During normal erythropoiesis, most orthochromatic erythroblasts have exited the cell cycle and entered G_0/G_1. The G_1 checkpoint integrates various intracellular signaling cascades, including pathways downstream of Ras, and either promotes or prevents DNA replication. Because loss of RASA3 function leads to increased active, GTP-bound Ras in *scat*, changes in Ras signaling pathways are likely influencing cell cycle progression. As mentioned above, the polychromatophilic to orthochromatic transition represents a key point of cell cycle exit during erythropoiesis that allows final terminal differentiation and enucleation. Prior work characterizing the erythroid

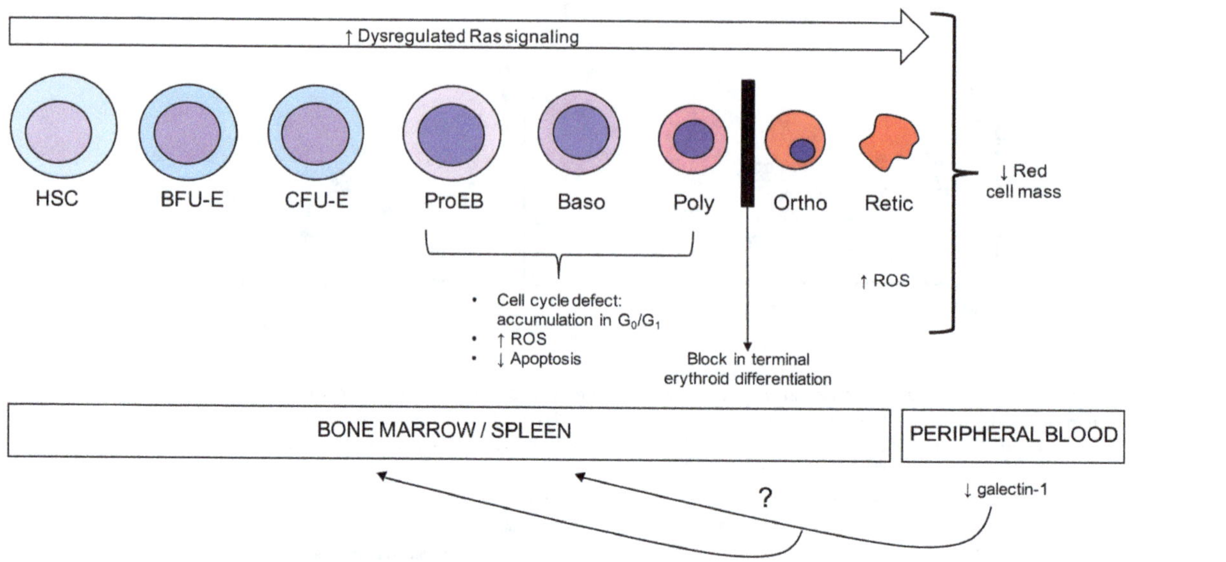

FIGURE 7 | Model of the mechanisms of anemia in the *scat* mouse model. Mutant RASA3 is rendered non-functional by its mislocalization to the cytosol, leading to dysregulated Ras signaling throughout erythroid differentiation. This dysregulated signaling is associated with an accumulation in the G_0/G_1 phase of the cell cycle in early erythroid precursors, impairing proper proliferation and differentiation and contributing to decreased red cell mass, despite decreased apoptosis in these populations. A block in terminal differentiation with an accumulation at the polychromatic/orthochromatic stages, as well as increased ROS accumulation in the reticulocyte stage further contribute to the anemia seen as a result of the loss of functional RASA3. Secreted factors, such as galectin-1, may contribute to mediating remission in the erythropoietic microenvironment while RASA3 remains mislocalized.

differentiation defect in *scat* demonstrated an accumulation specifically at the polychromatophilic/orthochromatic stages. This accumulation therefore aligns with and supports the notion of aberrant cell cycling in *scat* erythropoiesis. Finally, many inherited BMFS have a predisposition for hematologic malignancies that are characterized by dysregulated cell cycling (Al-Rahawan et al., 2008). Therefore, the altered cell cycle profiles observed in *scat* further support its characterization as a model of inherited bone marrow failure. Future work will characterize exactly which cell cycle regulators are being affected and how altered Ras signaling mediates these changes. We will notably investigate the role played by cyclins and CDKs in the regulation of the cell cycle. Due to the fragile nature of the *scat* mice in crisis, we were unable to inject Bromodeoxyuridine (BrdU) that would have allowed quantification of individual G_0/G_1, S, and G_2/M phases. However, even with our current methods, we were able to observe this consistent trend toward G_0/G_1 accumulation in *scat*.

We also identified increased ROS in *scat*, most notably the accumulation of superoxide in reticulocytes. ROS are known to negatively impact RBC health and lifespan, indicating that their increase likely contributes to the anemia of *scat* (Friedman et al., 2004). RASA3 is a known negative regulator of Ras activity, and previous studies have determined that upregulation of active Ras proteins can lead to increased intracellular ROS concentrations, further supporting a role for ROS in the *scat* phenotype (Zamkova et al., 2013). Impaired hemoglobin formation can also be a source of ROS. Accordingly, we previously documented hemoglobinization defects in *scat* (Blanc et al., 2012). Further studies will elucidate the mechanism(s) of increased ROS during erythropoiesis in *scat* by examining the activity of Ras isoforms, mitochondrial metabolism prior to proper removal, and hemoglobin synthesis. A surprising finding of the present work is the decrease in apoptosis seen in *scat* erythroid populations. Given the anemia and overall poor health of *scat*, one might expect to see an increase in apoptosis; however, this was not the case. Active H, K, and N-Ras are oncogenic proteins known to play a significant role in cell proliferation. Previous studies have shown that an overexpression of Ras isoforms leads to a block in terminal erythroid differentiation accompanied by increased proliferation of earlier erythroid populations (Zhang et al., 2003). Additionally, the same study demonstrated that the introduction of oncogenic Ras into erythroleukemia cells resulted in a block in terminal differentiation and extended proliferation with no effect on apoptosis (Zhang et al., 2003). This ability of precursor cells to survive and proliferate longer due to increased Ras signaling seen with loss of RASA3's negative regulation could potentially explain why apoptosis is decreased in *scat* compared to wild type mice. The mechanism of the interesting cyclic phenotype of the *scat* mouse has yet to be elucidated and likely holds key insights into general mechanisms of onset and resolution of BMFS. We hypothesized that secreted factors may be playing a role in mediating remission and thus compared the plasma cytokine profiles of *scat* crisis and wild type mice. Galectin-1 was consistently decreased in *scat* compared to wild type, but levels of common inflammatory mediators such as IL-6 and IL-1β were unchanged. Galectins, a family of β-galactoside binding proteins, have been shown to play key roles in the bone marrow niche and the erythroblastic island, indicating that these lectins have the capacity to modulate the maturation of hematopoietic cells. Within the bone marrow niche, galectins are known mediators of stromal cell-hematopoietic cell interactions (Rabinovich and Vidal, 2011). Galectin-5, a member of the same subfamily as galectin-1, has been specifically implicated in protein sorting and regulation of exosomal uptake in rat erythroblastic islands (Barres et al., 2010). Further, galectins are also known modulators of various mitogen-activated protein kinase (MAPK) signaling pathways in several cell types, including key pathways (PI3K/Akt, Raf/Mek/MAPK) downstream of Ras that are likely to be altered with loss of RASA3 (Masamune et al., 2006; Shimizu et al., 2009). In this context, the ability of galectin-1 to modulate these signaling pathways is of great interest. Though existing data is intriguing and suggestive of galectin-1's importance, future studies will be required to prove any mechanistic role for galectin-1 in the cyclic bone marrow failure phenotype, rather than its decrease simply being an effect of loss of RASA3 function across all cell types in the mouse, or a generic serum biomarker of disease.

AUTHOR CONTRIBUTIONS

EH and EB designed and performed the research, analyzed the data, and wrote the manuscript. JP, SC, and YZ performed the research, analyzed the data, and edited the manuscript. LP and LB designed the research, analyzed the data, and wrote the manuscript.

REFERENCES

Al-Rahawan, M. M., Alter, B. P., Bryant, B. J., and Elghetany, M. T. (2008). Bone marrow cell cycle markers in inherited bone marrow failure syndromes. *Leuk. Res.* 32, 1793–1799. doi: 10.1016/j.leukres.2008.05.020

Barres, C., Blanc, L., Bette-Bobillo, P., Andre, S., Mamoun, R., Gabius, H. J., et al. (2010). Galectin-5 is bound onto the surface of rat reticulocyte exosomes and modulates vesicle uptake by macrophages. *Blood* 115, 696–705. doi: 10.1182/blood-2009-07-231449

Blanc, L., Ciciotte, S. L., Gwynn, B., Hildick-Smith, G. J., Pierce, E. L., Soltis, K. A., et al. (2012). Critical function for the Ras-GTPase activating protein RASA3 in vertebrate erythropoiesis and megakaryopoiesis. *Proc. Natl. Acad. Sci. U.S.A.* 109, 12099–12104. doi: 10.1073/pnas.1204948109

Bodine, D., and Berliner, N. (2014). Introduction to the review series on "bone marrow failure". *Blood* 124:2755. doi: 10.1182/blood-2014-08-587394

de Jager, W., Bourcier, K., Rijkers, G. T., Prakken, B. J., and Seyfert-Margolis, V. (2009). Prerequisites for cytokine measurements in clinical trials with multiplex immunoassays. *BMC Immunol.* 10:52. doi: 10.1186/1471-2172-10-52

Friedman, J. S., Lopez, M. F., Fleming, M. D., Rivera, A., Martin, F. M., Welsh, M. L., et al. (2004). SOD2-deficiency anemia: protein oxidation and altered protein expression reveal targets of damage, stress response, and antioxidant responsiveness. *Blood* 104, 2565–2573. doi: 10.1182/blood-2003-11-3858

Fukuda, M., and Mikoshiba, K. (1996). Structure-function relationships of the mouse Gap1m. Determination of the inositol 1,3,4,5-tetrakisphosphate-binding domain. *J. Biol. Chem.* 271, 18838–18842. doi: 10.1074/jbc.271.31.18838

George, A., Pushkaran, S., Konstantinidis, D. G., Koochaki, S., Malik, P., Mohandas, N., et al. (2013). Erythrocyte NADPH oxidase activity modulated by Rac GTPases, PKC, and plasma cytokines contributes to oxidative stress in sickle cell disease. *Blood* 121, 2099–2107. doi: 10.1182/blood-2012-07-441188

Guinan, E. C. (2011). Diagnosis and management of aplastic anemia. *Hematology Am. Soc. Hematol. Educ. Program* 2011, 76–81. doi: 10.1182/asheducation-2011.1.76

Khincha, P. P., and Savage, S. A. (2013). Genomic characterization of the inherited bone marrow failure syndromes. *Semin. Hematol.* 50, 333–347. doi: 10.1053/j.seminhematol.2013.09.002

Lee, J. T., Lehmann, B. D., Terrian, D. M., Chappell, W. H., Stivala, F., Libra, M., et al. (2008). Targeting prostate cancer based on signal transduction and cell cycle pathways. *Cell Cycle* 7, 1745–1762. doi: 10.4161/cc.7.12.6166

Liu, F. T., and Rabinovich, G. A. (2010). Galectins: regulators of acute and chronic inflammation. *Ann. N. Y. Acad. Sci.* 1183, 158–182. doi: 10.1111/j.1749-6632.2009.05131.x

Liu, J., Zhang, J., Ginzburg, Y., Li, H., Xue, F., De Franceschi, L., et al. (2013). Quantitative analysis of murine terminal erythroid differentiation in vivo: novel method to study normal and disordered erythropoiesis. *Blood* 121, e43–e49. doi: 10.1182/blood-2012-09-456079

Masamune, A., Satoh, M., Hirabayashi, J., Kasai, K., Satoh, K., and Shimosegawa, T. (2006). Galectin-1 induces chemokine production and proliferation in pancreatic stellate cells. *Am. J. Physiol. Gastrointest. Liver Physiol.* 290, G729–G736. doi: 10.1152/ajpgi.00511.2005

Miano, M., and Dufour, C. (2015). The diagnosis and treatment of aplastic anemia: a review. *Int. J. Hematol.* 101, 527–535. doi: 10.1007/s12185-015-1787-z

Ney, P. A. (2011). Normal and disordered reticulocyte maturation. *Curr. Opin. Hematol.* 18, 152–157. doi: 10.1097/MOH.0b013e328345213e

Parmar, K., D'andrea, A., and Niedernhofer, L. J. (2009). Mouse models of Fanconi anemia. *Mutat. Res.* 668, 133–140. doi: 10.1016/j.mrfmmm.2009.03.015

Peters, L. L., Paw, B. H., and Blanc, L. (2013). The scat mouse model highlights RASA3, a GTPase activating protein, as a key regulator of vertebrate erythropoiesis and megakaryopoiesis. *Small GTPases* 4, 47–50. doi: 10.4161/sgtp.23013

Pop, R., Shearstone, J. R., Shen, Q., Liu, Y., Hallstrom, K., Koulnis, M., et al. (2010). A key commitment step in erythropoiesis is synchronized with the cell cycle clock through mutual inhibition between PU.1 and S-phase progression. *PLoS Biol.* 8:e1000484. doi: 10.1371/journal.pbio.1000484

Rabinovich, G. A., and Vidal, M. (2011). Galectins and microenvironmental niches during hematopoiesis. *Curr. Opin. Hematol.* 18, 443–451. doi: 10.1097/MOH.0b013e32834bab18

Rankin, E. B., Narla, A., Park, J. K., Lin, S., and Sakamoto, K. M. (2015). Biology of the bone marrow microenvironment and myelodysplastic syndromes. *Mol. Genet. Metab.* 116, 24–28. doi: 10.1016/j.ymgme.2015.07.004

Richardson, C., Yan, S., and Vestal, C. G. (2015). Oxidative stress, bone marrow failure, and genome instability in hematopoietic stem cells. *Int. J. Mol. Sci.* 16, 2366–2385. doi: 10.3390/ijms16022366

Sankaran, V. G., Orkin, S. H., and Walkley, C. R. (2008). Rb intrinsically promotes erythropoiesis by coupling cell cycle exit with mitochondrial biogenesis. *Genes Dev.* 22, 463–475. doi: 10.1101/gad.1627208

Scheinberg, P., and Chen, J. (2013). Aplastic anemia: what have we learned from animal models and from the clinic. *Semin. Hematol.* 50, 156–164. doi: 10.1053/j.seminhematol.2013.03.028

Shimamura, A., and Alter, B. P. (2010). Pathophysiology and management of inherited bone marrow failure syndromes. *Blood Rev.* 24, 101–122. doi: 10.1016/j.blre.2010.03.002

Shimizu, M., Khoshnoodi, J., Akimoto, Y., Kawakami, H., Hirano, H., Higashihara, E., et al. (2009). Expression of galectin-1, a new component of slit diaphragm, is altered in minimal change nephrotic syndrome. *Lab. Invest.* 89, 178–195. doi: 10.1038/labinvest.2008.125

Vasanthakumar, A., Arnovitz, S., Marquez, R., Lepore, J., Rafidi, G., Asom, A., et al. (2016). Brca1 deficiency causes bone marrow failure and spontaneous hematologic malignancies in mice. *Blood* 127, 310–313. doi: 10.1182/blood-2015-03-635599

Zamkova, M., Khromova, N., Kopnin, B. P., and Kopnin, P. (2013). Ras-induced ROS upregulation affecting cell proliferation is connected with cell type-specific alterations of HSF1/SESN3/p21Cip1/WAF1 pathways. *Cell Cycle* 12, 826–836. doi: 10.4161/cc.23723

Zhang, J., Randall, M. S., Loyd, M. R., Dorsey, F. C., Kundu, M., Cleveland, J. L., et al. (2009). Mitochondrial clearance is regulated by Atg7-dependent and -independent mechanisms during reticulocyte maturation. *Blood* 114, 157–164. doi: 10.1182/blood-2008-04-151639

Zhang, J., Socolovsky, M., Gross, A. W., and Lodish, H. F. (2003). Role of Ras signaling in erythroid differentiation of mouse fetal liver cells: functional analysis by a flow cytometry-based novel culture system. *Blood* 102, 3938–3946. doi: 10.1182/blood-2003-05-1479

7

Use of Laser Assisted Optical Rotational Cell Analyzer (LoRRca MaxSis) in the Diagnosis of RBC Membrane Disorders, Enzyme Defects and Congenital Dyserythropoietic Anemias: A Monocentric Study on 202 Patients

*Anna Zaninoni[1], Elisa Fermo[1], Cristina Vercellati[1], Dario Consonni[2], Anna P. Marcello[1], Alberto Zanella[1], Agostino Cortelezzi[1,3], Wilma Barcellini[1] and Paola Bianchi[1]**

[1] UOC Oncoematologia, UOS Fisiopatologia delle Anemie, Fondazione IRCCS Ca' Granda Ospedale Maggiore Policlinico, Milan, Italy, [2] UO Epidemiologia, Fondazione IRCCS Ca' Granda Ospedale Maggiore Policlinico, Milan, Italy, [3] Università degli Studi di Milano, Milan, Italy

***Correspondence:**
Paola Bianchi
paola.bianchi@policlinico.mi.it

Chronic hemolytic anemias are a group of heterogeneous diseases mainly due to abnormalities of red cell (RBC) membrane and metabolism. The more common RBC membrane disorders, classified on the basis of blood smear morphology, are hereditary spherocytosis (HS), elliptocytosis, and hereditary stomatocytoses (HSt). Among RBC enzymopathies, the most frequent is pyruvate kinase (PK) deficiency, followed by glucose-6-phosphate isomerase, pyrimidine 5′ nucleotidase P5′N, and other rare enzymes defects. Because of the rarity and heterogeneity of these diseases, diagnosis may be often challenging despite the availability of a variety of laboratory tests. The ektacytometer laser-assisted optical rotational cell analyser (LoRRca MaxSis), able to assess the RBC deformability in osmotic gradient conditions (Osmoscan analysis), is a useful diagnostic tool for RBC membrane disorders and in particular for the identification of hereditary stomatocytosis. Few data are so far available in other hemolytic anemias. We evaluated the diagnostic power of LoRRca MaxSis in a large series of 140 patients affected by RBC membrane disorders, 37 by enzymopathies, and 16 by congenital diserythropoietic anemia type II. Moreover, nine patients with paroxysmal nocturnal hemoglobinuria (PNH) were also investigated. All the hereditary spherocytoses, regardless the biochemical defect, showed altered Osmoscan curves, with a decreased Elongation Index (EI) max and right shifted Omin; hereditary elliptocytosis (HE) displayed a trapezoidal curve and decreased EImax. Dehydrated hereditary stomatocytosis (DHSt) caused by *PIEZO1* mutations was characterized by left-shifted curve, whereas *KCNN4* mutations were associated with a normal curve. Congenital diserythropoietic anemia type II and RBC enzymopathies had Osmoscan curve within the normal range except for glucosephosphate isomerase (GPI) deficient cases who displayed an enlarged curve associated with significantly increased Ohyper, offering a new diagnostic tool for this rare enzyme defect. The Osmoscan analysis performed by LoRRca MaxSis represents a useful and feasible first step screening test for specialized centers involved in the diagnosis of hemolytic anemias. However, the results should be interpreted by caution because different factors (i.e., splenectomy or coexistent diseases) may interfere with the analysis; additional tests or molecular investigations are therefore needed to confirm the diagnosis.

Keywords: red cell disorders, chronic hemolytic anemias, ektacytometer, LoRRca MaxSis, red cell membrane defects, red cell metabolism, differential diagnosis

INTRODUCTION

Hereditary red cell membrane disorders and defects of RBC metabolism are a group of rare and heterogeneous disorders eases characterized by chronic hemolytic anemia of variable degree, jaundice, and splenomegaly. The diagnostic workflow is based on laboratory tests, clinical examination, personal, and family history, and on the exclusion of other causes of hemolysis. However, because of their rarity and wide clinical heterogeneity, the diagnosis of these defects is often difficult, particularly in mild and atypical forms.

RBC membrane disorders are caused by defects of cytoskeleton proteins, which form a complex network providing the erythrocyte with its shape and deformability. Consequently, abnormalities of single proteins may impair the structural and functional integrity of the entire membrane causing an alteration of RBC shape. In general, defects in spectrin, ankyrin, protein band 3, and band 4.2 weaken the cohesion between the membrane lipid bilayer and cytoskeleton, leading to the release of microvesicles, loss of surface, and transformation of the discocyte into a spherocyte: these alterations result in hereditary spherocytosis (HS). Conversely, hereditary elliptocytosis (HE) is due to impaired interaction of spectrin dimers or defective spectrin-actin-protein 4.1 complex. If cytoskeleton weakening is excessive, red blood cells can undergo severe deformations resulting in hereditary pyropoikilocytosis (HPP), which mimicks cell fragmentation due to heat exposure (Mohandas and Gallagher, 2008; Perrotta et al., 2008).

The hereditary stomatocytoses (HSt) are caused by defects of membrane cation permeability and cell volume regulation; they are divided in two different entities: dehydrated hereditary stomatocytosis (DHSt) due to mutations in *PIEZO1* and *KCNN4* genes, and overhydrated hereditary stomatocytosis (OHS) associated with mutations in *RhAG* gene; additional more rare forms of stomatocytosis include defects in *ABCB6* (pseudohyperkaliemia) or *GLUT1* (cryohydrocytosis with neurological impairment) (Glogowska and Gallagher, 2015; Badens and Guizouarn, 2016).

The laboratory diagnosis of HS and other RBC membrane disorders is usually based on indirect assays that investigate the surface area-to-volume ratio, typically reduced in spherocytes, such as NaCl osmotic fragility tests (on fresh and incubated blood), Glycerol Lysis (GLT) and Acidified Glycerol Lysis tests (AGLT), and Pink test. These methods do not differentiate HS from secondary spherocytosis and may result falsely negative in some HS cases, particularly the mildest ones. The direct flow cytometric EMA-binding test (King et al., 2000), shows high sensitivity and specificity (Bianchi et al., 2012). In severe or atypical HS, the diagnostic workflow may require SDS-PAGE quantification of RBC membrane proteins (King et al., 2015) or more recently molecular characterization of the defect through NGS platforms (He et al., 2017). SDS-PAGE analysis is also necessary in differential diagnosis of congenital dyserythropoietic anemia type II (CDAII) (King and Zanella, 2013).

Chronic hereditary hemolytic anemias are also due to enzymatic defects of erythrocyte metabolism. Metabolic energy is needed to maintain the red cell shape, to keep the iron of hemoglobin in the divalent form, to pump ions against electrochemical gradients and to maintain the sulfydryl groups of proteins in the active, reduced forms. Pyruvate kinase (PK) deficiency is the most common ezymopathy associated with chronic hemolytic anemia, followed by glucosephosphate isomerase (GPI) and pyrimidine 5′-nucleotidase (P5′N) deficiencies (Koralkova et al., 2014). The diagnosis of these disorders relies on the exclusion of the more common hemolytic anemias, ultimately depending on the determination of red cell enzyme activity by quantitative assays and identification of the molecular defect in the causative genes. However, except for the rare enzymopathies whose causative genes have an ubiquitous expression leading to non-hematological signs (myopathy and neuromuscular abnormalities in triosephosphate isomerase (TPI) or phosphoglycerate kinase (PGK) deficiency), the clinical picture of these diseases is similar to the other congenital hemolytic anemias, making in some cases differential diagnosis tricking with possible misdiagnosis.

Osmotic gradient ektacytometry, which measures red cell deformability, osmotic fragility and cell hydration, has long been considered a reference technique for diagnosis of RBC membrane disorders, particularly HSt. Ektacytometry was however rarely used as a routine diagnostic tool due to the limited availability of the original device. Recently, a new generation ektacytometer has been made available, the Laser-assisted Optical Rotational Cell Analyzer (LoRRca), which is proposed as a simple laboratory method to detect red cell membrane abnormalities (Da Costa et al., 2013, 2016; Lazarova et al., 2017; Llaudet-Planas et al., 2018). Few data are so far available in other hemolytic anemias.

In this study we evaluated the performance and the diagnostic power of the LoRRca MaxSis in a large series of 202 consecutive patients with different forms of chronic hemolytic anemias referred to our Institution over the period 2014–2017, with the aim of ascertaining the possible role of this tool in the workflow of a laboratory specialized in the diagnosis of these diseases.

MATERIALS AND METHODS

Patients

A total of 202 consecutive patients with chronic hemolytic anemias (102 males and 100 females, median age 29 years, range 0.3–82 years) were diagnosed from 2014 to 2017. Peripheral blood was collected from patients and controls during diagnostic procedures after obtaining informed consent and approval from the Institutional Human Research Committee. The procedures followed were in accordance with the Helsinki international ethical standards on human experimentation. The great majority of samples were collected in our Institute; samples from other centers were shipped maintaining a temperature of 4°C and processed within 24 h. All tests were performed in a single site. None of the patients had been transfused within the 3 months preceding the study.

Testing for Diagnosis of Chronic Hemolytic Anemias

The diagnostic workflow for chronic hemolytic anemias includes RBC morphology, complete blood count, hemolysis markers, EMA binding test, osmotic fragility tests, and RBC enzymes activities. Confirmatory tests include SDS-PAGE analysis of red cell membrane proteins, and molecular testing for hereditary stomatocytosis, CDAII and enzymopathies.

Routine hematological investigations were carried out according to Dacie and Lewis (2001). The RBC morphology was assessed by two independent and expert operators. Red cell osmotic fragility was evaluated by the following tests: NaCl osmotic fragility test on both fresh and incubated blood, standard GLT, AGLT, and Pink test. EMA-binding test was performed as described by King et al. (2000) with minor modifications (Bianchi et al., 2012). Since 2014 Osmoscan LoRRca analysis was included in the diagnostic panel and performed in all the patients referred to our Institute to confirm the diagnosis of hemolytic anemia. The diagnostic workflow adopted for chronic hemolytic anemias is reported in **Figure 1**.

Red cell membrane proteins were analyzed by SDS-PAGE according to Fairbanks et al. (1971) and Laemmli (1970); on the basis of SDS-PAGE analysis HS patients were stratified according to their membrane defects on the following groups: deficiency of band 3, spectrin, ankyrin or combined spectrin/ankyrin, and no detectable defect (Mariani et al., 2008).

RBC enzymes activities were determined according to Beutler (1984); diagnosis of a red cell enzyme defect was confirmed at molecular level by DNA sequencing (*PK-LR* gene for PK deficiency, *GPI* gene for GPI deficiency, *NT5C3A* for P5′N, *TPI1* for TPI). Molecular testing was performed also in CDAII (*SEC23B* gene) and hereditary stomatocytosis patients (*PIEZO1* and *KCNN4* genes).

Osmotic Gradient Ektacytometry (Osmoscan Curve)

Two hundred and fifty microliters of EDTA sample suspended in 5 mL of polyvinylpyrrolidone buffer (PVP, Mechatronics, Hoorn, The Netherlands) were used for the analysis. Osmoscan was performed by means of Laser-assisted Optical Rotation Cell Analyzer (LoRRca MaxSis, Mechatronics, Hoorn, The Netherlands) according to the manufacturer's instructions and as reported in detail by Da Costa et al. (2013, 2016). The osmotic gradient curves reflect RBC deformability as a continuous function of suspending medium osmolality. The following parameters were evaluated: the Omin-value corresponds to the osmolality at which the deformability reaches its minimum and represents the 50% of the RBCs hemolysis in conventional osmotic fragility assays, reflecting mean cellular surface-to-volume ratio; the elongation index (EI) max corresponds to the maximal deformability or elongation obtained near the isotonic osmolality and is an expression of the membrane surface; the Ohyper (the osmolality in the hypertonic region corresponding to 50% of the EImax) reflects mean cellular hydration status; the area under the curve (AUC), is defined in the provided software as the AUC beginning from a starting point in the hypo-osmolar region and an ending point in the hyper-osmolar region (instrument settings 500 mOsm/kg; Baskurt and Meiselman, 2004; Baskurt et al., 2009). The corresponding parameters on the X or Y axis of Omin (EImin), EImax (Omax), and Ohyper (EIhyper), respectively, were also analyzed.

Osmoscan Analysis in Normal Subject

We evaluated Osmoscan curve of 170 healthy blood donors. All the main parameters of the curve showed a Gaussian distribution, therefore the area covered by all the control curves was considered as the reference range. Osmoscan profile obtained from each patient was compared with the reference range curve and with a daily normal control analyzed together with the sample.

Statistical Analysis

We calculated Sperman's rho correlation coefficients of osmoscan parameters and hematologic data either considering the total number of patients ($n = 202$), independently from the disease, either in HS/not HS patients. Osmoscan parameters across diseases were compared with Kruskal-Wallis tests. Receiver operating characteristic (ROC) analysis was used to calculate the Omin cut-off to discriminate HS between normal control and patients with other membrane defects. We also calculated sensitivity (Se) and specificity (Sp) at optimal cut-offs calculated according to the non-parametric approach proposed by Liu (2012), implemented in the Stata command "cutpt." Statistical analyses were performed with Stata 15 (StataCorp, 2017)

RESULTS

Patients

On the basis of these criteria 116 patients were diagnosed as HS and 86 as hemolytic anemias other than HS: 15 HE, 9 HSt (6 *PIEZO1* and 3 *KCNN4* variants), 37 erythroenzymopaties (27

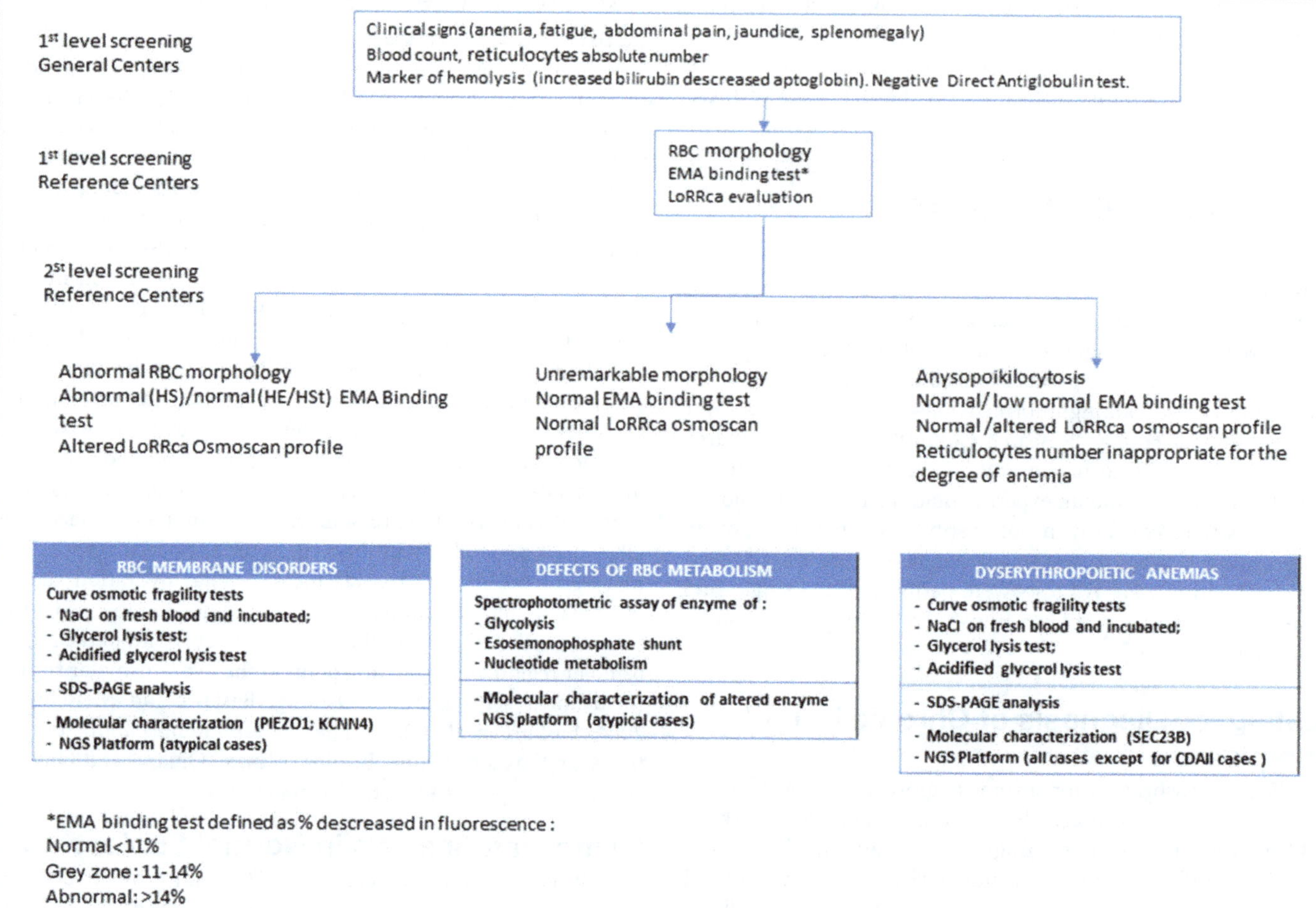

FIGURE 1 | Diagnostic workflow for chronic hemolytic anemias.

PK, 4 P5′N, 1 TPI, and 5 GPI deficiency), 16 CDAII. Nine patients underwent further investigations and were diagnosed as paroxysmal nocturnal hemoglobinuria (PNH). At the time of the study, 39 patients were splenectomized and 154 non-splenectomized. Hematologic and laboratory data of the patients grouped on the basis of their pathology and presence or not of spleen are reported in **Table 1**.

Osmoscan Curve in Chronic Hemolytic Anemias

Typical Osmoscan profiles obtained in different kind of hemolytic anemias are reported in **Figure 2**; the median values and range of specific parameters are summarized in **Table 2** for all the patients and normal controls. To reach a significant volume of data for statistical analysis some enzymopathies (PK, P5′N, and TPI deficiency) were grouped together since they didn't show significant differences of Osmoscan parameters (data not shown). Patients affected by GPI deficiency were separately considered due to typical abnormalities of Osmoscan curve.

Osmoscan curves were analyzed in splenectomized and non-splenectomized patients; significant differences in shape were observed particularly in enzyme deficiencies and CDAII patients (see below), therefore for these diseases only data from non-splenectomized patients are reported in **Table 2**.

The results of Osmoscan parameters were correlated with hematologic data, in particular RBC morphology (number of spherocytes, elliptocytes, or stomatocytes), red cell indexes (MVC, MCHC), osmotic fragility tests (GLT, AGLT), and EMA binding test (**Table 3** and **Supplementary Figure 1**). Omin showed a negative correlation with GLT, AGLT, and a positive one with EMA-binding test. Moreover, Omin was associated with results of incubated osmotic fragility test (NaCl inc) being 137 $\pm$ 28.7, 154 $\pm$ 11.5, and 166 $\pm$ 12.6 mOsm/kg in patients with decreased, normal or increased osmotic fragility, respectively ($p < 0.0001$). Interestingly, EImax was positively correlated with EMA binding test results; Ohyper showed a negative correlation with MCHC. Finally, AUC was correlated with RBC parameters and osmotic fragility tests, as expected being the resultant of Osmoscan parameters.

Hereditary Spherocytosis

The typical Osmoscan curve in HS patients is reported to be characterized by a decreased EImax, a shift to the right of Omin and to the left of Ohyper and, consequently, a

TABLE 1 | Hematological characteristics of 202 consecutive patients with chronic hemolytic anemias divided according to disease.

SPLENECTOMY		Hb (gr/dL)	Reticulocyte ($x10^9$/L)	MCV (fL)	MCH (pg/cell)	MCHC (gr/dL)	RDW (%)	Uncojugated bilirubin (mg/dL)	RBC morphology** (%)	EMA (% reduction)
		(F 12–16; M 13.5–17.5)	(24–84)	(78–99)	(25–35)	(31–37)	(11.8–14.8)	(<0.8)	Na	(<11%)
HS	NO	12	266	84	29.7	35.9	18.4	1.95	9	−29
	(N = 92)	(6.3/16.4)	(35/649)	(69/95.4)	(23.5/34.7)	(30.1/40.1)	(11.4/26.3)	(0.5/10.1)	(2/59)	(−62/+2)
	YES	15.7	145	86.6	32.3	35.7	13	0.71	7.5	−29
	(N = 16)	(9.3/17.6)	(51/362)	(75/97.3)	(30.4/33.1)	(29.4/38)	(11.1/19.7)	(0.2/9.3)	(1/19)	(−38/−16)
HE	NO	13.8	59	84	29.5	35	13.4	0.9	43	−8
	(N = 15)	(9.8/15.9)	(31/260)	(56.3*/92.2)	(19.3/32)	(33.1/36.4)	(11.8/17.5)	(0.4/1.4)	(10/90)	(−14/+4)
	YES	Na	Na	Na	Na	Na	Na	Na	Na	Na
	(N = 0)									
HSt	NO	9.9	260	102	36.7	35.7	16	3.2	8	+6
	(N = 5)	(8.3/13)	(104–273)	(71.9*/110)	(24.8/39.2)	(34.5/37.8)	(13.9/18.6)	(1.7/4.8)	(6/22)	(−5/+15)
	YES	11.7	272.5	105	37.5	35	16	1.7	13	+22
	(N = 4)	(11/13.2)	(166/654)	(101/109)	(34.1/40.1)	(33.5/38.3)	(15.1/19.7)	(0.8/6.7)	(6/33)	(+5/+30)
PK, P5′N,	NO	10.3	171	94	32.8	34.3	13.6	2.2	Na	+7
	(N = 26)	(5/14.5)	(53/727)	(67.6*/108)	(23.1/36.7)	(28.8/36.3)	(10.9/21.4)	(0.5/9.6)		(−9/+22)
TPI, GPI	YES	9.3	508	120	37.8	32.6	15.3	5.2	Na	+23
	(N = 11)	(7.5/12)	(88/1740)	(85.3/127)	(27.8/41.1)	(31.6/33.5)	(12.7/24.7)	(1.3/13.5)		(+19/+33)
CDAII	NO	10.7	92.5	86.4	30	35	19.4	2.2	Na	−13
	(N = 9)	(7.4/12.7)	(64/121)	(75.2/94)	(25.3/31.6)	(32.9/38.2)	(13.4/24)	(1/3.8)		(−19/+17)
	YES	10.1	40	94	33.6	33.7	20	1.7	Na	−20.5
	(N = 7)	(8.3/11.3)	(35/63)	(83.4/96.7)	(27.4/33.7)	(31.2/34.9)	(17.1/29.7)	(0.7/5.7)		(−28/−11)
PNH	NO	10.6	97	93.7	32	32.6	15.7	0.9	Na	+3
	(N = 9)	(7.9/13.6)	(52/248)	(81.3/111)	(27.7/34.4)	(31.1/34.9)	(12.8/20)	(0.5/1.4)		(+1/+16)
	YES	Na	Na	Na	Na	Na	Na	Na	Na	Na
	(N = 0)									

Values are expressed as median (range); Hb, hemoglobin, MCV, mean cell volume; MCH, mean corpuscular hemoglobin; MCHC, mean corpuscular hemoglobin concentration; RDW, red cell distribution width; RBC, red blood cell; EMA, EMAbinding test; Na, not available.
**beta-trait. ** % spherocytes for HS; % elliptocytes for HE; % stomatocytes for HSt.*

decreased AUC. As shown in **Table 2**, differences in all these parameters were observed when comparing HS patients with normal controls ($p < 0.001$). All the patients showed decreased AUC (referring to mean ± 2 SD of controls), all but two decreased Elmax, the majority (91%) had increased Omin, but only 31% had decreased Ohyper; 27 patients showed abnormalities in all the four parameters. Interestingly, 12/116 HS patients showed increased Ohyper generating a second kind of osmoscan profile for HS (**Figure 2A**). No differences were observed when patients were stratified according to splenectomy, to the type of biochemical defect (spectrin, spectrin/ankyrin, band 3, 4.2 protein deficiency), or to the severity of anemia.

Hereditary Elliptocytosis

Due to the elongated shape and decreased deformability, the resulting Osmoscan analysis in HE is characterized by a trapezoidal curve that is considered a typical finding in this disease. In the analyzed series (**Table 2**), HE patients (n = 15) displayed increased Omin (median 154, range 130–178), decreased Elmax (median 0.53, range 0.47–0.59), and AUC (median 119, range 106–157) ($p < 0.001$ for all). Typical trapezoidal shape was observed only in nine out of the 15 analyzed patients; in the remaining six cases (including the three patients with protein 4.1 defect) the curve fell in the area covered by HS patients (**Figure 2B**) making not possible a differential diagnosis among these two diseases by Osmoscan only. The shape of the curve was independent from the amount of ovalo/elliptocytes, ranging from 10 to 90%.

Hereditary Stomatocytosis

Six out of the nine HSt patients analyzed had mutations in *PIEZO1* gene and showed an Osmoscan curve characterized by

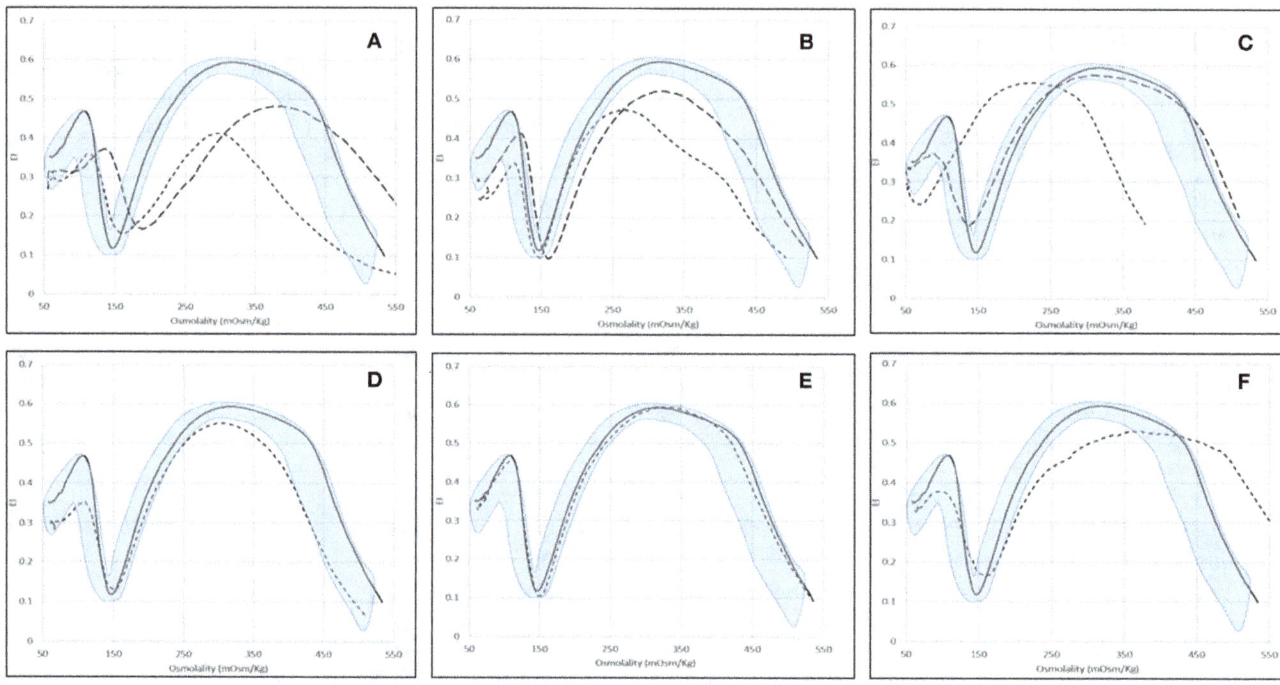

FIGURE 2 | Examples of typical osmoscan profiles in hemolytic anemias. Continuous line represents a daily control and shaded area the control range curve. **(A)** HS = hereditary spherocytosis: HS1 (- - -), HS2 (— — —); **(B)** HE = hereditary elliptocytosis: HE1 (- - -), HE2 (— — —); **(C)** HSt = hereditary stomatocytosis: HSt-PIEZO1 (- - -), HSt-KCNN4 (- - -); **(D)** CDAII (non-splenectomised) = congenital diserythropoietic anemia type II; **(E)** PKD (non-splenectomised) = pyruvate kinase deficiency; **(F)** GPI = glucosephosphate isomerase deficiency.

normal AUC and EImax, increased EImin (median 0.18, range 0.14–0.24) and significant left-shift of both Omin (median 98, range 71–136) and Ohyper (median 394, range 342–416, $p < 0.001$, for both) (**Figure 2C**). On the contrary, the remaining three patients, presenting R352H mutation in *KCNN4* gene, displayed Osmoscan parameters comparable to normal controls (**Table 2, Figure 2C**).

Congenital Dyserythropoietic Anemia Type II

The Osmoscan curve of the nine non-splenectomized cases showed increased Omin (median 152, range 133–164, $p < 0.05$), decreased EImax (0.58, range 0.55–0.59, $p < 0.001$), and AUC (median 133, range 119–146, $p < 0.001$); Ohyper-values were comparable with controls (**Table 2**). Despite of this, the Osmoscan curve falls for some parameters inside the normal control area (three patients had normal Omin and four normal EImax), not allowing to identify a diagnostic shape in CDAII (**Figure 2D**). Moreover, differences in Osmoscan parameters were observed in splenectomized patient (see below).

Enzyme Defects

The 24 non-splenectomized patients affected by PK (20 cases), Pyr5′N (3 cases), and TPI deficiency (1 case) displayed normal Osmoscan curve, with the only exception of increased Ohyper-values in some cases (median 482, range 427–565, $p < 0.001$; **Table 2**). Statistical differences were maintained in the PK deficient patients when separately analyzed. It is worth noting that all the five GPI deficient cases showed a striking enlargement of the right segment of the curve, which appears to be interrupted at 500 mOsm/Kg (**Figure 2F**). Although the number of patients is limited, a significantly increased Omin (median 157, range 146–176, $p < 0.001$) and, even more, Ohyper (median 552, range 500–579, $p < 0.001$) was observed; on the contrary, EImax was decreased compared to controls (median 0.56, range 0.51–0.58, $p < 0.05$) (**Table 2**).

Paroxysmal Nocturnal Hemoglobinuria

No differences were observed with normal controls except for increased OHyper-values (median 492, range 457–538, $p < 0.05$; **Table 2**).

Effect of Splenectomy and Concomitant Defects on Osmoscan Curve

For some diseases (i.e., enzyme defects and CDAII), Osmoscan curves of splenectomized patients fall into a defined area irrespective of the pathology, characterized by significantly decreased EImax and AUC and increased EImin and EIhyper ($p < 0.05$; **Table 4, Figures 3A–D**).

Moreover, concomitant defects may also interfere with Osmoscan analysis. In the analyzed series all the three cases carrying an additional β-thalassemia trait showed a left-shifted Osmoscan curve, representing a possible cause of misdiagnosis with dehydrated stomatocytosis.

TABLE 2 | Osmoscan parameters in normal controls and in patients with chronic hemolytic anemias (splenectomized patients with enzymopathies and CDAII were excluded)§.

	N	Omin (mOsm/kg)	Elmax	Ohyper (mOsm/kg)	Elmin	Omax (mOsm/kg)	Elhyper	AUC
HS	Total	166	0.53	444	0.12	334	0.26	108
	(*N* = 116)	(144–201)**	(0.41–0.59)**	(389–547)**	(0.08–0.19)*	(285–409)**	(0.21–0.29)**	(82–131)**
HE	Total	154	0.53	471	0.1	312	0.27	119
	(*N* = 15)	(130–178)**	(0.47–0.59)**	(428–526)	(0.08–0.19)*	(268–339)	(0.24–0.3)**	(106–157)**
HSt (PIEZO1)	Total	98	0.58	394	0.18	265	0.29	146
	(*N* = 6)	(71–136)**	(0.53–0.61)	(342–416)**	(0.14–0.24)**	(211–299)**	(0.27–0.3)	(130–153)
HSt (KCNN4)	Total	157	0.52	510	0.2	338	0.28	133
	(*N* = 3)	(146–161)	(0.51–0.58)*	(483–517)	(0.17–0.22)*	(303–341)	(0.26–0.29)	(126–144)
PK, P5′N, TPI	Not splenect	144	0.6	482	0.13	313	0.3	149
	(*N* = 24)	(122–173)	(0.56–0.61)	(427–565)**	(0.1–0.23)**	(253–368)	(0.28–0.31)	(138–161)
GPI	Total	157	0.56	552	0.16	372	0.28	132
	(*N* = 5)	(146–176)**	(0.51–0.58)*	(500–579)**	(0.11–0.2)*	(315–381)*	(0.26–0.3)*	(117–146)*
CDAII	Not splenect	152	0.58	458	0.13	327	0.29	133
	(*N* = 9)	(133–164)*	(0.55–0.59)**	(432–492)	(0.11–0.16)	(318–329)**	(0.28–0.3)**	(119–145)**
PNH	Total	150	0.6	492	0.13	323	0.3	146
	(*N* = 9)	(132–164)	(0.58–0.6)	(457–538)*	(0.11–0.15)*	(301–357)*	(0.29–0.3)	(132–156)
Controls	Total	142	0.6	464	0.12	311	0.3	148
	(*N* = 170)	(125–160)	(0.46–0.62)	(418–512)	(0.09–0.3)	(273–355)	(0.29–0.31)	(114–168)
	MEAN ± 1 SD	142 ± 6.8	0.6 ± 0.01	464.5 ± 15.45	0.12 ± 0.02	310.6 ± 12.15	0.3 ± 0.02	147.8 ± 6.6

*Values are expressed as median (range). *$p < 0.05$; **$p < 0.001$ vs. controls.*
§Only non-splenectomized patients affected by enzymopathies (PK and P5′N) and CDAII were considered due to differences in Osmoscan curve shape observed in the splenectomized ones.

Scatter Plot Analysis of Osmoscan Parameters

As reported in **Table 2**, overlaps are present among data obtained from HS, CDAII, and HE patients, doesn't allowing differential diagnosis by the analysis of the main Osmoscan parameters alone. A scatter plot analysis of Omin, EImax, and Ohyper coupled with the corresponding x-, y-axis-values (EImin, Omax, and EIhyper, respectively) was therefore performed in non-splenectomized patients and normal controls in the attempt to verify if Osmoscan coupled parameters differently clustered depending on diseases (**Figure 4**). Distinguishable clusters were observed for HS, HSt, GPI patients and normal controls. Also patients affected by CDAII and HE clustered, however falling in the normal/HS gates for Omin/EImin, and Ohyper/EIhyper regions and in the HS gate for the EImax/Omax.

Differential Diagnosis Between CDAII and HS

To establish the performance of the Osmoscan parameters in discriminating HS between normal controls and patients with other hemolytic anemias ROC curve analysis was performed for Omin, EImax, Omax, and AUC (**Table 5**).

From the analysis between HS and controls the best parameters were as follows: Omin (AUC 0.989, cut-off = 153), EImax (AUC 0.993, cut-off = 0.56), and AUC (AUC 0.997, cut-off = 114). Similar performances were observed between HS and all non-HS patients: Omin (AUC 0.960, cut-off = 157), and AUC (AUC 0.975, cut-off = 119).

As expected, the best parameters to discriminate HS from HSt were Omin (AUC 1.000, cut-off = 140), Ohyper (AUC 0.953, cut-off = 417), and AUC (AUC 0.991, cut-off = 130). On the contrary, a lower sensitivity and specificity was found in the analysis of HS/HE, thus not allowing establishing diagnostic cut-off. Considering the analysis between HS and CDAII we found that the best parameter to discriminate the two diseases was Omin (AUC 0.944, cut-off = 157).

Moreover, in the attempt to verify whether the combination of ektacytometric and hematologic parameters might improve differential diagnosis between HS and CDAII, we combined Osmoscan and hematologic parameters (data not shown). Omin and absolute reticulocyte number showed the best performances in discriminating the two diseases. We chose the cut-off value of 157 mOsm/kg for Omin as determined through the ROC curve, combined with the commonly used cut-off value of 150 × 10^9/L for reticulocytes (Russo et al., 2014; King et al., 2015; Bianchi et al., 2016). As reported in **Table 6**, we observed that when Omin and reticulocyte count were both high, none of patients had CDAII with a reasonably narrow confidence interval. When both indexes were low, all patients had CDAII, but with large uncertainty due the limited number of subjects. A high Omin with low reticulocyte count indicated a low probability (23%) of CDAII. Finally, we had only two patients with high reticulocytes count and low Omin, both with HS.

DISCUSSION

This is a monocentric study aimed to evaluate the diagnostic efficiency of the new generation LoRRca MaxSis ektacytometer in an extensive series of congenital hemolytic anemias of various type, including a substantial number of CDAII and enzyme deficiencies never or rarely investigated so far by this technique. The ektacytometric analysis was included in the diagnostic workflow, allowing correlating Osmoscan parameters with the results of all the routine laboratory investigations usually adopted for the diagnosis of hemolytic anemias (Bianchi et al., 2012; King et al., 2015).

Among the methods proposed for the diagnosis of hemolytic anemias, ektacytometry is certainly one of the most interesting due to its versatility, being able to discriminate different defects by a single analysis (Da Costa et al., 2013; King et al., 2015), and his repeatability and reproducibility, enabling an easy standardization in specialized laboratories, as recently reported by other groups (Da Costa et al., 2016; Lazarova et al., 2017; Llaudet-Planas et al., 2018).

Ektacytometry can detect with high sensitivity multiple changes in cellular properties, obtaining information that by conventional methods would require several different types of measurements. In particular, by studying normal cells in which water content and membrane surface area had been selectively modified, it was observed that the resulting curve was a balance in the adjustment of surface area-to-volume ratio (S/V) and intracellular viscosity: an inverse correlation was obtained between MCHC and Ohyper-values together with a tight correlation (correlation coefficient of 0.985) between Omin-values and the osmolality at which hemolysis reached 50% in an osmotic fragility assay (Clark et al., 1983). We therefore investigated correlation of single Osmoscan parameters with red cells indexes and the results of osmotic fragility tests and EMA binding. Omin-values obtained by all the patients, independently from the disease, showed a significant correlation with all the osmotic fragility tests and EMA-binding test. Moreover, MCHC was correlated with Ohyper-values. These data are

TABLE 3 | Correlation analysis among Osmoscan parameters, Osmotic fragility tests, EMA-binding and red blood cell indexes in patients with chronic hemolytic anemias.

		RDW	MCV	MCHC	Retic	AGLT	GLT	EMA
Omin	*r*	0.033	−0.236	0.308	0.266	**−0.658**	**−0.545**	**−0.589**
	P	0.72	0.008	0.0005	0.003	<0.0001	<0.0001	<0.0001
Eimax	*r*	−0.210	0.247	−0.167	−0.091	0.316	0.298	**0.419**
	P	0.02	0.006	0.06	0.31	0.0004	0.0008	<0.0001
Ohyper	*r*	0.075	0.160	**−0.585**	0.014	0.052	0.052	0.205
	P	0.40	0.08	<0.0001	0.875	0.57	0.57	0.022
AUC	*r*	−0.095	**0.416**	**−0.506**	−0.262	**0.554**	**0.542**	**0.648**
	P	0.30	<0.0001	<0.0001	0.003	<0.0001	<0.0001	<0.0001

Spearman' rho correlation analysis was performed in 124 patients for whom all the considered parameters were available.

r, correlation coefficient; P, p-values; GLT, standard glycerol lysis test; AGLT, acidified glycerol lysis test; EMA, eosin-5-maleimide. Highly significant correlations are reported in bold.

TABLE 4 | Osmoscan parameters in splenectomized and non-splenectomized patients.

	Splenectomy	Omin (mOsm/kg)	EImax	Ohyper (mOsm/kg)	EImin	Omax (mOsm/kg)	EIhyper	AUC
Enzyme defect	Total	146 (122–173)	0.59 (0.54–0.61)	485 (427–565)	0.13 (0.1–0.23)	311 (253–368)	0.3 (0.27–0.31)	147 (132–161)
	NO (*N* = 24)	144 (122–173)	0.6 (0.56–0.61)*	482 (427–565)	0.13 (0.1–0.23)*	313 (253–368)	0.3 (0.28–0.31)*	149 (138–161)*
	YES (*N* = 8)	147 (132–158)	0.56 (0.54–0.6)	490 (472–501)	0.17 (0.12–0.21)	309 (286–325)	0.28 (0.27–0.3)	144 (132–152)
CDAII	Total	148 (119–164)	0.55 (0.47–0.59)	456 (432–492)	0.16 (0.11–0.25)	319 (265–356)	0.28 (0.23–0.3)	130 (113–145)
	NO (*N* = 9)	152 (133–164)	0.58 (0.55–0.59)*	458 (432–492)	0.13 (0.11–0.16)*	327 (318–329)*	0.29 (0.28–0.30)*	133 (119–145)*
	YES (*N* = 7)	140 (119–156)	0.49 (0.47–0.51)	449 (438–466)	0.21 (0.18–0.25)	287 (235–306)	0.25 (0.23–0.26)	121 (113–131)

*Values are expressed as median (range). Enzyme defect included = PK, P5′N, and TPI deficiency. *p < 0.05 splenectomised vs. non-splenectomised.*

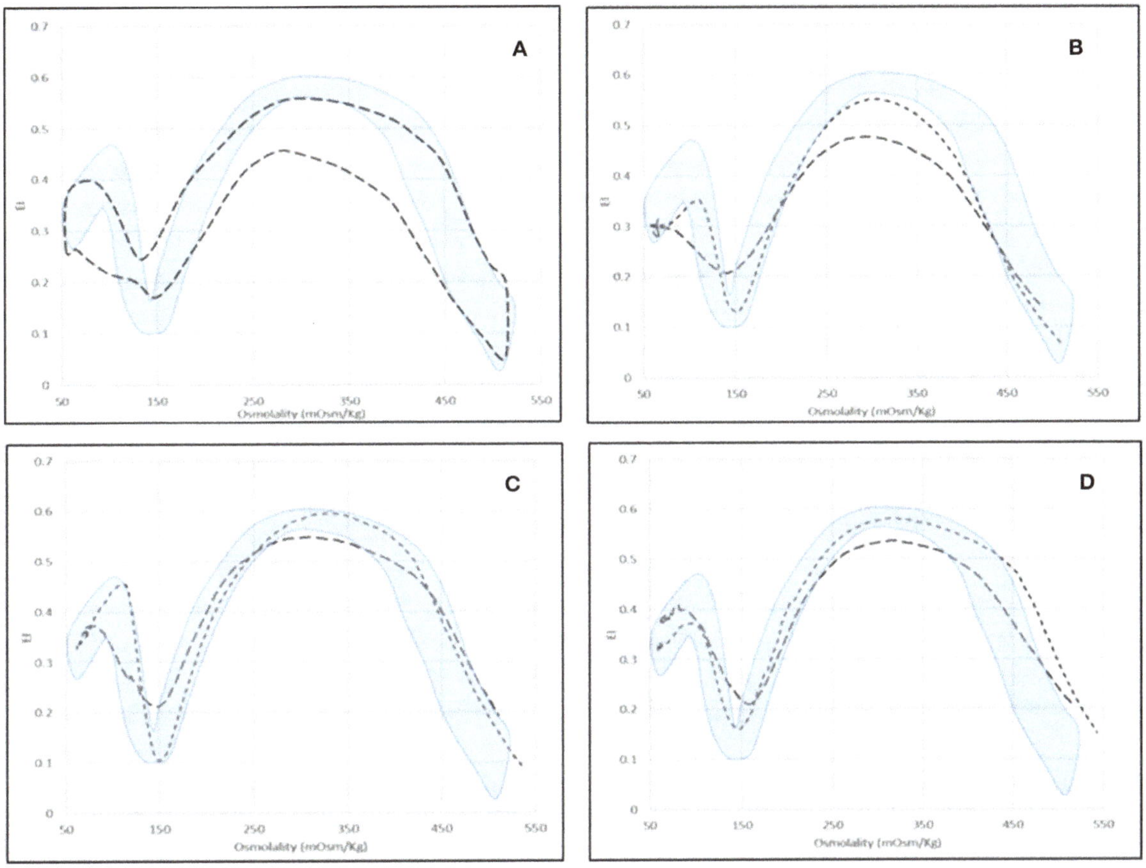

FIGURE 3 | Osmoscan profile in splenectomized patients. **(A)** Shaded area = control range curve; Dashed area = splenectomised patients (seven affected by PKD, two by Pyr5′N deficiency and seven by CDAII); **(B)** CDAII: non-splenectomised (▬ ▬ ▬), splenectomised (— — —); **(C)** PKD: non-splenectomised (▬ ▬ ▬), splenectomised (— — —); **(D)** Pyr5′N deficiency: non-splenectomised (▬ ▬ ▬), splenectomised (— — —).

particularly interesting because obtained from heterogeneous cell populations instead from *in vitro* artificially manipulated red cells (Clark et al., 1983). Despite the correlations observed, these data don't permit to establish diagnostic cut-offs for chronic hemolytic anemias.

To evaluate the diagnostic power of LoRRca MaxSis for hereditary hemolytic anemias, we established in each disease the range values of EImax, Omin, Ohyper, AUC, and their derived parameters (EImin, Omax, EIhyper). In most of the groups of diseases we detected statistically significant differences with normal controls, suggesting that the analysis of a single parameter could help in addressing the diagnosis, as already reported in previous series (Lazarova et al., 2017). This is particularly true for DHSt caused by mutation in *PIEZO1* gene where the typical shape of the curve gives precise diagnostic information, although a newly identified subgroup of stomatocytosis caused by R352H mutation in *KCNN4* gene displays a normal Osmoscan curve (Fermo et al., 2017). In line with previous studies (Llaudet-Planas et al., 2018), also ROC curve analysis led us to identify the osmoscan parameters with the best performance in discriminating HS from normal controls and other kind of hemolytic anemias. However, differences in optimal cut-off, sensitivity, and specificity for single parameters were observed. This could be partially explained by differences in the analyzed cohorts of patients. Inter-laboratory standardization would be useful to establish diagnostic cut-off.

On the contrary, overlaps in values were noted among other hemolytic anemias making not possible differential diagnosis by the analysis of Osmoscan parameters alone. In particular, in our series overlaps were present among data obtained from HS, CDAII, and HE patients.

As regards CDAII, it is worth mentioning that this disorder mimics HS both in terms of clinical presentation and laboratory features, and often requires SDS-PAGE analysis or molecular characterization to be identified (Bianchi et al., 2012; King et al., 2015). We analyzed for the first time a large group of CDAII patients by LoRRca MaxSis: the Osmoscan curve *per se* doesn't allow differential diagnosis, being normal in non-splenectomised CDAII patients and overlapping with HS in the splenectomised ones. We therefore performed the ROC curve of all the Osmoscan and hematologic data looking for the best combination of parameters capable of differentiating CDAII. The

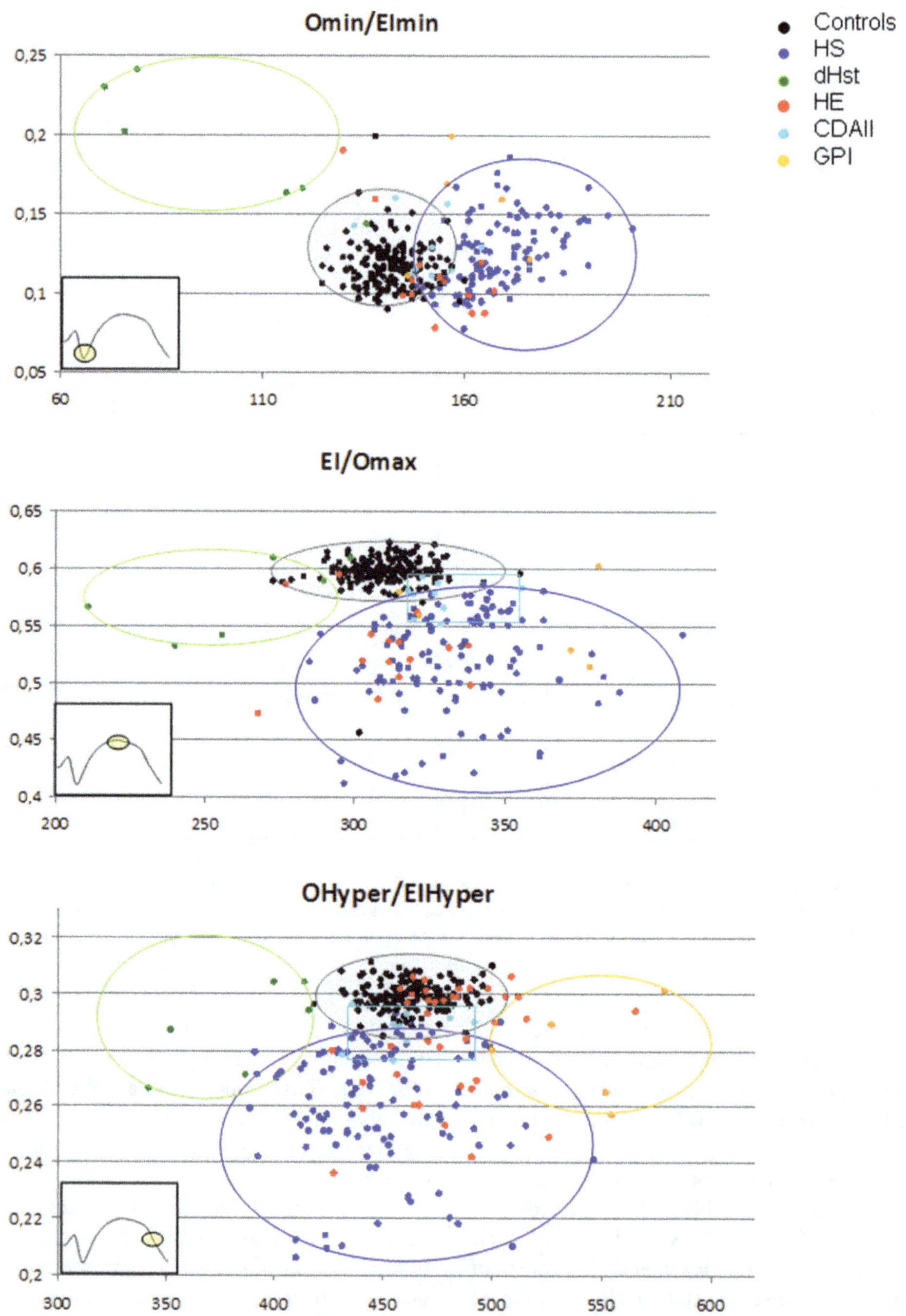

FIGURE 4 | Osmoscan coupled parameters differently clustered depending on diseases. Controls (●), HS (●), CDA II (●), HE (●), HSt (●), GPI (●).

cut-off values of 150 × 10^9/L absolute reticulocyte number and 157 mOsm/kg Omin showed the best performance. Interestingly by this approach we were able to discriminate HS from CDAII with a reasonably narrow confidence interval. The analysis of these parameters on larger series of patients will enable to verify the usefulness of this approach.

Osmoscan analysis of a very large group of different enzymopathies associated with chronic hemolytic anemia led us to identify an unexpected characteristic curve in all the GPI deficient patients tested, offering a first step laboratory screening for this rare enzyme defect. The reason why in GPI deficient patients Ohyper is drastically shifted to the right is unknown

TABLE 5 | Performance of the Osmoscan parameters in discriminating hereditary spherocytosis (HS) between normal control and patients with other membrane defects.

	HS vs. Normal 116/170	HS vs. All[§] 116/257	HS vs. Hst* 116/6	HS vs. HE 116/15	HS vs. CDAII 116/16
Omin	**AUC = 0.989**	**AUC = 0.960**	**AUC = 1.000**	AUC = 0.793	**AUC = 0.944**
	(0.980–0.998)	**(0.942–0.978)**	–	(0.657–0.929)	**(0.988–1.000)**
	Cut-off = 153	**Cut-off = 157**	**Cut-off = 140**	Cut-off = 155	**Cut-off = 157**
	Se = 0.95	**Se = 0.88**	**Se = 1.00**	Se = 0.89	**Se = 0.88**
	Sp = 0.94	**Sp = 0.93**	**Sp = 1.00**	Sp = 0.60	**Sp = 0.94**
Elmax	**AUC = 0.993**	AUC = 0.920	AUC = 0.840	AUC = 0.526	AUC = 0.607
	(0.983–1.000)	(0.893–0.947)	(0.671–1.000)	(0.378–0.674)	(0.417–0.797)
	Cut-off = 0.56	Cut-off = 0.54	Cut-off = 0.54	Cut-off = 0.54	Cut-off = 0.51
	Se = 0.84	Se = 0.61	Se = 0.61	Se = 0.59	Se = 0.35
	Sp = 0.99	Sp = 0.89	Sp = 0.67	Sp = 0.27	Sp = 0.56
Ohyper	AUC = 0.706	AUC = 0.718	**AUC = 0.953**	AUC = 0.731	AUC = 0.617
	(0.638–0.775)	(0.655–0.781)	**(0.899–1.000)**	(0.612–0.850)	(0.528–0.726)
	Cut-off = 475	Cut-off = 475	**Cut-off = 417**	Cut-off = 475	Cut-off = 461
	Se = 0.80	Se = 0.80	**Se = 0.85**	Se = 0.80	Se = 0.70
	Sp = 0.24	Sp = 0.33	**Sp = 1.00**	Sp = 0.40	Sp = 0.25
Area	**AUC = 0.997**	**AUC = 0.975**	**AUC = 0.991**	AUC = 0.740	AUC = 0.893
	0.994–1.000)	**(0.962–0.987)**	**(0.975–1.000)**	(0.619–0.861)	(0.817–0.968)
	Cut-off = 114	**Cut-off = 119**	**Cut-off = 130**	Cut-off = 112	Cut-off = 119
	Se = 0.66	**Se = 0.72**	**Se = 0.97**	Se = 0.56	Se = 0.72
	Sp = 0.99	**Sp = 0.95**	**Sp = 0.67**	Sp = 0.67	Sp = 0.75

AUC, area under the ROC curve; 95% confidence interval (in brackets), cut-off, optimal cut-off calculated by Liu's method; Se, sensitivity and Sp, specificity at the calculated cut-off. For Omin, values higher than cut-off were classified as "positive," for Elmax, Ohyper, and AREA, values lower than cut-off were classified as "positive." Significant analysis are reported in bold.

**PIEZO1 mutations; [§]All non-HS cases (normal subjects included).*

TABLE 6 | Combination of cut-off values of Omin and reticulocytes number for the differential diagnosis of HS and CDAII.

Reticulocyte number	Omin (mOsm/kg)	
	≥157	<157
≥150 × 10^9/L	0/72 = 0% 95% CI: 0–5%	0/2 = 0% 95% CI: 0–84%
<150 × 10^9/L	7/30 = 23% 95% CI: 10–42%	8/8 = 100% 95% CI: 63–100%

Automated reticulocyte number was available for 97 HS and 15 CDAII cases. CDAII/total number patients for each category is reported and expressed as %.

and can be only partially attributed to the increased MCV-values observed in these subjects (median MCV 112 fL, range 81–127).

Since Osmoscan curve results by the analysis of the entire red cell population, it is important to underline that concomitance of different defects, as the co-presence of beta-thalassemia trait and splenectomy, may alter the curve shape representing a possible cause of misdiagnosis.

In conclusion, the use of LoRRca MaxSis osmoscan, providing simultaneous information on the major RBC properties (cell geometry, viscosity, and deformability; Da Costa et al., 2016), is therefore particularly indicated in specialized laboratories to be performed as an intermediate step between the first screening (including clinical information, abnormal marker of hemolysis, and red cell morphology) and more specific diagnostic tests. Diagnostic cut-offs have been established, particularly for HS, in line with Llaudet-Planas et al. (2018). However, it is important to underline that in routine practice Osmoscan analysis alone is not sufficient to reach a diagnosis that have to be confirmed by specific second level tests.

AUTHOR CONTRIBUTIONS

AnZ performed the analysis, analyzed the results, and prepared the manuscript; CV and AM performed hematologic testings; DC performed statistical analysis; EF and PB performed molecular testing, analyzed the results, and prepared the manuscript; WB and AlZ clinical information of patients follow-up and critical revision of the manuscript; AC critical revision of the manuscript.

ACKNOWLEDGMENTS

The authors thank the STEM Onlus associations for supporting the acquisition of LoRRca MaxSis.

REFERENCES

Badens, C., and Guizouarn, H. (2016). Advances in understanding the pathogenesis of the red cell volume disorders. *Br. J. Haematol.* 174, 674–685. doi: 10.1111/bjh.14197

Baskurt, O. K., Hardeman, M. R., Uyuklu, M., Ulker, P., Cengiz, M., Nemeth, N., et al. (2009). Parameterization of red blood cell elongation index - shear stress curves obtained by ektacytometry, *Scand. J. Clin. Lab. Invest.* 69, 777–788. doi: 10.3109/00365510903266069

Baskurt, O. K., and Meiselman, H. J. (2004). Analyzing shear stress–elongation index curves: comparison of two approaches to simplify data presentation. *Clin. Hemorheol. Microcirc.* 31, 23–30.

Beutler, E. (1984). *Red Cell Metabolism: A Manual of Biochemical Methods*. New York, NY: Grune & Stratton, Inc.

Bianchi, P., Fermo, E., Vercellati, C., Marcello, A. P., Porretti, L., Cortelezzi, A., et al. (2012). Diagnostic power of laboratory tests for hereditary spherocytosis: a comparison study in 150 patients grouped according to molecular and clinical characteristics. *Haematologica* 97, 516–523. doi: 10.3324/haematol.2011.052845

Bianchi, P., Schwarz, K., Högel, J., Fermo, E., Vercellati, C., Grosse, R., et al. (2016). Analysis of a cohort of 101 CDAII patients: description of 24 new molecular variants and genotype-phenotype correlations. *Br. J. Haematol.* 175, 696–704. doi: 10.1111/bjh.14271

Clark, M. R., Mohandas, N., and Shohet, S. B. (1983). Osmotic gradient ektacytometry: comprehensive characterization of red cell volume and surface maintenance. *Blood* 61, 899–910.

Dacie, J. V., and Lewis, S. M. (2001). *Practical Haematology, 9th Edn*. London: Churchill Livingston.

Da Costa, L., Galimand, J., Fenneteau, O., and Mohandas, N. (2013). Hereditary spherocytosis, elliptocytosis, and other red cell membrane disorders. *Blood Rev.* 27, 167–178. doi: 10.1016/j.blre.2013.04.003

Da Costa, L., Suner, L., Galimand, J., Bonnel, A., Pascreau, T., Couque, N., et al. (2016). Diagnostic tool for red blood cell membrane disorders: assessment of a new generation ektacytometer. *Blood Cells Mol. Dis.* 56, 9–22. doi: 10.1016/j.bcmd.2015.09.001

Fairbanks, G., Steck, T. L., and Wallach, D. F. H. (1971). Electrophoretic analysis of bthe major polypeptides of the human erythrocyte membrane. *Biochemistry* 10, 2606–2617. doi: 10.1021/bi00789a030

Fermo, E., Bogdanova, A., Petkova-Kirova, P., Zaninoni, A., Marcello, A. P., Makhro, A., et al. (2017). 'Gardos Channelopathy': a variant of hereditary Stomatocytosis with complex molecular regulation. *Sci. Rep.* 7:1744. doi: 10.1038/s41598-017-01591-w

Glogowska, E., and Gallagher, P. G. (2015). Disorders of erythrocyte volume homeostasis. *Int. J. Lab. Hematol.* 37, 85–91. doi: 10.1111/ijlh.12357

He, Y., Jia, S., Dewan, R. K., and Liao, N. (2017). Novel mutations in patients with hereditary red blood cell membrane disorders using next-generation sequencing. *Gene* 627, 556–562. doi: 10.1016/j.gene.2017.07.009

King, M. J., Behrens, J., Rogers, C., Flynn, C., Greenwood, D., and Chambers, K. (2000). Rapid flow cytometric test for the diagnosis of membrane cytoskeleton-associated haemolytic anaemia. *Br. J. Haematol.* 111, 924–933. doi: 10.1111/j.1365-2141.2000.02416.x

King, M. J., Garçon, L., Hoyer, J. D., Iolascon, A., Picard, V., Stewart, G., et al. (2015). ICSH guidelines for the laboratory diagnosis of nonimmune hereditary red cell membrane disorders. *Int. J. Lab. Hematol.* 37, 304–325. doi: 10.1111/ijlh.12335

King, M. J., and Zanella, A. (2013). Hereditary red cell membrane disorders and laboratory diagnostic testing. *Int. J. Lab. Hematol.* 35, 237–243. doi: 10.1111/ijlh.12070

Koralkova, P., van Solinge, W. W., and van Wijk, R. (2014). Rare hereditary red blood cell enzymopathies associated with hemolytic anemia - pathophysiology, clinical aspects, and laboratory diagnosis. *Int. J. Lab. Hematol.* 36, 388–397. doi: 10.1111/ijlh.12223

Laemmli, U. K. (1970). Cleavage of structural proteins during the assembly of the head of bacteriophage T4. *Nature* 227, 680–685. doi: 10.1038/227680a0

Lazarova, E., Gulbis, B., Oirschot, B. V., and van Wijk, R. (2017). Next-generation osmotic gradient ektacytometry for the diagnosis of hereditary spherocytosis: interlaboratory method validation and experience. *Clin. Chem. Lab. Med.* 55, 394–402. doi: 10.1515/cclm-2016-0290

Liu, X. (2012). Classification accuracy and cut point selection. *Stat. Med.* 31, 2676–2686. doi: 10.1002/sim.4509

Llaudet-Planas, E., Vives-Corrons, J. L., Rizzuto, V., Gómez-Ramírez, P., Sevilla Navarro, J., Coll Sibina, M. T., et al. (2018). Osmotic gradient ektacytometry: a valuable screening test for hereditary spherocytosis and other red blood cell membrane disorders. *Int. J. Lab. Hematol.* 40, 94–102. doi: 10.1111/ijlh.12746

Mariani, M., Barcellini, W., Vercellati, C., Marcello, A. P., Fermo, E., Pedotti, P., et al. (2008). Clinical and hematologic features of 300 patients affected by hereditary spherocytosis grouped according to the type of the membrane protein defect. *Haematologica* 93, 1310–1317. doi: 10.3324/haematol.12546

Mohandas, N., and Gallagher, P. G. (2008). Red cell membrane: past, present, and future. *Blood* 112, 3939–3948. doi: 10.1182/blood-2008-07-161166

Perrotta, S., Gallagher, P. G., and Mohandas, N. (2008). Hereditary spherocytosis. *Lancet* 372, 1411–1426. doi: 10.1016/S0140-6736(08)61588-3

Russo, R., Gambale, A., Langella, C., Andolfo, I., Unal, S., and Iolascon, A. (2014). Retrospective cohort study of 205 cases with congenital dyserythropoietic anemia type II: definition of clinical and molecular spectrum and identification of new diagnostic scores. *Am. J. Hematol.* 89, E169–E175. doi: 10.1002/ajh.23800

StataCorp. (2017). *Stata Statistical Software: Release 15*. College Station, TX: StataCorp LP.

8

Low-Level Light Therapy Protects Red Blood Cells Against Oxidative Stress and Hemolysis During Extracorporeal Circulation

Tomasz Walski[1,2], Anna Drohomirecka[2,3], Jolanta Bujok[2,4], Albert Czerski[2,4], Grzegorz Wąż[2,5], Natalia Trochanowska-Pauk[1,2], Michał Gorczykowski[6], Romuald Cichoń[5] and Małgorzata Komorowska[1,2]*

[1] Department of Biomedical Engineering, Faculty of Fundamental Problems of Technology, Wrocław University of Science and Technology, Wrocław, Poland, [2] Regional Specialist Hospital in Wrocław, Research and Development Centre, Wrocław, Poland, [3] Institute of Cardiology, Warsaw, Poland, [4] Department of Animal Physiology and Biostructure, Faculty of Veterinary Medicine, Wrocław University of Environmental and Life Sciences, Wrocław, Poland, [5] Medinet Heart Center Ltd., Wrocław, Poland, [6] Department of Internal Medicine and Clinic of Diseases of Horses, Dogs and Cats, Faculty of Veterinary Medicine, Wrocław University of Environmental and Life Sciences, Wrocław, Poland

***Correspondence:**
Tomasz Walski
tomasz.walski@pwr.edu.pl

Aim: An activation of non-specific inflammatory response, coagulation disorder, and blood morphotic elements damage are the main side effects of the extracorporeal circulation (ECC). Red-to-near-infrared radiation (R/NIR) is thought to be capable of stabilizing red blood cell (RBC) membrane through increasing its resistance to destructive factors. We focused on the development of a method using low-level light therapy (LLLT) in the spectral range of R/NIR which could reduce blood trauma caused by the heart-lung machine during surgery.

Methods: R/NIR emitter was adjusted in terms of geometry and optics to ECC circuit. The method of extracorporeal blood photobiomodulation was tested during *in vivo* experiments in an animal, porcine model (1 h of ECC plus 23 h of animal observation). A total of 24 sows weighing 90–100 kg were divided into two equal groups: control one and LLLT. Blood samples were taken during the experiment to determine changes in blood morphology [RBC and white blood cell (WBC) counts, hemoglobin (Hgb)], indicators of hemolysis [plasma-free hemoglobin (PFHgb), serum bilirubin concentration, serum lactate dehydrogenase (LDH) activity], and oxidative stress markers [thiobarbituric acid reactive substances (TBARS) concentration, total antioxidant capacity (TAC)].

Results: In the control group, a rapid systemic decrease in WBC count during ECC was accompanied by a significant increase in RBC membrane lipids peroxidation, while in the LLLT group the number of WBC and TBARS concentration both remained relatively constant, indicating limitation of the inflammatory process. These results were consistent with the change in the hemolysis markers like PFHgb, LDH, and serum bilirubin concentration, which were significantly reduced in LLLT group. No differences in TAC, RBC count, and Hgb concentration were detected.

Conclusion: We presented the applicability of the LLLT with R/NIR radiation to blood trauma reduction during ECC.

Keywords: cardiopulmonary bypass (CPB), low-level light therapy (LLLT), red blood cell, extracorporeal circulation (ECC), near-infrared radiation (NIR), heart-lung machine, hemolysis, photobiomodulation

INTRODUCTION

Extracorporeal circulation (ECC) is a procedure routinely used in cardiac surgery (e.g., in coronary artery bypass grafting, valve surgery). During the procedures utilizing cardiopulmonary bypass (CPB) an extravasated blood comes into contact with the polymer surfaces of oxygenators, catheters, cannulas, pumps, and filters. It results in non-specific inflammatory response, destruction of blood cells, coagulation activation, and increase in oxidative stress. These factors may evoke a systemic inflammatory response syndrome which contributes to the morbidity and mortality of patients undergoing cardiac surgery (Hirai, 2003).

Hemolysis is one of the common problems occurring in the course of ECC but still requiring solution, as damaged red blood cells (RBCs) may induce toxic effects (Vercaemst, 2008). Even low concentrations of plasma-free hemoglobin (PFHgb) contribute to a significant increase in RBC aggregation in the presence of small shear stress (Ji and Undar, 2006; Cabrales, 2007). This, in turn, causes an increase in blood viscosity and thus a high resistance in capillaries. PFHgb also binds nitric oxide (NO) at the level of microcirculation after depletion of haptoglobin (Hp) stores (Cabrales, 2007). As a consequence, tissue hypoxia, in the presence of already reduced RBC count, is escalating.

Moreover, transfusion of RBC is associated with increased mortality and morbidity in patients undergoing cardiac surgery (Koch et al., 2008; van Straten et al., 2010), which is another argument to make effort to limit blood trauma.

There are several phenomena contributing to the hemolysis in ECC. One of the main factors leading to blood cells destruction during ECC is oxidative stress. The source of reactive oxygen species (ROS) are the phagocytes (mainly neutrophils and monocytes) (Boyle et al., 1997). Their activation results in a respiratory burst, which initiates oxidation of cell proteins and plasma membrane lipids and in consequence causes an inactivation of enzymes, cell membrane depolarization, changes in plasma membrane fluidity and permeability (Matés et al., 1999; Kirkham and Rahman, 2006). Another of the important factors responsible for enhanced RBC destruction during ECC is the altered hemodynamic conditions. Mechanical stress may lead to the complete destruction of the RBC. Depending on how big the stress is, how long it acts, and what the RBC condition is, hemolysis may occur immediately or with delay (Kameneva et al., 2004; Cabrales, 2007; Grygorczyk and Orlov, 2017). Non-physiological flow conditions cause a decrease in RBC deformability and membrane potential, promoting a high blood viscosity. Turbulent flow, cavitation, inappropriate flow rates, decreased oncotic pressure caused by dilution of plasma, and the absence of flow pulsatility also directly contribute to RBC destruction in ECC systems (Ji and Undar, 2006).

So far, methods reducing ECC side effects were focused on perfusion sets miniaturization, improvement of the biocompatibility of the materials that have direct contact with blood, and optimization of hemodynamic conditions generated by the device. Unfortunately, the results obtained are still insufficient, as evidenced by the numerous complications occurring both during and after the ECC.

Our method was based on beneficial effects of low-level light therapy (LLLT) in the red-to-near-infrared radiation (R/NIR) spectral region on blood cells, with special regard to erythrocytes. It was shown that direct blood photobiomodulation cause alterations of the membrane fluidity and membrane potential which results in RBC aggregability decrease (Komorowska et al., 2002; Korolevich et al., 2004; Mi et al., 2004; Chludzińska et al., 2005), increased cell membrane mechanical resistance (Itoh et al., 2000; Komorowska et al., 2002; Chludzińska et al., 2005), and it may act protectively against oxidative stress (Chludzińska et al., 2005). During the exposure of RBCs to R/NIR light, dehydration process induces the photochemical dissociation oxyhemoglobin to deoxyhemoglobin and decreases the amount of physiologically inactive methemoglobin (MetHgb) (Walski et al., 2015).

The aim of this study was to evaluate the effect of LLLT applied during the ECC on the RBCs in an animal model.

MATERIALS AND METHODS

Animals and Experimental Design

The study protocol was approved by a local II Ethical Review Board in Wrocław (II Lokalna Komisja Etyczna we Wrocławiu, approval No. 9/2013). Each animal was provided humane conditions and care according to the European Directive 2010/63/EU on the protection of animals used for scientific purposes.

The experiments were conducted on 24 clinically healthy female Polish Landrace pigs aged 5 months (mean weight 94.3 ± 3.2 kg) purchased from a single farm (The National Research Institute of Animal Production, Experimental Station in Pawłowice, Poland). The study was performed only in female pigs to preclude the impact of gender on the severity of hemolysis and oxidative stress (Kanias et al., 2016; Kander et al., 2017). After 1-week acclimatization period in the pens of the institutional vivarium, animals were randomly assigned into two experimental groups undergoing 1-h venoarterial ECC under general anesthesia: the control group and the LLLT group, in which the blood flowing through the oxygenator was exposed to R/NIR light. After decannulation, the animals were weaned from the ECC and transferred to the observation room for the following 23 h. During this time, several blood samples were collected to monitor the effects of ECC and R/NIR irradiation. At the end of the experiment, pigs were euthanized.

Extracorporeal Circulation Procedure

Animals were anesthetized with intramuscular injection of ketamine (10 mg/kg, Bioketan, Vetoquinol Biowet Puławy, Poland), dexmedetomidine (10 μg/kg, Dexdor, Orion, Espoo, Finland) and diazepam (20 mg/100 kg, Relanium, Polpharma SA, Poland). Pigs were intubated and connected to a respirator (Wowo 500 Veterinary Anesthesia Machine, China). Mechanical ventilation was used in case of respiratory arrest lasting over

1 min or PCO_2 in the exhaust phase exceeding 60 mmHg. Anesthesia was maintained with continuous rate infusion of propofol (0.2 mg/kg/min, Scanofol, ScanVet, Poland), fentanyl (50 μg/kg/10 min, Polfa SA, Poland), ketamine (10 mg/kg/30 min, IV), and diazepam (0.2 mg/kg/30 min, IV).

Prior to the ECC, a central venous catheter (11F/20 cm, dual-lumen polyurethane catheter, Medcomp®, United States) was inserted into the jugular vein to provide vascular access facilitating collection of subsequent blood samples scheduled for the experiment and drug administration. Jugular vein and carotid artery at the opposite side were surgically exposed and then cannulated with the ECC cannulas, which were connected to the drains of the perfusion set primed with 1500 ml crystalloid solution and 3000 IU unfractionated heparin (heparinum WZF®, Polfa Warszawa, Poland). When activated clotting time (ACT) was shorter than 200 s, additional doses of heparin were given to prevent extracorporeal blood clotting in the perfusion set. A single 1-h normothermic ECC was performed using Stoeckert 41-40-50 heart-lung machine (Sorin Group, Milan, Italy) with a roller pump and perfusion set Maquet VKMO 78000 (Maquet, Rastatt, Germany) in each animal. To complete the ECC set, an oxygenator Quadrox-i Adult, aortic filter, and a Dual Heater Cooler HCU-20 water pump (Maquet, Rastatt, Germany) were used. Main pump expenditure was maintained at 40–50% of the cardiac output and the air/oxygen mixer setting was 55%, with an oxygen flow of 2–3 L/min. Normal perfusion pressure and blood saturation were achieved in all animals. After weaning from ECC protamine sulfate was administered intravenously (Prosulf, Wockhardt, United Kingdom; 0.8 mg for every 100 units of previously given heparin) to normalize ACT. Afterward, the vascular cannulas were removed and the vessels were closed with an absorbable suture (4.0 PDS II, Ethicon LTD, Livingston, United Kingdom). The surgical wound was closed in two layers.

Extracorporeal Blood Low-Level Light Treatment

A module for blood irradiation during ECC was installed on the oxygenator. Light emitter consisted of two non-coherent sources of radiation each built of low-voltage halogen burners with IRR coating in glass reflector, an optical diffuser, and NIR filter (Schneider-Kreuznach NIR IFG 098, Germany). Finally, non-polarized R/NIR electromagnetic waves in the range 750÷1500 nm with a maximum intensity of 800 nm illuminated the inlet and outlet chambers of the oxygenator. The blood flowing through the oxygenator was exposed to an average irradiance of 12.8 mW/cm^2 throughout the whole ECC procedure. The dose of R/NIR radiation absorbed by the blood was 1.0 J/cm^3.

Blood Samples

Depending on the type of assays, venous blood was collected into test tubes containing 3.8% sodium citrate (FL Medical s.r.l., Torreglia, Italy) in a ratio of 1: 9 (anticoagulant: blood), K_2EDTA (Profilab sc, Warsaw, Poland), heparin or with poly(methyl methacrylate) for serum preparation (FL Medical s.r.l., Torreglia, Italy). The blood was withdrawn immediately before the surgery, after 30 min of ECC, directly after completion of ECC and protamine sulfate infusion as well as in the post-ECC period: in the 6th, 12th, and 24th hour of the experiment (after ECC initiation) (**Figure 1**).

Blood Analyses

Blood morphology measurements were performed using an automated hematology analyzer Scil Vet abc (Horiba, Kyoto, Japan) in K_2EDTA blood. Serum lactate dehydrogenase activity (LDH) and bilirubin were measured spectrophotometrically

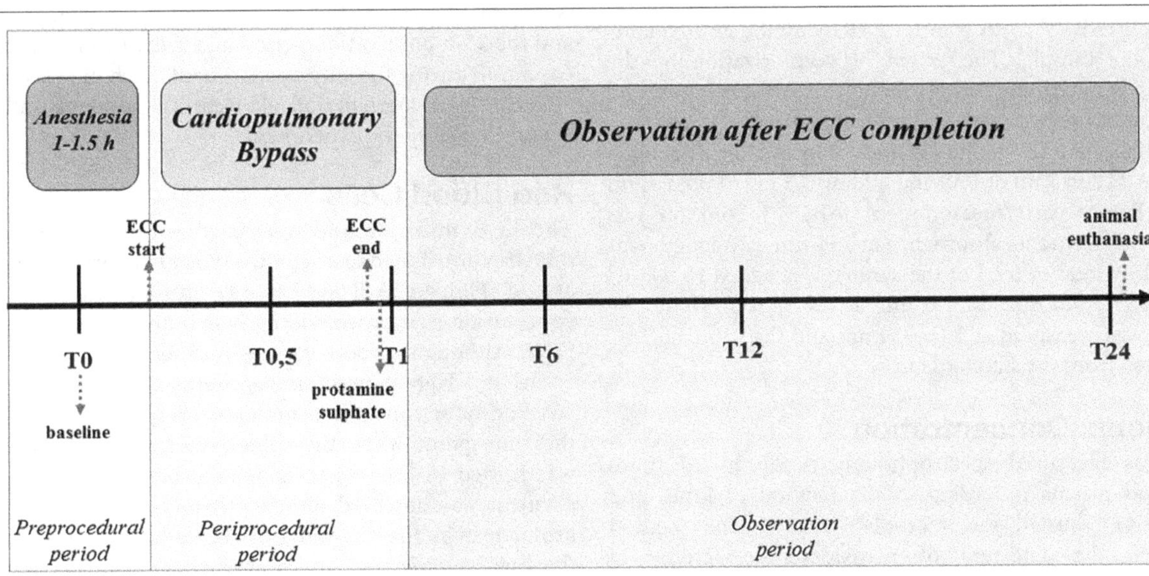

FIGURE 1 | Schedule of blood sampling during the experiment. T0 – before commencement of ECC (baseline), T0.5 – 30 min after ECC initiation, T1 – directly after 1 h of ECC, protamine sulfate infusion and normalization of the ACT, T6 – 6 h after completing ECC treatment, T12 – 12 h after initiation of ECC, and T24 – 24 h after initiation of ECC.

using a commercial reagent (Alpha Diagnostics, Warsaw, Poland).

Plasma-Free Hemoglobin Measurement

Plasma was obtained by centrifugation of citrated blood for 10 min at 1750 × *g*. Plasma free Hgb (PFHgb) was quantified in each sample through colorimetric assay using the Drabkin's reagent (Aqua-Med., Łódź, Poland). Each sample was measured in triplicate.

Peroxidation of Red Blood Cell Membrane Lipids

Lipid peroxidation was measured as the amount of malondialdehyde (MDA) determined by the thiobarbituric acid reactive substance (TBARS) (Heath and Packer, 1968) with little modification described in detail elsewhere (Oleszko et al., 2015). Trichloracetic acid [TCA, Chempur, Poland; 15% (wt/vol) TCA in 0.25 M HCl] and thiobarbituric acid [TBA, AppliChem, Germany; 0,37% (wt/vol) TBA in 0.25 M HCl] were used. Equal volumes of RBC suspension, TBA, and TCA were mixed together. Samples enclosed in small glass tubes were heated at 100°C for 15 min, then cooled and centrifuged for 10 min at 1750 × *g*. The absorbance of the supernatant was measured spectrophotometrically (Nicolet Evolution 60, Thermo Fisher Scientific, Waltham, MA, United States) at 535 nm and corrected for non-specific turbidity by subtracting the absorbance of the same sample at 600 nm. The content of TBARS was calculated using the extinction coefficient (155 mM^{-1} cm^{-1}).

Total Antioxidant Capacity

Total antioxidant capacity (TAC) was measured in plasma obtained by centrifugation of citrated blood as described by Re et al., 1999. Briefly, the method utilizes reduction of the bluish-green 2,2′-azinobis-(3-ethylbenzothiazoline-6-sulfonic acid) radical cation ($ABTS^{\bullet +}$) to colorless ABTS by the antioxidants present in the sample. The extent of decolorization by the antioxidants is determined as a function of concentration and time and calculated relative to the reactivity of Trolox as a standard. Stable $ABTS^{+}$ solution was prepared by dissolving 19.5 mg of ABTS in 7 ml of PBS and adding 3.3 mg of potassium persulfate. Before each measurement, $ABTS^{\bullet +}$ solution was diluted in PBS so that its absorbance at 734 nm wavelength was equal to 1.0. A total of 5 μl of the sample was added to 995 μl diluted $ABTS^{\bullet +}$ and mixed for 6 min at 500 rpm in 37°C. The absorbance was measured at $\lambda = 734$ nm and the value of TAC was calculated from the standard curve.

Haptoglobin Concentration

The Hp was measured spectrophotometrically in 10 times diluted blood plasma according to the method of Jones and Mould (1984) adjusted for microplate reader. The method is based on the detection of peroxidase-like activity of the haptoglobin-methemoglobin complex (Hp-MetHgb). The amount of hydrogen peroxide reduced by the Hp-MetHgb is proportional to the concentration of Hp. Breaking down of hydrogen peroxide leads to the oxidation of colorless guaiacol into yellowish-brown tetraguaiacol, which absorbance is measured at 492 nm.

Statistical Analysis

Longitudinal comparisons within groups were performed using bootstrap analysis of variance as described previously (Krishna Reddy et al., 2010; Walski et al., 2015). To test for differences between the groups at particular time points, the bootstrap *t*-test was used. The data were reported as a mean and standard deviation (SD). Although the groups were initially formed by random assignment, there were some differences in the RBC count and Hgb concentration at the baseline, so the results were presented as mean (SD) calculated from raw data as well as relative values to indicate the pattern of changes during experimental period (**Figures 2A,B** and **Table 1**). The results were considered significant for $p < 0.05$. Figures were performed using GraphPad[1] Prism version 5 for Windows (GraphPad Software, San Diego, CA, United States).

Analysis of the Reference Ranges

All the available reference ranges for pigs were from Latimer et al. (1981). Although there are no reference ranges for pigs for PFHgb, Hp, TBARS, and TAC, the 95% reference intervals for these parameters were acquired using baseline values (T0). When examined values showed a normal distribution in the Kolmogorov–Smirnov test, we acquired a 95% interval as the reference interval. When examined values did not show a normal distribution, a bootstrap methodology was applied (Horn et al., 1998; Horn and Pesce, 2003).

RESULTS

Animals

All animals survived the procedure of 1-h normothermic ECC and the 23-h observation period and remained in a good clinical condition during the entire experiment. Each pig was euthanized after the observation period. No technical problems with the ECC occurred during the experiment.

Red Blood Cells

The ECC initiation was associated with hemodilution which directly contributed to a significant drop in measured parameters at T0.5 (**Figures 2A,B** and **Table 1**). Both the RBC count and Hgb concentration decreased similarly in both groups throughout the ECC. Although in both groups postoperative changes in RBC count and Hgb showed similar trends – after initial return to baseline value constant drop in both parameters was observed – the time point when the values returned to the preoperative was shifted in time when compared between groups (in LLLT group it was observed directly after ECC while in the control group just in the 6th hour of the experiment). It resulted in the biggest difference of parameters value between groups at T6 – significantly lower values were measured in LLLT group (5.02×10^{12}/L vs. 6.06×10^{12}/L, $p < 0.001$, and 85 g/L vs. 102 g/L,

[1] www.graphpad.com

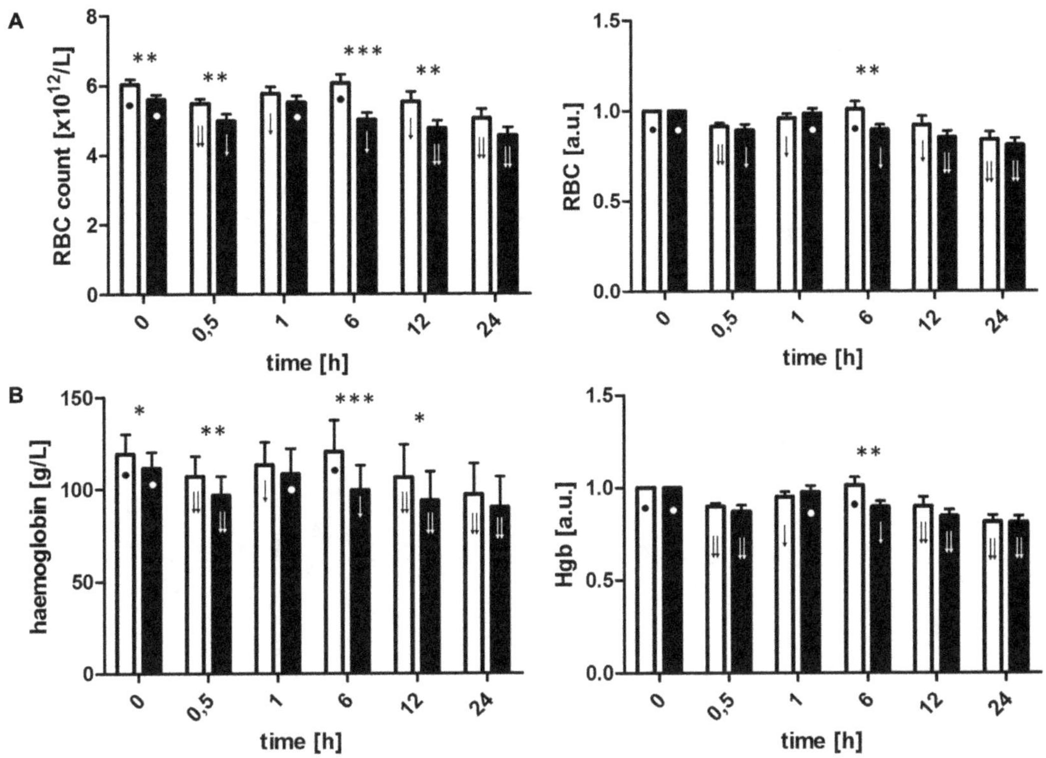

FIGURE 2 | Red blood cell count **(A)** and hemoglobin concentration **(B)** calculated from raw data and relative values of the baseline, before commencement of ECC (T0), 30 min after initiation of ECC (T0.5), post-circulation and normalization of ACT (T1), and 6 h (T6), 12 h (T12), and 24 h (T24) after commencement of ECC in the control group (□) and LLLT (■). Data are expressed as the mean (SD) ($n = 12$/group). *$p < 0.05$, **$p < 0.01$, ***$p < 0.001$, LLLT group compared with the control group at the sampling time. Changes in the values of the measurement points in a given group during the experiment were denoted by: ↓↓, ↓, •. Values marked with the same symbol do not differ significantly. The analysis was performed at confidence level $p < 0.05$.

$p < 0.001$, for RBC count and Hgb concentration, respectively). At the end of observation, both parameters were found to be comparable in study and control group. One of the possible causes associated with the decrease in RBC and Hgb during the study could be a relatively high volume of blood samples (c.a. 120 ml at each time point).

Hemolysis Parameters

The courses of PFHgb and bilirubin verified significant advantages in favor of LLLT (**Figures 3A,B**). The level of PFHgb decreased significantly after initiation of the ECC ($p < 0.05$) both in the control and in the LLLT groups. However, the decrease was significantly higher in the LLLT group (drop to the concentration of 0.10 g/L vs. 0.13 g/L, $p < 0.05$). Hemolysis increased after weaning from the ECC (rise in the level of PFHgb compared to T0.5). In the LLLT group in the observation period, both parameters were lower than before ECC and moreover lower than in the control group (levels of PFHgb in all postoperative time points, bilirubin at T1). Cell-free Hgb is released into the circulation in subjects undergoing ECC, so Hp showed the expected drop because of the binding of PFHgb (**Figure 3C**).

Not only PFHgb and serum bilirubin concentration but also serum LDH activity showed differences between the groups in favor of LLLT (**Figure 3D**). The activity of LDH increased significantly during the observation period ($p < 0.05$ for all) in the control group whereas in the LLLT group after an initial increase at T6 and T12 it was normalized at T24. In all time points (except baseline), LDH activity was higher in the control group compared to the LLLT group. No statistically significant differences between the groups were observed during the ECC, however, when the activity of LDH in the LLLT group decreased presumably due to hemodilution (T0.5 vs. T0, $p < 0.05$), whereas in the control group no drop in serum LDH activity was detected despite identical changes in plasma volume. Moreover, significantly lower serum LDH activity values in the LLLT group clearly demonstrate the persistence of LLLT effects during the observation period.

Inflammation and Oxidative Stress Markers

The ECC initiation resulted in white blood cells (WBCs) count decrease in the control group. Afterward, the values slowly increased until the end of the ECC (**Figure 4A**). In contrast, WBC count was constant during whole ECC procedure when blood photobiomodulation was applied. A sharp increase in the number of WBC released into the peripheral blood at the 6th hour of the experiment and a fall to the baseline level (control group) or below baseline level (LLLT group) at the end of observation were

TABLE 1 | Hematological and biochemical parameters assessed during entire experimental period.

Parameter	Group	T0		T0.5		T1		T6		T12		T24		Reference ranges
		Mean	***SD***	**Mean**	***SD***	**Mean**	***SD***	**Mean**	***SD***	**Mean**	***SD***	**Mean**	***SD***	
RBC count	CTR	6.02	0.49	5.49	0.43	5.78	0.63	6.06	0.83	5.53	0.91	5.05	0.85	5.00 ÷ 8.00
($\times 10^{12}$/L)	NIR	5.60	0.41	4.99$^{<}$	0.60	5.51	0.56	5.02	0.61	4.77$^{<}$	0.72	4.54$^{<}$	0.84	
Hgb	CTR	119	11	107	11	113	12	120	16	107	17	97	16	100 ÷ 160
(g/L)	NIR	111	9	97$^{<}$	10	108	13	100	13	94$^{<}$	15	90$^{<}$	16	
PFHgb	CTR	1.89	0.49	1.30	0.43	1.81	0.41	1.67	0.54	1.31	0.35	1.58	0.35	0.81 ÷ 2.9[a]
(mg/L)	NIR	1.83	0.50	0.96	0.29	1.33	0.43	1.04	0.34	0.95	0.34	1.17	0.47	
Bilirubin	CTR	4.25	1.90	–	–	5.47	1.90	3.83	1.51	4.22	2.61	3.36	1.00	0.00 ÷ 17.10
(μmol/L)	NIR	4.39	1.50			3.66	1.18	3.25	0.92	2.99	1.26	3.72	1.23	
Haptoglobin	CTR	0.49	0.50	0.31$^{<}$	0.42	0.31$^{<}$	0.37	0.29$^{<}$	0.42	0.35$^{<}$	0.35	1.01	0.23	0.37 ÷ 0.69[a]
(g/L)	NIR	0.57	0.49	0.44	0.46	0.37	0.44	0.38	0.42	0.61	0.41	1.26	0.16	
LDH	CTR	421	159	407	153	481	155	872$^{>}$	370	735$^{>}$	404	931$^{>}$	840	380 ÷ 634
(U/L)	NIR	526	73	435	98	560	127	616	180	608	117	524	89	
WBC count	CTR	16.02	4.63	12.54	5.66	14.13	6.82	22.38$^{>}$	5.29	19.43	5.76	16.54	4.75	11.0 ÷ 22.0
($\times 10^{9}$/L)	NIR	18.63	5.21	16.38	7.16	16.60	6.25	21.66	5.68	20.30	5.25	15.56	5.60	
TBARS	CTR	11.80	1.73	14.48	2.94	14.14	2.60	17.01$^{>}$	7.68	16.01$^{>}$	7.68	15.78$^{>}$	6.01	7.79 ÷ 15.72[a]
(nmol/gHgb)	NIR	11.72	2.02	12.28	2.26	10.58	1.47	14.31	3.51	14.58	3.42	13.42	3.63	
TAC	CTR	1.60	0.06	1.37	0.08	1.50	0.09	1.53	0.09	1.61	0.12	1.60	0.08	1.40 ÷ 1.77[a]
(mmol Trolox eq./L)	NIR	1.57	0.11	1.39	0.11	1.48	0.12	1.56	0.15	1.58	0.11	1.61	0.11	

[a] *Reference range estimated by the authors using baseline values.* $^{>}$ *Mean value above a reference range.* $^{<}$ *Mean value below a reference range.*

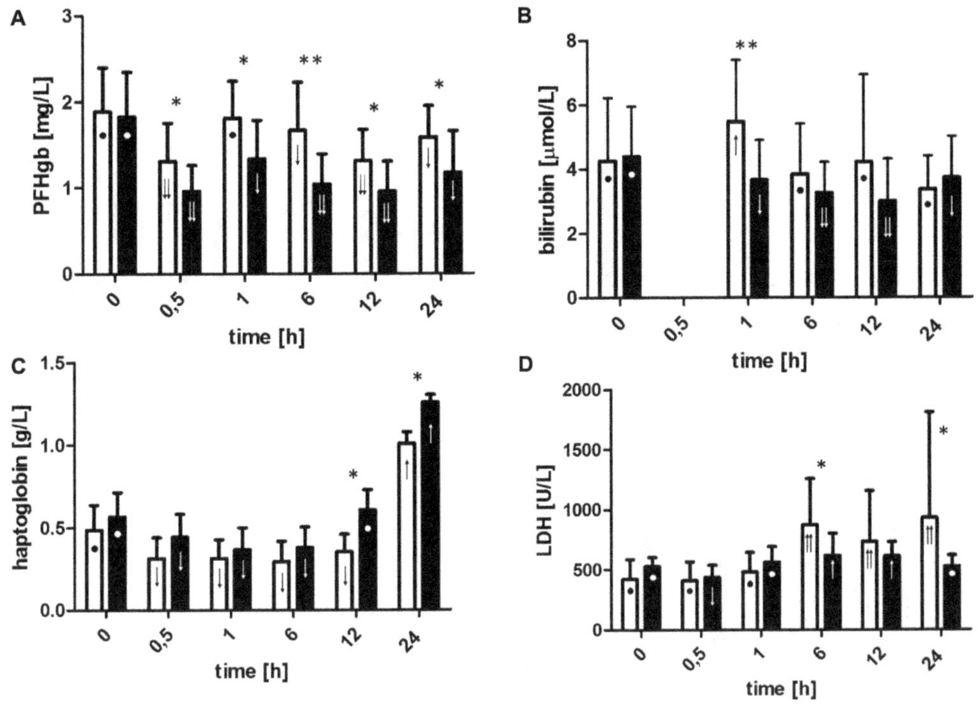

FIGURE 3 | Changes in plasma-free hemoglobin **(A)**, bilirubin **(B)**, haptoglobin **(C)**, and lactate dehydrogenase level **(D)**. For definition of time points, see **Figure 2** caption. Data are expressed as the mean (SD) (n = 12/group). *$p < 0.05$, **$p < 0.01$, ***$p < 0.001$, LLLT group compared with the control group at the sampling time. Changes in the values of the measurement points in a given group during the experiment were denoted by: ↓↓, ↓, •, ↑, ↑↑. Values marked with the same symbol do not differ significantly. The analysis was performed at confidence level $p < 0.05$.

noted. The patterns of WBC count changes were similar for both groups, however, the growth rate between the end of ECC (T1) and the peak value (T6) in the LLLT group was significantly lower when relative values are taken into an account (21.66×10^9/L vs. 22.38×10^9/L, ns. at T6, or increase by 30% vs. 58% at T6 in relation to T1, $p < 0.05$, for LLLT and control groups, respectively).

The concentrations of the TBARS increased significantly (for all time points, except for T1) in the control group with the peak at 6th hour post-circulation (17.01 nmol/gHgb vs. 11.80 nmol/gHgb when compared to the T0 value) and remained elevated over the upper reference limit throughout the whole observation period, while in the LLLT group RBC membrane lipid peroxidation slightly increased at T0.5 (12.28 nmol/L vs. 11.72 nmol/L when compared to the T0 value), returned to the baseline concentration at the end of ECC, furthermore, reached the maximum level at 12th hour (14.58 nmol/L), and finally declined to a moderately higher concentration than the baseline value (13.42 nmol/L) at the end of observation period (all described changes were significant at $p < 0.05$) (**Figure 4B**). TBARS concentration was significantly lower in the LLLT group during the whole ECC ($p < 0.05$ at T0.5, $p < 0.001$ at T1, with respect to the control group).

The ECC initiation was associated with TAC significant drop in both groups and gradual increase of the measured parameter up to the baseline achieved after 12 h of observation in the control group and after 6 h in the LLLT group, however, no significant differences between the groups were noted (**Figure 4C**).

DISCUSSION

To the best of our knowledge, our experiment is a first *in vivo* study which demonstrates that LLLT using R/NIR radiation may provide support for therapeutic procedures using ECC by limiting side effects associated with the activation and damage of extravasated blood cells.

During ECC, the primary cause of inflammation is blood contact with the non-physiological, polymer surfaces of the ECC system. Almost immediately after the beginning of ECC, plasma proteins are adsorbed on the biomaterials of ECC system. This coat consists mostly of fibrinogen and albumin, however, the content of individual proteins depends on their concentration in patients' plasma and the properties of biomaterial (Edmunds, 1995). Due to the conformational changes of the adhered proteins, receptors for circulating plasma proteins and blood cells are exposed. Finally, the activation of plasma cascade systems, endothelial cells, platelets, and leukocytes occurs (Edmunds, 1998).

Inflammatory response and oxidative stress are inherent disorders associated with ECC (Kawahito et al., 2000; Warren et al., 2009; Mamikonian et al., 2014; Zakkar et al., 2015), what was further confirmed by the results of our study. In the control

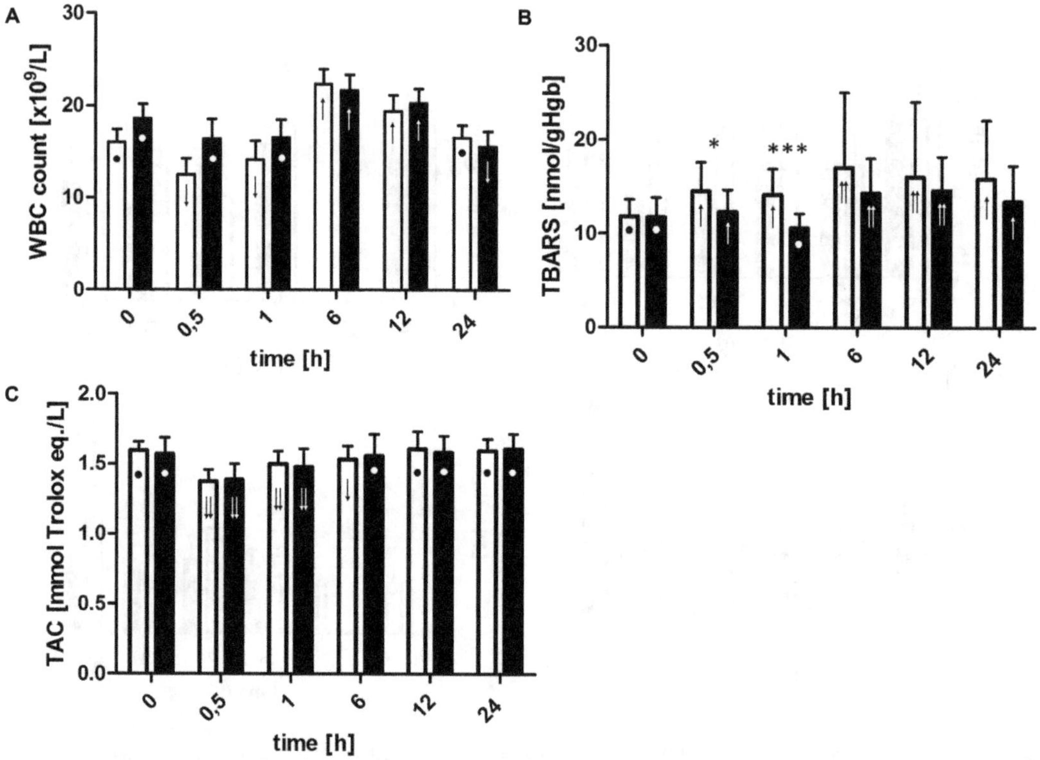

FIGURE 4 | Changes in White Blood Cell count **(A)**, thiobarbituric acid reactive substances concentration **(B)**, and plasma total antioxidant capacity **(C)**. For definition of time points, see **Figure 2** caption. Data are expressed as the mean (SD) (n = 12/group). *p < 0.05, ***p < 0.01, LLLT group compared with the control group at the sampling time. Changes in the values of the measurement points in a given group during the experiment were denoted by: ↓↓, ↓, •, ↑, ↑↑. Values marked with the same symbol do not differ significantly. The analysis was performed at confidence level p < 0.05.

group, a decrease in WBC count during ECC was accompanied by a significant increase in TBARS concentration. These changes result from two overlapping processes. On one hand, ECC is associated with hemodilution, on the other hand, neutrophils are activated by the contact with biomaterial and form platelet-leukocyte aggregates or they are sequestrated in the pulmonary vasculature as well as marginated to the tissues (mainly lungs and heart). In contrary, in the LLLT group, both WBC count and TBARS concentration remained relatively constant during ECC. Since hemodilution in both groups was comparable, it may be assumed that LLLT reduced generation of ROS, which contribute to the damage of RBCs plasma membranes. Moreover, photobiomodulation resulted in a limitation of the inflammatory response in the observation period as also evidenced by the significantly lower C-reactive protein (CRP) concentration (c.a. 60% lower at T6, $p < 0.05$, data not shown) in the postoperative period.

The impact of LLLT on oxidative stress in our study is consistent with the literature reports. It was previously shown that *in vitro* blood exposition to LLLT diminished platelet adhesion and aggregation when subjected to shear stress on subendothelial extracellular matrix-coated plates in time-dependent manner. The inhibitory effect was reversible up to 1 h after the termination of irradiation (Brill et al., 2000). More recently, Rola et al. (2017) confirmed decreased whole blood aggregation after LLLT exposure by the mechanisms independent of the NO metabolism and without significant effect on the release of platelet activation markers. It is important because platelet activation due to contact with biomaterial of ECC or alternating shear stress results in P-selectin expression, which binds to P-selectin glycoprotein ligand-1 in the plasma membranes of leukocytes. Platelet-leukocyte aggregates cause leucotrienes and proinflammatory cytokines release, thus stimulating inflammatory response. The activated polymorphonuclear leukocytes (mainly neutrophils) are believed to be a prime source of ROS during cardiac surgery, leading to peroxidation of erythrocytes plasma membrane lipids (Kamath et al., 2001; Zakkar et al., 2015). It can be concluded that the benefit of reversible inactivation of thrombocytes by LLLT may be a reduction of oxidative stress. However, direct suppression of the human neutrophils ROS production by NIR radiation was demonstrated by Shiraishi et al. (1999) and Fujimaki et al. (2003). Concomitantly, the serum opsonic activity was decreased, and this suppressive effect might be caused by inhibiting the activation of the classical and alternative complement pathway (Shiraishi et al., 1999). Since the primary mechanism of LLLT action is attributed to changes in hydrogen bond energy after absorption of R/NIR radiation and in consequence water molecules dissociation, that was firstly described by Goodall and Greenhow (1971), resulting in the mild conformational changes, the extent of the observed LLLT effects may be very broad (Goodall and Greenhow, 1971; Knight et al., 1979; Natzle et al., 1981; Walski et al., 2015). However, it is also important that the impact of LLLT during ECC persisted in the observation period limiting propagation of the inflammatory response, what was reflected in a significantly lower WBC count. In similar experimental models, neutrophil-free radical production was elevated 6 h after CPB compared to pre-CPB levels, accompanied by the highest neutrophil count, plasma TNF-α, IL-6, and IL-8 concentrations (Schwartz et al., 1998; Kawahito et al., 2000).

As a consequence of increased oxidative stress and hemodilution, a decrease in TAC was recorded. In the course of the ECC TAC dropped at a similar rate in both groups. As depicted in **Figure 4C**, the TAC values recovered initial levels during the postoperative period at 6th hour in LLLT group and at 12th hour in control group. Changes in TAC during CPB procedures have been widely discussed (Toivonen and Ahotupa, 1994; Clermont et al., 2002; Hadjinikolaou et al., 2003; Luyten et al., 2005). However, due to conflicting results, it was not possible to clearly demonstrate the mechanism responsible for TAC changes during and post ECC. In our opinion, initially, decrease of TAC during ECC is an indicator of a response to increased oxidative stress. Thus, to provide oxidative balance, scavengers of ROS are involved and utilized and till the new reserve of antioxidants is supplied, TAC is temporarily decreased. TAC return to baseline level is probably caused by a release (synthesis) of antioxidants into the blood plasma related to production of acute phase proteins (e.g., Hp, ceruloplasmin) and/or release of intracellular antioxidants (e.g., superoxide dismutase, catalase, glutathione, uric acid) from damaged cells (Hadjinikolaou et al., 2003).

Another consequence of ECC is morphotic blood elements damage resulting from their exposition to non-physiological mechanical (e.g., inappropriate flow rates, turbulence, cavitation) and environmental (e.g., decreased oncotic pressure by hemodilution, hypothermia) factors. It is manifested by immediate and delayed hemolysis and by changes in the mechanical properties of RBCs (Vercaemst, 2008; Olia et al., 2016). It is noteworthy that RBCs are much more resistant to mechanical stress than platelets and WBCs, and therefore, it is assumed that once RBCs are damaged, other blood elements have already been affected more severely (Vercaemst, 2008). The present study showed that LLLT using R/NIR radiation is capable to reduce RBC damage induced by ECC. In our experimental model, we were not able to see a severe hemolysis, as it is often the case during ECC procedures conducted in patients, in whom additional RBCs traumatization is related to surgery and ischemia-reperfusion episode (CPB with cardiac arrest and aortic clamping) (Pierangeli et al., 2001; Mamikonian et al., 2014). Although an increasing concentration of PFHgb always indicates hemolysis, normal values are not a necessary indicator of a healthy RBC (Vercaemst, 2008). Hemolysis associated with cardiovascular/circulation assist devices is assessed on the basis of criteria approved by the Interagency Registry for Mechanically Assisted Circulatory Support (INTERMACS). According to them, a minor hemolysis occurs when PFHgb concentration is greater than 20 mg/dl or LDH activity is greater than 2.5× the upper limit of the normal range (INTERMACS, 2016). In our experiment, none of the measured parameters exceeded the INTERMACS criteria, nevertheless, results of our study indicated the presence of blood trauma induced by ECC more severely in the control group. In the LLLT group, PFHgb concentration was significantly lower at each time point (except baseline) when compared to control group. Changes in LDH activity were more explicit because in the control group serum LDH activity strongly increased starting from T6 when it exceeded the upper limit of the reference range and remained elevated until the end of the experimental period. In contrast, in LLLT group LDH values were significantly lower in the observation period. Hp late increase might be associated with an inflammatory reaction as it acts as a moderate acute-phase protein, however, when blood is hemolytic, determination by Hgb binding assays may give unreliable results (Gruys et al., 2005). Our hemolytic parameters measurements are quite consistent with the results obtained by others (Cirri et al., 2001; Mamikonian et al., 2014; Vermeulen Windsant et al., 2014; Baumbach et al., 2016). Sublethal RBC damage results in decreased deformability and surface charge, and increased fragility and aggregability (Lee et al., 2007; Vercaemst, 2008) which subsequently lead to the early removal of the RBC from the circulation by the spleen or in the altered rheological proprieties of the blood followed by compromising efficient microcirculation and oxygen delivery to the surrounding tissues (Watanabe et al., 2007; Vercaemst, 2008; Ciana et al., 2017). Further blood trauma results in lethal damage of the ruptured, overstretched, or prematurely aged RBCs indicated by the intravascular hemolysis development (Olia et al., 2016). However, excessive increase in PFHb does not occur until Hp and NO scavenging capability is saturated. Even mild or transient hemolysis may provoke serious complications like thrombosis, postoperative kidney injury, and smooth muscle dystonia, vasculopathy, or endothelial dysfunction (Rother et al., 2005; Vercaemst, 2008; Vermeulen Windsant et al., 2014; Olia et al., 2016).

As we showed, LLLT application during ECC may significantly reduce the RBCs damage and thus limit hemolysis-related complications. Protective photochemical effect of R/NIR radiation on RBCs *in vitro* was demonstrated by Itoh et al. (1996, 2000) on ECC model. During the 4-h experiment, a dramatic decrease in erythrocytes intracellular ATP and deformability accompanied by the intense hemolysis was detected. LLLT irradiation limited the destructive impact of ECC on RBCs concomitantly, no significant difference was observed in the partial oxygen pressure, between the LLLT and control groups, indicating that erythrocyte oxygenation was maintained throughout the experiment. Moreover, SEM of the oxygenator membranes revealed a significantly higher number of discocytes in the laser treated sample compared with control (45 and 20%, respectively) (Itoh et al., 1996, 2000). Decreased hemolysis and reduced plasma lipid peroxidation resulting from exposure of erythrocytes to R/NIR radiation have also been demonstrated in experiments, in which samples pretreated with R/NIR radiation (700–2000 nm) were ozonated (Komorowska et al., 2002; Chludzińska et al., 2005). Changes in RBC osmotic fragility caused by R/NIR radiation also indicate plasma membrane stabilization and decreased hemolysis in the hypotonic environment (Iijima et al., 1991; Habodaszova et al., 2004). Furthermore, Walski et al. (2014) showed that osmotic properties of human erythrocytes subjected to NIR radiation are unified, what manifests as a change in slope of the hemolysis curve. Narrowing of population distribution suggests the strongest impact of NIR radiation on the most and least resistant cells.

An improvement of RBCs mechanical properties under the influence of LLLT using R/NIR may be explained by changes at the cellular and subcellular levels, mainly by an increase in overall activity of ATP-ases, especially sodium-potassium ATP-ase (Kujawa et al., 2004; Pasternak et al., 2012), which maintains resting membrane potential and is responsible for cell volume regulation (Lew and Tiffert, 2017). There are two mechanisms which explain changes in enzyme activity after R/NIR radiation: conformational changes in the protein structure, and indirect modification of the surrounding molecules. It has been shown that R/NIR radiation induces structural changes in the lipid bilayer. It causes a decrease in polarity of phospholipid hydrophilic fragments. Moreover, lower doses of LLLT diminished the order parameter, which is a measure of the relative fluidity in the membranes (Komorowska and Czyżewska, 1997). Higher RBC membrane fluidity after exposure to NIR radiation has also been confirmed in other studies (Kujawa et al., 2003; Chludzińska et al., 2005) and its macroscopic consequence is an improvement of the blood rheological properties related with increased erythrocytes deformability, which was observed both *in vitro* and *in vivo* (Iijima et al., 1993; Mi et al., 2004; Wang et al., 2016).

Furthermore, it has been demonstrated that R/NIR radiation causes an increase in electrokinetic potential and therefore may directly inhibit RBCs aggregation (Komorowska et al., 2002; Mi et al., 2004; Korolevich et al., 2004; Chludzińska et al., 2005). Erythrocytes are characterized by a tendency to form rouleaux and aggregates, thus influencing blood rheology (Steffen et al., 2011; Flormann et al., 2017). Pathological conditions such as cardiovascular disease (CVD) are accompanied by a presence of larger RBCs aggregates and a relative decrease in a number of singular erythrocytes. While in healthy individuals rouleaux are seen, in patients with CVD RBC agglutination occurs and irregular erythrocyte aggregates with a diameter up to 300 μm may be found (Korolevich et al., 2004; Brust et al., 2014; Flormann et al., 2017). The 5–15 min LLLT of the temporal region increased local microcirculation (measured as perfusion rate) almost twofold and caused a change in the aggregation characteristics of RBCs (Korolevich et al., 2004).

However, an improvement in microcirculation may result also from blood vessel relaxation in response to NO. It has been repeatedly reported, that R/NIR radiation leads to a partial photochemical dissociation of Hgb-ligand complexes (e.g., O_2, CO, NO) during radiation absorption (Komorowska et al., 2002; Vladimirov et al., 2004; Zalesskaya and Sambor, 2005; Walski et al., 2015). Moreover, Hgb deoxygenation causes tyrosine phosphorylation in band 3 protein. It results in its stronger binding with spectrin network of RBC. Erythrocyte membrane mechanical resistance increases and the rate of hemolysis decreases, suggesting greater resistivity to osmotic stress (Chludzińska et al., 2005).

Another important issue is the influence of photodynamic reactions induced by LLLT on the ability of blood to transport oxygen. On one hand, erythrocytes *in vitro* exposed to R/NIR light demonstrate a rapid increase of oxygen saturation (SpO_2) of Hgb and an increase of oxygen tension in the blood whereas both $PaCO_2$ and pH shows no significant changes after irradiation (Wąsik et al., 2007). An increase of oxy-Hgb concentration related with LLLT was also observed *in vivo* in humans during placebo-controlled studies (Tian et al., 2016; Wang et al., 2016). On the other hand, Yesman et al. (2016) observed the reduction in SpO_2 up to 5% which indicated the process of photodissociation of HbO_2 *in vivo*. However, despite the contradictory results, the final outcome of each study was an improvement of the tissue oxygenation as the LLLT can promote the release of oxygen from oxy-Hgb (Asimov et al., 2006; Tian et al., 2016; Wang et al., 2016; Yesman et al., 2016; Xu et al., 2018).

All in all, RBC modified by LLLT has a larger electrokinetic charge, higher plasma membrane fluidity and increased resistance to oxidative and mechanical stress. All these features may contribute to the reduction of hemolysis during ECC demonstrated in our study. Concomitantly, it is likely, that NO intravascular bioavailability increases after LLLT. Thus, the outcome in patients treated with ECC could theoretically be improved by LLLT as a factor at least partly eliminating toxic hemolysis-derived end products and rheological-altered blood cell characteristics. Although after the ECC hematocrit is not reduced only because of hemodilution or RBCs destruction but also as a result of erythropoiesis inhibition due to acute postoperative inflammation, LLLT application might accelerate erythropoiesis recovery and thus ensure a better outcome for patients undergoing cardiac surgery. However, this hypothesis should be validated in further studies which would include at least prolonged observation period.

Limitation of the Study

Our CPB animal model was quite free from bias related to other surgical trauma. To investigate the effect of ECC on RBCs and oxidative stress, we used a normal animal model to rule out the effect of other pathological factors on the experimental results. Additionally, animals were subjected to ECC without cardiac arrest, aortic clamping, or any cardiac surgery. On one hand, it enabled us to analyze the results as the pure effect of ECC, on the other hand, other pathological factors which are present during cardiac surgery were omitted so it is difficult to assess what meaning the changes we observed would have in real-life patients. Moreover, 1-h ECC may be too short to provoke extensive hemolysis and RBC damage. The decrease in RBC we noted after 6th hour of the experiment may be at least partially due to repeated blood collection. And the last but not least – it was previously determined that porcine RBC are less fragile to shear stress than human RBC and may, therefore, underestimate the impact of the ECC on the blood components (Chan et al., 2017), what is a common challenge of research results translation from model organisms to human (Minetti et al., 2013).

CONCLUSION

This study showed that ECC induces oxidative stress and blood cells destruction when performed in the porcine model of CPB even without ischemia/reperfusion injury or cardiac surgery. Our data clearly present that LLLT may significantly reduce blood trauma in this kind of treatment. The effect of extracorporeal blood photobiomodulation is both limited inflammatory response to ECC as well as RBCs damage and thus minimized hemolysis-related complications.

AUTHOR CONTRIBUTIONS

TW, AD, and MK defined the study and planned the experiments. AC, GW, and RC were responsible for the optimization of ECC protocol. TW, AD, JB, AC, GW, NT-P, and MG performed the acquisition and analysis. TW, AD, and MK interpreted the data. TW, AD, JB, and NT-P drafted the manuscript. AC, MK, and RC critically revised the manuscript. All authors approved the final version of the manuscript.

REFERENCES

Asimov, M. M., Asimov, R. M., Rubinov, A. N., Mamilov, S. A., and Plaksii, Y. S. (2006). Effect of temperature on the quantum yield of laser-induced photodissociation of oxyhemoglobin *in vivo*. *J. Appl. Spectrosc.* 73, 99–102. doi: 10.1007/s10812-006-0042-z

Baumbach, H., Rustenbach, C., Ahad, S., Nagib, R., Albert, M., Ratge, D., et al. (2016). Minimally invasive extracorporeal bypass in minimally invasive heart valve operations: a prospective randomized trial. *Ann. Thorac. Surg.* 102, 93–100. doi: 10.1016/j.athoracsur.2016.01.043

Boyle, E. M. Jr., Pohlman, T. H., Johnson, M. C., and Verrier, E. D. (1997). Endothelial cell injury in cardiovascular surgery: the systemic inflammatory response. *Ann. Thorac. Surg.* 63, 277–284.

Brill, A., Shenkman, B., Brill, G., Tamarin, I., Dardik, R., Kirichuk, V., et al. (2000). Blood irradiation by He-Ne laser induces a decrease in platelet responses to physiological agonists and an increase in platelet cyclic GMP. *Platelets* 11, 87–93. doi: 10.1080/09537100075698

Brust, M., Aouane, O., Thiébaud, M., Flormann, D., Verdier, C., Kaestner, L., et al. (2014). The plasma protein fibrinogen stabilizes clusters of red blood cells in microcapillary flows. *Sci. Rep.* 11:4348. doi: 10.1038/srep04348

Cabrales, P. (2007). Effects of erythrocyte flexibility on microvascular perfusion and oxygenation during acute anemia. *Am. J. Physiol. Heart Circ. Physiol.* 293, H1206–H1215. doi: 10.1152/ajpheart.00109.2007

Chan, C., Pieper, I., Robinson, C., Friedmann, Y., Kanamarlapudi, V., and Thornton, C. (2017). Shear stress-induced total blood trauma in multiple species. *Artif. Organs* 41, 934–947. doi: 10.1111/aor.12932

Chludzińska, L., Ananicz, E., Jarosławska, A., and Komorowska, M. (2005). Near-infrared radiation protects the red cell membrane against oxidation. *Blood Cells Mol. Dis.* 35, 74–79. doi: 10.1016/j.bcmd.2005.04.003

Ciana, A., Achilli, C., Gaur, A., and Minetti, G. (2017). Membrane remodelling and vesicle formation during ageing of human red blood cells. *Cell Physiol. Biochem* 42, 1127–1138. doi: 10.1159/000478768

Cirri, S., Negri, L., Babbini, M., Latis, G., Khlat, B., Tarelli, G., et al. (2001). Haemolysis due to active venous drainage during cardiopulmonary bypass: comparison of two different techniques. *Perfusion* 16, 313–318. doi: 10.1177/026765910101600408

Clermont, G., Vergely, C., Jazayeri, S., Lahet, J., Goudeau, J., Lecour, S., et al. (2002). Systemic free radical activation is a major event involved in myocardial oxidative stress related to cardiopulmonary bypass. *Anesthesiology* 96, 80–87. doi: 10.1097/00000542-200201000-00019

Edmunds, L. Jr. (1995). Why cardiopulmonary bypass makes patients sick: strategies to control the blood-synthetic surface interface. *Adv. Card. Surg.* 6, 131–167.

Edmunds, L. H. Jr. (1998). Inflammatory response to cardiopulmonary bypass. *Ann. Thorac. Surg.* 66, S12–S16. doi: 10.1016/S0003-4975(98)00967-9

Flormann, D., Aouane, O., Kaestner, L., Ruloff, C., Misbah, C., Podgorski, T., et al. (2017). The buckling instability of aggregating red blood cells. *Sci. Rep.* 7:7928. doi: 10.1038/s41598-017-07634-6

Fujimaki, Y., Shimoyama, T., Liu, Q., Umeda, T., Nakaji, S., and Sugawara, K. (2003). Low-level laser irradiation attenuates production of reactive oxygen species by human neutrophils. *J. Clin. Laser Med. Surg.* 21, 165–170. doi: 10.1089/104454703321895635

Goodall, D. M., and Greenhow, R. C. (1971). Ionization of water induced by vibrational excitation using a neodymium: glass laser. *Chem. Phys. Lett.* 9, 583–585. doi: 10.1016/0009-2614(71)85133-3

Gruys, E., Toussaint, M. J., Niewold, T. A., and Koopmans, S. J. (2005). Acute phase reaction and acute phase proteins. *J. Zhejiang Univ. Sci. B* 6, 1045–1056. doi: 10.1631/jzus.2005.B1045

Grygorczyk, R., and Orlov, S. N. (2017). Effects of hypoxia on erythrocyte membrane properties-implications for intravascular hemolysis and purinergic control of blood flow. *Front. Physiol.* 22:1110. doi: 10.3389/fphys.2017.01110

Habodaszova, D., Sikurova, L., Waczulikova, I., and Bryszewska, M. (2004). The osmotic fragility of human erythrocytes is inhibited by laser irradiation. *Acta Phys. Univ. Comen.* 4, 85–90.

Hadjinikolaou, L., Alexiou, C., Cohen, A., Standbridge Rde, L., McColl, A., and Richmond, W. (2003). Early changes in plasma antioxidant and lipid peroxidation levels following coronary artery bypass surgery: a complex response. *Eur. J. Cardiothorac. Surg.* 23, 969–975. doi: 10.1016/S1010-7940(03)00115-5

Heath, L., and Packer, L. (1968). Photoperoxidation in isolated chloroplasts. I. Kinetics and stoichiometry of fatty acid peroxidation. *Arch. Biochem. Biophys.* 125, 189–198. doi: 10.1016/0003-9861(68)90654-1

Hirai, S. (2003). Systemic inflammatory response syndrome after cardiac surgery under cardiopulmonary bypass. *Ann. Thorac. Cardiovasc. Surg.* 9, 365–370.

Horn, P. S., and Pesce, A. J. (2003). Reference intervals: an update. *Clin. Chim. Acta* 334, 5–23. doi: 10.1016/S0009-8981(03)00133-5

Horn, P. S., Pesce, A. J., and Copeland, B. E. (1998). A robust approach to reference interval estimation and evaluation. *Clin. Chem.* 44, 622–631.

Iijima, K., Shimoyama, N., Shimoyama, M., and Mizuguchi, T. (1991). Red and green low-powered He-Ne lasers protect human erythrocytes from hypotonic hemolysis. *J. Clin. Laser Med. Surg.* 9, 385–389.

Iijima, K., Shimoyama, N., Shimoyama, M., and Mizuguchi, T. (1993). Effect of low-power He-Ne laser on deformability of stored human erythrocytes. *J. Clin. Laser. Med. Surg.* 11, 185–189.

INTERMACS (2016). *Adverse Event Definitions: Adult and Pediatric patients, Approved by the INTERMACS Executive Committee.* Available at: https://www.uab.edu/medicine/intermacs/images/protocol_5.0/appendix_a/AE-Definitions-Final-02-4-2016.docx. May 15, 2013; AE Definitions 02/04/2016.

Itoh, T., Murakami, H., Orihashi, K., Sueda, T., Kusumoto, Y., Kakehashi, M., et al. (2000). Low power laser protects human erythrocytes In an In vitro model of artificial heart-lung machines. *Artif. Organs* 24, 870–873. doi: 10.1046/j.1525-1594.2000.06624.x

Itoh, T., Murakami, H., Orihashi, K., Sueda, T., and Matsuura, Y. (1996). The protective effect of low power He-Ne laser against erythrocytic damage caused by artificial heart-lung machines. *Hiroshima J. Med. Sci.* 45, 15–22.

Ji, B., and Undar, A. (2006). An evaluation of the benefits of pulsatile versus nonpulsatile perfusion during cardiopulmonary bypass procedures in pediatric and adult cardiac patients. *ASAIO J.* 52, 357–361. doi: 10.1097/01.mat.0000225266.80021.9b

Jones, G., and Mould, D. (1984). Adaptation of the guaiacol (peroxidase) test for haptoglobins to a microtitration plate system. *Res. Vet. Sci.* 37, 87–92.

Kamath, S., Blann, A., and Lip, G. (2001). Platelet activation: assessment and quantification. *Eur. Heart J.* 22, 1561–1571. doi: 10.1053/euhj.2000.2515

Kameneva, M., Burgreen, G., Kono, K., Repko, B., Antaki, J., and Umezu, M. (2004). Effects of turbulent stresses upon mechanical hemolysis: experimental and computational analysis. *ASAIO J.* 50, 418–423. doi: 10.1097/01.MAT.0000136512.36370.B5

Kander, M. C., Cui, Y., and Liucorresponding, Z. (2017). Gender difference in oxidative stress: a new look at the mechanisms for cardiovascular diseases. *J. Cell. Mol. Med.* 21, 1024–1032. doi: 10.1111/jcmm.13038

Kanias, T., Sinchar, D., Osei-Hwedieh, D., Baust, J., Jordan, A., Zimring, J. C., et al. (2016). Testosterone-dependent sex differences in red blood cell hemolysis in storage, stress and disease. *Transfusion* 56, 2571–2583. doi: 10.1111/trf.13745

Kawahito, K., Kobayashi, E., Ohmori, M., Harada, K., Kitoh, Y., Fujimura, A., et al. (2000). Enhanced responsiveness of circulatory neutrophils after cardiopulmonary bypass: increased aggregability and superoxide producing capacity. *Artif. Organs* 24, 37–42. doi: 10.1046/j.1525-1594.2000.06381.x

Kirkham, P., and Rahman, I. (2006). Oxidative stress in asthma and COPD: antioxidants as a therapeutic strategy. *Pharmacol. Ther.* 111, 476–494. doi: 10.1016/j.pharmthera.2005.10.015

Knight, B., Goodall, D. M., and Greenhow, R. C. (1979). Single-photon vibrational photochemistry. Part 1. Wavelength and temperature dependence of the quantum yield for the laser-induced ionization of water. *J. Chem. Soc. Faraday Trans. 2.* 75, 841–856. doi: 10.1039/F29797500841

Koch, C. G., Li, L., Sessler, D. I., Figueroa, P., Hoeltge, G. A., Mihaljevic, T., et al. (2008). Duration of red-cell storage and complications after cardiac surgery. *N. Engl. J. Med.* 358, 1229–1239. doi: 10.1056/NEJMoa070403

Komorowska, M., Cuissot, A., Czarnołeski, A., and Białas, W. (2002). Erythrocyte response to near-infrared radiation. *J. Photochem. Photobiol. B.* 68, 93–100. doi: 10.1016/S1011-1344(02)00361-5

Komorowska, M., and Czyżewska, H. (1997). The effect of near-infrared radiation on erythrocyte membranes: EPR study. *Nukleonika* 42, 379–386.

Korolevich, A., Dubina, N., Vecherinskii, S., and Belsley, M. (2004). Influence of low-intensity laser radiation on the rheological characteristics of human blood. *J. Appl. Spectrosc.* 71, 572–579. doi: 10.1023/B:JAPS.0000046301.36013.c5

Krishna Reddy, M., Naveen Kumar, B., and Ramu, Y. (2010). Bootstrap method for testing of equality of several means. *Inter Stat.* Available at: http://interstat.statjournals.net/YEAR/2010/articles/1004008.pdf

Kujawa, J., Zavodnik, L., Zavodnik, I., and Bryszewska, M. (2003). Low-intensity near-infrared laser radiation-induced changes of acetylcholinesterase activity of human erythrocytes. *J. Clin. Laser Med. Surg.* 21, 351–355. doi: 10.1089/104454703322650158

Kujawa, J., Zavodnik, L., Zavodnik, I., Buko, V., Lapshyna, A., and Bryszewska, M. (2004). Effect of low-intensity (3.75-25 J/cm2) near-infrared (810 nm) laser radiation on red blood cell ATPase activities and membrane structure. *J. Clin. Laser Med. Surg.* 22, 111–117. doi: 10.1089/104454704774076163

Latimer, K. S., Mahaffey, E. A., and Prasse, K. W. (1981). *Duncan and Prasse's Veterinary Laboratory Medicine: Clinical Pathology*. London: Wiley-Blackwell.

Lee, S., Antaki, J., Kameneva, M., Dobbe, J., Hardeman, M., Ahn, K., et al. (2007). Strain hardening of red blood cells by accumulated cyclic supraphysiological stress. *Artif. Organs* 31, 80–86. doi: 10.1111/j.1525-1594.2007.00344.x

Lew, V. L., and Tiffert, T. (2017). On the mechanism of human red blood cell longevity: roles of calcium, the sodium pump, PIEZO1, and gardos channels. *Front. Physiol.* 8:977. doi: 10.3389/fphys.2017.00977

Luyten, C., van Overveld, F., De Backer, L., Sadowska, A., Rodrigus, I., De Hert, S., et al. (2005). Antioxidant defence during cardiopulmonary bypass surgery. *Eur. J. Cardiothorac. Surg.* 27, 611–616. doi: 10.1016/j.ejcts.2004.12.013

Mamikonian, L., Mamo, L., Smith, P., Koo, J., Lodge, A., and Turi, J. (2014). Cardiopulmonary bypass is associated with hemolysis and acute kidney injury in neonates, infants, and children. *Pediatr. Crit. Care Med.* 15, 111–119. doi: 10.1097/PCC.0000000000000047

Matés, J., Pérez-Gómez, C., and Núñez de Castro, I. (1999). Antioxidant enzymes and human diseases. *Clin. Biochem.* 32, 595–603. doi: 10.1016/S0009-9120(99)00075-2

Mi, X., Chen, J., Cen, Y., Liang, Z., and Zhou, L. (2004). A comparative study of 632.8 and 532 nm laser irradiation on some rheological factors in human blood in vitro. *J. Photochem. Photobiol. B.* 74, 7–12. doi: 10.1016/j.jphotobiol.2004.01.003

Minetti, G., Egée, S., Mörsdorf, D., Steffen, P., Makhro, A., Achilli, C., et al. (2013). Red cell investigations: art and artefacts. *Blood Rev.* 27, 91–101. doi: 10.1016/j.blre.2013.02.002

Natzle, W. C., Moore, C. B., Goodall, D. M., Frisch, W., and Holzwarth, J. F. (1981). Dissociative ionization of water induced by single-photon vibrational excitation. *J. Phys. Chem.* 85, 2882–2884. doi: 10.1021/j150620a006

Oleszko, A., Olsztyńska-Janus, S., Walski, T., Grzeszczuk-Kuć, K., Bujok, J., Gałecka, K., et al. (2015). Application of FTIR-ATR spectroscopy to determine the extent of lipid peroxidation in plasma during haemodialysis. *Biomed. Res. Int.* 2015:245607. doi: 10.1155/2015/245607

Olia, S., Maul, T., Antaki, J., and Kameneva, M. (2016). Mechanical blood trauma in assisted circulation: sublethal RBC damage preceding hemolysis. *Int. J. Artif. Organs.* 39, 150–159. doi: 10.5301/ijao.5000478

Pasternak, K., Wróbel, D., Gworys, K., and Kujawa, J. (2012). Wpływ promieniowania MLS na aktywności ATPazowe błon erytrocytów ludzkich. *Kwart. Ortop.* 1, 74–82.

Pierangeli, A., Masieri, V., Bruzzi, F., De Toni, E., Grillone, G., Boni, P., et al. (2001). Haemolysis during cardiopulmonary bypass: how to reduce the free haemoglobin by managing the suctioned blood separately. *Perfusion* 16, 519–524. doi: 10.1177/026765910101600612

Re, R., Pellegrini, N., Proteggente, A., Pannala, A., Yang, M., and Rice-Evans, C. (1999). Antioxidant activity applying an improved ABTS radical cation decolorization assay. *Free Radic. Biol. Med.* 26, 1231–1237. doi: 10.1016/S0891-5849(98)00315-3

Rola, P., Doroszko, A., Szahidewicz-Krupska, E., et al. (2017). Low-level laser irradiation exerts antiaggregative effect on human platelets independently on the nitric oxide metabolism and release of platelet activation markers. *Oxid. Med. Cell. Longev.* 2017:6201797. doi: 10.1155/2017/6201797

Rother, R., Bell, L., Hillmen, P., and Gladwin, M. T. (2005). The clinical sequelae of intravascular hemolysis and extracellular plasma hemoglobin: a novel mechanism of human disease. *JAMA* 293, 1653–1662. doi: 10.1001/jama.293.13.1653

Schwartz, J., Shamamian, P., Schwartz, D., Grossi, E., Jacobs, C., Steiner, F., et al. (1998). Cardiopulmonary bypass primes polymorphonuclear leukocytes. *J. Surg. Res.* 75, 177–182. doi: 10.1006/jsre.1997.5287

Shiraishi, M., Suzuki, K., Nakaji, S., Sugawara, K., Sugita, N., Suzuki, K. J., et al. (1999). Effect of linear polarized near-infrared ray irradiation on the chemiluminescence of human neutrophils and serum opsonic activity. *Luminescence* 14, 239–243. doi: 10.1002/(SICI)1522-7243(199909/10)14:5<239::AID-BIO533>3.0.CO;2-N

Steffen, P., Jung, A., Nguyen, D. B., Müller, T., Bernhardt, I., Kaestner, L., et al. (2011). Stimulation of human red blood cells leads to Ca2+-mediated intercellular adhesion. *Cell Calcium* 50, 54–61. doi: 10.1016/j.ceca.2011.05.002

Tian, F., Hase, S. N., Gonzalez-Lima, F., and Liu, H. (2016). Transcranial laser stimulation improves human cerebral oxygenation. *Lasers Surg. Med.* 48, 343–349. doi: 10.1002/lsm.22471

Toivonen, H., and Ahotupa, M. (1994). Free radical reaction products and antioxidant capacity in arterial plasma during coronary artery bypass grafting. *J. Thorac. Cardiovasc. Surg.* 108, 140–147.

van Straten, A., Bekker, M., Soliman Hamad, M., van Zundert, A., Martens, E., Schönberger, J., et al. (2010). Transfusion of red blood cells: the impact on short-term and long-term survival after coronary artery bypass grafting, a ten-year follow-up. *Interact. Cardiovasc. Thorac. Surg.* 10, 37–42. doi: 10.1510/icvts.2009.214551

Vercaemst, L. (2008). Hemolysis in cardiac surgery patients undergoing cardiopulmonary bypass: a review in search of a treatment algorithm. *J. Extra Corpor. Technol.* 40, 257–267.

Vermeulen Windsant, I., de Wit, N., Sertorio, J., van Bijnen, A., Ganushchak, Y., Heijmans, J., et al. (2014). Hemolysis during cardiac surgery is associated with increased intravascular nitric oxide consumption and perioperative kidney and intestinal tissue damage. *Front. Physiol.* 5:340. doi: 10.3389/fphys.2014.00340

Vladimirov, Y., Osipov, A., and Klebanov, G. (2004). Photobiological principles of therapeutic applications of laser radiation. *Biochemistry (Mosc).* 69, 81–90. doi: 10.1023/B:BIRY.0000016356.93968.7e

Walski, T., Chludzińska, L., Komorowska, M., and Witkiewicz, W. (2014). Individual osmotic fragility distribution: a new parameter for determination of the osmotic properties of human red blood cells. *Biomed. Res. Int.* 2014:162102. doi: 10.1155/2014/162102

Walski, T., Dyrda, A., Dzik, M., Chludzińska, L., Tomków, T., Mehl, J., et al. (2015). Near infrared light induces post-translational modifications of human red blood cell proteins. *Photochem. Photobiol. Sci.* 14, 2035–2045. doi: 10.1039/c5pp00203f

Wang, H., Deng, J., Tu, W., Zhang, L., Chen, H., Wu, X., et al. (2016). The hematologic effects of low intensity 650 nm laser irradiation on hypercholesterolemia rabbits. *Am. J. Transl. Res.* 15, 2293–2300.

Warren, O., Smith, A., Alexiou, C., Rogers, P., Jawad, N., Vincent, C., et al. (2009). The inflammatory response to cardiopulmonary bypass: part 1-mechanisms of pathogenesis. *J. Cardiothorac. Vasc. Anesth.* 23, 223–231. doi: 10.1053/j.jvca.2008.08.007

Wąsik, M., Gorska, E., Modzelewska, M., Nowicki, K., Jakubczak, B., and Demkow, U. (2007). The influence of low-power helium-neon laser irradiation on function of selected peripheral blood cells. *J. Physiol. Pharmacol.* 58 Suppl 5(Pt 2), 729–737.

Watanabe, N., Sakota, D., Ohuchi, K., and Takatani, S. (2007). Deformability of red blood cells and its relation to blood trauma in rotary blood pumps. *Artif. Organs* 31, 352–358. doi: 10.1111/j.1525-1594.2007.00392.x

Xu, Y., Lin, Y., Gao, S., and Shen, J. (2018). Study on mechanism of release oxygen by photo-excited hemoglobin in low-level laser therapy. *Lasers Med. Sci.* 33, 135–139. doi: 10.1007/s10103-017-2363-y

Yesman, S. S., Mamilov, S. O., Veligotsky, D. V., and Gisbrecht, A. I. (2016). Local changes in arterial oxygen saturation induced by visible and near-infrared light radiation. *Lasers Med. Sci.* 31, 145–149. doi: 10.1007/s10103-015-1838-y

Zakkar, M., Guida, G., Suleiman, M.-S., and Angelini, G. (2015). Cardiopulmonary bypass and oxidative stress. *Oxid. Med. Cell. Longev.* 2015:189863. doi: 10.1155/2015/189863

Zalesskaya, G., and Sambor, E. (2005). Interaction of low-intensity laser radiation with blood and its components. *J. Appl. Spectrosc.* 72, 242–248. doi: 10.1007/s10103-014-1571-y

9

Effects of Hypoxia on Erythrocyte Membrane Properties—Implications for Intravascular Hemolysis and Purinergic Control of Blood Flow

Ryszard Grygorczyk [1]* *and Sergei N. Orlov* [2]

[1] Medicine, Université de Montréal, Montreal, QC, Canada, [2] Biology, M. V. Lomonosov Moscow State University, Moscow, Russia

Correspondence:
Ryszard Grygorczyk
ryszard.grygorczyk@umontreal.ca

Intravascular hemolysis occurs in hereditary, acquired, and iatrogenic hemolytic conditions but it could be also a normal physiological process contributing to intercellular signaling. New evidence suggests that intravascular hemolysis and the associated release of adenosine triphosphate (ATP) may be an important mechanism for *in vivo* local purinergic signaling and blood flow regulation during exercise and hypoxia. However, the mechanisms that modulate hypoxia-induced RBC membrane fragility remain unclear. Here, we provide an overview of the role of RBC ATP release in the regulation of vascular tone and prevailing assumptions on the putative release mechanisms. We show importance of intravascular hemolysis as a source of ATP for local purinergic regulation of blood flow and discuss processes that regulate membrane propensity to rupture under stress and hypoxia.

Keywords: red blood cell, red cell ATP release, intravascular hemolysis, purinergic signaling, red cell membrane fragility, hypoxia-induced ATP release

INTRODUCTION

During the last three decades it has become increasingly clear that in addition to passive uptake and release of oxygen and metabolically-derived gases, the red blood cells (RBC) also exhibit diverse oxygen-sensitive responses that autonomously regulate their own properties and functions. For example, changes in partial oxygen tension (PO_2) trigger a shift in glucose consumption from the pentose phosphate pathway (PPP) in oxygenated cells to glycolysis in deoxygenated cells (Messana et al., 1996). This shift is adaptive, since hemoglobin undergoes constant oxidation to methemoglobin in oxygenated cells, and its reduction back to hemoglobin would be facilitated by the enhanced production of NADPH in the PPP. Deoxygenation affects active Ca^{2+} transport and cytoplasmic Ca^{2+} buffering in human RBC (Tiffert et al., 1993). It was also shown that PO_2 has an impact on the activity of RBC monovalent ion transporters (Bogdanova et al., 2009). In RBC from several fish species, low PO_2 is required for β-adrenoceptor-mediated stimulation of Na^+/H^+ exchanger and elevation of hemoglobin affinity for O_2 via cytoplasm alkalization (Nikinmaa, 2002). In human RBC with mutated hemoglobin (HbS) K^+, Cl^- co-transport has an abnormal PO_2-dependence that probably contributes to the pathogenesis of sickle cell anemia (Brugnara et al., 1996). Apart from the above-listed enzymatic and ion transport pathways, mammalian RBC also show hypoxia-induced responses involved in regulation of blood flow. These include two different, likely complementary mechanisms: rapid reduction of blood viscosity via increased RBC deformability and, delayed but sustained increase of vessel's diameter via release of adenosine triphosphate (ATP) and purinergic receptor stimulated production of NO and other vasorelaxants in vascular endothelial cells.

Effects of Hypoxia on Blood Viscosity and RBC Deformability

Blood viscosity is determined by RBC flow properties that include adhesion, aggregation and deformability, i.e., ability to change shape under a given stress without hemolysing. Erythrocyte deformability affects blood flow in large blood vessels, due to the increased frictional resistance between fluid layers under laminar flow conditions. It also affects the microcirculatory blood flow significantly where erythrocytes are forced to pass through blood vessels with diameters smaller than their size. Numerous pathologies are associated with a decrease of RBC deformability. For our review it is important to note that increased blood viscosity in sickle cell anemia is caused by decreased RBC deformability due to gel formation of deoxygenated mutated hemoglobin HbS and its interaction with the cell membrane proteins determining membrane elasticity (for review see Yedgar et al., 2002; Diez-Silva et al., 2010; Viallat and Abkarian, 2014).

Modulation of blood viscosity by PO_2 may involve different processes depending on the duration and extent of oxygenation/deoxygenation. On the long time scale, these may include gradual changes of RBC membrane surface charges, mainly due to reduction in sialic acid content, and deformability that correlate with age (Huang et al., 2011) and markers of oxidative stress (Mehdi et al., 2012). On the other hand, the impact of prolonged hypoxia on RBC membrane properties remains poorly defined which contrasts with well documented, e.g., altered protein sialation in other cells types such as tumor cells. However, brief dips to a lower range of PO_2 as they occur in microcirculation, were recently found to have acute and significant impact on blood viscosity. Wei et al. (2016) reported that microinjection of O_2 scavengers resulted in vasoactive mediator-independent capillary hyperemia in mice cerebral microcirculation. In additional experiments, using microfluidic channels of small (5 μm) or large (20 μm) size they assessed effect of oxygenation on erythrocyte flow velocity and shear-induced deformability, respectively. These experiments revealed that O_2 depletion increased the velocity of erythrocyte flowing through the microfluidic channel due to increased RBC membrane deformability. Viewed collectively, these data demonstrate that in addition to the increment of vessel diameter (see below), elevation of blood flow in microcirculatory beds under hypoxic conditions might be achieved via PO_2-dependent regulation of erythrocyte deformability as a key determinant of blood viscosity (Wei et al., 2016).

Effects of Hypoxia on RBC ATP Release and Purinergic Regulation of Vascular Tone

Besides release of hemoglobin-associated nitric oxide (NO), hypoxia affects vascular tone via release of ATP from RBCs that, in turn, leads to activation of P2Y receptors on endothelial cells, stimulation of NO production and NO-mediated vasodilation (Dietrich et al., 2000; Wang et al., 2005; Ellsworth and Sprague, 2012; for review, see Ellsworth et al., 2009, 2016; Jensen, 2009; Luneva et al., 2015). *In vitro* studies have shown that shear stress, mechanical deformation and hypoxia are major stimuli of RBC ATP release (Bergfeld and Forrester, 1992; Sprague et al., 1996; Forsyth et al., 2012; Mairbäurl et al., 2013). These observations were confirmed using microbore capillaries (Fischer et al., 2003) and microfluidic channels (Price et al., 2004; Forsyth et al., 2011) demonstrating that shear stress *per se* is sufficient to trigger ATP release from RBC (Wan et al., 2011). Importantly, elevated ATP levels have also been found *in vivo* in venous effluent from exercising forearm muscle (Forrester, 1972; Ellsworth et al., 1995) and further augmented by exercise performed in hypoxia (Dietrich et al., 2000; González-Alonso et al., 2002). It has been demonstrated that only when the vessels were perfused with RBCs did venous effluent ATP level increase and the vessels dilate in response to low extraluminal PO_2 (Dietrich et al., 2000). Recent studies have shown that RBC-mediated ATP release is reduced in aging humans, which may contribute to impaired vasodilation and oxygen delivery to skeletal muscle during hypoxemia with advancing age (Kirby et al., 2012). Attenuated ATP production and release during deoxygenation was also found in banked RBCs, likely contributing to augmented microvascular adhesion of transfused RBCs *in vivo*. These alterations could be substantially corrected by restoring glycolysis-mediated ATP production (Kirby et al., 2014). To the best of our knowledge the comparative analysis of the action of hypoxia on ATP release under baseline conditions and in RBC subjected to shear stress has not been performed yet.

Search for Transporters Involved in ATP Release Triggered by Hypoxia

Since mature mammalian RBCs are devoid of intracellular organelles and unable to secrete ATP via endoplasmic reticulum-dependent exocytosis, it might be assumed that ATP release from RBC in hypoxic conditions is mediated by ATP-conducting channels (Praetorius and Leipziger, 2009). Cystic fibrosis transmembrane conductance regulator (CFTR), Pannexin-1 (Panex1), voltage dependent anion channel (VDAC), and other poorly defined VDAC-like maxi anion channels have been implicated in conductive ATP release in RBCs and in other cell types (Sprague et al., 1998; Sridharan et al., 2010, 2012).

Early reports have suggested that CFTR and other members of the superfamily of ATP-binding cassette transport proteins serve as a conductive pathway for ATP release, or regulate an associated ATP channels in several cell types, including RBCs (Reisin et al., 1994; Sugita et al., 1998). Since CFTR activity is regulated by cAMP-dependent PKA, it has been also hypothesized that shear stress- and hypoxia-induced ATP release involves activation of the cAMP signaling pathway (Sprague et al., 2007). Consistent with this hypothesis, ATP release has also been reported in response to other stimuli that elevate cAMP, such as agonists of prostacyclin (Montalbetti et al., 2011; Sridharan et al., 2012), or β-adrenergic receptors (Olearczyk et al., 2001; for review see Ellsworth and Sprague, 2012). However, subsequent studies by several independent groups with the patch clamp, lipid bilayer, and luminometry techniques, have not revealed any detectable CFTR-mediated or CFTR-regulated ATP release in several epithelial and non-epithelial cells (Grygorczyk et al., 1996; Li et al., 1996; Reddy et al., 1996; Grygorczyk and Hanrahan, 1997a,b; Watt et al., 1998; Hazama et al., 1999). In particular, it was also determined that CFTR protein is absent in the RBCs (Hoffman et al., 2004) and the role of cAMP signaling pathway in stimulating RBC ATP release was contradicted by recent studies (Sikora et al., 2014; Keller et al., 2017).

VDAC mediates ATP movement across the outer mitochondrial membrane (Rostovtseva and Colombini, 1997), and similar large conductance anion selective channels have occasionally been found in the plasma membrane of several cells (Báthori et al., 2000). However, these plasma membrane maxi anion channels and VDAC were shown to be unrelated proteins (Sabirov et al., 2006, 2017). VDAC pore selectivity favors the flow of adenine nucleotides (ATP, ADP) and anionic metabolites, over molecules of the same size and charge. The flow of small cations, including Ca^{2+}, proceeds at significant rates even for closed channel state (Colombini, 2012). Thus, presence of such large-conductance poorly selective channels in cell plasma membrane would perturb significantly cell homeostasis. Similar concerns may apply to other putative ATP channels (see below).

Connexins and the related pannexins, particularly Panx1 currently appear to be the most extensively investigated family of proteins reported to function as ATP conduits in a broad range of cell types (Romanello et al., 2001; Dando and Roper, 2009; Ma et al., 2009; Ransford et al., 2009; D'hondt et al., 2010; Lazarowski et al., 2011), including RBCs (Sridharan et al., 2010; Qiu et al., 2011; Chu et al., 2016). Nevertheless, several basic Panx1channel properties, including single channel conductance, selectivity and regulatory mechanisms still remain unclear (Chiu et al., 2014). Systematic electrophysiological studies revealed that Panx1 is a relatively low conductance anion channel (unitary conductance of 68 to 75 pS) with negligible permeability to large anions (aspartate, glutamate, gluconate), (Ma et al., 2012; Chiu et al., 2014). In particular, no measurable Panex1 permeability to ATP was detected in taste buds and several heterologous expression systems (HEK-293, CHO, and SK-N-SH cells) (Romanov et al., 2012). Thus, direct patch-clamp experiments to determine its selectivity so far did not provide convincing support for the involvement of these channels in ATP release. It has been suggested however, that permeability characteristics could change depending on how the channel was activated (Chiu et al., 2014).

Piezo 1 is a mechanosensitive non-selective cation channel expressed on RBC membrane. Gain-of-function mutations in Piezo 1 were linked to dehydrated hereditary stomatocytosis (Zarychanski et al., 2012; Albuisson et al., 2013). It was recently shown that Piezo 1 regulates mechanosensitive ATP release in RBCs by controlling the shear-induced Ca^{2+} influx (Cinar et al., 2015). Based on pharmacological data it was proposed that the release may involve CFTR and/or Pannexin 1 channels, but in the light of concerns discussed above, alternative pathways that might be modulated by intracellular Ca^{2+}-elevation should be also considered (see below).

Regardless of the molecular nature of ATP-conducting channels, the main conceptual difficulty with such a release mechanism is that ATP permeation requires pore of large dimensions (0.6–1.1 nm, Sabirov and Okada, 2005), resulting in poor selectivity and large conductance (hundreds of pS) for small ions such as K^+, Na^+, Cl^-, and Ca^{2+}, as exemplified by the well characterized VDAC channel. VDAC selectivity for ATP, ADP is based on steric constrains and charge distribution allowing to discriminate between large anions but it does not prevent permeation of small cations. Opening of such large, non-selective pores in the plasma membrane will result in significant influx of Na^+ and Ca^{2+} down their electrochemical gradients into the cytoplasm, posing an overwhelming challenge to normal cell homeostasis and survival (Akopova et al., 2012). Furthermore, in terms of energy expenditure, conductive ATP release would be a costly mechanism of intercellular signaling that requires action of energy-consuming transport processes to re-establish normal cellular Ca^{2+}, Na^+, and K^+ gradients. To the best of our knowledge, currently there is no example of a channel that on one hand would allow high permeability for anions as large as ATP and, on the other would prevent significant fluxes of small cations. None of the currently known putative plasma membrane ATP channels seems to be compatible with the requirement of preserving cell homeostasis. Therefore, the concept of such release mechanisms should be treated with caution.

ATP Release by Hemolysis

Hemolysis is an important source of extracellular ATP, and intravascular hemolysis occurs *in vivo* as a consequence of hypoxia and mechanical trauma to RBCs (Shaskey and Green, 2000; Mao et al., 2011; Mairbäurl, 2013). Although it has been also considered to be a potential factor contributing to stimulated ATP release in most previous *in vitro* investigations, its actual involvement has often not been assessed systematically. By paired measurements of ATP and free hemoglobin in each and every sample of human RBC supernatants Sikora et al. found that basal and stimulated ATP release not only correlated tightly with extracellular hemoglobin, but matched the levels expected from cell lysis and independently determined cell ATP content (Sikora et al., 2014, 2015). Unexpectedly, this was seen with all stimuli tested (hypotonic shock, shear stress, hypoxia) strongly indicating that, for each stimulus, the only source of extracellular ATP was cell lysis (Sikora et al., 2014; Luneva et al., 2016). Surprisingly, stimulation of cAMP pathway had no effect on RBC ATP release, which remained at the basal level observed with unstimulated cells. The report triggered a significant debate in the field with opposing views presented by Kirby et al. (2015) and Sikora et al. (2015). Absence of cAMP-regulated ATP release was recently confirmed by Keller et al. who also showed using Panex1$^{-/-}$ mice model that Panex1 has no role in exercise performance, challenging assumptions about Panex1 role in ATP-dependent blood perfusion to exercising skeletal muscle (Keller et al., 2017). In the study by Sikora et al. the primary role of hemolysis in hypotonic shock-induced ATP release was confirmed more directly by simultaneous luminescence ATP imaging and infrared imaging of substrate-attached RBCs

(Sikora et al., 2014). With luciferin-luciferase (LL) present in the extracellular solution these experiments identified single ATP-releasing cells and revealed that only lysing cells contributed to the release. This was seen as a flash of ATP-dependent LL luminescence around the cell followed, after some delay, with cell ghosting due to Hb leakage, **Figure 1A**. Individual cells showed variable duration of ATP release as might be expected for different number and/or size of lytic pores in the membrane, **Figure 1B**. Interestingly, time-course of ATP release correlated with time delay of cell ghosting, i.e., cells showing slower ATP release also displayed longer delay before ghosting, consistent with slower Hb leakage. This is in agreement with 3-to 4-fold difference of their diffusion coefficients in water, supporting the view that release of Hb and ATP proceeds through the common pathway. The study demonstrated that at least in the case of hypotonic shock and cAMP/forskolin stimulation hemolysis is likely the only mechanism of RBC ATP release, and therefore processes that control RBC susceptibility to lysis will also contribute to modulation of ATP release (Sikora et al., 2014). In the light of this finding there is an urgent need to understand mechanisms underlying the hemolysis (Thomas, 2014).

RBC fragility, or propensity to hemolyse under osmotic or mechanical stress, is determined by properties of the cell membrane. It is comprised of a phospholipid bilayer and an underlying two-dimensional cytoskeleton, a network of

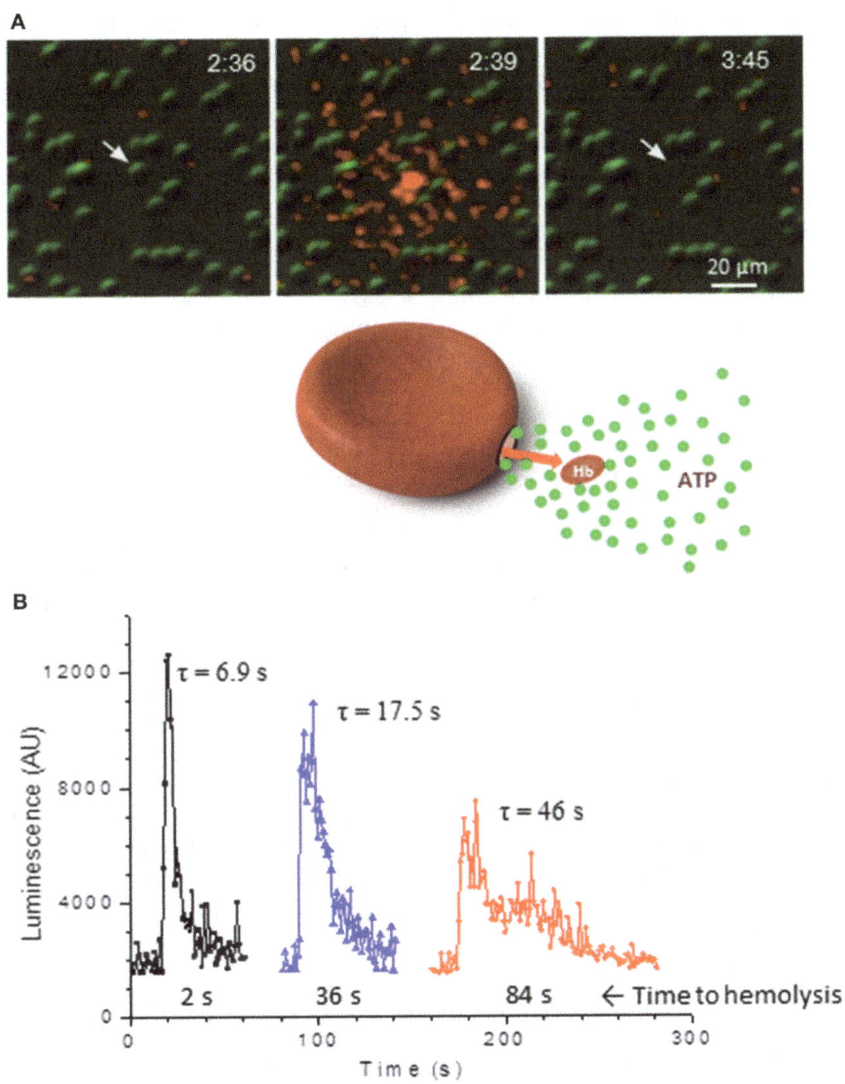

FIGURE 1 | ATP release due to lysis of single RBCs. **(A)**, sequential infrared images of RBCs (green) that are overlaid with extracellular ATP-dependent bioluminescence from luciferin-luciferase reaction (red). Elapsed time is indicated in the right-upper corners (min:s). Twenty percent of hypotonic solution was introduced at time 0 and hypotonic shock-induced ATP release is shown on the center image. Ghosting of the RBC (indicated by arrow) due to Hb leakage occurred with a delay of about 66 s. No ATP release from intact RBCs is evident. **(B)**, three examples of ATP release time-course due to lysis of single RBCs such as shown in A. Duration of ATP release τ (in s) is indicated for each trace and corresponding delay from peak ATP release until cell ghosting is shown below. Adapted from Sikora et al. (2014).

actin and α- and β-spectrin molecules that are held together by ankyrin. The membrane is stabilized by interactions of ankyrin with band 3, the major RBC membrane integral protein (Mohandas and Gallagher, 2008). The composite properties of the phospholipid bilayer and 2D cytoskeleton are responsible for the biconcave discocyte morphology of healthy RBC and membrane elastic and rheological properties. Disruptions of interactions between cytoskeletal components and/or integral membrane proteins change spectrin network density causing cell morphological changes and membrane fluctuations, affecting RBC deformability and fragility (Diez-Silva et al., 2010).

Under shear stress the RBC cell membrane deforms until the membrane reaches its "yield point." Beyond this threshold point, additional stress results in irreversible plastic deformation of the membrane, which accelerates with accumulation of microdefects in the membrane, leading to the cell destruction (Orbach et al., 2017). However stressed cells do not rupture immediately, the time-course of this process depends on the duration and extent of the stimuli. Li et al. (2013) showed that after exposure to brief pulse of cavitation-induced shear stress (i.e., during air bubble formation and collapse) RBC lysis is a 2-step process. It involves formation of nanopores followed by colloidal osmotic cell swelling until cell bursts. To reach that point, the nanopores in the membrane must remain for a sufficient time. In erythrocyte membrane the brush-like glycocalyx molecules by steric interactions may contribute to stabilization of nanopores. In their study pores of up to 1.6 μm effective size were formed at rupture site that allowed diffusion of cellular content. Lysis occurred within few seconds to several tenths of seconds. Interestingly, in these experiments cells that ruptured showed irregular shape, indicating that changes in the 2D spectrin network and/or anchor points to plasma membrane are important factors enabling lytic pore formation (Li et al., 2013).

Role of RBC Aging and Membrane Vesiculation

The circulating RBCs undergo a natural aging process occurring throughout their lifespan of about 120 days. The aged "senescent" cells are characterized by loss of cell surface area, cell morphology alterations, increased cell rigidity and aggregability, reduced level of cell membrane stomatin (band 7 protein), and translocation of phosphatidylserine (PS) to the cell surface. The surface membrane content of sialoglycoproteins and sialic acids which accounts for majority of the negative surface charge of RBC membrane is also reduced in aged RBC contributing to altered RBC membrane mechanical and electrical properties, receptor-mediated cellular interactions, immune responses and survival (Durocher et al., 1975; Huang et al., 2011). The aging of RBCs are also characterized by the formation and accumulation of microdefects in the RBC membrane which as mentioned above, makes them susceptible to stress. Indeed, Orbach et al. found that the cells that were destroyed under low mechanical stress were characterized by low deformability, high level of surface PS, and reduced level of membrane stomatin, all properties consistent with aged senescent cells possessing augmented macrovesicle formation terminated by RBC lysis (Orbach et al., 2017).

The molecular mechanisms underlying the formation of the plasma membrane macrovesicles remain poorly understood. Changes in metabolic status and decrease of cellular ATP levels during prolonged deoxygenation induce RBC shape changes and increase membrane fluctuations. Membrane fluctuations are directly linked to binding of membrane bilayer to spectrin network which is actively controlled by ATP (Diez-Silva et al., 2010; Park et al., 2010). Low ATP-induced morphological changes are reversible upon restoration of normal cellular ATP levels. Thus, metabolic status of RBC might be important factor affecting RBC susceptibility to membrane vesiculation and RBC lysis. It was also well documented that RBC vesiculation is sharply potentiated by elevation of intracellular Ca^{2+} concentration ($[Ca^{2+}]_i$) via activation of scramblase and inhibition of flipase. These $[Ca^{2+}]_i$-dependent events results in a collapse of membrane phospholipid asymmetry and cytoskeleton detachment (for review see (Greenwalt, 2006; Alaarg et al., 2013). In early studies, Tiffert and co-workers observed that brief deoxygenation results in elevation of $[Ca^{2+}]_i$ up to 70% that was probably caused by Ca^{2+}-ATPase inhibition (Tiffert et al., 1993).

Intravascular vesiculation process and associated hemolysis of senescent cells in healthy subjects was reassessed in recent study by Ciana et al. (2017). They showed that contrary to some earlier *in vitro* investigations vesiculation process of senescent RBCs removes membrane in a balanced way as a lipid bilayer vesicles containing membrane cytoskeleton. Moreover, the study suggests that *in vivo* vesiculation almost entirely occurs by active processing in the spleen producing progressively smaller but otherwise viable discoid shape cells. This agrees with the view that vesiculation is a self-protective mechanism to remove damaged membrane patches containing removal proteins, thereby postponing untimely elimination of healthy RBCs (Willekens et al., 2008). The study implies that in healthy subjects under normal conditions contribution of intravascular hemolysis to RBC clearance may be negligible. Therefore, intravascular hemolysis may occur only under particular conditions in the localized regions of the vasculature where elevated shear and hypoxia may arise, such as in the microvessels of skeletal muscle during intense exercise. It should be noted, however, that due to high ATP content of RBCs (1–5 mM) even negligibly small intravascular hemolysis may readily produce local ATP concentrations reaching ~1 μM, sufficient for purinergic control of blood flow. For example, lysis of a single erythrocyte will result in ATP concentration of 1 μM within 2–10 mm long segment of a capillary with a diameter comparable to RBC size (7 μm). Thus, a miniscule fraction of the circulating pre-senescent cells, e.g., those prior to their processing in the splenic system could constitute a sufficient pool of RBCs available for intravascular hemolytic ATP release and blood flow control. Contribution of the oldest RBCs showing so called terminal density reversal and the role of the nonselective cationic channels in the sustained elevation of Ca^{2+} and triggering of hemolysis should be also considered (Lew and Tiffert, 2013; Thomas, 2014).

Search for Upstream PO_2 Sensors and Downstream Intermediates of PO_2-Dependent Signaling

Hemoglobin is the only known O_2-binding protein in erythrocytes. Keeping this in mind, the reversible association of oxygenated and/or deoxygenated hemoglobin (oxyHb and deoxyHb, respectively) with downstream intermediates of intracellular signaling might be considered as a mechanism of triggering PO_2-dependent erythrocyte responses. Indeed, in cell-free experiments it was shown that hemoglobin binds to the cytoplasmic domain of band 3 (cdb3) (Cassoly, 1983; Low et al., 1984) also known as anion exchanger (AE1, SLC4A1), i.e., the major integral protein of erythrocytes membrane, playing a key role in anion transport and the organization of membrane cytoskeleton (Reithmeier et al., 2016). Importantly, both in human and mice the affinity of cdb3 for deoxyHb is much higher than for oxyHb (Walder et al., 1984; Sega et al., 2012, 2015).

Downstream intermediates of PO_2-dependent erythrocyte responses remain poorly understood (**Figure 2**). Stefanovic and co-workers has demonstrated that oxygentation strengthens band 3-ankyrin interactions, thereby stabilizing the erythrocyte membrane during turbulent flow from the lungs to the capillary beds (Stefanovic et al., 2013). Deoxygenation displaces ankyrin from band 3 releasing the spectrin/actin cytoskeleton from the membrane. This weakening of membrane-cytoskeleton interactions could increase RBC deformability enabling deoxygenated RBCs move more efficiently through narrow capillaries. Prolonged deoxygenation, on the other hand, could increase membrane propensity to rupture due to diminished mechanical support by the cytoskeleton. Indeed, theoretical considerations of membrane stability and pore formation in a lipid bilayer showed importance of cytoskeletal network in stabilizing the membrane against pore growth by reducing the surface tension (Sung and Park, 1997).

It is important to note that when oxygenated RBCs enter a region of low PO_2 the full-scale saturation of hemoglobin deoxygenation occurs within 25 ms (Ellsworth et al., 2016). Therefore, we constructed a special chamber allowing isolation of RBC ghosts in control and deoxygenated conditions and found a ~2-fold elevation of ~60 kDa membrane-bound protein content under deoxygenated conditions (Luneva et al., 2016). Currently, we employ proteomics technology for identification of full set of proteins whose interaction with RBC membrane is affected by hypoxia. This approach should lead to

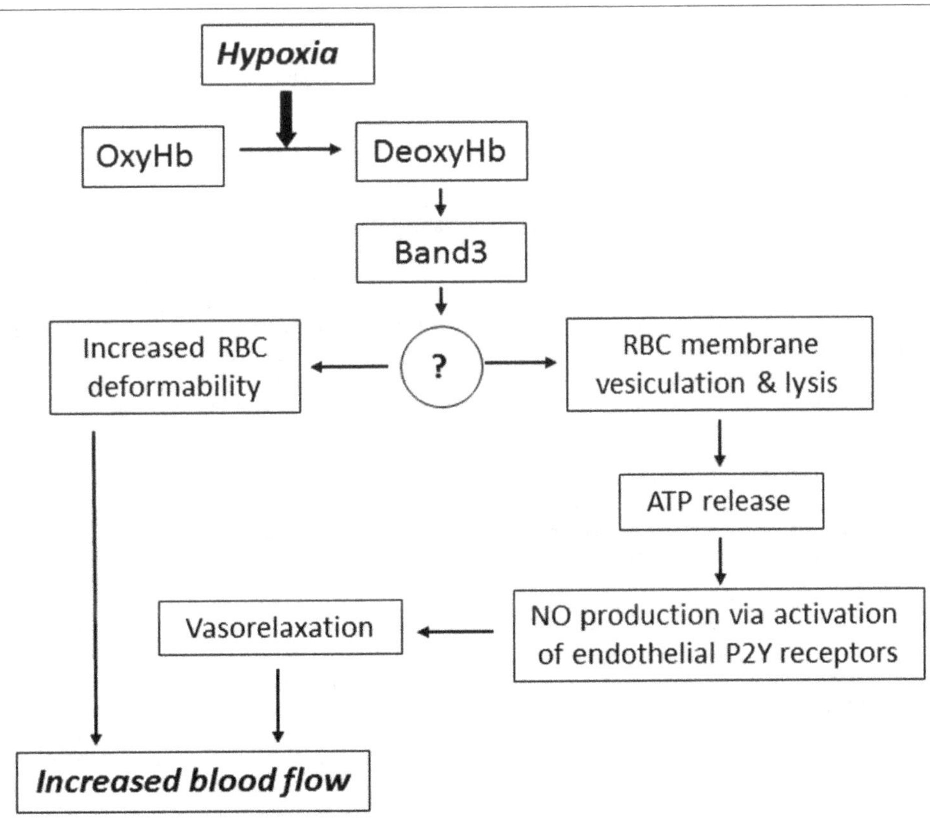

FIGURE 2 | Mechanisms underlying the implication of RBC in blood flow regulation. Hypoxia leads to accumulation of deoxyhemoglobin (DeoxyHb) and its interaction with cytoplasmic domain of anion exchanger (Band 3 protein). This interaction triggers signaling via changes in the content of unknown membrane-bound proteins (?) resulting in increased RBC deformability, membrane vesiculation and ATP release via hemolysis. For more details, see text.

identification of downstream intermediates involved in hypoxia-induced ATP release mediated by diminished RBC membrane integrity.

FUTURE RESEARCH DIRECTIONS

Several issues remain unsettled and require further investigations. Among them the question remains if besides hemolysis as the primary release mechanisms, are there conditions or stimuli that would induce regulated non-lytic ATP release from RBC and what pathway it could involve? What might be the contribution of young immature erythrocytes (reticulocytes) to such release? With their residual intracellular structures could they release ATP via exocytosis? While modest in relative terms (0.5–2.5%) these cells constitute a significant cellular pool (~4.5 × 10^4 cells/μl) with plenty of ATP for local purinergic signaling. If conductive release pathway would be involved what could be the mechanism allowing selective permeation of ATP but preventing massive influx of Ca^{2+} and Na^+? Finally, much remains to be learned about the downstream intermediates involved in hypoxia-induced membrane fragility, membrane microdefects, lytic pore formation and associated ATP release.

AUTHOR CONTRIBUTIONS

All authors listed have made a substantial, direct and intellectual contribution to the work, and approved it for publication.

ACKNOWLEDGMENTS

This work was supported by grants from the Canadian Institutes of Health Research (MOP64364 to RG) and the Russian Scientific Foundation (RNF #16-15-10026 to SO).

REFERENCES

Akopova, I., Tatur, S., Grygorczyk, M., Luchowski, R., Gryczynski, I., Gryczynski, Z., et al. (2012). Imaging exocytosis of ATP-containing vesicles with TIRF microscopy in lung epithelial A549 cells. *Purinergic Signal.* 8, 59–70. doi: 10.1007/s11302-011-9259-2

Alaarg, A., Schiffelers, R. M., van Solinge, W. W., and van Wijk, R. (2013). Red blood cell vesiculation in hereditary hemolytic anemia. *Front. Physiol.* 4:365. doi: 10.3389/fphys.2013.00365

Albuisson, J., Murthy, S. E., Bandell, M., Coste, B., Louis-Dit-Picard, H., Mathur, J., et al. (2013). Dehydrated hereditary stomatocytosis linked to gain-of-function mutations in mechanically activated PIEZO1 ion channels. *Nat. Commun.* 4:1884. doi: 10.1038/ncomms2899

Báthori, G., Parolini, I., Szabó, I., Tombola, F., Messina, A., Oliva, M., et al. (2000). Extramitochondrial porin: facts and hypotheses. *J. Bioenerg. Biomembr.* 32, 79–89. doi: 10.1023/A:1005516513313

Bergfeld, G. R., and Forrester, T. (1992). Release of ATP from human erythrocytes in response to a brief period of hypoxia and hypercapnia. *Cardiovasc. Res.* 26, 40–47. doi: 10.1093/cvr/26.1.40

Bogdanova, A., Berenbrink, M., and Nikinmaa, M. (2009). Oxygen-dependent ion transport in erythrocytes. *Acta Physiol.* 195, 305–319. doi: 10.1111/j.1748-1716.2008.01934.x

Brugnara, C., Gee, B., Armsby, C. C., Kurth, S., Sakamoto, M., Rifai, N., et al. (1996). Therapy with oral clotrimazole induces inhibition of the Gardos channel and reduction of erythrocytes dehydration in patients with sicle cell disease. *J. Clin. Invest.* 97, 1227–1234. doi: 10.1172/JCI118537

Cassoly, R. (1983). Quantitative analysis of the association of human hemoglobin with the cytoplasmic fragment of band 3 protein. *J. Biol. Chem.* 258, 3859–3864.

Chiu, Y. H., Ravichandran, K. S., and Bayliss, D. A. (2014). Intrinsic properties and regulation of Pannexin 1 channel. *Channels* 8, 103–109. doi: 10.4161/chan.27545

Chu, H., McKenna, M. M., Krump, N. A., Zheng, S., Mendelsohn, L., Thein, S. L., et al. (2016). Reversible binding of hemoglobin to band 3 constitutes the molecular switch that mediates O2 regulation of erythrocyte properties. *Blood* 128, 2708–2716. doi: 10.1182/blood-2016-01-692079

Ciana, A., Achilli, C., Gaur, A., and Minetti, G. (2017). Membrane Remodelling and vesicle formation during ageing of human red blood cells. *Cell. Physiol. Biochem.* 42, 1127–1138. doi: 10.1159/000478768

Cinar, E., Zhou, S., DeCourcey, J., Wang, Y., Waugh, R. E., and Wan, J. (2015). Piezo1 regulates mechanotransductive release of ATP from human RBCs. *Proc. Natl. Acad. Sci. U.S.A.* 112, 11783–11788. doi: 10.1073/pnas.1507309112

Colombini, M. (2012). VDAC structure, selectivity, and dynamics. *Biochim. Biophys. Acta* 1818, 1457–1465. doi: 10.1016/j.bbamem.2011.12.026

Dando, R., and Roper, S. D. (2009). Cell-to-cell communication in intact taste buds through ATP signalling from pannexin 1 gap junction hemichannels. *J. Physiol.* 587(Pt 24), 5899–5906. doi: 10.1113/jphysiol.2009.180083

D'hondt, C., Ponsaerts, R., De Smedt, H., Vinken, M., De Vuyst, E., De Bock, M., et al. (2010). Pannexin channels in ATP release and beyond: An unexpected rendezvous at the endoplasmic reticulum. *Cell Signal* 23, 305–316. doi: 10.1016/j.cellsig.2010.07.018

Dietrich, H. H., Ellsworth, M. L., Sprague, R. S., and Dacey, R. G. Jr. (2000). Red blood cell regulation of microvascular tone through adenosine triphosphate. *Am. J. Physiol. Heart Circ. Physiol.* 278, H1294–H1298. doi: 10.1152/ajpheart.2000.278.4.H1294

Diez-Silva, M., Dao, M., Han, J., Lim, C. T., and Suresh, S. (2010). Shape and biomechanical characteristics of human red blood cells in health and disease. *MRS Bull.* 35, 382–388. doi: 10.1557/mrs2010.571

Durocher, J. R., Payne, R. C., and Conrad, M. E. (1975). Role of sialic acid in erythrocyte survival. *Blood* 45, 11–20.

Ellsworth, M. L., Ellis, C. G., Goldman, D., Stephenson, A. H., Dietrich, H. H., and Sprague, R. S. (2009). Erythrocytes: oxygen sensors and modulators of vascular tone. *Physiology* 24, 107–116. doi: 10.1152/physiol.00038.2008

Ellsworth, M. L., Ellis, C. G., and Sprague, R. S. (2016). Role of erythrocyte-released ATP in the regulation of microvascular oxygen supply in skeletal muscle. *Acta Physiol.* 216, 265–276. doi: 10.1111/apha.12596

Ellsworth, M. L., Forrester, T., Ellis, C. G., and Dietrich, H. H. (1995). The erythrocyte as a regulator of vascular tone. *Am. J. Physiol.* 269(6 Pt 2), H2155–H2161.

Ellsworth, M. L., and Sprague, R. S. (2012). Regulation of blood flow distribution in skeletal muscle: role of erythrocyte-released ATP. *J. Physiol.* 590(Pt 20), 4985–4991. doi: 10.1113/jphysiol.2012.233106

Fischer, D. J., Torrence, N. J., Sprung, R. J., and Spence, D. M. (2003). Determination of erythrocyte deformability and its correlation to cellular ATP release using microbore tubing with diameters that approximate resistance vessels *in vivo*. *Analyst* 128, 1163–1168. doi: 10.1039/b308225n

Forrester, T. (1972). An estimate of adenosine triphosphate release into the venous effluent from exercising human forearm muscle. *J. Physiol.* 224, 611–628. doi: 10.1113/jphysiol.1972.sp009915

Forsyth, A. M., Braunmüller, S., Wan, J., Franke, T., and Stone, H. A. (2012). The effects of membrane cholesterol and simvastatin on red blood cell deformability and ATP release. *Microvasc. Res.* 83, 347–351. doi: 10.1016/j.mvr.2012.02.004

Forsyth, A. M., Wan, J., Owrutsky, P. D., Abkarian, M., and Stone, H. A. (2011). Multiscale approach to link red blood cell dynamics, shear viscosity, and ATP release. *Proc. Natl. Acad. Sci. U.S.A.* 108, 10986–10991. doi: 10.1073/pnas.1101315108

González-Alonso, J., Olsen, D. B., and Saltin, B. (2002). Erythrocyte and the regulation of human skeletal muscle blood flow and oxygen delivery: role of circulating ATP. *Circ. Res.* 91, 1046–1055. doi: 10.1161/01.RES.0000044939.73286.E2

Greenwalt, T. J. (2006). The how and why of exocytic vesicles. *Transfusion* 46, 143–152. doi: 10.1111/j.1537-2995.2006.00692.x

Grygorczyk, R., and Hanrahan, J. W. (1997a). CFTR-independent ATP release from epithelial cells triggered by mechanical stimuli. *Am. J. Physiol.* 272(3 Pt 1), C1058–C1066.

Grygorczyk, R., and Hanrahan, J. W. (1997b). Cystic fibrosis transmembrane conductance regulator and adenosine triphosphate [response]. *Science* 275, 1325–1326.

Grygorczyk, R., Tabcharani, J. A., and Hanrahan, J. W. (1996). CFTR channels expressed in CHO cells do not have detectable ATP conductance. *J. Membr. Biol.* 151, 139–148. doi: 10.1007/s002329900065

Hazama, A., Shimizu, T., Ando-Akatsuka, Y., Hayashi, S., Tanaka, S., Maeno, E., et al. (1999). Swelling-induced, CFTR-independent ATP release from a human epithelial cell line: lack of correlation with volume-sensitive Cl- channels. *J. Gen. Physiol.* 114, 525–533. doi: 10.1085/jgp.114.4.525

Hoffman, J. F., Dodson, A., Wickrema, A., and Dib-Hajj, S. D. (2004). Tetrodotoxin-sensitive Na^+ channels and muscarinic and purinergic receptors identified in human erythroid progenitor cells and red blood cell ghosts. *Proc. Natl. Acad. Sci. U.S.A.* 101, 12370–12374. doi: 10.1073/pnas.0404228101

Huang, Y. X., Wu, Z. J., Mehrishi, J., Huang, B. T., Chen, X. Y., Zheng, X. J., et al. (2011). Human red blood cell aging: correlative changes in surface charge and cell properties. *J. Cell. Mol. Med.* 15, 2634–2642. doi: 10.1111/j.1582-4934.2011.01310.x

Jensen, F. B. (2009). The dual roles of red blood cells in tissue oxygen delivery: oxygen carriers and regulator of local blood flow. *J. Exp. Biol.* 212, 3387–3393. doi: 10.1242/jeb.023697

Keller, A. S., Diederich, L., Panknin, C., DeLalio, L. J., Drake, J. C., Sherman, R., et al. (2017). Possible roles for ATP release from RBCs exclude the cAMP-mediated Panx1 pathway. *Am. J. Physiol. Cell Physiol.* 313, C593–C603. doi: 10.1152/ajpcell.00178.2017

Kirby, B. S., Crecelius, A. R., Voyles, W. F., and Dinenno, F. A. (2012). Impaired skeletal muscle blood flow control with advancing age in humans: attenuated ATP release and local vasodilation during erythrocyte deoxygenation. *Circ. Res.* 111, 220–230. doi: 10.1161/CIRCRESAHA.112.269571

Kirby, B. S., Hanna, G., Hendargo, H. C., and McMahon, T. J. (2014). Restoration of intracellular ATP production in banked red blood cells improves inducible ATP export and suppresses RBC-endothelial adhesion. *Am. J. Physiol. Heart Circ. Physiol.* 307, H1737–H1744. doi: 10.1152/ajpheart.00542.2014

Kirby, B. S., Schwarzbaum, P. J., Lazarowski, E. R., Dinenno, F. A., and McMahon, T. J. (2015). Liberation of ATP secondary to hemolysis is not mutually exclusive of regulated export. *Blood* 125, 1844–1845. doi: 10.1182/blood-2014-11-609610

Lazarowski, E. R., Sesma, J. I., Seminario-Vidal, L., and Kreda, S. M. (2011). Molecular mechanisms of purine and pyrimidine nucleotide release. *Adv. Pharmacol.* 61, 221–261. doi: 10.1016/B978-0-12-385526-8.00008-4

Lew, V. L., and Tiffert, T. (2013). The terminal density reversal phenomenon of aging human red blood cells. *Front. Physiol.* 4:171. doi: 10.3389/fphys.2013.00171

Li, C., Ramjeesingh, M., and Bear, C. E. (1996). Purified cystic fibrosis transmembrane conductance regulator (CFTR) does not function as an ATP channel. *J. Biol. Chem.* 271, 11623–11626. doi: 10.1074/jbc.271.20.11623

Li, F., Chan, C. U., and Ohl, C. D. (2013). Yield strength of human erythrocyte membranes to impulsive stretching. *Biophys. J.* 105, 872–879. doi: 10.1016/j.bpj.2013.06.045

Low, P. S., Westfall, M. A., Allen, D. P., and Appel, K. C. (1984). Characterization of the reversible conformational equilibrium of the cytoplasmic domain of erythrocyte membrane band 3. *J. Biol. Chem.* 259, 13070–13076.

Luneva, O. G., Sidorenko, S. V., Maksimov, G. V., Grygorczyk, R., and Orlov, S. N. (2015). Erythrocytes as regulators of blood vessel tone. *Biochem. Suppl. Ser. A Membr. Cell Biol.* 9, 161–171. doi: 10.1134/S1990747815040078

Luneva, O. G., Sidorenko, S. V., Ponomarchuk, O. O., Tverskoy, A. M., Cherkashin, A. A., Rodnenkov, O. V., et al. (2016). Deoxygenation affects composition of membrane-bound proteins in human erythrocytes. *Cell. Physiol. Biochem.* 39, 81–88. doi: 10.1159/000445607

Ma, W., Compan, V., Zheng, W., Martin, E., North, R. A., Verkhratsky, A., et al. (2012). Pannexin 1 forms an anion-selective channel. *Pflugers Arch.* 463, 585–592. doi: 10.1007/s00424-012-1077-z

Ma, W., Hui, H., Pelegrin, P., and Surprenant, A. (2009). Pharmacological characterization of pannexin-1 currents expressed in mammalian cells. *J. Pharmacol. Exp. Ther.* 328, 409–418. doi: 10.1124/jpet.108.146365

Mairbäurl, H. (2013). Red blood cells in sports: effects of exercise and training on oxygen supply by red blood cells. *Front. Physiol.* 4:332. doi: 10.3389/fphys.2013.00332

Mairbäurl, H., Ruppe, F. A., and Bärtsch, P. (2013). Role of hemolysis in red cell adenosine triphosphate release in simulated exercise conditions *in vitro*. *Med. Sci. Sports Exerc.* 45, 1941–1947. doi: 10.1249/MSS.0b013e318296193a

Mao, T. Y., Fu, L. L., and Wang, J. S. (2011). Hypoxic exercise training causes erythrocyte senescence and rheological dysfunction by depressed Gardos channel activity. *J. Appl. Physiol. (1985)* 111, 382–391. doi: 10.1152/japplphysiol.00096.2011

Mehdi, M. M., Singh, P., and Rizvi, S. I. (2012). Erythrocyte sialic acid content during aging in humans: correlation with markers of oxidative stress. *Dis. Markers* 32, 179–186. doi: 10.1155/2012/293429

Messana, I., Orlando, M., Cassiano, M., Pennacchietti, L., Zuppi, C., Castagnola, M., et al. (1996). Human erythrocyte metabolism is modulated by the O_2-linked transition of hemoglobin. *FEBS Lett.* 390, 25–28. doi: 10.1016/0014-5793(96)00624-2

Mohandas, N., and Gallagher, P. G. (2008). Red cell membrane: past, present, and future. *Blood* 112, 3939–3948. doi: 10.1182/blood-2008-07-161166

Montalbetti, N., Leal Denis, M. F., Pignataro, O. P., Kobatake, E., Lazarowski, E. R., and Schwarzbaum, P. J. (2011). Homeostasis of extracellular ATP in human erythrocytes. *J. Biol. Chem.* 286, 38397–38407. doi: 10.1074/jbc.M111.221713

Nikinmaa, M. (2002). Oxygen-dependent cellular functions - why fishes and aquatic envirinment are a prime choice of study. *Comp. Biochem. Physiol. A Mol. Integr. Physiol.* 2133, 1–16. doi: 10.1016/S1095-6433(02)00132-0

Olearczyk, J. J., Stephenson, A. H., Lonigro, A. J., and Sprague, R. S. (2001). Receptor-mediated activation of the heterotrimeric G-protein Gs results in ATP release from erythrocytes. *Med. Sci. Monit.* 7, 669–674.

Orbach, A., Zelig, O., Yedgar, S., and Barshtein, G. (2017). Biophysical and biochemical markers of red blood cell fragility. *Transfus. Med. Hemother.* 44, 183–187. doi: 10.1159/000452106

Park, Y., Best, C. A., Auth, T., Gov, N. S., Safran, S. A., Popescu, G., et al. (2010). Metabolic remodeling of the human red blood cell membrane. *Proc. Natl. Acad. Sci. U.S.A.* 107, 1289–1294. doi: 10.1073/pnas.0910785107

Praetorius, H. A., and Leipziger, J. (2009). ATP release from non-excitable cells. *Purinergic Signal.* 5, 433–446. doi: 10.1007/s11302-009-9146-2

Price, A. K., Fischer, D. J., Martin, R. S., and Spence, D. M. (2004). Deformation-induced release of ATP from erythrocytes in a poly(dimethylsiloxane)-based microchip with channels that mimic resistance vessels. *Anal. Chem.* 76, 4849–4855. doi: 10.1021/ac0495992

Qiu, F., Wang, J., Spray, D. C., Scemes, E., and Dahl, G. (2011). Two non-vesicular ATP release pathways in the mouse erythrocyte membrane. *FEBS Lett.* 585, 3430–3435. doi: 10.1016/j.febslet.2011.09.033

Ransford, G. A., Fregien, N., Qiu, F., Dahl, G., Conner, G. E., and Salathe, M. (2009). Pannexin 1 Contributes to ATP Release in airway epithelia. *Am. J. Respir. Cell Mol. Biol.* 41, 525–534. doi: 10.1165/rcmb.2008-0367OC

Reddy, M. M., Quinton, P. M., Haws, C., Wine, J. J., Grygorczyk, R., Tabcharani, J. A., et al. (1996). Failure of the cystic fibrosis transmembrane conductance regulator to conduct ATP. *Science* 271, 1876–1879.

Reisin, I. L., Prat, A. G., Abraham, E. H., Amara, J. F., Gregory, R. J., Ausiello, D. A., et al. (1994). The cystic fibrosis transmembrane conductance regulator is a dual ATP and chloride channel. *J. Biol. Chem.* 269, 20584–20591.

Reithmeier, R. A., Casey, J. R., Kalli, A. C., Sansom, M. S. P., Alguel, Y., and Iwata, S. (2016). Band 3, the human red cell chloride/bicarbonate exchanger (AE1, SLC4A1), in a structural context. *Biochim. Biophys. Acta* 1858, 1507–1532. doi: 10.1016/j.bbamem.2016.03.030

Romanello, M., Pani, B., Bicego, M., and D'Andrea, P. (2001). Mechanically induced ATP release from human osteoblastic cells. *Biochem. Biophys. Res. Commun.* 289, 1275–1281. doi: 10.1006/bbrc.2001.6124

Romanov, R. A., Bystrova, M. F., Rogachevskaya, O. A., Sadovnikov, V. B., Shestopalov, V. I., and Kolesnikov, S. S. (2012). The ATP permeability of pannexin 1 channels in a heterologous system and in mammalian taste cells is dispensable. *J. Cell Sci.* 125(Pt 22), 5514–5523. doi: 10.1242/jcs.111062

Rostovtseva, T., and Colombini, M. (1997). VDAC channels mediate and gate the flow of ATP: implications for the regulation of mitochondrial function. *Biophys. J.* 72, 1954–1962. doi: 10.1016/S0006-3495(97)78841-6

Sabirov, R. Z., Merzlyak, P. G., Okada, T., Islam, M. R., Uramoto, H., Mori, T., et al. (2017). The organic anion transporter SLCO2A1 constitutes the core component of the Maxi-Cl channel. *EMBO J.* 36, 3309–3324. doi: 10.15252/embj.201796685

Sabirov, R. Z., and Okada, Y. (2005). ATP release via anion channels. *Purinergic Signal.* 1, 311–328. doi: 10.1007/s11302-005-1557-0

Sabirov, R. Z., Sheiko, T., Liu, H., Deng, D., Okada, Y., and Craigen, W. J. (2006). Genetic demonstration that the plasma membrane maxianion channel and voltage-dependent anion channels are unrelated proteins. *J. Biol. Chem.* 281, 1897–1904. doi: 10.1074/jbc.M509482200

Sega, M. F., Chu, H., Christian, J. A., and Low, P. S. (2015). Fluorescence assay of the interaction between hemoglobin and the cytoplasmic domain of erythrocyte membrane band 3. *Blood Cells Mol. Dis.* 55, 266–271. doi: 10.1016/j.bcmd.2015.07.004

Sega, M. F., Chu, H., Christian, J., and Low, P. S. (2012). Interaction of deoxyhemoglobin with the cytoplasmic domain of murine erythrocyte band 3. *Biochemistry* 51, 3264–3272. doi: 10.1021/bi201623v

Shaskey, D. J., and Green, G. A. (2000). Sports haematology. *Sports Med.* 29, 27–38. doi: 10.2165/00007256-200029010-00003

Sikora, J., Orlov, S. N., Furuya, K., and Grygorczyk, R. (2014). Hemolysis is a primary ATP-release mechanism in human erythrocytes. *Blood* 124, 2150–2157. doi: 10.1182/blood-2014-05-572024

Sikora, J., Orlov, S. N., Furuya, K., and Grygorczyk, R. (2015). Response: hemolysis is a primary and physiologically relevant ATP release mechanism in human erythrocytes. *Blood* 125, 1845–1846. doi: 10.1182/blood-2015-01-622159

Sprague, R. S., Ellsworth, M. L., Stephenson, A. H., Kleinhenz, M. E., and Lonigro, A. J. (1998). Deformation-induced ATP release from red blood cells requires CFTR activity. *Am. J. Physiol.* 275(5 Pt 2), H1726–H1732.

Sprague, R. S., Ellsworth, M. L., Stephenson, A. H., and Lonigro, A. J. (1996). ATP: the red blood cell link to NO and local control of the pulmonary circulation. *Am. J. Physiol.* 271(6 Pt 2), H2717–H2722.

Sprague, R. S., Stephenson, A. H., and Ellsworth, M. L. (2007). Red not dead: signaling in and from erythrocytes. *Trends Endocrinol. Metab.* 18, 350–355. doi: 10.1016/j.tem.2007.08.008

Sridharan, M., Adderley, S. P., Bowles, E. A., Egan, T. M., Stephenson, A. H., Ellsworth, M. L., et al. (2010). Pannexin 1 is the conduit for low oxygen tension-induced ATP release from human erythrocytes. *Am. J. Physiol. Heart Circ. Physiol.* 299, H1146–H1152. doi: 10.1152/ajpheart.00301.2010

Sridharan, M., Bowles, E. A., Richards, J. P., Krantic, M., Davis, K. L., Dietrich, K. A., et al. (2012). Prostacyclin receptor-mediated ATP release from erythrocytes requires the voltage-dependent anion channel. *Am. J. Physiol. Heart Circ. Physiol.* 302, H553–H559. doi: 10.1152/ajpheart.00998.2011

Stefanovic, M., Puchulu-Campanella, E., Kodippili, G., and Low, P. S. (2013). Oxygen regulates the band 3-ankyrin bridge in the human erythrocyte membrane. *Biochem. J.* 449, 143–150. doi: 10.1042/BJ20120869

Sugita, M., Yue, Y., and Foskett, J. K. (1998). CFTR Cl- channel and CFTR-associated ATP channel: distinct pores regulated by common gates. *EMBO J.* 17, 898–908. doi: 10.1093/emboj/17.4.898

Sung, W., and Park, P. J. (1997). Dynamics of pore growth in membranes and membrane stability. *Biophys. J.* 73, 1797–1804. doi: 10.1016/S0006-3495(97)78210-9

Thomas, S. L. (2014). Intravascular hemolysis: the sacrifice of few. *Blood* 124, 2011–2012. doi: 10.1182/blood-2014-08-595447

Tiffert, T., Etzion, Z., Bookchin, R. M., and Lew, V. L. (1993). Effects of deoxygenation on active and passive Ca^{2+} transport and cytoplasmic Ca^{2+} buffering in normal human red cells. *J. Physiol.* 464, 529–544. doi: 10.1113/jphysiol.1993.sp019649

Viallat, A., and Abkarian, M. (2014). Red blood cell: from its mechanics to its motion in shear flow. *Int. J. Lab. Hematol.* 36, 237–243. doi: 10.1111/ijlh.12233

Walder, J. A., Chatterjee, R., Steck, T. L., Low, P. S., Musso, G. F., Kaiser, E. T., et al. (1984). The interaction of hemoglobin with the cytoplasmic domain of band 3 of the human eyrthrocyte membrabe. *J. Biol. Chem.* 259, 10238–10246.

Wan, J., Forsyth, A. M., and Stone, H. A. (2011). Red blood cell dynamics: from cell deformation to ATP release. *Integr. Biol.* 3, 972–981. doi: 10.1039/c1ib00044f

Wang, L., Olivecrona, G., Götberg, M., Olsson, M. L., Winzell, M. S., and Erlinge, D. (2005). ADP acting on P2Y13 receptors is a negative feedback pathway for ATP release from human red blood cells. *Circ. Res.* 96, 189–196. doi: 10.1161/01.RES.0000153670.07559.E4

Watt, W. C., Lazarowski, E. R., and Boucher, R. C. (1998). Cystic fibrosis transmembrane regulator-independent release of ATP. Its implications for the regulation of P2Y2 receptors in airway epithelia. *J. Biol. Chem.* 273, 14053–14058. doi: 10.1074/jbc.273.22.14053

Wei, H. S., Kang, H., Rasheed, I. Y., Zhou, S., Lou, N., Gershteyn, A., et al. (2016). Erythrocytes are oxygen-sensing regulators of the cerebral microcirculation. *Neuron* 91, 851–862. doi: 10.1016/j.neuron.2016.07.016

Willekens, F. L., Werre, J. M., Groenen-Döpp, Y. A., Roerdinkholder-Stoelwinder, B., de Pauw, B., and Bosman, G. J. (2008). Erythrocyte vesiculation: a self-protective mechanism? *Br. J. Haematol.* 141, 549–556. doi: 10.1111/j.1365-2141.2008.07055.x

Yedgar, S., Koshkaryev, A., and Barshtein, G. (2002). The red blood cell in vascular occlusion. *Pathophysiol. Haemost. Thromb.* 32, 263–268. doi: 10.1159/000073578

Zarychanski, R., Schulz, V. P., Houston, B. L., Maksimova, Y., Houston, D. S., Smith, B., et al. (2012). Mutations in the mechanotransduction protein PIEZO1 are associated with hereditary xerocytosis. *Blood* 120, 1908–1915. doi: 10.1182/blood-2012-04-422253

10

RNA Binding Proteins and Regulation of mRNA Translation in Erythropoiesis

*Kat S. Moore and Marieke von Lindern**

Department of Hematopoiesis, Sanquin Research, and Landsteiner Laboratory, Amsterdam UMC, Amsterdam, Netherlands

***Correspondence:**
Marieke von Lindern
m.vonlindern@sanquin.nl

Control of gene expression in erythropoiesis has to respond to signals that may emerge from intracellular processes or environmental factors. Control of mRNA translation allows for relatively rapid modulation of protein synthesis from the existing transcriptome. For instance, the protein synthesis rate needs to be reduced when reactive oxygen species or unfolded proteins accumulate in the cells, but also when iron supply is low or when growth factors are lacking in the environment. In addition, regulation of mRNA translation can be important as an additional layer of control on top of gene transcription, in which RNA binding proteins (RBPs) can modify translation of a set of transcripts to the cell's actual protein requirement. The 5′ and 3′ untranslated regions of mRNA (5′UTR, 3′UTR) contain binding sites for general and sequence specific translation factors. They also contain secondary structures that may hamper scanning of the 5′UTR by translation complexes or may help to recruit translation factors. In addition, the term 5′UTR is not fully correct because many transcripts contain small open reading frames in their 5′UTR that are translated and contribute to regulation of mRNA translation. It is becoming increasingly clear that the transcriptome only partly predicts the proteome. The aim of this review is (i) to summarize how the availability of general translation initiation factors can selectively regulate transcripts because the 5′UTR contains secondary structures or short translated sequences, (ii) to discuss mechanisms that control the length of the mRNA poly(A) tail in relation to mRNA translation, and (iii) to give examples of sequence specific RBPs and their targets. We focused on transcripts and RBPs required for erythropoiesis. Whereas differentiation of erythroblasts to erythrocytes is orchestrated by erythroid transcription factors, the production of erythrocytes needs to respond to the availability of growth factors and nutrients, particularly the availability of iron.

Keywords: erythropoiesis, mRNA translation, translation initiation factors, eIF4E, eIF2, CSDE1, polyadenylation

GENE EXPRESSION AND SIGNAL TRANSDUCTION SET THE STAGE FOR ERYTHROPOIESIS

Erythrocytes circulate through human peripheral blood for approximately 120 days. Every day, the human body produces 10^{11} new erythrocytes to replenish the cells that are taken out of the circulation by macrophages. This requires a tight balance between progenitor proliferation and maturation, in conjunction with erythropoietin (Epo) dependent cell survival. Erythroid homeostasis is controlled by a cascade of transcription factors and by signaling pathways triggered by environmental factors.

Several transcription factors that are specifically expressed in erythroid progenitors, are essential for determining the erythroid program of gene expression (**Figure 1**). For instance, GATA-1 (GATA-binding factor 1) functions as one of the master regulators of erythropoiesis, inducing for instance (i) the expression of the Epo receptor (EpoR), (ii) commitment to the erythroid lineage, and (iii) transcription of the β-globin locus (Gregory et al., 1999; Ferreira et al., 2005; Kim and Bresnick, 2007; Ribeil et al., 2013). GATA1 protein synthesis is reduced in Diamond-Blackfan anemia (DBA), a congenital red cell aplasia caused by reduced biosynthesis of ribosomes, and mutations in GATA1 can cause a DBA-like phenotype (Ludwig et al., 2014; Vlachos et al., 2014; Paolini et al., 2016). Also of importance, particularly during terminal erythroid differentiation, is KLF1 (Kruppel-like factor 1, or E-KLF: erythroid KLF), a transcription factor involved in many cellular changes required for the maturation of erythroblasts to erythrocytes, including expression of β-globin (Dzierzak and Philipsen, 2013; Perkins et al., 2016). Haploinsufficiency in KLF1 causes hereditary persistence of fetal hemoglobin (HPFH) (Borg et al., 2010), and a specific mutation in the DNA-binding domain of KLF1 causes type IV congenital dyserythropoietic anemia (CDA) (Iolascon et al., 2013).

Signaling cascades allow for the adaption of the gene expression program laid down by transcription factors such as GATA1 and KLF1 during erythropoietic expansion and differentiation upon demand (**Figure 1**). For instance, during hypoxic stress, Epo production in the kidneys is dramatically increased (Sposi, 2015). The binding of Epo to its cognate receptor (EpoR) activates the cytoplasmic tyrosine kinase JAK2 (Witthuhn et al., 1993), which triggers a downstream signaling cascade via the signal transducer and activator of transcription 5 (STAT5), phosphoinositide-3-kinase (PI3K), and protein kinase B (PKB) pathways to support the proliferation and differentiation of erythropoietic progenitors (Sui et al., 2000; Menon et al., 2006; Fang et al., 2007; Socolovsky et al., 2007). STAT5 induces the expression of, for instance, anti-apoptotic B-cell lymphoma-extra large (BCL-X_L) to maintain viability during terminal maturation (Gregory et al., 1999). Recently, many erythroid specific STAT5 targets were identified (Gillinder et al., 2017). Stem cell factor (SCF), the ligand for the SCF receptor KIT, acts in conjunction with Epo to repress differentiation and promote expansion of the population of erythroid progenitors (Broudy et al., 1996). SCF signaling is enacted via the PI3K pathway, resulting in the activation of PKB (Sui et al., 2000; van Dijk et al., 2000). PI3K/PKB signaling has two major effector pathways in erythroblasts. On the one hand, it prevents nuclear localization of the Forkhead box O3 (FOXO3) transcription factor that otherwise induces erythroid differentiation (Bakker et al., 2004). Concurrently, the PI3K/PKB signaling pathway activates mammalian target of rapamycin (mTOR), which interacts with translation initiation factors to promote the translation of a specific set of transcripts (Gingras et al., 1999; Grech et al., 2008).

Studies on gene expression have historically focused on transcription as the primary regulatory mechanism. However, it has become increasingly clear that protein levels correlate poorly with transcript expression, and that translation is a major determinant of protein abundance in the cell (Schwanhäusser et al., 2011; Brar and Weissman, 2015). In other words, DNA transcription determines whether a given gene is expressed and determines the fundamentals of the gene expression program. Subsequently, mRNA translation has this program at

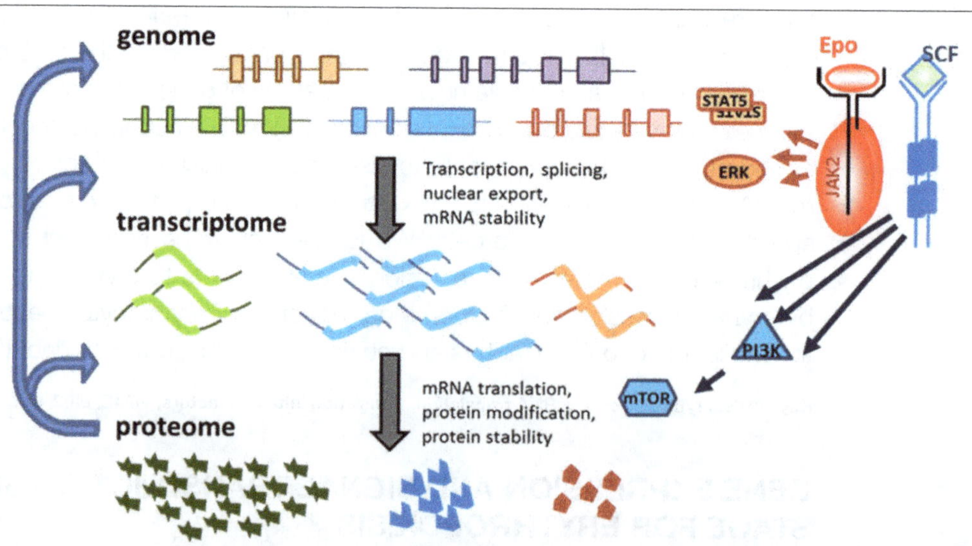

FIGURE 1 | Different levels of regulation of gene expression in erythropoiesis. Cell-specific transcription factors control which genes are expressed. Transcript levels per gene differ because of transcription rate, but also due to mRNA stability. Transcript levels poorly predict protein expression. Translation factors and mRNA structure control protein synthesis efficiency. Transcript and protein expression is partly cell intrinsically regulated as a cascade of subsequent gene expression regulation (left hand arrows). In addition, signal transduction (Epo and SCF in erythroid progenitors) can modify signaling molecules to activate transcription and translation. For instance, phosphorylation of STAT5 causes dimerization and activates the transcription activity, ERK phosphorylation cause nuclear location and phosphorylation of transcription factors. PI3K activates mTOR, a critical factor in protein synthesis.

its disposal for control of protein synthesis. Finally, protein modification and degradation also control protein expression (**Figure 1**). This review focusses on specificity in control of translation, which is generated by the combination of nucleotide sequences in the 5′ and 3′ untranslated regions (5′UTR, 3′UTR), together with expression levels and posttranslational control of constitutive translation factors and RNA binding proteins (RBPs). Control of mRNA translation is mediated by a complex web of overlapping mechanisms, including, but not limited to, regulation of translation initiation and the length of the poly(A) tail, by the presence of short upstream open reading frames (uORFs), and by sequence-specific association with RBPs. In this review, a brief overview of these topics of selective mRNA translation as pertains to erythropoiesis will be presented.

TRANSLATION INITIATION FACTORS IN CAP-DEPENDENT PROTEIN SYNTHESIS

Canonically, translation is initiated via an interaction between the 5′ 7-methylguanylate (^{7m}G) cap structure of the mRNA and the cap-binding protein eukaryotic initiation factor 4E (eIF4E) (Kong and Lasko, 2012). Interaction of eIF4E with the cap is the major rate limiting step, which is followed by binding of scaffolding protein eIF4G, and the RNA helicase eIF4A to form the eIF4F complex. The scaffolding protein eIF4G in this complex interacts with poly-A binding protein (PABP) to form a closed-loop structure between the 5′ and 3′ end of the mRNA (**Figure 2**). Concurrently, the ternary complex (TC), consisting of the methionine loaded initiator tRNA (tRNA$_i^{met}$) and the GTP-loaded GTPase eIF2 associates with the 40S ribosomal subunit and with translation factors eIF1, -1A, -3, and -5 to form the 43S pre-initiation complex (**Figure 2**; Hinnebusch, 2014). The preinitiation scanning complex, also referred to as the 48S initiation complex, is subsequently formed via an interaction between eIF4G and eIF3. The preinitiation scanning complex scans the bound mRNA until encountering an initiation codon, at which point recognition of the initiation codon triggers the hydrolysis of eIF2-bound GTP by eIF5 and the recruitment of the 60S large ribosomal subunit, marking the end of initiation phase and the beginning of elongation (**Figure 2**).

Next to eIF4E, the availability of GTP-loaded eIF2 is an important rate limiting factor of translation initiation (Proud, 2005). Once translation initiation starts, the TC dissociates upon hydrolysis of GTP to GDP. To reassociate with the TC and rejoin the scanning complex, eIF2 must be reloaded before a new round of translational initiation can begin. This is accomplished via GDP-GTP exchange factor eIF2B, allowing the pre-initiation complex containing eIF2-GTP and tRNA$_i^{met}$ to reform. This mechanism is subject to control by phosphorylation of the α subunit of eIF2, which prevents the GDP-GTP exchange, resulting in the inhibition of cap-dependent translation (**Figure 2**).

The control of rate-limiting factors eIF4E and eIF2 in erythropoiesis and the corresponding signaling pathways are discussed in the next two paragraphs.

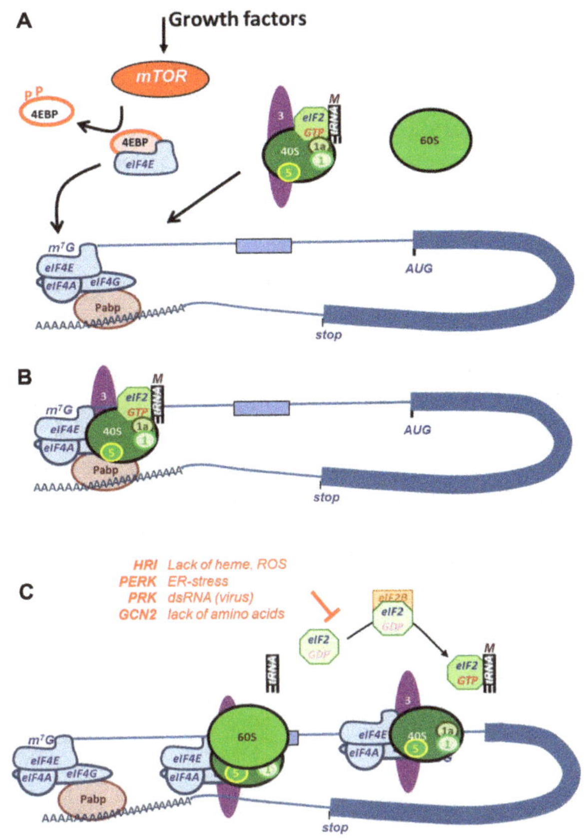

FIGURE 2 | Mechanism and regulation of cap-dependent translation initiation. **(A)** Growth factor signaling activates phosphorylation of 4EBP by mTOR, which releases the cap-binding factor eIF4E. Upon binding to the mRNA cap, eIF4E associates with helicase eIF4A and scaffold protein eIF4G to form the eIF4F complex. The interaction between the poly(A)-tail binding protein PABP with eIF4G forms a closed loop between cap and tail. Concurrently, the ternary complex, existing of eIF2:GTP and tRNA$_i^{met}$, associates with the 40S ribosomal subunit and eIF1, -1A, -3, and -5 (labeled numerically in the figure). This assembly is referred to as that 43S pre-initiation complex. **(B)** eIF3 interacts with eIF4G in the eIF4F complex. After docking with the ribosome, the 48S pre-initiation scanning complex is formed, and the transcript is scanned until encountering a start codon, upon which eIF2-bound GTP is hydrolyzed and the 60S ribosomal subunit is recruited. At this stage, initiation of translation is complete, and translational elongation begins. **(C)** Cap-dependent translation is regulated by the phosphorylation of eIF2. After a round of translation initiation, eIF2 must be recharged with GTP by eIF2B in order for the ternary complex to be reformed and for the 60S ribosomal subunit to be recruited in subsequent cycles of translational initiation. Under stress conditions, eIF2 is phosphorylated by, for example, HRI (heme regulated inhibitor, during heme scarcity), PKR (Protein kinase R, upon recognition of viral dsRNA), PERK (PRK-like endoplasmic reticulum kinase, upon aggregation of malfolded proteins), or GCN (General control non-derepressible, during amino acid starvation), preventing eIF2B from exchanging eIF2-bound GDP for GTP. The lack of unphosphorylated eIF2 leads to translational arrest.

Epo and SCF Controlled Translational Initiation in Erythroblasts

Stem cell factor (SCF) cooperates with Epo to expand erythroblast numbers *in vivo* and *in vitro*, whereas erythroblasts mature to erythrocytes in presence of Epo only (Wessely et al., 1999).

The crucial pathway activated by SCF is the mTOR-dependent release of the cap binding factor eIF4E from its binding protein 4EBP (Blázquez-Domingo et al., 2005). Overexpression of eIF4E inhibits erythroid differentiation (Blázquez-Domingo et al., 2005; **Figure 3**). This is in part due to SCF-independent proliferation of erythroblasts, but also due to a block in erythroid differentiation (Chung et al., 2015). Upon release from 4EBP, eIF4E binds the mRNA cap-structure, allowing the formation of the pre-initiation scanning complex (Hinnebusch, 2014; Siddiqui and Sonenberg, 2015). In addition to release of eIF4E, PI3K dependent phosphorylation of eIF4B increases its association with the helicase eIF4A and enhances eIF4A activation, which facilitates scanning of the 5′UTR (Shahbazian et al., 2010). Thus, PI3K activation increases formation of the preinitiation complex at the cap, but also increases the capacity of the complex to unwind structures in the 5′UTR. The increased scanning capacity controls overall translation initiation, but transcripts with a TOP (terminal oligopyrimidine tract) or secondary structures are hypersensitive to PI3K activity and eIF4E availability (Graff and Zimmer, 2003; Modelska et al., 2015).

One such transcript is *immunoglobulin binding protein* (*IGBP1*), which is constitutively expressed in erythroblasts, but selectively translated only upon SCF-induced eIF4E release (Grech et al., 2008). IGBP1 is more suitably known as the alpha4 subunit of protein phosphatase 2A (PP2A) (Nanahoshi et al., 1998). As a regulatory subunit, it inhibits the catalytic activity of PP2A on 4EBP (**Figure 3**). Therefore, expression of IGBP1/Alpha4 enhances the effect of low levels mTOR activation on mRNA translation. SCF-induced expression of IGBP1 acts as a positive feedback mechanism in the polysome recruitment of multiple eIF4E-sensitive mRNAs, resulting in SCF-independent proliferation of erythroblasts and attenuation of erythroid differentiation (Grech et al., 2008). Another transcript subject to the mTOR/eIF4E pathway and crucial for erythroid differentiation encodes USE1 (Unusual SNARE protein in the ER 1), which controls retrograde vesicle transport between the Golgi apparatus and the endoplasmic

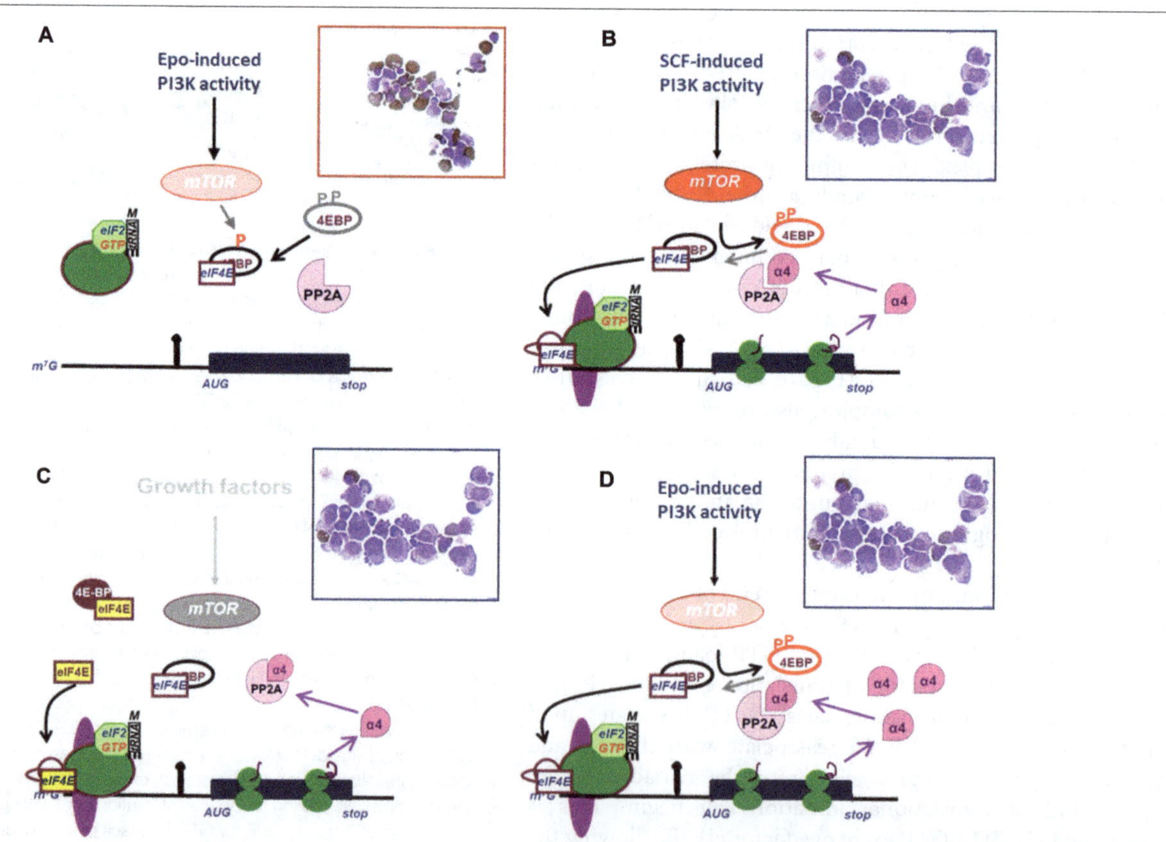

FIGURE 3 | Release of eIF4E and expression of IGBP1/alpha4 are effectors of mTOR activation. **(A)** Epo induces weak PI3K/mTOR signaling which causes only partial phosphorylation of 4EBP and fails to release eIF4E. The protein phosphatase PP2A dephosphorylates 4EBP and thereby inhibits eIF4E. In absence of eIF4E, 43 kD complex (see legend **Figure 2**) cannot associate with mRNA. As a result, erythroid progenitors differentiate (hemoglobin is stained brown in cytospin). **(B)** Epo plus SCF induces full phosphorylation of 4EBP and release ofeIF4E, which enables asembly of the preinitiation scanning complex at the mRNA cap, and translation of *IGBP1* mRNA to produce IGBP1 also known as the alpha4 inhibitory subunit of PP2A. **(C)** Overexpression of eIF4E out-titrates 4EBP and enables translation of *IGBP1* in absence of mTOR activation. **(D)** Constitutive expression of IGBP1/Alpha4 inhibits dephosphorylation of 4EBP and enables weak PI3K/mTOR activation to result in full phosphorylation of 4EBP, release of eIF4E and translation of IGBP1/Alpha4. **(B–D)** IGBP1 is an example representing many other transcripts with highly structured 5′UTRs. Cytospins indicate that translation of IGBP1 is associated with proliferation of erythroid progenitors in absence of differentiation.

reticulum (Grech et al., 2008; Nieradka et al., 2014). Finally, also mitochondrial biogenesis is under control of the mTOR/eIF4E pathway in erythroblasts (Liu et al., 2017).

eIF2 Phosphorylation in Erythropoiesis

Regulation of translation initiation is of particular importance in hemoglobin synthesis. Erythrocytes carry approximately 250 million hemoglobin molecules, each consisting of 4 globin peptides and 4 iron-containing heme molecules. Iron deficiency reduces heme availability and presents a risk of cell damage from the accumulation of free α- and β-globins that form toxic precipitates known as Heinz bodies (Jacob and Winterhalter, 1970). Therefore, in- and export of iron in erythroblasts, and the synthesis of heme and globin needs to be tightly coupled (Chen, 2014). Heme acts as a signaling molecule which binds to eIF2 associated kinase (eIF2ak1), also called HRI (Heme Regulated Inhibitor) (Han et al., 2005). During heme deficiency, HRI phosphorylates the α-chain of trimeric eIF2, preventing the exchange of eIF2-bound GDP for GTP by eIF2B and therefore also preventing the reassociation of the TC and the preinitiation scanning complex (**Figure 2**; Chen, 2007; Chung et al., 2012). This results in a global inhibition of protein synthesis (Liu et al., 2008). This mechanism is similar to eIF2 alpha phosphorylation resulting from detection of (viral) double-stranded RNA via eIF2ak2 (PKR), ER-stress via eIF2ak3 (PERK), and amino acid starvation via eIF2ak4 (GCN2) (Wek et al., 2006). Control of eIF2 phosphorylation is crucial during erythroid differentiation. Mice carrying alleles in which control of eIF2 phosphorylation is disturbed suffer from anemia. Phosphorylation of eIF2 induces translation of *ATF4* (Activating transcriptional factor 4), and expression of its target *PPR15a* (*Protein phosphatase 1, regulatory subunit 15A,* also known as *GADD34*). GADD34 enhances the enzyme activity of the catalytic PP1 subunit PPR15b (Harding et al., 2009). Mice that lack ATF4 suffer from mild compensated anemia, whereas mice lacking HRI or GADD34 are anemic with inefficient erythropoiesis (Masuoka, 2002; Patterson et al., 2006; Zhang et al., 2018). Mice lacking the PP1 catalytic subunit die perinatally with severe anemia (Harding et al., 2009).

Upstream Open Reading Frames

Increased sensitivity to translation factors, and particularly to eIF2, is predicted by the presence of uORFs in the 5′UTR of the transcript. The uORFs render mRNA translation hypersensitive to translation initiation factors at the level of (i) start codon recognition, (ii) interaction of the peptide or the uORF sequence with the ribosome, and (iii) reinitiation of the TC (eIF2:GTP and $tRNA_i^{met}$) with the scanning complex (Hinnebusch, 2014; Young et al., 2015). Translation of the uORF first requires recognition of the start codon. The better a start codon is embedded in a Kozak consensus sequence, the longer the scanning complex pauses, and the higher the chance that the GTPase activity of eIF2 is activated and translation is initiated (Kozak, 1986). Not only the local nucleotide sequence, also a downstream secondary structure may delay the scanning while the eIF4A helicase activity unfolds the transient obstacle. Finally, the activity of the eIF2 GTPase activity is controlled by eIF1 and eIF5 that regulate eIF2 activity and specificity. Interestingly, expression of eIF1 and −5 is controlled by SCF and during erythroid differentiation (Grech et al., 2008). Translation of the uORF causes eIF2 to dissociate from the complex, and requires reassociation of a new TC with the scanning complex before the scanning complex reaches the start codon of the next ORF. Fast reassociation depends on eIF2 expression and phosphorylation (**Figure 2C**). In cases where the uORFs overlaps with the protein-coding ORF (indicated as CDS, coding sequence), start codon recognition is mostly in a less favorable Kozak consensus sequence, whereas the presence of multiple uORFs in the 5′UTR typically renders translation dependent on the distance between uORFs and between the uORF and the CDS.

Whereas translation is generally inhibited upon eIF2 phosphorylation, the translation of specific transcripts may be enhanced under these conditions. One such transcript is *ATF4,* which is essential for erythroid differentiation and for reduction of oxidative stress during the basophilic erythroblast stage (Suragani et al., 2012). ATF4 contains two uORFs, the second of which overlaps with the CDS (Vattem and Wek, 2004). Translation of the second uORF inhibits ATF4 protein expression by overwriting the CDS (Lu et al., 2004). Phosphorylation of eIF2 decreases translation of the second uORF and increases translation of the *ATF4* CDS ORF. Whether uORFs are translated, has to be determined experimentally. Ribosome footprint analysis is a novel breakthrough in this field, because it provides the position of ribosomes on a transcript, and can identify which uORFs are actually translated (Ingolia, 2014). Treatment of erythroblasts with tunicamycin to induce eIF2 phosphorylation via PERK reduces the overall density of ribosomes on the transcriptome (Paolini et al., 2018). The ribosome density increases, however, on at least 140 transcripts among which *ATF4,* but also *PNRC2* (*proline rich nuclear receptor coactivator 2,* involved in RNA stability) and *IFDR1* (*interferon-related developmental regulator 1,* involved in cellular stress resistance) (Paolini et al., 2018). Other uORF-containing transcripts, instead, are hypersensitive to eIF2 phosphorylation and translation decreases more than average upon eIF2 phosphorylation in erythroblasts, among which *CSDE1* (*Cold shock domain protein e1,* see below), *PABPC1* (*PolyA binding protein c1*), and *PAPOLA,* [*poly(A) polymerase alpha*], which suggests that eIF2 phosphorylation may result in shortening of mRNA polyA-tails. The response to eIF2 phosphorylation is cell type specific, as indicated by a comparison between ribosome footprints in erythroblasts and HEK293 cells (Andreev et al., 2015; Paolini et al., 2018).

The analysis of uORF translation in erythroblasts indicates that uORFs are involved in eIF2-dependent translational regulation, but they do not predict eIF2-dependent translational regulation. This characterizes the advances of the field. We increasingly understand how general translation factors act together to control cap-dependent translation in commonly used cell models. For specific transcripts we understand the interplay of general translation initiation factors and specific sequences or structural elements in the 5′UTR of the transcript. However, when this information is used to make general predictions, the predictions are often wrong. For instance, Mfold is a well-known program for making structural predictions (Zuker, 2003). This is a useful tool, but chaperones and RBPs present in specific cell types may be more important determinants of structures and the energy required to unfold these structures. Therefore, we need to increase our understanding on the role of sequences and structures in the 5′UTR that have often been neglected when promoter studies were performed to understand gene expression and only the protein coding ORF of a transcript was used to study the role of the encoded protein.

Alternative 5′UTR Through Erythroid Specific Promoters or Alternative Splicing

The use of erythroid specific promoters and alternative splicing of the 5′UTR is common and has largely been ignored when it does not affect protein identity. It has been estimated that up to one third of all genes expressed in erythroid progenitors may be expressed from an alternative promoter (Tan et al., 2006; Cheng et al., 2014). The presence of an alternative 5′UTR can include or exclude structural elements (stem-loop structures or uORFs), with major consequence for translation initiation. RBP involved in alternative splicing of the 5′UTR are also modifiers of translation. Notably, erythroid differentiation is associated with extensive alternative splicing (Pimentel et al., 2014), with a prominent role for the RBP Muscleblind (Cheng et al., 2014). Alternative splicing mainly involves coding sequences (Cheng et al., 2014), but may specifically alter translation regulation in the 5′UTR. For instance, translation and stability of *Heme Oxygenase-1* (*HO1*) is regulated by hemin as part of feedback control. Alternative splicing generates a hemin resistant alternative transcript (Kramer et al., 2013). Similarly, transcript variants of *Ferroportin* are expressed during erythropoiesis that vary in their 5′UTR to enable iron responsive and non-responsive translation (Cianetti et al., 2005). In case of the SNARE-complex protein USE1, a predicted G-quadruplex in an alternatively spliced 5′UTR results in USE1 protein expression mainly from the small ratio of transcripts with intron retention (Nieradka et al., 2014). Alternative splicing can also alter the translation initiation codon that is used. Detection of alternative translation start sites can be established by ribosome footprinting or by mass spectrometry, in which case novel predicted N-termini must first be added to the reference library (Van Damme et al., 2014; Floor and Doudna, 2016).

IRES TRANS-ACTIVATING FACTORS

In addition to cap-dependent translation, ribosomes can associate on a subset of transcripts that carries an internal ribosomal entry site (IRES) (Komar and Hatzoglou, 2011). While there is no consensus sequence or universal structural motifs for IRESs, they typically contain complex structural elements which include stem loops and pseudoknots (Komar and Hatzoglou, 2005; Baird et al., 2007). The majority of IRESs are found within the 5′UTR directly upstream of the initiation codon, though they can also exist within the coding region, causing synthesis of a truncated protein (Komar et al., 2003; Grover et al., 2009). IRES-mediated translation is preferred under conditions of decreased availability of cap-dependent translation (Lewis and Holcik, 2008; Spriggs et al., 2008), due, for example, to eIF2 phosphorylation (Gerlitz et al., 2002; Tinton et al., 2005) or cleavage of scaffolding protein eIF4G (Komar and Hatzoglou, 2005). This includes, but is not limited to, viral infection, hypoxia, nutrient starvation, ER stress, and cell differentiation (Komar and Hatzoglou, 2005; Graber and Holcik, 2007).

Translation via an IRES requires the binding of IRES *trans*-activating factors (ITAFs) such as Polypyrimidine Tract Binding protein (PTB) (Bushell et al., 2006; Cobbold et al., 2010) and CSDE1 (Hunt et al., 1999; Mitchell et al., 2003; Cornelis et al., 2005). Some ITAFs are required to unfold the secondary structure, which subsequently enables other ITAFs to bind to specific sequence elements, and to recruit the ribosomal subunits. IRES-mediated translation initiation is less competitive in ribosome recruitment. Compared to the ^{7m}G cap structure, IRES elements are less competitive to recruit ribosomes. It is probably for that reason that primarily IRES-dependent translation initiation is suppressed when less ribosomes are present, which is a hallmark of DBA (Horos et al., 2012). The induction of severe anemia due to loss of ribosomes indicates that IRES-mediated translation is of particular importance in erythropoiesis.

Several genes involved in hematopoiesis are subject to IRES-mediated translation. BCL2-associated athanogen 1 (BAG1) and Heat Shock Protein 70 (HSP70) cochaperone are required for terminal differentiation of erythroblasts (Horos et al., 2012). All three BAG1 isoforms are produced from a single transcript dependent upon the involvement of either cap-dependent or IRES-mediated translation (Coldwell et al., 2001). Two ITAFs are involved in this process: PCBP1 [poly(rC) binding protein 1], which remodels the RNA to allow ribosomal entry, and PTB, which is necessary for the recruitment of the ribosome to the *BAG1* transcript (Pickering et al., 2004). Bag1 deficiency is lethal at day E13.5 in mice because of a complete lack of definitive erythropoiesis (Götz et al., 2005). shRNA-mediated knockdown of BAG1 in erythroblasts results in the production of fewer hemoglobinated daughter cells under differentiation conditions.

Another example of IRES-mediated translation is transcription factor RUNX1, which is essential for fetal liver hematopoiesis (Okuda et al., 1996). The *RUNX1* gene has two promoters that yield RUNX1 transcripts with two distinct 5′UTRs, one of which contains an IRES (Pozner et al., 2000; Levanon and Groner, 2004). The absence of the IRES in Runx1 causes embryonic fatality due to disordered proliferation and differentiation of hematopoietic cells in the fetal liver (Nagamachi et al., 2010).

Internal ribosomal entry sites have a unique role in circular RNAs that are generated by backsplicing. Without head and tail, these circular RNAs are hardly degraded, and lack the potential of being translated by cap-dependent mRNA translation. Interestingly, some circular RNAs encode proteins because translation initiation of circular RNA can be initiated from an IRES (Legnini et al., 2017; Pamudurti et al., 2017; Begum et al., 2018).

RBPs CONTROL mRNA STABILITY AND TRANSLATION THROUGH THE mRNA POLY(A) TAIL

Almost all protein coding mRNAs (except histones) are polyadenylated at their 3′ end. The poly(A) tail protects from degradation, and the length of the poly(A) tail also affects translation initiation (**Figure 2**). The length of the poly(A) tail is determined by the recruitment of polyadenylating and deadenylating enzymes to the transcript. Polyadenylation initially occurs in the nucleus where mRNA cleavage and polyadenylation are coupled (Charlesworth et al., 2013). Upon cleavage site recognition, a nuclear poly(A) polymerase is recruited to synthesize the poly(A) tail. Typically this is carried out by PAPOLA, but depending on the cell type and specific transcript, another, non-canonical polymerase may be involved (Charlesworth et al., 2013). Upon export to the cytoplasm, RBP binding to the 3′UTR may recruit polyadenylating or deadenylating proteins that may enhance or repress translation of the mRNA transcript. A broad array of RNA-binding proteins governs this process. Here, an overview of some of the larger families of poly(A)-interacting proteins and their influence on erythropoiesis will be presented (**Figure 4**).

PABPs Promote Translational Initiation and Stabilize Transcripts via poly(A) Binding

Essential to the initiation of translation is the binding of poly(A) binding proteins (PABPs) to the poly(A) tail. PABPs directly interact with the eIF4G scaffold protein of the eIF4F cap-binding complex (Hinnebusch and Lorsch, 2012). This brings the mRNA tail close to the cap, and forms a mRNA loop conformation that is believed to optimize recycling of translation initiation and elongating factors (Wakiyama et al., 2000). The interaction of PABP with eIF4G stabilizes pre-initiation scanning complexes on the 5′UTR (Kahvejian et al., 2005; **Figure 2**). A longer poly(A) tail increases PABP affinity for target transcripts, which enhances the stabilization of multiple preinitiation scanning complexes and thereby enhances translation initiation efficiency. Additionally, the binding of PABP to the poly(A) tail protects the transcript from deadenylation and degradation (Norbury, 2013), a process which is discussed in more detail below.

The most common PABP is PABPC1. In erythroid MEL (mouse erythroid leukemia) cells, however, there is a prominent role for Pabpc4 (Kini et al., 2014). Pabpc4 binds to a specific subset of transcripts with short poly(A) tails containing an AU-rich motif, including α-globin, and protects them from further degradation. Depletion of Pabpc4 blocks induced terminal differentiation of MEL cells by altering the expression of five genes associated with erythroid maturation. Receptor tyrosine kinase c-Kit is strongly upregulated in Pabpc4-depleted MEL cells. This activity is specific to Pabpc4 and not redundant with Pabpc1. Given that downregulation of c-Kit is essential for terminal differentiation (Munugalavadla et al., 2005; Dzierzak and Philipsen, 2013), the rescue of c-Kit expression is likely responsible for the inability of Pabpc4-depleted MEL cells to mature (Kini et al., 2014). Also induced were c-Myb, c-Myc, CD44, and Stat5a, all well-studied genes which promote erythroblast maintenance at the expense of differentiation (Hattangadi et al., 2011).

CPEBs Control poly(A) Tail Length

Among the proteins able to recruit cytoplasmic polyadenylation enzymes are the cytoplasmic polyadenylation element binding proteins (CPEBs). CPEBs, however, are promiscuous proteins

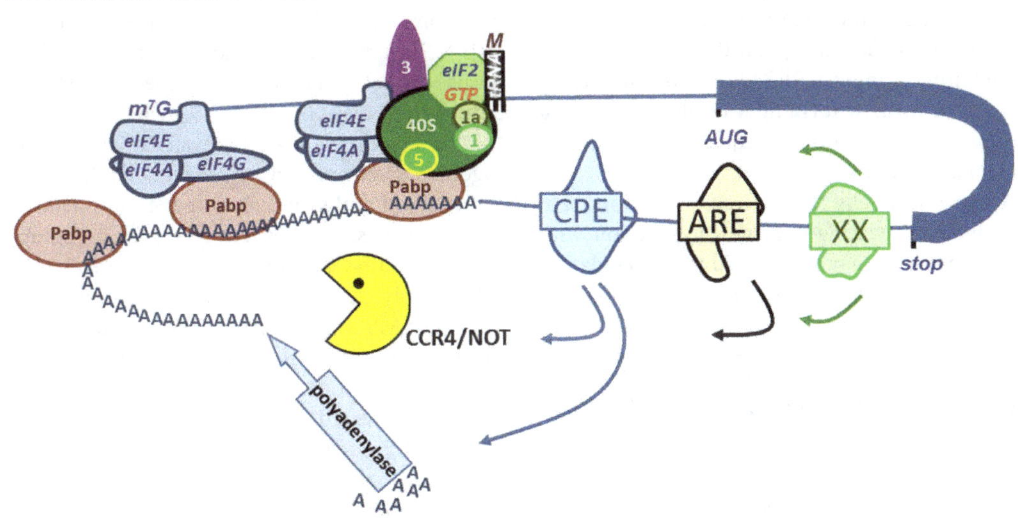

FIGURE 4 | RNA binding proteins (RBP) control mRNA stability and translation. Interaction of eIF4G in the eIF4F complex with PABP results in a closed loop model of mRNA translation (see legend **Figure 2**). Binding of PABPs to the poly(A) tail enhances mRNA stability and translation. A variety of RBP binding to e.g., the cytoplasmic polyadenylation element (CPE), AU-rich Elements (ARE) or other element represented as XX. These RPB interact with polyadenylases or with the CCR4/NOT deadenylating complex.

able to recruit either cytoplasmic poly(A) polymerases such as the Drosophila GLD2 protein (Germ Line Development 2; TENT2, terminal nucleotidyltransferase 2, in man; PAPD4, PAP associated domain containing 4 in mouse), which promotes mRNA stability and translation, or the deadenylating CCR4/NOT complex (Barnard et al., 2004; Ogami et al., 2014; **Figure 4**). Whether binding of CPEBs increases the length of the poly(A) tail or causes deadenylation depends on the interaction with additional RBP such as PUMILIO, or on phosphorylation of CPEB, for instance by Aurora kinase A (AURA) (Charlesworth et al., 2013). Deadenylation by CPEB depends on recruitment of the CCR4/NOT complex that is composed of several CNOT subunits, which individually have varying roles in a myriad of physiological processes. CAF1 and CCR4 are subunits with deadenylation activity (Shirai et al., 2014). In particular, CNOT9 was identified as an erythropoietin-responsive gene, indicating a role for the complex in erythropoiesis (Gregory et al., 2000). Deadenylation initially represses translation, because less PABP can bind and connect to eIF4G proteins in preinitiation complexes. Ultimately, deadenylation results in silencing of gene expression via mRNA degradation (Shirai et al., 2014).

Of the CPEB family members, CPEB4 is specifically induced during erythroid differentiation (Bakker et al., 2007; Hu et al., 2014). Erythroid expression of CPEB4 is regulated via the transcription factors GATA1 and TAL1 (Hu et al., 2014), its strong upregulation late in differentiation depends on FOXO3 (Bakker et al., 2007; Kerenyi and Orkin, 2010; Hattangadi et al., 2011). Because the recruitment of polyadenylating or deadenylating complexes depends on the context of the transcripts, i.e., on the complexes formed with RBP that bind to nearby elements in the 3′UTR, CPEB4 enhances or decreases mRNA translation with transcript-specific regulation. In erythroblasts, CPEB4 also associates with the eIF3 complex and the major mechanism appears to be repression of translation via the interaction with eIF3 (Hu et al., 2014). Both over- and underexpression of CPEB4 impairs the terminal differentiation of erythroblasts to reticulocytes, indicating that the level of CPEB4 needs to be controlled. Interestingly, CPEB4 is capable of binding to and repressing its own mRNA, forming a feedback loop that maintains CPEB4 levels within a range required for terminal erythropoiesis (Hu et al., 2014).

Although CPEBs are generally considered as factors that recruit adenylating or deadenylating enzymes, interaction with other general translation factors may also contribute to regulation of translation. Whereas CPEB4 binds eIF3, CPEB1 is known to increase mRNA stability by binding to PABPC1 and PABPC1L (Seli et al., 2005; Guzeloglu-Kayisli et al., 2008).

Musashi-Mediated Translational Control in Hematopoiesis

In addition to CPEB and PABP, cytoplasmic polyadenylation is regulated by MUSASHI-1 and -2 (MSI1 and MSI2). These proteins do not specifically control erythropoiesis, but they are very important for hematopoietic stem- and progenitor cells (HSPC) from which erythropoiesis develops. MSI1 and MSI2 interact with mRNA via the MSI-binding element (MBE) (Charlesworth et al., 2013). The MBE element is known to confer cytoplasmic polyadenylation in the absence of CPEB activity (Charlesworth et al., 2006). The poly(A) polymerase GLD2 interacts with MSI in Xenopus oocytes, but interactions between MSI proteins and the polyadenylation machinery have been described in mammalian cells (Charlesworth et al., 2013; Cragle and MacNicol, 2014).

The majority of studies done on MUSASHI-mediated translational repression have been done with MSI1. MSI1 represses the translation of target transcripts by competing with eIF4G for binding with PABP, preventing the formation of the 80S ribosome subunit (Kerwitz et al., 2003). Transcripts silenced by Msi1 include cell cycle regulators such as Numb, an inhibitor of the NOTCH pathway, and the cell cycle inhibitor p21 (Bardwell et al., 1990; Topalian et al., 2001). RNA binding domains between MSI1 and MSI2 are largely homologous (85–95%), but MSI2 has no PABP-binding domain (de Andrés-Aguayo et al., 2012). However, there is evidence to suggest that MSI2 alters NOTCH localization and upregulates HES1, a NOTCH reporter protein (Kharas et al., 2010), suggesting that MSI1 and MSI2 overlap in regulating common targets.

MSI2 is abundantly expressed in primitive LSK cells of the hematopoietic lineage, where MSI1 expression is nearly absent (Kharas et al., 2010; de Andrés-Aguayo et al., 2011; Hope and Sauvageau, 2011). The expression of MSI2 is subsequently downregulated during differentiation. Downregulation of MSI2 alters the balance between self-renewal and differentiation of HSCs via regulation of the NOTCH pathway (Kharas et al., 2010; Hope and Sauvageau, 2011). This effect is achieved without influencing apoptotic rates or homing behavior. A mouse line expressing a truncated MSI2 gene ($Msi2^{Gt/Gt}$) results in a marked decrease in short term hematopoietic stem cells (ST-HSCs) and multipotent progenitors (MPPs) while the effect on long term hematopoietic stem cells (LT-HSCs) was nominal (de Andrés-Aguayo et al., 2011). MSI2-defective LSKs display impaired proliferation, and the LT-HSC population is decreased following non-competitive bone marrow transplantation (Kharas et al., 2010). In addition, a doxycycline-inducible MSI2 transgenic mouse model observed an increase in ST-HSC/MPP populations and a decrease in LT-HSC, whereas MSI2 overexpression increased LT-HSC self-renewal in transplanted mice. Taken together, these findings suggest that MSI2 is important for HSPC self-renewal and stem cell homeostasis particularly during stress hematopoiesis. Studies on MSI2 in hematopoiesis have been largely functional in focus and do not mechanistically investigate mRNA polyadenylation via MSI2. Although the direct molecular targets of MSI2 in hematopoiesis are unknown, gene expression profiling indicates a regulatory function for pathways involved in HSC proliferation, including MEIS1, HOXA9, HOXA10 (Hope and Sauvageau, 2011), RAS, MAPK, CyclinD1, and MYC (Kharas et al., 2010; de Andrés-Aguayo et al., 2011). The role of MSI2 in Hematopoiesis has been extensively reviewed in de Andrés-Aguayo et al. (2012).

AUBPs in Hematopoiesis

The AAU1/HNRPD family of AU-rich element binding proteins (AUBPs) are oppositely regulated from the MSI proteins (Sakakibara et al., 2002). AU-rich elements (AREs) are sequence motifs (typically AUUUA) in the 3′UTR that recruit a large family of AU-binding proteins (AUBPs) that regulate translation (**Figure 4**). They were among the first sequence elements known to affect stability of mRNA (Shaw and Kamen, 1986). Translational regulation via AUBPs can occur via a number of mechanisms including deadenylation, and transcript sequestration to P-bodies and stress granules (Baou et al., 2011). AUBPs key to erythropoiesis include the tristetraprolin (TTP) family members (ZFP36, ZFP36L1, and ZFP36L2) and HuR/ELAV1.

TTP family members interact with NOT1 to promote the rapid deadenylation by the CCR4/NOT complex (Sandler et al., 2011; Fabian et al., 2013). Interestingly, ZFP36L1 and ZFP36L2 demonstrate opposite regulation in erythropoiesis. ZFP36L2 is expressed in erythroid progenitors in response to glucocorticoids and downregulated during terminal differentiation. ZFPL1, instead, is only expressed in more mature erythroblasts (Zhang et al., 2013; MvL unpublished data). Concordantly, ZFP36L2 is required for burst-forming unit-erythrocyte (BFU-E) renewal (Zhang et al., 2013), whereas ZFP36L1 downregulates STAT5B expression, reducing the formation of erythroid colonies (Vignudelli et al., 2010). Why these highly homologous factors have such opposite effects in erythropoiesis, and how they regulate the transcripts to which they are bound, is unclear. In keratinocytes, ZFP36L1 and ZFP36L2 also have non-redundant roles in the regulation of growth factor expression, but in T cells, both ZFP36L1 and ZFP36L2 inhibit cell proliferation by inhibiting the expression of cell cycle genes, particularly D Cyclins (Galloway et al., 2016; Prenzler et al., 2016).

ELAV1, also known as HuR, is a ubiquitously expressed AUBP with thousands of direct and functional targets (Lebedeva et al., 2011; Mukherjee et al., 2011). Relevant transcripts bound by ELAV1 encode proteins that control cell cycle progression, apoptosis, signal transduction, and lineage specific transcription factors (reviewed in Baou et al., 2011). Interestingly, ZFP36L1 is a functional target of ELAV1 in cells exposed to oxidative stress, wherein ionizing radiation decreases *ZFP36L1* transcript binding by ELAV1, resulting in a decreased recruitment of *ZFP36L1* to polysomes (Mazan-Mamczarz et al., 2011). This suggests that ZFP36L1 may synergize with ZFP36L1 in regulating erythropoiesis under some conditions.

Alternative Polyadenylation Controls mRNA Stability and Translation

The examples mentioned above are only a brief and incomplete overview of how proteins binding to the 3′UTR may control mRNA stability and translation through recruitment of polyadenylases or the deadenylating complex. It is long known that the nuclear cleavage and polyadenylation complex may recognize alternative sites for mRNA cleavage resulting in alternative length of the 3′UTR. The exclusion of binding sites for RBPs can have major consequences for mRNA stability and translation (Mayr, 2016). The implications of single transcripts have been studied, but systematic analysis of alternative polyadenylation (APA) and their consequences for mRNA stability are scarce (Sun et al., 2012). Novel methods are available to determine APA sites, but it is difficult to combine for instance ribosome footprint analysis with APA because the output of ribosome footprinting exists of short ribosome protected fragments that cannot be attributes to distinct transcripts. To date only few examples of APA are known in erythropoiesis but nothing is known about the relation of APA and control of gene expression by RBPs (Kudo et al., 1994; Boehmelt et al., 1998).

RBPs INVOLVED IN ADDITIONAL CONTROL OF TRANSLATION

In addition to general translation initiation factors and RBP that control the poly(A), mRNAs contain secondary structures and specific sequences that bind RBP to specifically control their translation. An important posttranscriptional mechanism of gene expression is mediated by microRNAs. Argonaut proteins are the miRNA-binding RBPs that associate with RNA. Mice deficient in Argonaut 2 (Ago2) suffer from severe anemia, which is caused by the failure of miR-144/451 to act on its targets (Rasmussen et al., 2010). However, Ago2 is the Argonaut protein with slicing activity and appears to control mRNA stability more than translation (Jee et al., 2018). We therefore focus our discussion on the role of a few selected RBP that are important for erythropoiesis, rather than on miRs.

Translational Control of Iron Homeostasis

Iron homeostasis in erythroid cells is achieved via a balanced regulation of iron import via transferrin receptor 1 (TfR1), storage in ferritin and export via ferroportin (Kühn et al., 2015). Posttranscriptional control over these proteins is enacted by iron regulatory proteins (IRPs). IRPs are recruited to *ferritin* mRNA via a conserved sequence that forms a hairpin structure in the 5′UTR (Aziz and Munro, 1986; Hentze et al., 1987). Binding of the IRP to the IRE (Iron Response Element) prevents the association of the 43S preinitiation complex to the mRNA transcript (Gray and Hentze, 1994). The presence of iron blocks the IRE-IRP interaction, allowing translation of the formerly repressed ferritin transcript. A similar mechanism governs the translation of *ferroportin* (Abboud and Haile, 2000). Interestingly, a splice variant of *ferroportin* lacking the IRE is expressed in duodenum and erythroid cells permits the escape of IRP-mediated translational control (Cianetti et al., 2005). By contrast, the TfR1 transcript possesses 5 IREs in the 3′UTR rather than the 5′UTR (Koeller et al., 1989; Müllner et al., 1989). Binding of IRPs to *TfR1* confers increased mRNA stability to the transcript, resulting in an inverse relationship between TfR1 protein expression and iron abundancy (Owen and Kühn, 1987; Müllner and Kühn, 1988).

Both IRPs cooperate to control iron homeostasis, yet they are regulated via different mechanisms. IRP1 is a bifunctional protein with both enzymatic and RNA-binding activity. Its possesses the capacity to act as an aconitase in the catalyzation of citrate to isocitrate (Kennedy et al., 1983). The catalytic activity is dependent upon the assimilation of an additional iron atom in the active site, with the result that IRP1 functions as an enzyme when iron is abundant, and as an RNA-binding protein when iron is depleted (Haile et al., 1992; Emery-Goodman et al., 1993; Hirling et al., 1994). Because the formation of the iron-sulfur cluster in the active site requires an oxygen-free environment (Beinert and Kennedy, 1993), the RNA-binding form is preferentially induced in the presence of the vasodilating agent nitrous oxide (Drapier et al., 1993).

Although IRP2 is 57% homologous with IRP1 in humans, it does not function as an aconitase under iron-rich conditions (Guo et al., 1994). Unlike IRP1, IRP2 is rapidly degraded by the proteasome when iron and oxygen levels are high (Guo et al., 1994, 1995). Degradation of IRP2 is prevented by low oxygen pressure (Hanson et al., 2003). Taken together, IRP1 and IRP2 are capable of controlling iron homeostasis under both low and high iron and oxygen supply, allowing a proportional response to environmental stimuli (Kühn et al., 2015).

The RBP Csde1 Is Essential for Erythropoiesis

CSDE1, originally called UNR (upstream of N-ras) is an RNA-binding protein with five cold-shock domains (Triqueneaux et al., 1999). CSDE1/UNR was initially shown to silence *MSL* (*Male Sex Lethal)* during sex determination of *Drosophila melanogaster* (Jacquemin-Sablon et al., 1994; Gebauer et al., 1999; Grskovic et al., 2003; Abaza et al., 2006; Duncan et al., 2006; Abaza and Gebauer, 2008). Repression of *MSL2* occurs via a direct interaction between CSDE1 and 3′UTR-bound PABP, resulting in the prevention of PABP-mediated recruitment of the 43S complex (Duncan et al., 2009). Paradoxically, the CSDE1-PABP complex has also been reported to stimulate translation by stabilizing the interaction between PABP and eIF4G (Ray and Anderson, 2016).

CSDE1 is implicated in both endogenous and viral IRES-mediated translation in mammalian cells. Both rhinovirus and poliovirus contain IRES elements that require an interaction between CSDE1 and PTB (Hunt et al., 1999; Boussadia et al., 2003). Early studies indicated that all five of CSDE1's cold-shock domains were necessary for maintenance of CSDE1's affinity for rhinovirus IRESs, whereas cold-shock domains 1 and 2 had the most impact on CSDE1's binding to *MSL-2* (Brown and Jackson, 2004; Abaza and Gebauer, 2008), and cold-shock domains 2 and 4 were the only required elements for stimulation of translation via PABP (Ray and Anderson, 2016).

CSDE1 and PTB also cooperate in IRES binding of the *CSDE1* transcript itself, resulting in repression of translation of *CSDE1* (Cornelis et al., 2005; Dormoy-Raclet et al., 2005; Schepens et al., 2007). IRES-mediated translation is promoted during mitosis and apoptosis at the expense of cap-dependent translation (Komar and Hatzoglou, 2005; Tinton et al., 2005). The CSDE1 IRES activity is strongly upregulated during mitosis due to increased binding of hnRNPC1/C2 proteins with simultaneous release of CSDE1 and PTB (Schepens et al., 2007). The resultant increase in Csde1 expression during the G2/M phase of the cell cycle facilitates the IRES-mediated translation of cyclin-dependent PITSLRE kinases, which are essential for centrosome maturation and mitotic spindle formation (Tinton et al., 2005; Petretti et al., 2006). During apoptosis, CSDE1 and PTB upregulate APAF1 (apoptotic protease-activating factor 1) (Mitchell et al., 2001). Binding of CSDE1 and PTB changes the conformation of the APAF1 IRES, granting access for ribosomal recruitment and thereby permitting the translation of the transcript (Mitchell et al., 2003).

CSDE1 is also implicated as a regulator of mRNA stability via poly(A) deadenylation. CSDE1 binds to *cFOS* in conjunction with PABP (Chang et al., 2004). In contrast to the stabilizing influence of PABP when interacting with CPEB, the CSDE1-PABP complex promotes transcript degradation via recruitment of the deadenylase CCR4. Given that binding of PABP and CSDE1 to the poly(A) tail can also increase transcript stability, Chang et al. propose a model in which the CSDE1-PABP complex initially protects the poly(A) tail from deadenylation by CCR4 prior to initiation of translation. Upon ribosomal transit of the mCRD, a conformational change is triggered that forms a landing pad for CCR4, resulting in transcript repression by deadenylation.

CSDE1 also interacts with the 4E-Transporter (4E-T), itself a translational regulator with a wide breadth of functions. 4E-T competitively binds to cap-binding protein eIF4E, preventing its association with scaffolding protein eIF4G (Sonenberg and Hinnebusch, 2009; Kamenska et al., 2016), while simultaneously reducing ribosomal access to the 5′ cap via interaction with RNA-binding proteins at the 3′UTR (Rhoads, 2009; Kamenska et al., 2014b). Furthermore, 4E-T is a component of the CPEB translation repressor complex (Minshall et al., 2007), the CCR4/NOT complex (Kamenska et al., 2014a), and enhances decay of transcripts containing AREs (Ferraiuolo et al., 2005; Chang et al., 2014; Nishimura et al., 2015). 4E-T is directly bound by CSDE1 (Kamenska et al., 2016). 4E-T binding to CSDE1 and CNOT4 is mutually exclusive, which predicts that Csde1 abrogates 4E-Ts role as a bridge between CNOT1 and CNOT4 complex subunits (Kamenska et al., 2016). Due to the complexity of the overlapping pathways associated with 4E-T, it is unclear precisely how CSDE1 cooperates with 4E-T in the regulation of translation. The authors suggest that CSDE1 and DDX6, an RNA helicase component of the CPEB repressor complex, simultaneously bind 4E-T to either redundantly repress translation or to selectively affect specific translational stages. Another possibility is that CSDE1 acts as a competitive inhibitor of 4E-T binding to other, unknown cofactors/repressors, disruption of which unravels a network of interactions necessary for translational repression.

Notably, CSDE1 expression is decreased in erythroblasts with a haploinsufficiency in ribosomal proteins. Expression of CSDE1 is >100-fold upregulated in erythroblasts compared to early progenitors, and expression of Csde1 is required for erythroblast proliferation and differentiation in mouse erythroblasts (Horos et al., 2012). Csde1-bound transcripts and associated proteins that are identified using Csde1 pulldown, encode proteins involved in ribogenesis, mRNA translation and protein degradation, but also proteins associated with the mitochondrial respiratory chain and mitosis (Moore et al., 2018). RNA expression and/or protein expression of Csde1-bound transcripts are deregulated in MEL clones in which the first cold-shock domain of Csde1 is deleted by Crispr/Cas9. For instance, protein expression of Pabpc1 was enhanced while *Pabpc1* mRNA expression was reduced indicating more efficient translation of *Pabpc1* followed by negative feedback on mRNA stability (Moore et al., 2018). Under the conditions used for Csde1 pull down experiments, Csde1 associates most prominently with Strap (serine threonine kinase receptor associated protein). Strap does not affect Csde1/mRNA association, but it alters expression of some transcripts and/or proteins (Moore et al., 2017). In addition to Strap, also Pabpc1 and Pabpc4 associate with Csde1 in MEL cells.

Heterogeneous Nuclear Ribonucleoproteins hnRNPK and GRSF1

Among the first RBP that were identified and characterized are members of the large superfamily of heterogeneous nuclear ribonucleoproteins (hnRNPs). Within this superfamily four different RNA binding domains and several auxiliary domains are discerned, on basis of which 16 independent families are identified by capital letters (Geuens et al., 2016). The hnRNP family members do not specifically control translation. They are involved in many levels of gene expression regulation including gene transcription, mRNA splicing, mRNA nuclear-cytoplasmic transport, mRNA stability, and translation.

The RBPs hnRNPE1 and hnRNPK are important for late erythroid maturation. Together they control translation of the reticulocyte enzyme 15-lipoxygenase (r15-LOX) (Ostareck et al., 2001). This enzyme is at the base of mitochondrial degradation through dioxygenation of phospholipids in mitochondrial membranes (Grüllich et al., 2001). The silencing of *r15-LOX* translation by hnRNPK involves association of *r15-LOX* with DDX6 in P-bodies, and is regulated by SRC kinase through an intricate feed-back control of hnRNPK and SRC (Naarmann et al., 2008). Translational regulation of mitochondrial degradation in late erythroblasts and reticulocytes is not limited to control of *r15-LOX* translation. Expression of Non-muscle myosin heavy chain IIA (NmhcIIA), involved in intracellular vesicle transport, is also regulated by hnRNPK (Naarmann-de Vries et al., 2016). Thus, the maturation of reticulocytes depends on hnRNPE1 and hnRNPK. These are the only two subtypes of the hnRNP superfamily that carry the unique RNA binding domain indicated as a K-homology domain (KH) (Geuens et al., 2016).

The subfamilies hnRNPF and hnRNPH share a high degree of homology and contain 3 QRRM domains (Quasi RNA recognition motif) (Geuens et al., 2016). Interestingly, hnRNPF/H members were prominently detected among G-quadruplex binding proteins (von Hacht et al., 2014). Similar to hnRNP proteins, the G-quadruplex structure that can occur in DNA and RNA is widely employed to control gene expression, mRNA splicing, transport, stability, and translation (Song et al., 2016). In translational control, they are mainly detected in transcripts expressed during mitosis, and particularly in transcripts that are well expressed in tumor cells (Wolfe et al., 2014). The Guanine-rich RNA sequence binding factor 1 (GRSF1) contains three RNA binding domains and is a member of the heterogeneous nuclear ribonucleoprotein F/H family (hnRNPF/H) (Ufer, 2012; Sofi et al., 2018). GRSF1 binds a G-rich element in *Glutathione Peroxidase 4* (*GPX4*), and in the transcript encoding *Unusual SNARE protein in the ER-1* (*USE1*) (Ufer et al., 2008; Nieradka et al., 2014). Translation of *USE1* depends on the PI3K/mTOR pathway, and on the availability of eIF4E in erythroblasts. Constitutive expression of a truncated USE1 isoform inhibits erythroid differentiation, whereas clones expressing full length USE1 could not be established (Grech et al., 2008). This suggests that regulation of USE1 expression during erythropoiesis is critical. Differential splicing creates transcripts with a long and short 5′UTR. Although most transcripts are spliced and contain a short 5′UTR, the unspliced *USE1* transcript is predominantly present in polyribosomes (Nieradka et al., 2014). This is due to the presence of a G-rich element that scores high in G-quadruplex prediction models. Both USE1 and GRSF1 are expressed in proliferating erythroblasts and are downregulated during differentiation. Suppression of USE1 and GRSF1 expression in erythroblasts decreases the capacity to undergo renewal divisions, and induces terminal erythroid differentiation instead (Nieradka et al., 2014). Thus, the RBP GRSF1 is crucial to erythropoiesis, either through regulation of *USE1* translation or through regulation of other G-Quadruplex containing transcripts.

More RBPs and Methods to Decipher Translation Efficiency

Transcripts that are subject to control of translation can be identified by density centrifugation to separate subpolysomal from polyribosomal transcripts. In erythroblasts, this resulted in the identification of numerous transcripts that are dependent on for instance growth factors Epo and SCF for their translation (Joosten et al., 2004; Grech et al., 2008). Detailed mRNA translation, at the nucleotide level, can be determined using ribosome footprinting technology (Ingolia et al., 2011). This technology uncovered changes in mRNA translation efficiency in response to tunicamycin-induced phosphorylation of eIF2 (paragraphs 2.2 and 2.3; Paolini et al., 2018). Ribosome footprinting during terminal differentiation of erythroblasts to reticulocytes revealed several classes of transcripts subject to regulated translation (Alvarez-Dominguez et al., 2017). RNA binding motif 38 (RBM38) is an RBP that is prominently expressed in erythroblast. Its expression steadily increases from basophilic erythroblasts to the reticulocyte stage. Interestingly, a polymorphism in RBM38 is associated with erythrocyte volume (van der Harst et al., 2012). RBM38 is known to be associated with erythroid differentiation through control of mRNA splicing (Heinicke et al., 2013; Ulirsch et al., 2016). Of interest, Rbm38 serves as a tumor suppressor gene, and mice that lack Rbm38 are prone to cancer development. In addition, however, they suffer from anemia (Zhang et al., 2014). RBM38 binds to a UGUGU element in the 3′UTR of its target transcripts and interacts with the scaffold protein eIF4G in the eIF4F cap-binding complex. Therefore, Alvarez-Dominguez et al. (2017) hypothesize that RBM38 interferes with the closed loop model of mRNA translation and thereby decreases the efficiency of translation.

Finally, ribosome profiling also showed that ribosomes fail to be recovered in reticulocytes and therefore accumulate in the 3′UTR (Mills et al., 2016). This is due to loss of ABCE1. This loss of ribosome recovery may be the start of total RNA degradation which characterizes the maturation of reticulocytes to erythrocytes during the first 2 days after release of reticulocytes in the peripheral circulation.

CONCLUSION

This review presents a general overview of distinct mechanisms and major players that control mRNA translation in erythropoiesis. However, it is clear that there is still much we have yet to understand regarding mechanisms in mRNA translation. The advent of novel molecular and biochemical technologies has revolutionized the large-scale identification of RBPs and their transcripts. Technologies such as iCLIP (Individual-nucleotide resolution UV crosslinking and immunoprecipitation) and ribosome profiling have the exciting potential to rapidly advance the field.

After transcription, translation functions as an additional regulatory layer of gene expression. Precise translational control enables coordinated protein synthesis in response to environmental signals, or the differentiation stage of cells. It also enables the dissociation of gene transcription and protein synthesis in time, which is of particular importance once gene transcription has ceased in late erythroblasts and reticulocytes undergoing terminal erythropoiesis. We expect that the coming years will provide exciting new insights in selective translation of mRNA during erythropoiesis.

AUTHOR CONTRIBUTIONS

All authors listed have made a substantial, direct and intellectual contribution to the work, and approved it for publication.

REFERENCES

Abaza, I., Coll, O., Patalano, S., and Gebauer, F. (2006). Drosophila UNR is required for translational repression of male-specific lethal 2 mRNA during regulation of X-chromosome dosage compensation. *Genes Dev.* 20, 380–389. doi: 10.1101/gad.371906

Abaza, I., and Gebauer, F. (2008). Functional domains of Drosophila UNR in translational control. *RNA* 14, 482–490. doi: 10.1261/rna.802908

Abboud, S., and Haile, D. J. (2000). A novel mammalian iron-regulated protein involved in intracellular iron metabolism. *J. Biol. Chem.* 275, 19906–19912. doi: 10.1074/jbc.M000713200

Alvarez-Dominguez, J. R., Zhang, X., and Hu, W. (2017). Widespread and dynamic translational control of red blood cell development. *Blood* 129, 619–629. doi: 10.1182/blood-2016-09-741835

Andreev, D. E., O'Connor, P. B., Fahey, C., Kenny, E. M., Terenin, I. M., Dmitriev, S. E., et al. (2015). Translation of 5' leaders is pervasive in genes resistant to eIF2 repression. *eLife* 4:e03971. doi: 10.7554/eLife.03971

Aziz, N., and Munro, H. N. (1986). Both subunits of rat liver ferritin are regulated at a translational level by iron induction. *Nucleic Acids Res.* 14, 915–927. doi: 10.1093/nar/14.2.915

Baird, S. D., Lewis, S. M., Turcotte, M., and Holcik, M. (2007). A search for structurally similar cellular internal ribosome entry sites. *Nucleic Acids Res.* 35, 4664–4677. doi: 10.1093/nar/gkm483

Bakker, W. J., Blázquez-Domingo, M., Kolbus, A., Besooyen, J., Steinlein, P., Beug, H., et al. (2004). FoxO3a regulates erythroid differentiation and induces BTG1, an activator of protein arginine methyl transferase 1. *J. Cell Biol.* 164, 175–184. doi: 10.1083/jcb.200307056

Bakker, W. J., van Dijk, T. B., Parren-van Amelsvoort, M., Kolbus, A., Yamamoto, K., Steinlein, P., et al. (2007). Differential regulation of Foxo3a target genes in erythropoiesis. *Mol. Cell. Biol.* 27, 3839–3854. doi: 10.1128/MCB.01662-06

Baou, M., Norton, J. D., and Murphy, J. J. (2011). AU-rich RNA binding proteins in hematopoiesis and leukemogenesis. *Blood* 118, 5732–5740. doi: 10.1182/blood-2011-07-347237

Bardwell, V. J., Zarkower, D., Edmonds, M., and Wickens, M. (1990). The enzyme that adds poly(A) to mRNAs is a classical poly(A) polymerase. *Mol. Cell. Biol.* 10, 846–849. doi: 10.1128/MCB.10.2.846

Barnard, D. C., Ryan, K., Manley, J. L., and Richter, J. D. (2004). Symplekin and xGLD-2 are required for CPEB-mediated cytoplasmic polyadenylation. *Cell* 119, 641–651. doi: 10.1016/j.cell.2004.10.029

Begum, S., Yiu, A., Stebbing, J., and Castellano, L. (2018). Novel tumour suppressive protein encoded by circular RNA, *circ-SHPRH*, in glioblastomas. *Oncogene.* doi: 10.1038/s41388-018-0230-3

Beinert, H., and Kennedy, M. C. (1993). Aconitase, a two-faced protein: enzyme and iron regulatory factor. *FASEB J.* 7, 1442–1449. doi: 10.1096/fasebj.7.15.8262329

Blázquez-Domingo, M., Grech, G., and von Lindern, M. (2005). Translation initiation factor 4E inhibits differentiation of erythroid progenitors. *Mol. Cell. Biol.* 25, 8496–8506. doi: 10.1128/MCB.25.19.8496-8506.2005

Boehmelt, G., Antonio, L., and Iscove, N. N. (1998). Cloning of the murine transcriptional corepressor component SAP18 and differential expression of its mRNA in the hematopoietic hierarchy. *Gene* 207, 267–275. doi: 10.1016/S0378-1119(97)00648-3

Borg, J., Papadopoulos, P., Georgitsi, M., Gutiérrez, L., Grech, G., Fanis, P., et al. (2010). Haploinsufficiency for the erythroid transcription factor KLF1 causes hereditary persistence of fetal hemoglobin. *Nat. Genet.* 42, 801–805. doi: 10.1038/ng.630

Boussadia, O., Niepmann, M., Créancier, L., Prats, A.-C., Dautry, F., and Jacquemin-Sablon, H. (2003). Unr is required in vivo for efficient initiation of translation from the internal ribosome entry sites of both rhinovirus and poliovirus. *J. Virol.* 77, 3353–3359. doi: 10.1128/jvi.77.6.3353-3359.2003

Brar, G. A., and Weissman, J. S. (2015). Ribosome profiling reveals the what, when, where and how of protein synthesis. *Nat. Rev. Mol. Cell Biol.* 16, 651–664. doi: 10.1038/nrm4069

Broudy, V. C., Lin, N. L., Priestley, G. V., Nocka, K., and Wolf, N. S. (1996). Interaction of stem cell factor and its receptor c-kit mediates lodgment and acute expansion of hematopoietic cells in the murine spleen. *Blood* 88, 75–81.

Brown, E. C., and Jackson, R. J. (2004). All five cold-shock domains of unr (upstream of N-ras) are required for stimulation of human rhinovirus RNA translation. *J. Gen. Virol.* 85, 2279–2287. doi: 10.1099/vir.0.80045-0

Bushell, M., Stoneley, M., Kong, Y. W., Hamilton, T. L., Spriggs, K. A., Dobbyn, H. C., et al. (2006). Polypyrimidine tract binding protein regulates IRES-mediated gene expression during apoptosis. *Mol. Cell* 23, 401–412. doi: 10.1016/j.molcel.2006.06.012

Chang, S.-H., Elemento, O., Zhang, J., Zhuang, Z. W., Simons, M., and Hla, T. (2014). ELAVL1 regulates alternative splicing of eIF4E transporter to promote postnatal angiogenesis. *Proc. Natl. Acad. Sci. U.S.A.* 111, 18309–18314. doi: 10.1073/pnas.1412172111

Chang, T. C., Yamashita, A., Chen, C. Y. A., Yamashita, Y., Zhu, W., Durdan, S., et al. (2004). UNR, a new partner of poly(A)-binding protein, plays a key role in translationally coupled mRNA turnover mediated by the c-fos major coding-region determinant. *Genes Dev.* 18, 2010–2023. doi: 10.1101/gad.1219104

Charlesworth, A., Meijer, H. A., and de Moor, C. H. (2013). Specificity factors in cytoplasmic polyadenylation. *Wiley Interdiscip. Rev. RNA* 4, 437–461. doi: 10.1002/wrna.1171

Charlesworth, A., Wilczynska, A., Thampi, P., Cox, L. L., and MacNicol, A. M. (2006). Musashi regulates the temporal order of mRNA translation during Xenopus oocyte maturation. *EMBO J.* 25, 2792–2801. doi: 10.1038/sj.emboj.7601159

Chen, J.-J. (2007). Regulation of protein synthesis by the heme-regulated eIF2alpha kinase: relevance to anemias. *Blood* 109, 2693–2699. doi: 10.1182/blood-2006-08-041830

Chen, J.-J. (2014). Translational control by heme-regulated eIF2α kinase during erythropoiesis. *Curr. Opin. Hematol.* 21, 172–178. doi: 10.1097/MOH.0000000000000030

Cheng, A. W., Shi, J., Wong, P., Luo, K. L., Trepman, P., Wang, E. T., et al. (2014). Muscleblind-like 1 (Mbnl1) regulates pre-mRNA alternative splicing during terminal erythropoiesis. *Blood* 124, 598–610. doi: 10.1182/blood-2013-12-542209

Chung, J., Bauer, D. E., Ghamari, A., Nizzi, C. P., Deck, K. M., Kingsley, P. D., et al. (2015). The mTORC1/4E-BP pathway coordinates hemoglobin production with L-leucine availability. *Sci. Signal.* 8:ra34. doi: 10.1126/scisignal.aaa5903

Chung, J., Chen, C., and Paw, B. H. (2012). Heme metabolism and erythropoiesis. *Curr. Opin. Hematol.* 19, 156–162. doi: 10.1097/MOH.0b013e328351c48b

Cianetti, L., Segnalini, P., Calzolari, A., Morsilli, O., Felicetti, F., Ramoni, C., et al. (2005). Expression of alternative transcripts of ferroportin-1 during human erythroid differentiation. *Haematologica* 90, 1595–1606.

Cobbold, L. C., Wilson, L. A., Sawicka, K., King, H. A., Kondrashov, A. V., Spriggs, K. A., et al. (2010). Upregulated c-myc expression in multiple myeloma by internal ribosome entry results from increased interactions with and expression of PTB-1 and YB-1. *Oncogene* 29, 2884–2891. doi: 10.1038/onc.2010.31

Coldwell, M. J., deSchoolmeester, M. L., Fraser, G. A., Pickering, B. M., Packham, G., and Willis, A. E. (2001). The p36 isoform of BAG-1 is translated by internal ribosome entry following heat shock. *Oncogene* 20, 4095–4100. doi: 10.1038/sj.onc.1204547

Cornelis, S., Tinton, S. A., Schepens, B., Bruynooghe, Y., and Beyaert, R. (2005). UNR translation can be driven by an IRES element that is negatively regulated by polypyrimidine tract binding protein. *Nucleic Acids Res.* 33, 3095–3108. doi: 10.1093/nar/gki611

Cragle, C., and MacNicol, A. M. (2014). Musashi protein-directed translational activation of target mRNAs is mediated by the poly(A) polymerase, germ line development defective-2. *J. Biol. Chem.* 289, 14239–14251. doi: 10.1074/jbc.M114.548271

de Andrés-Aguayo, L., Varas, F., and Graf, T. (2012). Musashi 2 in hematopoiesis. *Curr. Opin. Hematol.* 19, 268–272. doi: 10.1097/MOH.0b013e328353c778

de Andrés-Aguayo, L., Varas, F., Kallin, E. M., Infante, J. F., Wurst, W., Floss, T., et al. (2011). Musashi 2 is a regulator of the HSC compartment identified by a retroviral insertion screen and knockout mice. *Blood* 118, 554–564. doi: 10.1182/blood-2010-12-322081

Dormoy-Raclet, V., Markovits, J., Jacquemin-Sablon, A., and Jacquemin-Sablon, H. (2005). Regulation of Unr expression by 5'- and 3'-untranslated regions of its mRNA through modulation of stability and IRES mediated translation. *RNA Biol.* 2, e27–e35. doi: 10.4161/rna.2.3.2203

Drapier, J. C., Hirling, H., Wietzerbin, J., Kaldy, P., and Kühn, L. C. (1993). Biosynthesis of nitric oxide activates iron regulatory factor in macrophages. *EMBO J.* 12, 3643–3649.

Duncan, K., Grskovic, M., Strein, C., Beckmann, K., Niggeweg, R., Abaza, I., et al. (2006). Sex-lethal imparts a sex-specific function to UNR by recruiting it to the msl-2 mRNA 3': UTR: translational repression for dosage compensation. *Genes Dev.* 20, 368–379. doi: 10.1101/gad.371406

Duncan, K. E., Strein, C., and Hentze, M. W. (2009). The SXL-UNR corepressor complex uses a PABP-mediated mechanism to inhibit ribosome recruitment to msl-2 mRNA. *Mol. Cell* 36, 571–582. doi: 10.1016/j.molcel.2009.09.042

Dzierzak, E., and Philipsen, S. (2013). Erythropoiesis: development and differentiation. *Cold Spring Harb. Perspect. Med.* 3:a011601. doi: 10.1101/cshperspect.a011601

Emery-Goodman, A., Hirling, H., Scarpellino, L., Henderson, B., and Kühn, L. C. (1993). Iron regulatory factor expressed from recombinant baculovirus: conversion between the RNA-binding apoprotein and Fe-S cluster containing aconitase. *Nucleic Acids Res.* 21, 1457–1461. doi: 10.1093/nar/21.6.1457

Fabian, M. R., Frank, F., Rouya, C., Siddiqui, N., Lai, W. S., Karetnikov, A., et al. (2013). Structural basis for the recruitment of the human CCR4–NOT deadenylase complex by tristetraprolin. *Nat. Struct. Mol. Biol.* 20, 735–739. doi: 10.1038/nsmb.2572

Fang, J., Menon, M., Kapelle, W., Bogacheva, O., Bogachev, O., Houde, E., et al. (2007). EPO modulation of cell-cycle regulatory genes, and cell division, in primary bone marrow erythroblasts. *Blood* 110, 2361–2370. doi: 10.1182/blood-2006-12-063503

Ferraiuolo, M. A., Basak, S., Dostie, J., Murray, E. L., Schoenberg, D. R., and Sonenberg, N. (2005). A role for the eIF4E-binding protein 4E-T in P-body formation and mRNA decay. *J. Cell Biol.* 170, 913–924. doi: 10.1083/jcb.200504039

Ferreira, R., Ohneda, K., Yamamoto, M., and Philipsen, S. (2005). GATA1 function, a paradigm for transcription factors in hematopoiesis. *Mol. Cell. Biol.* 25, 1215–1227. doi: 10.1128/MCB.25.4.1215-1227.2005

Floor, S. N., and Doudna, J. A. (2016). Tunable protein synthesis by transcript isoforms in human cells. *eLife* 5:e10921. doi: 10.7554/eLife.10921

Galloway, A., Saveliev, A., Łukasiak, S., Hodson, D. J., Bolland, D., Balmanno, K., et al. (2016). RNA-binding proteins ZFP36L1 and ZFP36L2 promote cell quiescence. *Science* 352, 453–459. doi: 10.1126/science.aad5978

Gebauer, F., Corona, D. F., Preiss, T., Becker, P. B., and Hentze, M. W. (1999). Translational control of dosage compensation in Drosophila by Sex-lethal: cooperative silencing via the 5' and 3' UTRs of msl-2 mRNA is independent of the poly(A) tail. *EMBO J.* 18, 6146–6154. doi: 10.1093/emboj/18.21.6146

Gerlitz, G., Jagus, R., and Elroy-Stein, O. (2002). Phosphorylation of initiation factor-2 alpha is required for activation of internal translation initiation during cell differentiation. *Eur. J. Biochem.* 269, 2810–2819. doi: 10.1046/j.1432-1033.2002.02974.x

Geuens, T., Bouhy, D., and Timmerman, V. (2016). The hnRNP family: insights into their role in health and disease. *Hum. Genet.* 135, 851–867. doi: 10.1007/s00439-016-1683-5

Gillinder, K. R., Tuckey, H., Bell, C. C., Magor, G. W., Huang, S., Ilsley, M. D., et al. (2017). Direct targets of pSTAT5 signalling in erythropoiesis. *PLoS One* 12:e0180922. doi: 10.1371/journal.pone.0180922

Gingras, A. C., Gygi, S. P., Raught, B., Polakiewicz, R. D., Abraham, R. T., Hoekstra, M. F., et al. (1999). Regulation of 4E-BP1 phosphorylation: a novel two-step mechanism. *Genes Dev.* 13, 1422–1437. doi: 10.1101/gad.13.11.1422

Götz, R., Wiese, S., Takayama, S., Camarero, G. C., Rossoll, W., Schweizer, U., et al. (2005). Bag1 is essential for differentiation and survival of hematopoietic and neuronal cells. *Nat. Neurosci.* 8, 1169–1178. doi: 10.1038/nn1524

Graber, T. E., and Holcik, M. (2007). Cap-independent regulation of gene expression in apoptosis. *Mol. Biosyst.* 3, 825–834. doi: 10.1039/b708867a

Graff, J. R., and Zimmer, S. G. (2003). Translational control and metastatic progression: enhanced activity of the mRNA cap-binding protein eIF-4E selectively enhances translation of metastasis-related mRNAs. *Clin. Exp. Metastasis* 20, 265–273. doi: 10.1023/A:1022943419011

Gray, N. K., and Hentze, M. W. (1994). Iron regulatory protein prevents binding of the 43S translation pre-initiation complex to ferritin and eALAS mRNAs. *EMBO J.* 13, 3882–3891.

Grech, G., Blázquez-Domingo, M., Kolbus, A., Bakker, W. J., Müllner, E. W., Beug, H., et al. (2008). Igbp1 is part of a positive feedback loop in stem cell factor–dependent, selective mRNA translation initiation inhibiting erythroid differentiation. *Blood* 112, 2750–2760. doi: 10.1182/blood-2008-01-133140

Gregory, R. C., Lord, K. A., Panek, L. B., Gaines, P., Dillon, S. B., and Wojchowski, D. M. (2000). Subtraction cloning and initial characterization of novel epo-immediate response genes. *Cytokine* 12, 845–857. doi: 10.1006/cyto.2000.0686

Gregory, T., Yu, C., Ma, A., Orkin, S. H., Blobel, G. A., and Weiss, M. J. (1999). GATA-1 and erythropoietin cooperate to promote erythroid cell survival by regulating bcl-xL expression. *Blood* 94, 87–96.

Grover, R., Candeias, M. M., Fåhraeus, R., and Das, S. (2009). p53 and little brother p53/47: linking IRES activities with protein functions. *Oncogene* 28, 2766–2772. doi: 10.1038/onc.2009.138

Grskovic, M., Hentze, M. W., and Gebauer, F. (2003). A co-repressor assembly nucleated by Sex-lethal in the 3'UTR mediates translational control of Drosophila msl-2 mRNA. *EMBO J.* 22, 5571–5581. doi: 10.1093/emboj/cdg539

Grüllich, C., Duvoisin, R. M., Wiedmann, M., and van Leyen, K. (2001). Inhibition of 15-lipoxygenase leads to delayed organelle degradation in the reticulocyte. *FEBS Lett.* 489, 51–54. doi: 10.1016/S0014-5793(01)02080-4

Guo, B., Phillips, J. D., Yu, Y., and Leibold, E. A. (1995). Iron regulates the intracellular degradation of iron regulatory protein 2 by the proteasome. *J. Biol. Chem.* 270, 21645–21651. doi: 10.1074/jbc.270.37.21645

Guo, B., Yu, Y., and Leibold, E. A. (1994). Iron regulates cytoplasmic levels of a novel iron-responsive element-binding protein without aconitase activity. *J. Biol. Chem.* 269, 24252–24260.

Guzeloglu-Kayisli, O., Pauli, S., Demir, H., Lalioti, M. D., Sakkas, D., and Seli, E. (2008). Identification and characterization of human embryonic poly(A) binding protein (EPAB). *MHR Basic Sci. Reprod. Med.* 14, 581–588. doi: 10.1093/molehr/gan047

Haile, D. J., Rouault, T. A., Tang, C. K., Chin, J., Harford, J. B., and Klausner, R. D. (1992). Reciprocal control of RNA-binding and aconitase activity in the regulation of the iron-responsive element binding protein: role of the iron-sulfur cluster. *Proc. Natl. Acad. Sci. U.S.A.* 89, 7536–7540. doi: 10.1073/pnas.89.16.7536

Han, A.-P., Fleming, M. D., and Chen, J.-J. (2005). Heme-regulated eIF2alpha kinase modifies the phenotypic severity of murine models of erythropoietic protoporphyria and beta-thalassemia. *J. Clin. Invest.* 115, 1562–1570. doi: 10.1172/JCI24141

Hanson, E. S., Rawlins, M. L., and Leibold, E. A. (2003). Oxygen and iron regulation of iron regulatory protein 2. *J. Biol. Chem.* 278, 40337–40342. doi: 10.1074/jbc.M302798200

Harding, H. P., Zhang, Y., Scheuner, D., Chen, J., Kaufman, R. J., and Ron, D. (2009). Ppp1r15 gene knockout reveals an essential role for translation initiation factor 2 alpha (eIF2alpha) dephosphorylation in mammalian development. *Proc. Natl. Acad. Sci. U.S.A.* 106, 1832–1837. doi: 10.1073/pnas.0809632106

Hattangadi, S. M., Wong, P., Zhang, L., Flygare, J., and Lodish, H. F. (2011). From stem cell to red cell: regulation of erythropoiesis at multiple levels by multiple proteins, RNAs, and chromatin modifications. *Blood* 118, 6258–6268. doi: 10.1182/blood-2011-07-356006

Heinicke, L. A., Nabet, B., Shen, S., Jiang, P., van Zalen, S., Cieply, B., et al. (2013). The RNA binding protein RBM38 (RNPC1) regulates splicing during late erythroid differentiation. *PLoS One* 8:e78031. doi: 10.1371/journal.pone.0078031

Hentze, M. W., Caughman, S. W., Rouault, T. A., Barriocanal, J. G., Dancis, A., Harford, J. B., et al. (1987). Identification of the iron-responsive element for the translational regulation of human ferritin mRNA. *Science* 238, 1570–1573. doi: 10.1126/science.3685996

Hinnebusch, A. G. (2014). The scanning mechanism of eukaryotic translation initiation. *Annu. Rev. Biochem.* 83, 779–812. doi: 10.1146/annurev-biochem-060713-035802

Hinnebusch, A. G., and Lorsch, J. R. (2012). The mechanism of eukaryotic translation initiation: new insights and challenges. *Cold Spring Harb. Perspect. Biol.* 4, 1–25. doi: 10.1101/cshperspect.a011544

Hirling, H., Henderson, B. R., and Kühn, L. C. (1994). Mutational analysis of the [4Fe-4S]-cluster converting iron regulatory factor from its RNA-binding form to cytoplasmic aconitase. *EMBO J.* 13, 453–461.

Hope, K. J., and Sauvageau, G. (2011). Roles for MSI2 and PROX1 in hematopoietic stem cell activity. *Curr. Opin. Hematol.* 18, 203–207. doi: 10.1097/MOH.0b013e328347888a

Horos, R., Ijspeert, H., Pospisilova, D., Sendtner, R., Andrieu-Soler, C., Taskesen, E., et al. (2012). Ribosomal deficiencies in Diamond-Blackfan anemia impair translation of transcripts essential for differentiation of murine and human erythroblasts. *Blood* 119, 262–272. doi: 10.1182/blood-2011-06-358200

Hu, W., Yuan, B., and Lodish, H. F. (2014). Cpeb4-mediated translational regulatory circuitry controls terminal erythroid differentiation. *Dev. Cell* 30, 660–672. doi: 10.1016/j.devcel.2014.07.008

Hunt, S. L., Hsuan, J. J., Totty, N., and Jackson, R. J. (1999). unr, a cellular cytoplasmic RNA-binding protein with five cold-shock domains, is required for internal initiation of translation of human rhinovirus RNA. *Genes Dev.* 13, 437–448. doi: 10.1101/gad.13.4.437

Ingolia, N. T. (2014). Ribosome profiling: new views of translation, from single codons to genome scale. *Nat. Rev. Genet.* 15, 205–213. doi: 10.1038/nrg3645

Ingolia, N. T., Lareau, L. F., and Weissman, J. S. (2011). Ribosome profiling of mouse embryonic stem cells reveals the complexity and dynamics of mammalian proteomes. *Cell* 147, 789–802. doi: 10.1016/j.cell.2011.10.002

Iolascon, A., Heimpel, H., Wahlin, A., and Tamary, H. (2013). Congenital dyserythropoietic anemias: molecular insights and diagnostic approach. *Blood* 122, 2162–2166. doi: 10.1182/blood-2013-05-468223

Jacob, H., and Winterhalter, K. (1970). Unstable hemoglobins: the role of heme loss in Heinz body formation. *Proc. Natl. Acad. Sci. U.S.A.* 65, 697–701. doi: 10.1073/pnas.65.3.697

Jacquemin-Sablon, H., Triqueneaux, G., Deschamps, S., le Maire, M., Doniger, J., and Dautry, F. (1994). Nucleic acid binding and intracellular localization of unr, a protein with five cold shock domains. *Nucleic Acids Res.* 22, 2643–2650. doi: 10.1093/nar/22.13.2643

Jee, D., Yang, J.-S., Park, S.-M., Farmer, D. T., Wen, J., Chou, T., et al. (2018). Dual strategies for argonaute2-mediated biogenesis of erythroid miRNAs underlie conserved requirements for slicing in mammals. *Mol. Cell* 69, 265.e–278.e. doi: 10.1016/j.molcel.2017.12.027

Joosten, M., Blázquez-Domingo, M., Lindeboom, F., Boulmé, F., Van Hoven-Beijen, A., Habermann, B., et al. (2004). Translational control of putative protooncogene Nm23-M2 by cytokines via phosphoinositide 3-kinase signaling. *J. Biol. Chem.* 279, 38169–38176. doi: 10.1074/jbc.M401283200

Kahvejian, A., Svitkin, Y. V., Sukarieh, R., M'Boutchou, M.-N., and Sonenberg, N. (2005). Mammalian poly(A)-binding protein is a eukaryotic translation initiation factor, which acts via multiple mechanisms. *Genes Dev.* 19, 104–113. doi: 10.1101/gad.1262905

Kamenska, A., Lu, W.-T., Kubacka, D., Broomhead, H., Minshall, N., Bushell, M., et al. (2014a). Human 4E-T represses translation of bound mRNAs and enhances microRNA-mediated silencing. *Nucleic Acids Res.* 42, 3298–3313. doi: 10.1093/nar/gkt1265

Kamenska, A., Simpson, C., and Standart, N. (2014b). eIF4E-binding proteins: new factors, new locations, new roles. *Biochem. Soc. Trans.* 42, 1238–1245. doi: 10.1042/BST20140063

Kamenska, A., Simpson, C., Vindry, C., Broomhead, H., Bénard, M., Ernoult-Lange, M., et al. (2016). The DDX6-4E-T interaction mediates translational repression and P-body assembly. *Nucleic Acids Res.* 44, 6318–6334. doi: 10.1093/nar/gkw565

Kennedy, M. C., Emptage, M. H., Dreyer, J. L., and Beinert, H. (1983). The role of iron in the activation-inactivation of aconitase. *J. Biol. Chem.* 258, 11098–11105.

Kerenyi, M. A., and Orkin, S. H. (2010). Networking erythropoiesis. *J. Exp. Med.* 207, 2537–2541. doi: 10.1084/jem.20102260

Kerwitz, Y., Kühn, U., Lilie, H., Knoth, A., Scheuermann, T., Friedrich, H., et al. (2003). Stimulation of poly(A) polymerase through a direct interaction with the nuclear poly(A) binding protein allosterically regulated by RNA. *EMBO J.* 22, 3705–3714. doi: 10.1093/emboj/cdg347

Kharas, M. G., Lengner, C. J., Al-Shahrour, F., Bullinger, L., Ball, B., Zaidi, S., et al. (2010). Musashi-2 regulates normal hematopoiesis and promotes aggressive myeloid leukemia. *Nat. Med.* 16, 903–908. doi: 10.1038/nm.2187

Kim, S.-I., and Bresnick, E. H. (2007). Transcriptional control of erythropoiesis: emerging mechanisms and principles. *Oncogene* 26, 6777–6794. doi: 10.1038/sj.onc.1210761

Kini, H. K., Kong, J., and Liebhaber, S. A. (2014). Cytoplasmic poly(A) binding protein C4 serves a critical role in erythroid differentiation. *Mol. Cell. Biol.* 34, 1300–1309. doi: 10.1128/MCB.01683-13

Koeller, D. M., Casey, J. L., Hentze, M. W., Gerhardt, E. M., Chan, L. N., Klausner, R. D., et al. (1989). A cytosolic protein binds to structural elements within the iron regulatory region of the transferrin receptor mRNA. *Proc. Natl. Acad. Sci. U.S.A.* 86, 3574–3578. doi: 10.1073/pnas.86.10.3574

Komar, A. A., and Hatzoglou, M. (2005). Internal ribosome entry sites in cellular mrnas: mystery of their existence. *J. Biol. Chem.* 280, 23425–23428. doi: 10.1074/jbc.R400041200

Komar, A. A., and Hatzoglou, M. (2011). Cellular IRES-mediated translation: the war of ITAFs in pathophysiological states. *Cell Cycle* 10, 229–240. doi: 10.4161/cc.10.2.14472

Komar, A. A., Lesnik, T., Cullin, C., Merrick, W. C., Trachsel, H., and Altmann, M. (2003). Internal initiation drives the synthesis of Ure2 protein lacking the prion domain and affects [URE3] propagation in yeast cells. *EMBO J.* 22, 1199–1209. doi: 10.1093/emboj/cdg103

Kong, J., and Lasko, P. (2012). Translational control in cellular and developmental processes. *Nat. Rev. Genet.* 13, 383–394. doi: 10.1038/nrg3184

Kozak, M. (1986). Influences of mRNA secondary structure on initiation by eukaryotic ribosomes. *Proc. Natl. Acad. Sci. U.S.A.* 83, 2850–2854. doi: 10.1073/pnas.83.9.2850

Kramer, M., Sponholz, C., Slaba, M., Wissuwa, B., Claus, R. A., Menzel, U., et al. (2013). Alternative 5' untranslated regions are involved in expression regulation of human heme oxygenase-1. *PLoS One* 8:e77224. doi: 10.1371/journal.pone.0077224

Kudo, S., Onda, M., and Fukuda, M. (1994). Characterization of glycophorin A transcripts: control by the common erythroid-specific promoter and alternative usage of different polyadenylation signals. *J. Biochem.* 116, 183–192. doi: 10.1093/oxfordjournals.jbchem.a124492

Kühn, L. C., Samuelsson, T., Bottke, W., Laftah, A. H., Takeuchi, K., Halliday, N., et al. (2015). Iron regulatory proteins and their role in controlling iron metabolism. *Metallomics* 7, 232–243. doi: 10.1039/C4MT00164H

Lebedeva, S., Jens, M., Theil, K., Schwanhäusser, B., Selbach, M., Landthaler, M., et al. (2011). Transcriptome-wide analysis of regulatory interactions of the RNA-binding protein HuR. *Mol. Cell* 43, 340–352. doi: 10.1016/j.molcel.2011.06.008

Legnini, I., Di Timoteo, G., Rossi, F., Morlando, M., Briganti, F., Sthandier, O., et al. (2017). Circ-ZNF609 is a circular RNA that can be translated and functions in myogenesis. *Mol. Cell* 66, 22.e–37.e. doi: 10.1016/j.molcel.2017.02.017

Levanon, D., and Groner, Y. (2004). Structure and regulated expression of mammalian RUNX genes. *Oncogene* 23, 4211–4219. doi: 10.1038/sj.onc.1207670

Lewis, S. M., and Holcik, M. (2008). For IRES trans-acting factors, it is all about location. *Oncogene* 27, 1033–1035. doi: 10.1038/sj.onc.1210777

Liu, S., Bhattacharya, S., Han, A., Suragani, R. N. V. S., Zhao, W., Fry, R. C., et al. (2008). Haem-regulated eIF2alpha kinase is necessary for adaptive gene expression in erythroid precursors under the stress of iron deficiency. *Br. J. Haematol.* 143, 129–137. doi: 10.1111/j.1365-2141.2008.07293.x

Liu, X., Zhang, Y., Ni, M., Cao, H., Signer, R. A. J., Li, D., et al. (2017). Regulation of mitochondrial biogenesis in erythropoiesis by mTORC1-mediated protein translation. *Nat. Cell Biol.* 19, 626–638. doi: 10.1038/ncb3527

Lu, P. D., Harding, H. P., and Ron, D. (2004). Translation reinitiation at alternative open reading frames regulates gene expression in an integrated stress response. *J. Cell Biol.* 167, 27–33. doi: 10.1083/jcb.200408003

Ludwig, L. S., Gazda, H. T., Eng, J. C., Eichhorn, S. W., Thiru, P., Ghazvinian, R., et al. (2014). Altered translation of GATA1 in Diamond-Blackfan anemia. *Nat. Med.* 20, 748–753. doi: 10.1038/nm.3557

Masuoka, H. C. (2002). Targeted disruption of the activating transcription factor 4 gene results in severe fetal anemia in mice. *Blood* 99, 736–745. doi: 10.1182/blood.V99.3.736

Mayr, C. (2016). Evolution and Biological Roles of Alternative 3'UTRs. *Trends Cell Biol.* 26, 227–237. doi: 10.1016/j.tcb.2015.10.012

Mazan-Mamczarz, K., Hagner, P. R., Zhang, Y., Dai, B., Lehrmann, E., Becker, K. G., et al. (2011). ATM regulates a DNA damage response posttranscriptional RNA operon in lymphocytes. *Blood* 117, 2441–2450. doi: 10.1182/blood-2010-09-310987

Menon, M. P., Karur, V., Bogacheva, O., Bogachev, O., Cuetara, B., and Wojchowski, D. M. (2006). Signals for stress erythropoiesis are integrated via an erythropoietin receptor-phosphotyrosine-343-Stat5 axis. *J. Clin. Invest.* 116, 683–694. doi: 10.1172/JCI25227

Mills, E. W., Wangen, J., Green, R., and Ingolia, N. T. (2016). Dynamic regulation of a ribosome rescue pathway in erythroid cells and platelets. *Cell Rep.* 17, 1–10. doi: 10.1016/j.celrep.2016.08.088

Minshall, N., Reiter, M. H., Weil, D., and Standart, N. (2007). CPEB interacts with an ovary-specific eIF4E and 4E-T in early *Xenopus* oocytes. *J. Biol. Chem.* 282, 37389–37401. doi: 10.1074/jbc.M704629200

Mitchell, S. A., Brown, E. C., Coldwell, M. J., Jackson, R. J., and Willis, A. E. (2001). Protein factor requirements of the Apaf-1 internal ribosome entry segment: roles of polypyrimidine tract binding protein and upstream of N-ras. *Mol. Cell. Biol.* 21, 3364–3374. doi: 10.1128/MCB.21.10.3364-3374.2001

Mitchell, S. A., Spriggs, K. A., Coldwell, M. J., Jackson, R. J., and Willis, A. E. (2003). The Apaf-1 internal ribosome entry segment attains the correct structural conformation for function via interactions with PTB and unr. *Mol. Cell* 11, 757–771. doi: 10.1016/S1097-2765(03)00093-5

Modelska, A., Turro, E., Russell, R., Beaton, J., Sbarrato, T., Spriggs, K., et al. (2015). The malignant phenotype in breast cancer is driven by eIF4A1-mediated changes in the translational landscape. *Cell Death Dis.* 6, e1603. doi: 10.1038/cddis.2014.542

Moore, K. S., Yagci, N., van Alphen, F., Meijer, A. B., t' Hoen, P. A. C., and von Lindern, M. M. (2017). Csde1 cooperates with Strap to control translation of erythroid transcripts. *bioRxiv.* doi: 10.1101/203539 [Preprint].

Moore, K. S., Yagci, N., van Alphen, F., Paolini, N. A., Horos, R., Held, N. M., et al. (2018). Csde1 binds transcripts involved in protein homeostasis and controls their expression in an erythroid cell line. *Sci. Rep.* 8:2628. doi: 10.1038/s41598-018-20518-7

Mukherjee, N., Corcoran, D. L., Nusbaum, J. D., Reid, D. W., Georgiev, S., Hafner, M., et al. (2011). Integrative regulatory mapping indicates that the RNA-binding protein HuR Couples Pre-mRNA processing and mRNA stability. *Mol. Cell* 43, 327–339. doi: 10.1016/j.molcel.2011.06.007

Müllner, E. W., and Kühn, L. C. (1988). A stem-loop in the 3' untranslated region mediates iron-dependent regulation of transferrin receptor mRNA stability in the cytoplasm. *Cell* 53, 815–825. doi: 10.1016/0092-8674(88)90098-0

Müllner, E. W., Neupert, B., and Kühn, L. C. (1989). A specific mRNA binding factor regulates the iron-dependent stability of cytoplasmic transferrin receptor mRNA. *Cell* 58, 373–382. doi: 10.1016/0092-8674(89)90851-9

Munugalavadla, V., Dore, L. C., Tan, B. L., Hong, L., Vishnu, M., Weiss, M. J., et al. (2005). Repression of c-kit and its downstream substrates by GATA-1 inhibits cell proliferation during erythroid maturation. *Mol. Cell. Biol.* 25, 6747–6759. doi: 10.1128/MCB.25.15.6747-6759.2005

Naarmann, I. S., Harnisch, C., Flach, N., Kremmer, E., Kühn, H., Ostareck, D. H., et al. (2008). mRNA silencing in human erythroid cell maturation: heterogeneous nuclear ribonucleoprotein K controls the expression of its regulator c-Src. *J. Biol. Chem.* 283, 18461–18472. doi: 10.1074/jbc.M710328200

Naarmann-de Vries, I. S., Brendle, A., Bähr-Ivacevic, T., Benes, V., Ostareck, D. H., and Ostareck-Lederer, A. (2016). Translational control mediated by hnRNP K links NMHC IIA to erythroid enucleation. *J. Cell Sci.* 129, 1141–1154. doi: 10.1242/jcs.174995

Nagamachi, A., Htun, P. W., Ma, F., Miyazaki, K., Yamasaki, N., Kanno, M., et al. (2010). A 5' untranslated region containing the IRES element in the Runx1 gene is required for angiogenesis, hematopoiesis and leukemogenesis in a knock-in mouse model. *Dev. Biol.* 345, 226–236. doi: 10.1016/j.ydbio.2010.07.015

Nanahoshi, M., Nishiuma, T., Tsujishita, Y., Hara, K., Inui, S., Sakaguchi, N., et al. (1998). Regulation of protein phosphatase 2A catalytic activity by alpha4 protein and its yeast homolog Tap42. *Biochem. Biophys. Res. Commun.* 251, 520–526. doi: 10.1006/bbrc.1998.9493

Nieradka, A., Ufer, C., Thiadens, K., Grech, G., Horos, R., van Coevorden-Hameete, M., et al. (2014). Grsf1-induced translation of the SNARE protein Use1 is required for expansion of the erythroid compartment. *PLoS One* 9:e104631. doi: 10.1371/journal.pone.0104631

Nishimura, T., Padamsi, Z., Fakim, H., Milette, S., Dunham, W. H., Gingras, A.-C., et al. (2015). The eIF4E-Binding Protein 4E-T Is a Component of the mRNA Decay Machinery that Bridges the 5' and 3', Termini of Target mRNAs. *Cell Rep.* 11, 1425–1436. doi: 10.1016/j.celrep.2015.04.065

Norbury, C. J. (2013). Cytoplasmic RNA: a case of the tail wagging the dog. *Nat. Rev. Mol. Cell Biol.* 14, 643–653. doi: 10.1038/nrm3645

Ogami, K., Hosoda, N., Funakoshi, Y., and Hoshino, S. (2014). Antiproliferative protein Tob directly regulates c-myc proto-oncogene expression through cytoplasmic polyadenylation element-binding protein CPEB. *Oncogene* 33, 55–64. doi: 10.1038/onc.2012.548

Okuda, T., van Deursen, J., Hiebert, S. W., Grosveld, G., and Downing, J. R. (1996). AML1, the target of multiple chromosomal translocations in human leukemia, is essential for normal fetal liver hematopoiesis. *Cell* 84, 321–330. doi: 10.1016/S0092-8674(00)80986-1

Ostareck, D. H., Ostareck-Lederer, A., Shatsky, I. N., and Hentze, M. W. (2001). Lipoxygenase mRNA silencing in erythroid differentiation: The 3'UTR regulatory complex controls 60S ribosomal subunit joining. *Cell* 104, 281–290. doi: 10.1016/S0092-8674(01)00212-4

Owen, D., and Kühn, L. C. (1987). Noncoding 3' sequences of the transferrin receptor gene are required for mRNA regulation by iron. *EMBO J.* 6, 1287–1293.

Pamudurti, N. R., Bartok, O., Jens, M., Ashwal-Fluss, R., Stottmeister, C., Ruhe, L., et al. (2017). Translation of CircRNAs. *Mol. Cell* 66, 9.e–21.e. doi: 10.1016/j.molcel.2017.02.021

Paolini, N. A., MacInnes, A. W., von Lindern, M., Paolini, N. A., MacInnes, A. W., and Lindern, M. (2016). *Diamond-Blackfan Anaemia: From Genotype to Phenotype in eLS.* Chichester: John Wiley & Sons, Ltd, 1–8. doi: 10.1002/9780470015902.a0024471

Paolini, N. A., Moore, K. S., di Summa, F. M., Fokkema, I. F. A. C., 't Hoen, P. A. C., and von Lindern, M. (2018). Ribosome profiling uncovers selective mRNA translation associated with eIF2 phosphorylation in erythroid progenitors. *PLoS One* 13:e0193790. doi: 10.1371/journal.pone.0193790

Patterson, A. D., Hollander, M. C., Miller, G. F., and Fornace, A. J. Jr. (2006). Gadd34 requirement for normal hemoglobin synthesis Gadd34 requirement for normal hemoglobin synthesis. *Mol. Cell. Biol.* 26, 1644–1653. doi: 10.1128/MCB.26.5.1644

Perkins, A., Xu, X., Higgs, D. R., Patrinos, G. P., Arnaud, L., Bieker, J. J., et al. (2016). Krüppeling erythropoiesis: an unexpected broad spectrum of human red blood cell disorders due to *KLF1* variants. *Blood* 127, 1856–1862. doi: 10.1182/blood-2016-01-694331

Petretti, C., Savoian, M., Montembault, E., Glover, D. M., Prigent, C., and Giet, R. (2006). The PITSLRE/CDK11p58 protein kinase promotes centrosome maturation and bipolar spindle formation. *EMBO Rep.* 7, 418–424. doi: 10.1038/sj.embor.7400639

Pickering, B. M., Mitchell, S. A., Spriggs, K. A., Willis, A. E., and Stoneley, M. (2004). Bag-1 Internal Ribosome Entry Segment Activity Is Promoted by Structural Changes Mediated by Poly (rC) Binding Protein 1 and Recruitment of Polypyrimidine Tract Binding Protein 1.. *Mol. Cell. Biol.* 24, 5595–5605. doi: 10.1128/MCB.24.12.5595

Pimentel, H., Parra, M., Gee, S., Ghanem, D., An, X., Li, J., et al. (2014). A dynamic alternative splicing program regulates gene expression during terminal erythropoiesis. *Nucleic Acids Res.* 42, 4031–4042. doi: 10.1093/nar/gkt1388

Pozner, A., Goldenberg, D., Negreanu, V., Le, S. Y., Elroy-Stein, O., Levanon, D., et al. (2000). Transcription-coupled translation control of AML1/RUNX1 is mediated by cap- and internal ribosome entry site-dependent mechanisms. *Mol. Cell. Biol.* 20, 2297–2307. doi: 10.1128/MCB.20.7.2297-2307.2000

Prenzler, F., Fragasso, A., Schmitt, A., and Munz, B. (2016). Functional analysis of ZFP36 proteins in keratinocytes. *Eur. J. Cell Biol.* 95, 277–284. doi: 10.1016/j.ejcb.2016.04.007

Proud, C. G. (2005). eIF2 and the control of cell physiology. *Semin. Cell Dev. Biol.* 16, 3–12. doi: 10.1016/j.semcdb.2004.11.004

Rasmussen, K. D., Simmini, S., Abreu-Goodger, C., Bartonicek, N., Di Giacomo, M., Bilbao-Cortes, D., et al. (2010). The miR-144/451 locus is required for erythroid homeostasis. *J. Exp. Med.* 207, 1351–1358. doi: 10.1084/jem.20100458

Ray, S., and Anderson, E. C. (2016). Stimulation of translation by human Unr requires cold shock domains 2 and 4, and correlates with poly(A) binding protein interaction. *Sci. Rep.* 6:22461. doi: 10.1038/srep22461

Rhoads, R. E. (2009). eIF4E: new family members, new binding partners, new roles. *J. Biol. Chem.* 284, 16711–16715. doi: 10.1074/jbc.R900002200

Ribeil, J.-A., Arlet, J.-B., Dussiot, M., Cruz Moura, I., Courtois, G., and Hermine, O. (2013). Ineffective Erythropoiesis in Beta-Thalassemia. *Sci. World J.* 2013, 1–11. doi: 10.1155/2013/394295

Sakakibara, S., Nakamura, Y., Yoshida, T., Shibata, S., Koike, M., Takano, H., et al. (2002). RNA-binding protein Musashi family: roles for CNS stem cells and a subpopulation of ependymal cells revealed by targeted disruption and antisense ablation. *Proc. Natl. Acad. Sci. U.S.A.* 99, 15194–15199. doi: 10.1073/pnas.232087499

Sandler, H., Kreth, J., Timmers, H. T. M., and Stoecklin, G. (2011). Not1 mediates recruitment of the deadenylase Caf1 to mRNAs targeted for degradation by tristetraprolin. *Nucleic Acids Res.* 39, 4373–4386. doi: 10.1093/nar/gkr011

Schepens, B., Tinton, S. A., Bruynooghe, Y., Parthoens, E., Haegman, M., Beyaert, R., et al. (2007). A role for hnRNP C1/C2 and Unr in internal initiation of translation during mitosis. *EMBO J.* 26, 158–169. doi: 10.1038/sj.emboj.7601468

Schwanhäusser, B., Busse, D., Li, N., Dittmar, G., Schuchhardt, J., Wolf, J., et al. (2011). Global quantification of mammalian gene expression control. *Nature* 473, 337–342. doi: 10.1038/nature10098

Seli, E., Lalioti, M. D., Flaherty, S. M., Sakkas, D., Terzi, N., and Steitz, J. A. (2005). An embryonic poly(A)-binding protein (ePAB) is expressed in mouse oocytes and early preimplantation embryos. *Proc. Natl. Acad. Sci. U.S.A.* 102, 367–372. doi: 10.1073/pnas.0408378102

Shahbazian, D., Parsyan, A., Petroulakis, E., Hershey, J. W. B., and Sonenberg, N. (2010). eIF4B controls survival and proliferation and is regulated by proto-oncogenic signaling pathways. *Cell Cycle* 9, 4106–4109. doi: 10.4161/cc.9.20.13630

Shaw, G., and Kamen, R. (1986). A conserved AU sequence from the 3' untranslated region of GM-CSF mRNA mediates selective mRNA degradation. *Cell* 46, 659–667. doi: 10.1016/0092-8674(86)90341-7

Shirai, Y.-T., Suzuki, T., Morita, M., Takahashi, A., and Yamamoto, T. (2014). Multifunctional roles of the mammalian CCR4-NOT complex in physiological phenomena. *Front. Genet.* 5:286. doi: 10.3389/fgene.2014.00286

Siddiqui, N., and Sonenberg, N. (2015). Signalling to eIF4E in cancer. *Biochem. Soc. Trans.* 43, 763–772. doi: 10.1042/BST20150126

Socolovsky, M., Murrell, M., Liu, Y., Pop, R., Porpiglia, E., and Levchenko, A. (2007). Negative autoregulation by FAS mediates robust fetal erythropoiesis. *PLoS Biol.* 5:e252. doi: 10.1371/journal.pbio.0050252

Sofi, S., Fitzgerald, J. C., Jähn, D., Dumoulin, B., Stehling, S., Kuhn, H., et al. (2018). Functional characterization of naturally occurring genetic variations of the human guanine-rich RNA sequence binding factor 1 (GRSF1). *Biochim. Biophys. Acta* 1862, 866–876. doi: 10.1016/j.bbagen.2017.12.008

Sonenberg, N., and Hinnebusch, A. G. (2009). Regulation of translation initiation in eukaryotes: mechanisms and biological targets. *Cell* 136, 731–745. doi: 10.1016/j.cell.2009.01.042

Song, J., Perreault, J.-P., Topisirovic, I., and Richard, S. (2016). RNA G-quadruplexes and their potential regulatory roles in translation. *Translation* 4:e1244031. doi: 10.1080/21690731.2016.1244031

Sposi, N. M. (2015). "Interaction between Erythropoiesis and Iron Metabolism in Human β-thalassemia - Recent Advances and New Therapeutic Approaches," in *Inherited Hemoglobin Disorders*, ed. A. Munshi (Rijeka: InTech), doi: 10.5772/61716

Spriggs, K. A., Stoneley, M., Bushell, M., and Willis, A. E. (2008). Re-programming of translation following cell stress allows IRES-mediated translation to predominate. *Biol. Cell* 100, 27–38. doi: 10.1042/BC20070098

Sui, X., Krantz, S. B., and Zhao, Z. J. (2000). Stem cell factor and erythropoietin inhibit apoptosis of human erythroid progenitor cells through different signalling pathways. *Br. J. Haematol.* 110, 63–70. doi: 10.1046/j.1365-2141.2000.02145.x

Sun, Y., Fu, Y., Li, Y., and Xu, A. (2012). Genome-wide alternative polyadenylation in animals: insights from high-throughput technologies. *J. Mol. Cell Biol.* 4, 352–361. doi: 10.1093/jmcb/mjs041

Suragani, R. N. V. S., Zachariah, R. S., Velazquez, J. G., Liu, S., Sun, C.-W., Townes, T. M., et al. (2012). Heme-regulated eIF2α kinase activated Atf4 signaling pathway in oxidative stress and erythropoiesis. *Blood* 119, 5276–5284. doi: 10.1182/blood-2011-10-388132

Tan, J. S., Mohandas, N., and Conboy, J. G. (2006). High frequency of alternative first exons in erythroid genes suggests a critical role in regulating gene function. *Blood* 107, 2557–2561. doi: 10.1182/blood-2005-07-2957

Tinton, S. A., Schepens, B., Bruynooghe, Y., Beyaert, R., and Cornelis, S. (2005). Regulation of the cell-cycle-dependent internal ribosome entry site of the PITSLRE protein kinase: roles of Unr (upstream of N-ras) protein and phosphorylated translation initiation factor eIF-2alpha. *Biochem. J.* 385, 155–163. doi: 10.1042/BJ20040963

Topalian, S. L., Kaneko, S., Gonzales, M. I., Bond, G. L., Ward, Y., and Manley, J. L. (2001). Identification and functional characterization of neo-poly(A) polymerase, an RNA processing enzyme overexpressed in human tumors. *Mol. Cell. Biol.* 21, 5614–5623. doi: 10.1128/MCB.21.16.5614-5623.2001

Triqueneaux, G., Velten, M., Franzon, P., Dautry, F., and Jacquemin-Sablon, H. (1999). RNA binding specificity of Unr, a protein with five cold shock domains. *Nucleic Acids Res.* 27, 1926–1934. doi: 10.1093/nar/27.8.1926

Ufer, C. (2012). The biology of the RNA binding protein guanine-rich sequence binding factor 1. *Curr. Protein Pept. Sci.* 13, 347–357. doi: 10.2174/138920312801619457

Ufer, C., Wang, C. C., Fähling, M., Schiebel, H., Thiele, B. J., Billett, E. E., et al. (2008). Translational regulation of glutathione peroxidase 4 expression through guanine-rich sequence-binding factor 1 is essential for embryonic brain development. *Genes Dev.* 22, 1838–1850. doi: 10.1101/gad.466308

Ulirsch, J. C., Nandakumar, S. K., Wang, L., Giani, F. C., Zhang, X., Rogov, P., et al. (2016). Systematic functional dissection of common genetic variation affecting red blood cell traits. *Cell* 165, 1530–1545. doi: 10.1016/j.cell.2016.04.048

Van Damme, P., Gawron, D., Van Criekinge, W., and Menschaert, G. (2014). N-terminal proteomics and ribosome profiling provide a comprehensive view of the alternative translation initiation landscape in mice and men. *Mol. Cell. Proteomics* 13, 1245–1261. doi: 10.1074/mcp.M113.036442

van der Harst, P., Zhang, W., Mateo Leach, I., Rendon, A., Verweij, N., Sehmi, J., et al. (2012). Seventy-five genetic loci influencing the human red blood cell. *Nature* 492, 369–375. doi: 10.1038/nature11677

van Dijk, T. B., van Den Akker, E., Amelsvoort, M. P., Mano, H., Löwenberg, B., and von Lindern, M. (2000). Stem cell factor induces phosphatidylinositol 3'-kinase-dependent Lyn/Tec/Dok-1 complex formation in hematopoietic cells. *Blood* 96, 3406–3413.

Vattem, K. M., and Wek, R. C. (2004). Reinitiation involving upstream ORFs regulates ATF4 mRNA translation in mammalian cells. *Proc. Natl. Aead. Sci. U.S.A.* 101, 11269–11274. doi: 10.1073/pnas.0400541101

Vignudelli, T., Selmi, T., Martello, A., Parenti, S., Grande, A., Gemelli, C., et al. (2010). ZFP36L1 negatively regulates erythroid differentiation of CD34 + hematopoietic stem cells by interfering with the Stat5b pathway. *Mol. Biol. Cell* 21, 3340–3351. doi: 10.1091/mbc.E10-01-0040

Vlachos, A., Blanc, L., and Lipton, J. M. (2014). Diamond Blackfan anemia: a model for the translational approach to understanding human disease. *Expert Rev. Hematol.* 7, 359–372. doi: 10.1586/17474086.2014.897923

von Hacht, A., Seifert, O., Menger, M., Schütze, T., Arora, A., Konthur, Z., et al. (2014). Identification and characterization of RNA guanine-quadruplex binding proteins. *Nucleic Acids Res.* 42, 6630–6644. doi: 10.1093/nar/gku290

Wakiyama, M., Imataka, H., Sonenberg, N., Fukunaga, R., Hunter, T., and Sonenberg, N. (2000). Interaction of eIF4G with poly(A)-binding protein stimulates translation and is critical for Xenopus oocyte maturation. *Curr. Biol.* 10, 1147–1150. doi: 10.1016/S0960-9822(00)00701-6

Wek, R. C., Jiang, H.-Y., and Anthony, T. G. (2006). Coping with stress: eIF2 kinases and translational control. *Biochem. Soc. Trans.* 34, 7–11. doi: 10.1042/BST20060007

Wessely, O., Bauer, A., Quang, C. T., Deiner, E. M., von Lindern, M., Mellitzer, G., et al. (1999). A novel way to induce erythroid progenitor self renewal: cooperation of c-Kit with the erythropoietin receptor. *Biol. Chem.* 380, 187–202. doi: 10.1515/BC.1999.027

Witthuhn, B. A., Quelle, F. W., Silvennoinen, O., Yi, T., Tang, B., Miura, O., et al. (1993). JAK2 associates with the erythropoietin receptor and is tyrosine phosphorylated and activated following stimulation with erythropoietin. *Cell* 74, 227–236. doi: 10.1016/0092-8674(93)90414-L

Wolfe, A. L., Singh, K., Zhong, Y., Drewe, P., Rajasekhar, V. K., Sanghvi, V. R., et al. (2014). RNA G-quadruplexes cause eIF4A-dependent oncogene translation in cancer. *Nature* 513, 65–70. doi: 10.1038/nature13485

Young, S. K., Willy, J. A., Wu, C., Sachs, M. S., and Wek, R. C. (2015). Ribosome reinitiation directs gene-specific translation and regulates the integrated stress response. *J. Biol. Chem.* 290, 28257–28271. doi: 10.1074/jbc.M115.693184

Zhang, J., Xu, E., Ren, C., Yan, W., Zhang, M., Chen, M., et al. (2014). Mice deficient in Rbm38, a target of the p53 family, are susceptible to accelerated aging and spontaneous tumors. *Proc. Natl. Acad. Sci. U.S.A.* 111, 18637–18642. doi: 10.1073/pnas.1415607112

Zhang, L., Prak, L., Rayon-Estrada, V., Thiru, P., Flygare, J., Lim, B., et al. (2013). ZFP36L2 is required for self-renewal of early burst-forming unit erythroid progenitors. *Nature* 499, 92–96. doi: 10.1038/nature12215

Zhang, S., Macias-Garcia, A., Velazquez, J., Paltrinieri, E., Kaufman, R. J., and Chen, J.-J. (2018). HRI coordinates translation by eIF2αP and mTORC1 to mitigate ineffective erythropoiesis in mice during iron deficiency. *Blood* 131, 450–461. doi: 10.1182/blood-2017-08-799908

Zuker, M. (2003). Mfold web server for nucleic acid folding and hybridization prediction. *Nucleic Acids Res.* 31, 3406–3415. doi: 10.1093/nar/gkg595

11

Red Blood Cell Homeostasis: Mechanisms and Effects of Microvesicle Generation in Health and Disease

*Joames K. F. Leal, Merel J. W. Adjobo-Hermans and Giel J. C. G. M. Bosman**

Department of Biochemistry, Radboud University Medical Center, Nijmegen, Netherlands

Correspondence:
Giel J. C. G. M. Bosman
Giel.Bosman@radboudumc.nl

Red blood cells (RBCs) generate microvesicles to remove damaged cell constituents such as oxidized hemoglobin and damaged membrane constituents, and thereby prolong their lifespan. Damage to hemoglobin, in combination with altered phosphorylation of membrane proteins such as band 3, lead to a weakening of the binding between the lipid bilayer and the cytoskeleton, and thereby to membrane budding and microparticle shedding. Microvesicle generation is disturbed in patients with RBC-centered diseases, such as sickle cell disease, glucose 6-phosphate dehydrogenase deficiency, spherocytosis or malaria. A disturbance of the membrane-cytoskeleton interaction is likely to be the main underlying mechanism, as is supported by data obtained from RBCs stored in blood bank conditions. A detailed proteomic, lipidomic and immunogenic comparison of microvesicles derived from different sources is essential in the identification of the processes that trigger vesicle generation. The contribution of RBC-derived microvesicles to inflammation, thrombosis and autoimmune reactions emphasizes the need for a better understanding of the mechanisms and consequences of microvesicle generation.

Keywords: red blood cell, microvesicles, membrane, aging, inflammation, autoimmunity, hemoglobin, oxidation

INTRODUCTION

Generation of microvesicles, i.e., extracellular vesicles that are shed from the plasma membrane (Raposo and Stoorvogel, 2013), constitutes an integral part of red blood cell (RBC) homeostasis, and is responsible for the loss of 20% of the hemoglobin and the cell membrane during physiological RBC aging *in vivo*, and the accompanying decrease in cell volume and increase in cell density (Willekens et al., 2003, 2008). The blood of healthy subjects contains approximately 1000 RBC-derived vesicles per microliter of plasma (Berckmans et al., 2001; Hron et al., 2007; Westerman et al., 2008; Willekens et al., 2008). The microvesicle hemoglobin composition suggests an enrichment of the irreversibly modified hemoglobins HbA1c and HbA1e2. Microvesicles contain various immunological recognition and removal signals (Willekens et al., 2008), that are responsible for a rapid elimination – probably within minutes – from the circulation (Willekens et al., 2005, 2008). Shedding of damaged cellular components by vesiculation prevents untimely removal of otherwise functional RBCs, as well as unwanted reactions of the hemostasis and immune systems. Thus, vesiculation couples general aging processes such as oxidation and glycation to organismal homeostasis. On the other hand, RBC-centered hemoglobinopathies such as sickle cell disease and thalassemia are accompanied by a substantial increase in microvesicle levels (Ferru et al., 2014; Camus et al., 2015). Also, infection of RBC with the malaria parasite *Plasmodium* induces vesicle formation. However, the underlying mechanism is likely to be strongly influenced by parasite-derived proteins, and therefore beyond the scope of this review (e.g., Mantel et al., 2013). Increased vesiculation is associated with systemic inflammation, which may be directly responsible for hemolysis and anemia (Dinkla et al., 2012b, 2016). Thus, microvesicles are part of the complex of interactions between RBCs and the organism (Bosman, 2016a,b). In this review, we aim to integrate the newest data on microvesicle composition and production in various conditions, in order to obtain more insight into the basic mechanisms underlying microvesicle generation, and the involvement of RBC-derived microvesicles in pathophysiology.

MICROVESICLES *IN VIVO*

Immunochemical analyses together with a proteomic inventory of RBC-derived microvesicles from the plasma of healthy individuals show the almost exclusive presence of the membrane proteins band 3 and actin (Bosman et al., 2012). Microvesicles are enriched in enzymes involved in redox homeostasis, i.e., glutathione S-transferase, thioredoxin and peroxiredoxin-1 and peroxiredoxin-2, and in ubiquitin. The hemoglobin composition of microvesicles isolated from plasma resembles that of the oldest cells, with an enrichment in irreversibly modified hemoglobins HbA1c and HbA1e2 (Willekens et al., 1997). Microvesicles display removal signals such as phosphatidylserine in the outer membrane layer and senescent cell-specific band 3 epitopes that are mainly found in the oldest RBCs (Willekens et al., 2008). Also, microvesicles contain the glycosylphosphatidylinositol (GPI)-anchored, complement-inhibiting proteins CD55 and CD59. These may not be in a functional configuration, as recently shown for the, similarly GPI-anchored enzyme acetylcholinesterase (Willekens et al., 2008; Freitas Leal et al., 2017). The striking absence of spectrin and ankyrin in microvesicles, together with immunoblot and proteomic patterns indicating extensive protein degradation in the oldest RBCs, as well as the aging-related increase in membrane-associated proteasome components (Bosman et al., 2012), all support a role for proteolytic breakdown of the band 3-ankyrin connection between the cytoskeleton and the lipid bilayer in the vesiculation process. However, the absence of especially spectrin in microvesicles isolated from the blood has led to alternative explanations for the aging-associated changes in RBC cell volume and density (Ciana et al., 2017a,b). The breakage of the band 3-ankyrin binding is predicted to cause a relaxation of the cytoskeletal spring and thereby spontaneous buckling of the lipid bilayer, resulting in evagination and vesiculation (Sens and Gov, 2007; Bosman et al., 2012) (**Figure 1**). Proteomic analysis of aging RBCs and RBC-derived microvesicles purified from the plasma support this model (Bosman et al., 2012), but do not provide many clues for the upstream processes, or for the relatively high concentration of actin in the microvesicles. The hemoglobin data, together with the accumulation of redox status-regulating enzymes, indicate that damage to hemoglobin may be such an upstream process, if not the primary trigger for vesiculation. A role for damaged hemoglobin in vesiculation is supported by the finding that the concentration of RBC-derived microvesicles is increased in the blood of patients with hemoglobinopathies (Westerman et al., 2008). The microvesicles from the blood of thalassemia patients contain high concentrations of oxidized, denatured alpha globin chains (Ferru et al., 2014). Also, these microvesicles contain enzymes involved in the maintenance of redox status such as catalase and peroxiredoxin-2, as well as large amounts of complement proteins and immunoglobulins (Ferru et al., 2014).

The protein composition of microvesicles from patients with membranopathies, i.e., abnormal RBCs such as elliptocytes and stomatocytes due to genetic aberrations in membrane proteins, is likely to differ from those of control RBCs. Actual data are lacking, but this prediction can be deduced from the effects of splenectomy on the membrane protein composition of spectrin/ankyrin-deficient and band 3-deficient spherocytes (Reliene et al., 2002; Alaarg et al., 2013). In RBCs from patients with thalassemia intermedia, hemoglobin damage may induce the formation of band 3 polymers, associated with increased phosphorylation that leads to a weakening of the band 3-ankyrin connection, resulting in microvesicle formation (Ferru et al., 2014). These observations, together with the vesiculation-reducing effect of p72Syk kinase inhibitors, not only support a central role for the binding of modified hemoglobin, possibly especially to oxidized and/or proteolytically degraded band 3 (Arashiki et al., 2013; Lange et al., 2014) in the vesiculation process (**Figure 1**), but also show the involvement of phosphorylation networks in RBC homeostasis. The involvement of various signaling pathways in RBC vesiculation was supported by the relative large numbers of signaling proteins in microvesicles obtained from the plasma of a healthy donor (Bosman et al., 2012), and in a pharmacological screening *in vitro* (Kostova et al., 2015).

THE INVOLVEMENT OF MICROVESICLES IN COAGULATION AND INFLAMMATION

Most RBC-derived microvesicles from healthy donors as well as from various patients expose phosphatidylserine, which promotes not only phagocytosis but also coagulation.

In vitro, thrombin generation through the intrinsic pathway has been shown to be induced by RBC-derived microvesicles derived from sickle cell patients, storage units, or after treatment with a calcium ionophore (van Beers et al., 2009; van der Meijden et al., 2012; Rubin et al., 2013). In addition, correlations have been reported between the number of phosphatidylserine-exposing, RBC-derived microvesicles, and thrombin generation in sickle cell patients (van Beers et al., 2009; Gerotziafas et al., 2012). Microvesicles may also disturb anticoagulation reactions of the protein C system, possibly through binding of protein S (e.g.,

Koshiar et al., 2014). Increases in RBC-derived microvesicles in sickle cell disease and thalassemia patients is often accompanied by a decrease in deformability and hemolysis, which may as such constitute a risk factor for thrombosis.

Phagocytosis-triggered monocyte activation may induce proinflammatory and procoagulant endothelial cell responses (Straat et al., 2016). Thrombin may promote inflammation by activation of the complement system, e.g., by acting as C3 or C5 convertase (Zecher et al., 2014). RBCs of patients with paroxysmal nocturnal hemoglobinuria (PNH) lack the GPI-anchored proteins CD55 and CD59 that protect against complement activation-associated hemolysis. GPI-anchored proteins may be involved in raft formation (Salzer and Prohaska, 2001), and their absence may be directly responsible for the release of relatively high numbers of RBC-derived microvesicles with procoagulant activity in PNH patients *in vitro* (Hugel et al., 1999; Kozuma et al., 2011; Devalet et al., 2014). In addition, microvesicles scavenge NO almost as fast as free hemoglobin and much faster than RBCs, which may impair vasodilation (Donadee et al., 2011). This effect is already detectable with the number of microvesicles present in one transfusion unit (Liu et al., 2013).

THE ROLE OF THE SPLEEN

The spleen facilitates vesiculation, as apparent from the retention of microvesicles in RBCs in asplenic individuals. In these individuals, the normal aging-related decrease in total RBC hemoglobin is absent, due to an increase in HbA1c (Willekens et al., 2003). In patients with spherocytosis, splenectomy increased RBC deformability *in vitro*, probably by inhibiting spleen-mediated microvesicle shedding (Reliene et al., 2002). The molecular mechanism underlying vesiculation in the spleen is unknown, but may involve a combination of biochemical and biophysical stress. Recent model simulations support the involvement of degraded hemoglobin in reducing the cytoskeleton/membrane connection, thereby promoting microvesicle shedding during splenic flow (Zhu et al., 2017). Thus, the mechanical and biochemical circumstances in the spleen, together with the presence of specialized macrophages, may make the spleen a microvesicle-based quality control and repair system. This emphasizes the importance of establishing the functionality of the spleen, especially in the study of diabetic control (Willekens et al., 2003). Also, the notable paucity of data for microvesicles generated *in vivo* warrants a more detailed investigation on the fundamental and clinical relationship between splenectomy or functional asplenia, RBC-derived microvesicles and RBC homeostasis (Wernick et al., 2017).

MICROVESICLES *IN VITRO*

Vesiculation also occurs during storage of RBCs in the blood bank. Storage microvesicles contain removal signals such as phosphatidylserine in the outer layer of their membrane and degraded as well as aggregated band 3 molecules, similar to microvesicles in the circulation (Bosman et al., 2008; Willekens et al., 2008). In blood bank microvesicles, the number of carbonyl groups is increased relative to RBC membranes, possibly due to the accumulation of oxidized membrane proteins band 3, actin and protein 4.1 (Bosman et al., 2008; Kriebardis et al., 2008; Delobel et al., 2016). This is accompanied by a correlation between oxidized cell constituents and vesiculation during storage (D'Alessandro et al., 2017). Blood bank microvesicles are immunologically active, as they contain immunoglobulins and complement factors, derived from the plasma fraction of the storage fluid (Bosman et al., 2008; Kriebardis et al., 2008). Also, storage microvesicles are readily recognized by pathological autoantibodies from patients with autoimmune hemolytic anemia (Dinkla et al., 2012a). These data indicate that the coupling of removal of damaged components from the RBC to their removal from the circulation is a general phenomenon for RBC-derived microvesicles. The enrichment of the GPI-anchored proteins acetylcholinesterase and CD55, as well as raft-associated forms of stomatin and the flotillins in storage microvesicles, indicates that lipid-related changes in membrane organization are involved in vesiculation during storage (Bosman et al., 2008; Salzer et al., 2008). The underlying mechanism has been proposed to be revolving around membrane budding and fission. This could be triggered by the loss of binding between cytoskeletal and membrane proteins, followed by large-scale separation of various lipid phases that may be formed by membrane protein-stabilized microdomains (Salzer et al., 2008). The loss of interaction between the cytoskeleton and cell membrane may be triggered by oxidized hemoglobin, similar to what may happen *in vivo*. Indeed, accumulation of oxidized hemoglobin residues during storage is accompanied by their enrichment in microvesicles (Wither et al., 2016). This role of hemoglobin in microvesicle formation is supported by the observation that, in the early phase of storage, a significant amount of hemoglobin is associated with the lipid bilayer in microvesicles (Szigyártó et al., 2018). There is a shortage of detailed quantitative and qualitative information on the primary triggers driving microvesicle production *in vitro*. The available data, albeit mostly showing associations, support a role of phosphorylation and rearrangement of band 3. For example, inhibition of tyrosine dephosphorylation not only induces RBC shapes such as echinocytes, which indicates a loss of interaction between the cytoskeleton and the lipid bilayer but also stimulates microvesicle production *in vitro* (Ferru et al., 2011, 2014; Cluitmans et al., 2016). In the misshapen cells found in patients with neuroacanthocytosis, disturbed phosphorylation and altered cell morphology are accompanied by disturbed microvesicle generation (Bosman and De Franceschi, 2008). Phosphorylation of band 3 is associated with clustering and correlates with microvesicle formation during storage and in the RBCs of patients with thalassemia intermedia (Ferru et al., 2014; Azouzi et al., 2018). Similar effects are observed upon treatment of RBCs with agents that induce aggregation of band 3 (Ferru et al., 2011; Cluitmans et al., 2016). A well-known stimulus for microvesicle formation *in vitro* is an artificial increase in intracellular calcium concentration. However, the protein composition of calcium-induced microvesicles differs

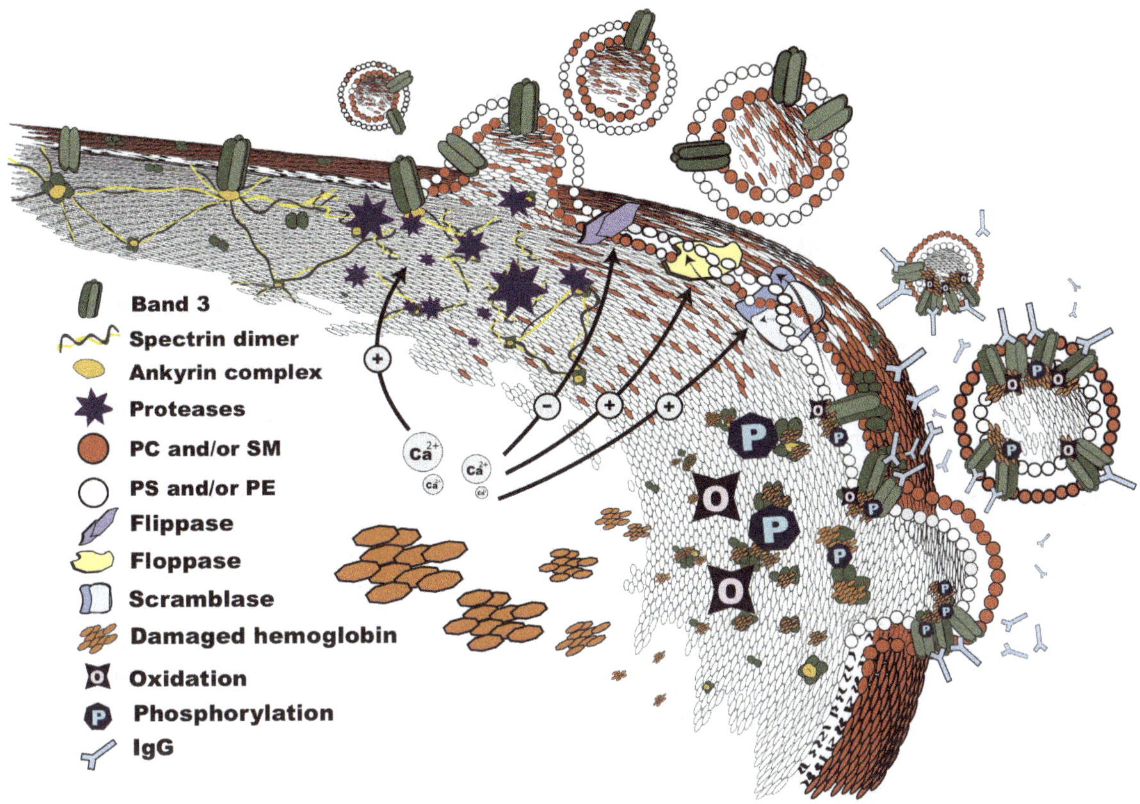

FIGURE 1 | Vesiculation in progress. Structure of the RBC membrane during vesiculation, showing mechanisms involved in microvesicle shedding: breakdown of the cytoskeleton by calcium-dependent proteases; lipid bilayer rearrangement due to altered phospholipid transporter activities, which results in phosphatidylserine exposure; changes in band 3 configuration and distribution due to oxidation, binding of damaged hemoglobin, and phosphorylation, leading to loss of binding to the cytoskeleton at the ankyrin complex, recognition by IgG, and vesiculation. The order and interdependence of these processes are discussed in the text. PC, phosphatidylcholine; SM, sphingomyelin; PS, phosphatidylserine; PE, phosphatidylethanolamine.

from storage or blood microvesicles, e.g., the content of membrane proteins, the presence of band 3 aggregates and breakdown products, and of raft-associated proteins (Bosman et al., 2008; Salzer et al., 2008; Prudent et al., 2015). This indicates that alterations in intracellular calcium concentrations are not primary factors in microvesicle generation *in vivo*, nor in the blood bank.

MECHANISMS OF VESICULATION: INVOLVEMENT OF LIPIDS

The few data that are available indicate that disturbances of the organization of the lipid part of the cell membrane may play a role in the vesiculation process. The RBC membrane contains sphingomyelin/cholesterol-enriched as well as cholesterol-enriched domains that are associated with high-curvature areas. Since these domains become associated with budding membrane areas during storage at 4°C, they have been speculated to be specific sites of microvesicle generation (Leonard et al., 2017). However, RBCs and microvesicles obtained during storage in blood bank conditions showed no significant differences in the main phospholipid classes (Laurén et al., 2018). This included the lack of enrichment of the raft-associated lipids cholesterol and sphingomyelin. Thus, lipid-involving reorganizations in the RBC membrane may be instrumental in microvesicle generation, but they do not seem to result in significant alterations in microvesicle lipid composition. Changes in membrane lipid organization, such as an increase in exposure of phosphatidylserine and/or phosphatidylethanolamine, may promote vesiculation during storage (Verhoeven et al., 2006; Larson et al., 2017). However, severe disruptions of the protein-protein interactions, that are associated with altered RBC morphology, may induce increased microvesicle generation, but are not always accompanied by increased phosphatidylserine exposure (Cluitmans et al., 2016) (**Figure 1**). In this context, it should be emphasized that not all RBC-derived microvesicles expose detectable amounts of phosphatidylserine (Willekens et al., 2008; Nielsen et al., 2014). Disruption of the lipid bilayer, e.g., by treating RBCs with sphingomyelinase, strongly catalysed microvesicle generation *in vitro*. This process was accompanied by the appearance of CD59 and stomatin clusters in the RBCs, supporting a role for lipid rearrangement in microvesicle formation. The sphingomyelinase-induced microvesicles were much more heterogeneous in phosphatidylserine exposure and glycophorin

A content than the microvesicles generated by spontaneous vesiculation, indicating the involvement of different mechanisms (Dinkla et al., 2012b). Thus, changes in lipid organization may facilitate microvesicle formation, but may not constitute the primary mechanism in most physiological conditions.

MECHANISMS OF VESICULATION: COMPARISON WITH EXOSOME FORMATION

All reports on RBC-derived microvesicle composition, especially in combination with the aging-associated changes in the RBC membrane proteome, indicate the involvement of proteins that are involved in the release of exosomes as well (Raposo and Stoorvogel, 2013). This includes small GTPases, lipid raft-associated proteins such as acetylcholinesterase and flotillins, and annexins (Bosman et al., 2012; Raposo and Stoorvogel, 2013; Prudent et al., 2015). Although it is not clear how cytosolic components end up in exosomes, the mechanisms by which cytosolic molecules are recruited into RBC-derived microvesicles may be similar to those involved in exosome generation, as indicated by the presence of various chaperone proteins (Bosman et al., 2012; Raposo and Stoorvogel, 2013). The molecular details of the mechanisms underlying microvesicle generation in other cell types are largely unknown. Incorporation of the available data on RBC-derived microvesicles into the catalog 'Vesiclepedia' (Kalra et al., 2012) may be a worthwhile first step toward further elucidation of the mechanism of microvesicle in RBCs, as well as in other cell types. A comparison of RBC microvesicle data with the already available data on RBC exosomes that are shed by reticulocytes from human cord blood (Chu et al., 2018) will facilitate the identification of the molecular mechanisms involved in various types of vesiculation *in vivo*. Already, endocytosis and autophagy have been involved in the disappearance of CD71 and other membrane proteins during reticulocyte maturation *in vitro* (Griffiths et al., 2012). Such an approach profits from the possibility that RBCs create to study exosome as well as microvesicle formation during differentiation and aging in the same cell, that has a relatively homogeneous and well-charted membrane system.

FROM MECHANISM TO MARKER TO MEDICINE

Red blood cells form microvesicles in response to a variety of physiological and pathological triggers. Although the inventory of the composition of microvesicles generated in different circumstances is far from complete, the available data indicate that they all are enriched in damaged RBC components, depending on the various stimuli (**Figure 1**). This suggests that an exhaustive study of RBC-derived microvesicles will offer insights into the molecular mechanisms of their generation *in vivo*, and thereby into the physiological and pathological triggers. Also, RBC-derived microvesicles may constitute a model for the study of the biological, biophysical and clinical properties of microvesicles in general. This model will benefit from the comparison of the composition and characteristics of RBC-derived microvesicles with microvesicles generated by other cell types, and with exosomes. RBC-derived microvesicles are potentially sensitive and specific biomarkers for the clinical severity of RBC-centered diseases such as sickle cell disease, thalassemia or spherocytosis (Reliene et al., 2002; Hebbel and Key, 2016; Kittivorapart et al., 2018). Also, microvesicles may reveal the activity as well as the clinical consequences, such as anemia or thrombosis, of systemic processes, such as inflammation. In addition, RBC-derived microvesicles may be useful in the transfer of surface proteins, as has been shown in the 'painting' of RBCs of PNH patients with the complement-protecting proteins CD55 and CD59 (Sloand et al., 2004).

Where RBC-derived microvesicles may be actively involved in pathology, e.g., by their procoagulant, proinflammatory or autoimmune activity (Sadallah et al., 2008), pharmacological prevention of the formation of harmful microvesicles may become of clinical importance. The recent finding that inhibition of sphingomyelinase attenuated lung inflammation caused by infusion of stored RBC-derived microvesicles (Hoehn et al., 2017), supports this notion. Thus, on one hand, microvesicle shedding may prevent the untimely removal of functional RBCs in physiological conditions. On the other hand, in pathological conditions, prevention of vesiculation following splenectomy may have beneficial effects, or prevent a pathological immune reaction, for example after massive or frequent RBC transfusion in compromised, transfusion-dependent patients.

AUTHOR CONTRIBUTIONS

GB conceived the topic and wrote the final version. GB, JL, and MA-H wrote parts of the manuscript.

REFERENCES

Alaarg, A., Schiffelers, R. M., Van Solinge, W. W., and Van Wijk, R. (2013). Red blood cell vesiculation in hereditary hemolytic anemia. *Front. Physiol.* 4:365. doi: 10.3389/fphys.2013.00365

Arashiki, N., Kimata, N., Manno, S., Mohandas, N., and Takakuwa, Y. (2013). Membrane peroxidation and methemoglobin formation are both necessary for band 3 clustering: mechanistic insights into human erythrocyte senescence. *Biochemistry* 52, 5760–5769. doi: 10.1021/bi400405p

Azouzi, S., Romana, M., Arashiki, N., Takakuwa, Y., El Nemer, W., Peyrard, T., et al. (2018). Band 3 phosphorylation induces irreversible alterations of stored red blood cells. *Am. J. Hematol.* 93, E110–E112. doi: 10.1002/ajh.25044

Berckmans, R. J., Nieuwland, R., Boing, A. N., Romijn, F. P., Hack, C. E., and Sturk, A. (2001). Cell-derived microparticles circulate in healthy humans and support low grade thrombin generation. *Thromb. Haemost.* 85, 639–646. doi: 10.1055/s-0037-1615646

Bosman, G. (2016a). The proteome of the red blood cell: an auspicious source of new insights into membrane-centered regulation of homeostasis. *Proteomes* 4:35. doi: 10.3390/proteomes4040035

Bosman, G. J. (2016b). The involvement of erythrocyte metabolism in organismal homeostasis in health and disease. *Proteom. Clin. Appl.* 10, 774–777. doi: 10.1002/prca.201500129

Bosman, G. J., Lasonder, E., Groenen-Döpp, Y. A., Willekens, F. L., and Werre, J. M. (2012). The proteome of erythrocyte-derived microparticles from plasma: new clues for erythrocyte aging and vesiculation. *J. Proteomics.* 76, 203–210. doi: 10.1016/j.jprot.2012.05.031

Bosman, G. J., Lasonder, E., Luten, M., Roerdinkholder-Stoelwinder, B., Novotný, V. M., Bos, H., et al. (2008). The proteome of red cell membranes and vesicles during storage in blood bank conditions. *Transfusion.* 48, 827–835. doi: 10.1111/j.1537-2995.2007.01630.x

Bosman, G. J. C. G. M., and De Franceschi, L. (2008). "Neuroacanthocytosis-related changes in erythrocyte membrane organization and function," in *Neuroacanthocytosis Syndromes II*, ed. R. H. Walker et al. (Berlin: Springer-Verlag), 133–142. doi: 10.1007/978-3-540-71693-8_10

Camus, S. M., De Moraes, J. A., Bonnin, P., Abbyad, P., Le Jeune, S., Lionnet, F., et al. (2015). Circulating cell membrane microparticles transfer heme to endothelial cells and trigger vasoocclusions in sickle cell disease. *Blood* 125, 3805–3814. doi: 10.1182/blood-2014-07-589283

Chu, T. T. T., Sinha, A., Malleret, B., Suwanarusk, R., Park, J. E., Naidu, R. et al. (2018). Quantitative mass spectrometry of human reticulocytes reveal proteome-wide modifications during maturation. *Br. J. Haematol.* 180, 118–133. doi: 10.1111/bjh.14976

Ciana, A., Achilli, C., Gaur, A., and Minetti, G. (2017a). Membrane remodelling and vesicle formation during ageing of human red blood cells. *Cell. Physiol. Biochem.* 42, 1127–1138. doi: 10.1159/000478768

Ciana, A., Achilli, C., and Minetti, G. (2017b). Spectrin and other membrane-skeletal components in human red blood cells of different age. *Cell. Physiol. Biochem.* 42, 1139–1152. doi: 10.1159/000478769

Cluitmans, J. C., Gevi, F., Siciliano, A., Matte, A., Leal, J. K., De Franceschi, L., et al. (2016). Red blood cell homeostasis: pharmacological interventions to explore biochemical, morphological and mechanical properties. *Front. Mol. Biosci.* 3:10. doi: 10.3389/fmolb.2016.00010

D'Alessandro, A., Nemkov, T., Reisz, J., Dzieciatkowska, M., Wither, M. J., and Hansen, K. C. (2017). Omics markers of the red cell storage lesion and metabolic linkage. *Blood Transfus.* 15, 137–144. doi: 10.2450/2017.0341-16

Delobel, J., Prudent, M., Crettaz, D., ElHajj, Z., Riederer, B., Tissot, J.-D., et al. (2016). Cysteine redox proteomics of the hemoglobin-depleted cytosolic fraction of stored red blood cells. *Proteomics Clin. Appl.* 10, 883–893. doi: 10.1002/prca.201500132

Devalet, B., Mullier, F., Chatelain, B., Dogne, J.-M., and Chatelain, C. (2014). The central role of extracellular vesicles in the mechanisms of thrombosis in paroxysmal nocturnal haemoglobinuria: a review. *J. Extracell. Vesicles.* 3, 1–8. doi: 10.3402/jev.v3.23304

Dinkla, S., Novotný, V. M. J., Joosten, I., and Bosman, G. J. C. G. M. (2012a). Storage-induced changes in erythrocyte membrane proteins promote recognition by autoantibodies. *PLoS One* 7:e42250. doi: 10.1371/J.pone.0042250

Dinkla, S., van Eijk, L. T., Fuchs, B., Schiller, J., Joosten, I., Brock, R. et al. (2016). Inflammation-associated changes in lipid composition and the organization of the erythrocyte membrane. *BBA Clin.* 5, 186–192. doi: 10.1016/j.bbacli.2016.03.007

Dinkla, S., Wessels, K., Verdurmen, W. P. R., Tomelleri, C., Cluitmans, J. C. A., Fransen, J., et al. (2012b). Functional consequences of sphingomyelinase-induced changes in erythrocyte membrane structure. *Cell. Death Dis.* 3, 410–412. doi: 10.1038/cddis.2012.143

Donadee, C., Raat, N. J. H., Kanias, T., Tejero, J., Lee, J. S., Kelley, E. E., et al. (2011). Nitric oxide scavenging by red blood cell microparticles and cell-free hemoglobin as a mechanism for the red cell storage lesion. *Circulation* 124, 465–476. doi: 10.1161/CIRCULATIONAHA.110.008698

Ferru, E., Giger, K., Pantaleo, A., Campanella, E., Grey, J., Ritchie, K., et al. (2011). Regulation of membrane-cytoskeletal interactions by tyrosine phosphorylation of erythrocyte band 3. *Blood* 117, 5998–6006. doi: 10.1182/blood-2010-11-317024

Ferru, E., Pantaleo, A., Carta, F., Mannu, F., Khadjavi, A., Gallo, V., et al. (2014). Thalassemic erythrocytes release microparticles loaded with hemichromes by redox activation of p72Syk kinase. *Haematologica* 99, 570–578. doi: 10.3324/haematol.2013.084533

Freitas Leal, J. K., Adjobo-Hermans, M. J. W., Brock, R., and Bosman, G. J. C. G. M. (2017). Acetylcholinesterase provides new insights into red blood cell ageing *in vivo* and *in vitro*. *Blood Transfus.* 15, 232–238. doi: 10.2450/2017.0370-16

Gerotziafas, G. T., Van Dreden, P., Chaari, M., Galea, V., Khaterchi, A., Lionnet, F., et al. (2012). The acceleration of the propagation phase of thrombin generation in patients with steady-state sickle cell disease is associated with circulating erythrocyte-derived microparticles. *Thromb. Haemost.* 107, 1044–1052. doi: 10.1160/TH11-10-0689

Griffiths, R. E., Kupzig, S., Cogan, N., Mankelow, T. J., Betin, V. M., Trakarnsanga, K., et al. (2012). Maturing reticulocytes internalize plasma membrane in glycophorin A-containing vesicles that fuse with autophagosomes before exocytosis. *Blood* 119, 6296–62306. doi: 10.1182/blood-2011-09-376475

Hebbel, R. P., and Key, N. S. (2016). Microparticles in sickle cell anaemia: promise and pitfalls. *Br. J. Haematol.* 174, 16–29. doi: 10.1111/bjh.14112

Hoehn, R. S., Jernigan, P. L., Japtok, L., Chang, A. L., Midura, E. F., Caldwell, C. C., et al. (2017). Acid sphingomyelinase inhibition in stored erythrocytes reduces transfusion-associated lung inflammation. *Ann. Surg.* 265, 218–226. doi: 10.1097/SLA.0000000000001648

Hron, G., Kollars, M., Weber, H., Sagaster, V., Quehenberger, P., Eichinger, S., et al. (2007). Tissue factor-positive microparticles: cellular origin and association with coagulation activation in patients with colorectal cancer. *Thromb. Haemost.* 97, 119–123.

Hugel, B., Socié, G., Vu, T., Toti, F., Gluckman, E., Freyssinet, J. M., et al. (1999). Elevated levels of circulating procoagulant microparticles in patients with paroxysmal nocturnal hemoglobinuria and aplastic anemia. *Blood* 93, 3451–3456.

Kalra, H., Simpson, R. J., Ji, H., Aikawa, E., Altevogt, P., Askenase, P., et al. (2012). Vesiclepedia: a compendium for extracellular vesicles with continuous community annotation. *PLoS Biol.* 10:e1001450. doi: 10.1371/journal.pbio.1001450

Kittivorapart, J., Crew, V. K., Wilson, M. C., Heesom, K. J., Siritanaratkul, N., and Toye, A. M. (2018). Quantitative proteomics of plasma vesicles identify novel biomarkers for hemoglobin E/β-thalassemic patients. *Blood Adv.* 2, 95–104. doi: 10.1182/bloodadvances.2017011726

Koshiar, R. L., Somajo, S., Norström, E., and DahlBäck, B. (2014). Erythrocyte-derived microparticles supporting activated protein C-mediated regulation of blood coagulation. *PLoS One* 9:e104200. doi: 10.1371/journal.pone.0104200

Kostova, E. B., Beuger, B. M., Klei, T. R. L., Halonen, P., Lieftink, C., Beijersbergen, R., et al. (2015). Identification of signalling cascades involved in red blood cell shrinkage and vesiculation. *Biosci. Rep.* 35:e00187. doi: 10.1042/BSR20150019

Kozuma, Y., Sawahata, Y., Takei, Y., Chiba, S., and Ninomiya, H. (2011). Procoagulant properties of microparticles released from red blood cells in paroxysmal nocturnal haemoglobinuria. *Br. J. Haematol.* 152, 631–639. doi: 10.1111/j.1365-2141.2010.08505.x

Kriebardis, A. G., Antonelou, M. H., Stamoulis, K. E., Economou-Petersen, E., Margaritis, L. H., and Papassideri, I. S. (2008). RBC-derived vesicles during storage: ultrastructure, protein composition, oxidation, and signaling components. *Transfusion.* 48, 1943–1953. doi: 10.1111/j.1537-2995.2008.01794.x

Lange, P. F., Huesgen, P. F., Nguyen, K., and Overall, C. M. (2014). Annotating N termini for the human proteome project: N termini and Nα-acetylation status differentiate stable cleaved protein species from degradation remnants in the human erythrocyte proteome. *J. Proteome Res.* 13, 2028–2044. doi: 10.1021/pr401191w

Larson, M. C., Karafin, M. S., Hillery, C. A., and Hogg, N. (2017). Phosphatidylethanolamine is progressively exposed in RBCs during storage. *Transfus. Med.* 27, 136–141. doi: 10.1111/tme.12382

Laurén, E., Tigistu-Sahle, F., Valkonen, S., Westberg, M., Valkeajärvi, A., Eronen, J., et al. (2018). Phospholipid composition of packed red blood cells and that of extracellular vesicles show a high resemblance and stability during storage. *Biochim. Biophys. Acta.* 1863, 1–8. doi: 10.1016/j.bbalip.2017.09.012

Leonard, C., Conrard, L., Guthmann, M., Pollet, H., Carquin, M., Vermylen, C., et al. (2017). Contribution of plasma membrane lipid domains to red blood cell (re)shaping. *Sci. Rep.* 7:4264. doi: 10.1038/s41598-017-04388-z

Liu, C., Zhao, W., Christ, G. J., Gladwin, M. T., and Kim-Shapiro, D. B. (2013). Nitric oxide scavenging by red cell microparticles. *Free Radic. Biol. Med.* 65, 1164–1173. doi: 10.1016/j.freeradbiomed.2013.09.002

Mantel, P. Y., Hoang, A. N., Goldowitz, I., Potashnikova, D., Hamza, B., Vorobjev, I., et al. (2013). Malaria-infected erythrocyte-derived microvesicles mediate cellular communication between the parasite population and with the host immune system. *Cell Host Microbe* 13, 521–534. doi: 10.1016/j.chom.2013.04.009

Nielsen, M. H., Beck-Nielsen, H., Andersen, M. N., and Handberg, A. (2014). A flow cytometric method for characterization of circulating cell-derived microparticles in plasma. *J. Extracell. Vesicles.* 3, 1–12. doi: 10.3402/jev.v3.20795

Prudent, M., Crettaz, D., Delobel, J., Seghatchian, J., Tissot, J. D., and Lion, N. (2015). Differences between calcium-stimulated and storage-induced erythrocyte-derived microvesicles. *Transfus. Apher. Sci.* 53, 153–158. doi: 10.1016/j.transci.2015.10.012

Raposo, G., and Stoorvogel, W. (2013). Extracellular vesicles: Exosomes, microvesicles, and friends. *J. Cell Biol.* 200, 373–383. doi: 10.1083/jcb.201211138

Reliene, R., Mariani, M., Zanella, A., Reinhart, W. H., Ribeiro, M. L., del Giudice, E. M., et al. (2002). Splenectomy prolongs in vivo survival of erythrocytes differently in spectrin/ankyrin- and band 3-deficient hereditary spherocytosis. *Blood* 100, 2208–2215.

Rubin, O., Delobel, J., Prudent, M., Lion, N., Kohl, K., Tucker, E. I., et al. (2013). Red blood cell-derived microparticles isolated from blood units initiate and propagate thrombin generation. *Transfusion* 53, 1744–1754. doi: 10.1111/trf.12008

Sadallah, S., Eken, C., and Schifferli, J. A. (2008). Erythrocyte-derived ectosomes have immunosuppressive properties. *J. Leukoc. Biol.* 84, 1316–1325. doi: 10.1189/jlb.0108013

Salzer, U., and Prohaska, R. (2001). Stomatin, flotillin-1, and flotillin-2 are major integral proteins of erythrocyte lipid rafts. *Blood* 97, 1141–1143. doi: 10.1182/blood.V97.4.1141

Salzer, U., Zhu, R., Luten, M., Isobe, H., Pastushenko, V., Perkmann, T., et al. (2008). Vesicles generated during storage of red cells are rich in the lipid raft marker stomatin. *Transfusion* 48, 451–462. doi: 10.1111/j.1537-2995.2007.01549.x

Sens, P., and Gov, N. (2007). Force balance and membrane shedding at the red-blood-cell surface. *Phys. Rev. Lett.* 98:018102. doi: 10.1103/PhysRevLett.98.018102

Sloand, E. M., Mainwaring, L., Keyvanfar, K., Chen, J., Maciejewski, J., Klein, H. G., et al. (2004). Transfer of glycosylphosphatidylinositol-anchored proteins to deficient cells after erythrocyte transfusion in paroxysmal nocturnal hemoglobinuria. *Blood* 104, 3782–3788. doi: 10.1182/blood-2004-02-0645

Straat, M., van Hezel, M. E., Böing, A., Tuip-De Boer, A., Weber, N., Nieuwland, R., et al. (2016). Monocyte-mediated activation of endothelial cells occurs only after binding to extracellular vesicles from red blood cell products, a process mediated by β-integrin. *Transfusion* 56, 3012–3020. doi: 10.1111/trf.13851

Szigyártó, I. C., Deák, R., Mihály, J., Rocha, S., Zsila, F., Varga, Z., et al. (2018). Flow alignment of extracellular vesicles: structure and orientation of membrane-associated bio-macromolecules studied with polarized light. *ChemBioChem.* 19, 545–551. doi: 10.1002/cbic.201700378

van Beers, E. J., Schaap, M. C., Berckmans, R. J., Nieuwland, R., Sturk, A., van Doormaal, F. F., et al. (2009). Circulating erythrocyte-derived microparticles are associated with coagulation activation in sickle cell disease. *Haematologica* 94, 1513–1519. doi: 10.3324/haematol.2009.008938

van der Meijden, P. E., van Schilfgaarde, M., van Oerle, R., Renné, T., ten Cate, H., and Spronk, H. M. (2012). Platelet- and erythrocyte-derived microparticles trigger thrombin generation via factor XIIa. *J. Thromb. Haemost.* 10, 1355–1362. doi: 10.1111/j.1538-7836.2012.04758.x

Verhoeven, A. J., Hilarius, P. M., Dekkers, D. W. C., Lagerberg, J. W. M., and De Korte, D. (2006). Prolonged storage of red blood cells affects aminophospholipid translocase activity. *Vox Sang.* 91, 244–251. doi: 10.1111/j.1423-0410.2006.00822.x

Wernick, B., Cipriano, A., Odom, S. R., MacBean, U., Mubang, R. N., Wojda, T. R., et al. (2017). Temporal changes in hematologic markers after splenectomy, splenic embolization, and observation for trauma. *Eur. J. Trauma Emerg. Surg.* 43, 399–409. doi: 10.1007/s00068-016-0679-0

Westerman, M., Pizzey, A., Hirschman, J., Cerino, M., Weil-Weiner, Y., Ramotar, P., et al. (2008). Microvesicles in haemoglobinopathies offer insights into mechanisms of hypercoagulability, haemolysis and the effects of therapy. *Br. J. Haematol.* 142, 126–135. doi: 10.1111/j.1365-2141.2008.07155.x

Willekens, F. L., Bosch, F. H., Roerdinkholder-Stoelwinder, B., Groenen-Döpp, Y. A., and Werre, J. M. (1997). Quantification of loss of haemoglobin components from the circulating red blood cell in vivo. *Eur. J. Haematol.* 58, 246–250. doi: 10.1111/j.1600-0609.1997.tb01662.x

Willekens, F. L., Roerdinkholder-Stoelwinder, B., Groenen-Döpp, Y. A., Bos, H. J., Bosman, G. J., Van den Bos, A. G., et al. (2003). Hemoglobin loss from erythrocytes in vivo results from spleen-facilitated vesiculation. *Blood* 101, 747–751. doi: 10.1182/blood-2002-02-0500

Willekens, F. L., Werre, J. M., Groenen-Döpp, Y. A., Roerdinkholder-Stoelwinder, B., De Pauw, B., and Bosman, G. J. (2008). Erythrocyte vesiculation: a self-protective mechanism? *Br. J. Haematol.* 141, 549–556. doi: 10.1111/j.1365-2141.2008.07055.x

Willekens, F. L., Werre J. M., Kruijt, J. K., Roerdinkholder-Stoelwinder, B., Groenen-Döpp, Y. A., van den Bos A. G., et al. (2005). Liver Kupffer cells rapidly remove red blood cell-derived vesicles from the circulation by scavenger receptors. *Blood* 105, 2141–2145. doi: 10.1182/blood-2004-04-1578

Wither, M., Dzieciatkowska, M., Nemkov, T., Strop, P., D'Alessandro, A., and Hansen, K. C. (2016). Hemoglobin oxidation at functional amino acid residues during routine storage of red blood cells. *Transfusion* 56, 421–426. doi: 10.1111/trf.13363

Zecher, D., Cumpelik, A., and Schifferli, J. A. (2014). Erythrocyte-derived microvesicles amplify systemic inflammation by thrombin-dependent activation of complement. *Arterioscler. Thromb. Vasc. Biol.* 34, 313–320. doi: 10.1161/ATVBAHA.113.302378

Zhu, Q., Salehyar, S., Cabrales, P., and Asaro, R. J. (2017). Prospects for human erythrocyte skeleton-bilayer dissociation during splenic flow. *Biophys. J.* 113, 900–912. doi: 10.1016/j.bpj.2017.05.052

12

Neocytolysis: How to Get Rid of the Extra Erythrocytes Formed by Stress Erythropoiesis Upon Descent from High Altitude

*Heimo Mairbäurl**

Medical Clinic VII, Sports Medicine, Translational Lung Research Center, German Center for Lung Research, University Hospital Heidelberg, Heidelberg, Germany

Correspondence:
Heimo Mairbäurl
heimo.mairbaeurl@med.uni-heidelberg.de

Neocytolysis is the selective destruction of those erythrocytes that had been formed during stress-erythropoiesis in hypoxia in order to increase the oxygen transport capacity of blood. Neocytolysis likely aims at decreasing this excess amount of erythrocytes and hemoglobin (Hb) when it is not required anymore and to decrease blood viscosity. Neocytolysis seems to occur upon descent from high altitude. Similar processes seem to occur in microgravity, and are also discussed to mediate the replacement of erythrocytes containing fetal hemoglobin (HbF) with those having adult hemoglobin (HbA) after birth. This review will focus on hypoxia at high altitude. Hemoglobin concentration and total hemoglobin in blood increase by 20–50% depending on the altitude (i.e., the degree of hypoxia) and the duration of the sojourn. Upon return to normoxia hemoglobin concentration, hematocrit, and reticulocyte counts decrease faster than expected from inhibition of stress-erythropoiesis and normal erythrocyte destruction rates. In parallel, an increase in haptoglobin, bilirubin, and ferritin is observed, which serve as indirect markers of hemolysis and hemoglobin-breakdown. At the same time markers of progressing erythrocyte senescence appear even on reticulocytes. Unexpectedly, reticulocytes from hypoxic mice show decreased levels of the hypoxia-inducible factor HIF-1α and decreased activity of the BCL2/adenovirus E1B 19 kDa protein-interacting protein 3 (BNIP3), which results in elevated mitochondrial activity in these cells. Furthermore, hypoxia increases the expression of miR-21, which inhibits the expression of catalase and thus decreases one of the most important mechanisms protecting against oxygen free radicals in erythrocytes. This unleashes a series of events which likely explain neocytolysis, because upon re-oxygenation systemic and mitochondrial oxygen radical formation increases and causes the selective destruction of those erythrocytes having impaired anti-oxidant capacity.

Keywords: high altitude medicine, erythropoiesis, reticulocytes, hemoglobins, total hemoglobin mass, antioxidant capacity, hypoxia

INTRODUCTION

Adjusting amount and function of erythrocytes is required in a variety of situations, the most obvious being the decrease in Hb after birth and the slow replacement of erythrocytes containing HbF with ones with HbA after birth (Terrenato et al., 1981). Altered blood distribution among compartments seems to induce a reduction in the total mass of erythrocytes in microgravity (Alfrey et al., 1996). Many diseases are associated with anemia by removing damaged erythrocytes (e.g., Rifkind, 1966). Although destruction likely occurs by different mechanisms, all might be classified into the non-specific term "erythrolysis." Yet another mechanism might explain the destruction of erythrocytes when highly polycythemic high altitude natives descent from high altitude (Merino, 1950). This review addresses targeted destruction of erythrocytes upon return to sea level, which lowlanders form during staying at high altitude for a limited time. Because in particular these newly formed cells seem to be removed, their destruction is called "neocytolysis" (Alfrey et al., 1997). For better understanding selectivity of destruction, biochemical characteristics, and mechanisms of cell destruction of erythrocytes formed under normal and stress conditions will be summarized.

ADJUSTMENTS OF OXYGEN TRANSPORT TO HYPOXIA AT HIGH ALTITUDE

Oxygen supply to tissues is impaired at high altitude because decreased oxygen content of inspired air resulting in a mild decrease in arterial oxygen saturation (SaO_2) at moderate altitudes (~92% at 2,500 m) but much more pronounced at higher altitudes (~83% at 4,500 m) because of the sigmoidal shape of the oxygen dissociation curve (Mairbäurl and Weber, 2012).

Arterial oxygen content (CaO_2) varies during a sojourn at high altitude (Rasmussen et al., 2013): CaO_2 is decreased upon acute ascent to high altitude, increases slightly within a few hours because of ventilatory acclimatization and respiratory alkalosis, increases further within days because of decreased plasma volume and increased hematocrit, and increases even further within weeks to months at high altitude because stimulated erythropoiesis increases total hemoglobin (tHb) reaching even pre-altitude values (Calbet et al., 2003).

Importantly, only CaO_2 gets normalized but not PaO_2, which is the main driving-force for oxygen diffusion to tissues, which therefore remain to some extent oxygen-limited. This seems to be well tolerated because at some point during a long-term stay at high altitude tHb reaches a stably-elevated value (Hurtado et al., 1945; Merino, 1950; Reynafarje et al., 1959). Performance is not improved equally because of impaired O_2-diffusion (Calbet et al., 2003; Bärtsch and Swenson, 2014).

Stimulation of erythropoiesis at high altitude depends on HIF-2α and erythropoietin (EPO) (Haase, 2013) and adjustments of iron metabolism (Hentze et al., 2010). EPO increases rapidly upon exposure to hypoxia; the magnitude depends on the degree of hypoxia (Eckardt et al., 1989) following a semi-logarithmic function (Wenger and Kurtz, 2011). After this initial increase EPO decreases significantly to reach a steady state level that remains significantly above normoxic values, while one is still exposed to hypoxia (Wenger and Kurtz, 2011). Yet, the rate of formation of new erythrocytes stays elevated provided there is sufficient supply with iron. Iron uptake seems to peak after approximately 4 days at high altitude, reticulocytes have their highest values after approximately 7 days in hypoxia (Siri et al., 1966). This pattern of changes has been named the "EPO-paradox" (Milledge and Bärtsch, 2014). It is likely caused by a shift from hematopoietic stem cells toward erythroid progenitor cells associated with up-regulation of the erythroid transcription factor GATA-1, which stimulates EPO-receptor expression (Li et al., 2011), resulting in an increased EPO-sensitivity and sustained erythropoiesis even at lower EPO. EPO receptors on progenitor cells are gradually lost during differentiation, and EPO-receptor density is very low in circulating mouse erythrocytes (Mihov et al., 2009).

The rapid increase in reticulocyte count, which is commonly observed, is likely caused by increased bone marrow blood flow and immature release of red cells (Aoki and Tavassoli, 1981). These immature cells differ in properties from reticulocytes produced under stress-free conditions, similar to what has been found in thalassemia (Rivella, 2009).

At moderate altitudes 2 weeks do not result in an increase in Hb in athletes (Friedmann et al., 1999), and stays longer than 3 weeks seem to increase total red cell volume by 60–250 ml/week (Sawka et al., 2000). Natives to high altitudes in the Andes have an increased total Hb, and their blood volume in increased by approximately 20% (Hurtado, 1964; Sánchez et al., 1970). Similar values are observed in sojourners after weeks to months at high altitude.

MATURATION OF ERYTHROID PRECURSORS

The viability of committed erythroid progenitor cells downstream of the erythroid differentiation depends on the presence of EPO by supporting survival of erythroid precursors, which stimulates proliferation (Kimura et al., 2000). This process depends on cKit and EPO-receptors on the progenitor cells (Fisher et al., 1994; Wenger and Kurtz, 2011) and other growth factors all of which cause tyrosine-phosphorylation by Janus-kinase JAK2 (Klingmüller, 1997). JAK2 phosphorylates the EPO-receptor and the signal transducer and activator of transcription 5 (STAT5), which blocks apoptosis by inhibiting the Forkhead-Box-Protein O3 (FOXO3)-dependent pro-apoptotic pathways (Wojchowski et al., 2006). There is also an inhibition of the death receptor Fas and its ligand FasL in splenic erythroid cells, which promotes survival (Koulnis et al., 2011). The BNIP3-ligand (BNIP3L; Nix) controls mitochondrial autophagy (Sandoval et al., 2008). Thus, by the action of EPO, dividing progenitor cells are not destroyed resulting in increased production of normoblasts and release of reticulocytes into circulation (Wenger and Kurtz, 2011). In addition, phosphorylation of STAT3 increases the expression of antioxidant enzymes such as superoxide dismutase (SOD) and glutamin-cystein antiporter xCT while at the same time decreases the expression of proteins of the mitochondrial electron transfer chain (Linher-Melville and Singh, 2017). Together these two processes protect from hypoxia-induced mitochondrial oxygen radicals (ROS) (Chandel and Schumacker, 2000), which might impair erythropoiesis. Hypoxia also causes a HIF-1α and BNIP3-dependent decrease in mitochondrial activity, which further reduces ROS formation (Semenza, 2008). Therefore, during acute hypoxia, when mitochondrial adjustments have not yet been established, hypoxia likely increases mitochondrial ROS production, whereas hypoxia-adapted cells seem to produce less ROS (Chandel et al., 1997). However, there is also evidence that hypoxia might down-regulate the expression of anti-oxidant enzymes such as catalase (Song et al., 2015). If this were the case, then one might speculate on a decreased anti-oxidant activity in hypoxia-adjusted cells and increased vulnerability to oxidant damage. This issue requires clarification.

STRESS-ERYTHROPOIESIS

While normal steady-state erythropoiesis produces cells at a nearly constant rate, situations of acute tissue hypoxia such as blood loss, hemolysis, and elevated erythropoietin dramatically increase the rate of erythrocyte production and the rapid appearance of newly formed cells in circulation ("stress-erythropoiesis"). Most experimental evidence comes from work on mice, whereas evidence for human equivalents is sparse. It has to be noted that the mouse model most often used is phenylhydrazine-induced lipid-peroxydation and hemolytic anemia (Jain and Subrahmanyam, 1978), a quite "un-physiological" system.

In the acutely anemic mouse some of the EPO-induced progenitors migrate to the spleen (there may also be resident, self-renewing ones), with much enhanced maturation (Paulson et al., 2011). This is based on the finding that erythroid burst forming units (BFU-E) from the spleen differ from bone marrow BFU-E in that they form larger colonies and that the only growth factor required is EPO, whereas in the bone marrow additional burst-promoting factors are required (Valtieri et al., 1989). Bone morphogenic protein-4 (BMP4), who's expression depends on HIF-2α (Wu and Paulson, 2010), induces the expansion of BFU-E in the spleen to produce specialized resident stress erythroid progenitors (Paulson et al., 2011). It is interesting to note that hypoxia strongly stimulates the expansion of spleen-derived BFU-E (Perry et al., 2007). There is only indirect evidence for similarities between murine and human stress erythropoiesis. In acute anemia human stress erythropoiesis exhibits similarities to fetal erythropoiesis (Paulson et al., 2011), because a higher proportion of blood progenitor cells than typical bone marrow derived cells contains HbF. Hypoxia of cultured progenitor cells from patients with sickle cell disease and thalassemia also induces the production of HbF cells. A moderate increase in HbF-containing erythrocytes has also been found in humans after a 17-day stay at altitudes above 3,100 m (Risso et al., 2012). Thus it was speculated that this type of stress progenitors resemble the spleen-derived stress BFU-Es of the mouse model.

The marrow transit time of ^{59}Fe was shortened in mice made anemic by phlebotomy, and there was an inverse relation between transit time and the degree of anemia (Hillman, 1969). Cells appear to be released immaturely indicated by larger size, increased reticulum content, iron uptake, membrane ion transporter activity, and increased density of transferrin receptors (TfR; CD71) on the plasma membrane (summary in Rhodes et al., 2016). TfR could be detected on circulating erythrocytes longer than during normal erythropoiesis. This indicates that the rate of maturation is similar in stress and normal erythropoiesis, but that maturation of circulating stress reticulocytes takes longer because of their immature release (Al-Huniti et al., 2005; Rhodes et al., 2016).

NEOCYTOLYSIS

Neocytolysis is the selective destruction of the youngest population of erythrocytes in blood, just after they had left the bone marrow, and it is thought to bring an elevated erythrocyte mass (e.g., after a stay at high altitude) back to normal (Alfrey et al., 1997). It seems to occur in a variety of different situations (Alfrey et al., 1997; Harris and Epstein, 2001; Song et al., 2017). Neocytolysis appears to be caused not simply by discontinuing stress erythropoiesis but by "controlled" processes (for a recent review see Risso et al., 2014). However, indications for neocytolysis after return from high altitude hypoxia are weak.

Merino noted disappearance of polycythemia within a few days after return from high altitude and explained it by reduced erythropoiesis (Merino, 1950), which has been indicated experimentally by decreased iron incorporation in high altitude natives on traveling to low altitude (Huff et al., 1951). Also the reticulocyte number decreased. Greater "blood destruction" was indicated by increased plasma bilirubin and urobilinogen excretion (Merino, 1950).

Pace et al. based the discussion of neocytolysis (Pace et al., 1956) on a normal erythrocyte disappearance rate of 0.0083 per day (experimentally determined from the rate of removal of transfused erythrocytes; Callender et al., 1945). Erythrocyte count and Hb decreased at a rate of 0.011 per day upon return to sea level after an expedition to the Himalayas (Pace et al., 1956). This was interpreted to be caused by decreased rate of erythropoiesis and increased "erythrolysis," but also by restoring the decrease in plasma volume that occurs at high altitude (Siebenmann et al., 2017).

Rice et al. studied polycythemic residents of Cerre de Pasco (4,380 m) upon travel to sea level and found a decrease by 9% in erythrocyte mass within 3–7 days after descent, a rapid decrease in EPO, and increased bilirubin. Changes did not occur in three subjects receiving EPO upon descent (Rice et al., 2001).

Polycythemia by itself shortens erythrocyte survival (Bogdanova et al., 2007). Risso et al. (Risso et al., 2007) separated age-fractions of erythrocytes by density gradient centrifugation from blood of mountaineers 1 day after return from a mountaineering expedition and found that the youngest fraction had disappeared. Cells had acquired a "senescent phenotype" indicated by decreased levels of expression of the integrin associated protein (CD47), of the complement decay accelerating factor (DAF; CD55), and of protectin (membrane inhibitor of reactive lysis; CD59), which may be an indication of increased susceptibility to phagocytosis (Risso et al., 2007). However, only one time-point had been studied, and results may be flawed by the fact that the descent itself had lasted almost 1 week.

Mechanisms Causing Neocytolysis

Results on three subjects (Rice et al., 2001) suggest that the withdrawal of EPO might be responsible for the destruction of erythrocytes produced in hypoxia. It is thought that increased EPO favors the expression of CD55 and CD59 such as observed in EPO-treated patients with renal anemia (Ohi et al., 2003), which protects from destruction by macrophages, whereas EPO withdrawal decreases expression and coincides with reappearance of anemia (Ohi et al., 2003), resulting in a picture comparable to that observed with EPO-withdrawal and treatment upon descent (Trial and Rice, 2004; Risso et al., 2014). This seems to be in line with the dependency of erythrocyte destruction on EPO and EPO-receptors in polycythemia of a gain-of-function mutation of the EPO-receptor (Divoky et al., 2016).

Another line of evidence suggests a role for altered antioxidant capacity. Erythrocytes exposed to anoxia have a decreased antioxidant capacity, indicated by decreased glutathione, nicotine-adenine dinucleotide (phosphate) (GSH, NADPH, and NADH, resp.) redox couples and reduced membrane thiols (Rogers et al., 2009). This has been explained with a re-direction of glycolytic flux toward the synthesis of 2,3-diphosphoglycerate (2,3-DPG) and binding to deoxygenated Hb, as well as altered glycolytic activity caused by competition of binding between deoxygenated Hb and glycolytic enzymes to band 3 (Weber et al., 2004), which also results in decreased NADPH and GSH formation (Rogers et al., 2009). Though this mechanism might adversely affect erythrocyte survival during high altitude hypoxia, it should rapidly be reversed upon descent thus protecting mature erythrocytes from oxidative stress. Erythropoiesis in hypoxic mice results in erythrocytes with a decreased anti-oxidative capacity because of decreased expression of catalase due to elevated levels of the micro-RNA miR-21 (Song et al., 2015). Anti-oxidative enzymes are typically high in young erythrocytes and decrease rapidly with aging (Bartosz and Bartkowiak, 1981). In the mouse model hypoxia during maturation increases mitochondrial activity in erythroid precursors due to suppression of HIF-1α and decreased BNIP3L. It was argued that mitochondrial ROS production would increase in normoxia and cause neocyte destruction (Song et al., 2015). This is in sharp contradiction to results showing HIF-1α-induced increase in mitophagy and reduction of mitochondrial mass in a variety of cell types thought to protect from increased ROS formation and cell destruction (Zhang et al., 2008) because hypoxic mitochondria produce more ROS than normoxic ones (Chandel et al., 1998; Chandel and Schumacker, 2000; Levraut et al., 2003). This issue awaits clarification.

Interestingly, it was found that treating mice with polyethylene glycol-conjugated catalase, which is not taken up by reticulocytes and mature erythrocytes, as well as treatment with the anti-oxidant N-acety-cysteine increased reticulocyte half-life and prevented the reduction in hematocrit (Song et al., 2015). This result contradicts the above described argument for a role for elevated mitochondrial but argues for systemic elevation of ROS which damage hypoxia-derived neocytes, a mechanism similar to re-oxygenation injury known from many organs, e.g., the lung (Pak et al., 2017).

DESTRUCTION OF SENESCENT ERYTHROCYTES

The average life-span of mature erythrocytes is 100–130 days. The destruction rate amounts to approximately 1% per day. Senescent erythrocytes are removed by the reticulo-endothelial system, mainly in the spleen, where cells are tested for functionality and are sequestered "if they don't pass the test" (Rifkind, 1966). Random hemolysis of pre-senescent erythrocytes is negligible in humans but amounts to 0.5–1% per day in mice and rat (Landaw, 1988). Loss of erythrocytes is balanced by a production rate of $\sim 160 \times 10^6$ erythrocytes per minute in humans.

Interestingly, erythrocytes produced in hypoxic stress appear to have a shortened life span in some species, which is caused by increased random hemolysis and accelerated senescence (Fryers and Berlin, 1952). Every doubling of the erythrocyte production rate resulted in a 3.5% reduction in survival in rat (Landaw, 1988). Mechanisms seem to be intrinsic to erythrocytes, because cross-transfusion of newly formed cells into normoxic animals did not improve survival (Landaw, 1988). This is in line with reports on elevated levels of breakdown-products of heme in high altitude residents (Merino, 1950). It is further supported by an approximately 25% increase in the ^{59}Fe disappearance rate from blood in Peruvian high altitude relative to sea-level residents (Huff et al., 1951) indicating increased production due to accelerated sequestration to maintain stably elevated Hb.

CONSEQUENCES OF NEOCYTOLYSIS AND ACCELERATED SENESCENCE

If in fact erythrocytes produced by hypoxic marrow have characteristics limiting their survival upon return to normoxia, then hemolysis will affect different age-cohorts of erythrocytes depending on the duration of the sojourn and on the altitude (Rasmussen et al., 2013). After a sojourn at moderately high altitude for a few weeks as done by athletes for continuous or intermittent altitude training with the goal of increasing oxygen transport capacity and sea-level performance (Levine and Stray-Gundersen, 1997; Stray-Gundersen and Levine, 2008), only a small fraction of newly released erythrocytes will be found in circulation (Rasmussen et al., 2013; Garvican-Lewis et al., 2016). In fact, athletes had an elevated fraction of immature reticulocytes with high expression of TfR after returning from training at 1,905 m, which fell to sub-baseline values by day 9, and returned to baseline on day 16 after the training camp (Nadarajan et al., 2010). Similarly, increased ferritin levels were found post-altitude-training (Garvican et al., 2012). These changes are consistent with neocytolysis. However, there were no or only minor changes in tHb within 1 or 2 weeks after return from training at 2,300 m, during which total Hb had increased by ∼8% (Prommer et al., 2010; Garvican et al., 2012; Wachsmuth et al., 2013a,b), which may indicate decrease in erythrocyte mass by decreasing erythropoietic activity and by random loss, but a minor contribution of neocytolysis. In contrast, polycythemia after a stay at 5,260 m was reverted already within 1 week after descent indicating neocytolysis (Ryan et al., 2014). This may indicate that neocytolysis plays a minor role after a stay at moderate altitude, and that athletes performing altitude training may take advantage of a slightly increased oxygen carrying capacity at low altitudes for several weeks.

The situation is different for long-term sojourners and high altitude residents returning to low altitudes, because all their erythrocytes in circulation may have a decreased anti-oxidant capacity. Thus, elevated ROS will not only lyze young erythrocytes, but also random destruction might be increased and shorten erythrocyte life span. Hemolysis will progress until all erythrocytes with high altitude characteristics will be replaced by normoxic ones having increased antioxidant capacity. This process might cause a severe hemolytic strain, which might be even more pronounced in polycythemic individuals with chronic mountain sickness.

CONCLUSION AND PERSPECTIVES

There are indications of destruction of erythrocytes formed during exposure to hypoxia upon return to normoxia. Mechanisms are unclear and might include withdrawal of EPO and impaired defense against increased ROS. Experiments are needed to better define the mechanisms causing the fast and selective removal of neocytes formed in situations of stress erythropoiesis and to clearly distinguish between selective destruction and random loss.

Another aspect to be clarified concerns the use of the term "neocytolysis," which implies the destruction selectively of erythrocytes formed in an acute and transient situation of stress erythropoiesis. Thus this term cannot be used to describe the destruction of a fraction of erythrocytes produced during long-term or even life-long exposure to such a stress environment such as fetal life and being an altitude native. In those situations it needs to be sorted out whether just erythrocytes newly released from the marrow are removed, or whether all circulating cells are more susceptible to random loss, and why.

AUTHOR CONTRIBUTIONS

The author confirms being the sole contributor of this work and approved it for publication.

REFERENCES

Alfrey, C. P., Rice, L., Udden, M. M., and Driscoll, T. B. (1997). Neocytolysis: physiological down-regulator of red-cell mass. *Lancet* 349, 1389–1390. doi: 10.1016/S0140-6736(96)09208-2

Alfrey, C. P., Udden, M. M., Leach-Huntoon, C., Driscoll, T., and Pickett, M. H. (1996). Control of red blood cell mass in spaceflight. *J. Appl. Physiol.* 81, 98–104. doi: 10.1152/jappl.1996.81.1.98

Al-Huniti, N. H., Widness, J. A., Schmidt, R. L., and Veng-Pedersen, P. (2005). Pharmacodynamic analysis of changes in reticulocyte subtype distribution in phlebotomy-induced stress erythropoiesis. *J. Pharmacokinet. Pharmacodyn.* 32, 359–376. doi: 10.1007/s10928-005-0009-3

Aoki, M., and Tavassoli, M. (1981). Dynamics of red cell egress from bone marrow after blood letting. *Br. J. Haematol.* 49, 337–347. doi: 10.1111/j.1365-2141.1981.tb07235.x

Bartosz, G., and Bartkowiak, A. (1981). Aging of the erythrocyte. II. Activities of peroxide-detoxifying enzymes. *Experientia* 37, 722–723. doi: 10.1007/BF01967944

Bärtsch, P., and Swenson, E. R. (2014). *High Altitude: Human Adaptation to Hypoxia.* New York, NY: Springer.

Bogdanova, A., Mihov, D., Lutz, H., Saam, B., Gassmann, M., and Vogel, J. (2007). Enhanced erythro-phagocytosis in polycythemic mice overexpressing erythropoietin. *Blood* 110, 762–769. doi: 10.1182/blood-2006-12-063602

Calbet, J. A., Boushel, R., Radegran, G., Sondergaard, H., Wagner, P. D., and Saltin, B. (2003). Why is VO_{2max} after altitude acclimatization still reduced despite normalization of arterial O_2 content? *Am. J. Physiol.* 284, R304–R316. doi: 10.1152/ajpregu.00156.2002

Callender, S. T., Powell, E. O., and Witts, L. J. (1945). The life-span of the red cell in man. *J. Path. Bact.* 57, 129–139. doi: 10.1002/path.1700570116

Chandel, N., Budinger, G. R. S., Choe, S. H., and Schumacker, P. T. (1997). Cellular respiration during hypoxia. *J. Biol. Chem.* 272, 18808–18816. doi: 10.1074/jbc.272.30.18808

Chandel, N. S., Maltepe, E., Goldwasser, E., Mathieu, C. E., Simon, M. C., and Schumacker, P. T. (1998). Mitochondrial reactive oxygen species trigger hypoxia- induced transcription. *Proc. Natl. Acad. Sci. U.S.A.* 95, 11715–11720. doi: 10.1073/pnas.95.20.11715

Chandel, N. S., and Schumacker, P. T. (2000). Cellular oxygen sensing by mitochondria: old questions, new insight. *J. Appl. Physiol.* 88, 1880–1889. doi: 10.1152/jappl.2000.88.5.1880

Divoky, V., Song, J., Horvathova, M., Kralova, B., Votavova, H., Prchal, J. T., et al. (2016). Delayed hemoglobin switching and perinatal neocytolysis in mice with gain-of-function erythropoietin receptor. *J. Mol. Med.* 94, 597–608. doi: 10.1007/s00109-015-1375-y

Eckardt, K. U., Boutellier, U., Kurtz, A., Schopen, M., Koller, E. A., and Bauer, C. (1989). Rate of erythropoietin formation in humans in response to acute hypobaric hypoxia. *J. Appl. Physiol.* 66, 1785–1788. doi: 10.1152/jappl.1989.66.4.1785

Fisher, M. J., Prchal, J. F., Prchal, J. T., and D'Andrea, A. D. (1994). Anti-erythropoietin (EPO) receptor monoclonal antibodies distinguish EPO-dependent and EPO-independent erythroid progenitors in polycythemia vera. *Blood* 84, 1982–1991.

Friedmann, B., Jost, J., Rating, T., Weller, E., Werle, E., Eckardt, K. U., et al. (1999). Effects of iron supplementation on total body hemoglobin during endurance training at moderate altitude. *Int. J. Sports Med.* 20, 78–85. doi: 10.1055/s-2007-971097

Fryers, G. R., and Berlin, N. I. (1952). Mean red cell life of rats exposed to reduced barometric pressure. *Am. J. Physiol.* 171, 465–470. doi: 10.1152/ajplegacy.1952.171.2.465

Garvican, L., Martin, D., Quod, M., Stephens, B., Sassi, A., and Gore, C. (2012). Time course of the hemoglobin mass response to natural altitude training in elite endurance cyclists. *Scand. J. Med. Sci. Sports* 22, 95–103. doi: 10.1111/j.1600-0838.2010.01145.x

Garvican-Lewis, L. A., Sharpe, K., and Gore, C. J. (2016). Time for a new metric for hypoxic dose? *J. Appl. Physiol.* 121, 352–355. doi: 10.1152/japplphysiol.00579.2015

Haase, V. H. (2013). Regulation of erythropoiesis by hypoxia-inducible factors. *Blood Rev.* 27, 41–53. doi: 10.1016/j.blre.2012.12.003

Harris, B. A. Jr., and Epstein, P. E. (2001). Out of thin air: the evolving enigma of erythropoietin and neocytolysis. *Ann. Intern. Med.* 134, 710–712. doi: 10.7326/0003-4819-134-8-200104170-00015

Hentze, M. W., Muckenthaler, M. U., Galy, B., and Camaschella, C. (2010). Two to tango: regulation of Mammalian iron metabolism. *Cell* 142, 24–38. doi: 10.1016/j.cell.2010.06.028

Hillman, R. S. (1969). Characteristics of marrow production and reticulocyte maturation in normal man in response to anemia. *J. Clin. Invest.* 48, 443–453. doi: 10.1172/JCI106001

Huff, R. L., Lawrence, J. H., Siri, W. E., Wasserman, L. R., and Hennessy, T. G. (1951). Effects of changes in altitude on hematopoietic activity. *Medicine (Baltimore).* 30, 197–217. doi: 10.1097/00005792-195109000-00001

Hurtado, A. (1964). "Some physiological and clinical aspectsof life at high altitudes," in *Aging of the Lung*, eds L. Cander and J. H. Moyer (New York, NY: Grune & Stratton), 257.

Hurtado, A., Merino, C., and Delgado, E. (1945). Influence of anoxaemia on the hematopoietic acitvity. *Arch. Intern. Med.* 75, 284–323. doi: 10.1001/archinte.1945.00210290007002

Jain, S. K., and Subrahmanyam, D. (1978). On the mechanism of phenylhydrazine-induced hemolytic anemia. *Biochem. Biophys. Res. Commun.* 82, 1320–1324. doi: 10.1016/0006-291X(78)90332-7

Kimura, T., Sonoda, Y., Iwai, N., Satoh, M., Yamaguchi-Tsukio, M., Izui, T., et al. (2000). Proliferation and cell death of embryonic primitive erythrocytes. *Exp. Hematol.* 28, 635–641. doi: 10.1016/S0301-472X(00)00156-9

Klingmüller, U. (1997). The role of tyrosine phosphorylation in proliferation and maturation of erythroid progenitor cells–signals emanating from the erythropoietin receptor. *Eur. J. Biochem.* 249, 637–647. doi: 10.1111/j.1432-1033.1997.t01-1-00637.x

Koulnis, M., Liu, Y., Hallstrom, K., and Socolovsky, M. (2011). Negative autoregulation by Fas stabilizes adult erythropoiesis and accelerates its stress response. *PLoS ONE* 6:e21192. doi: 10.1371/journal.pone.0021192

Landaw, S. A. (1988). Factors that accelerate or retard red blood cell senescence. *Blood Cells* 14, 47–59.

Levine, B. D., and Stray-Gundersen, J. (1997). "Living high-training low": effect of moderate-altitude acclimatization with low-altitude training on performance. *J. Appl. Physiol.* 83, 102–112. doi: 10.1152/jappl.1997.83.1.102

Levraut, J., Iwase, H., Shao, Z. H., Vandenhoek, T. L., and Schumacker, P. T. (2003). Cell death during ischemia: relationship to mitochondrial depolarization and ROS generation. *Am. J. Physiol.* 284, H549–H558. doi: 10.1152/ajpheart.00708.2002

Li, P., Huang, J., Tian, H. J., Huang, Q. Y., Jiang, C. H., and Gao, Y. Q. (2011). Regulation of bone marrow hematopoietic stem cell is involved in high-altitude erythrocytosis. *Exp. Hematol.* 39, 37–46. doi: 10.1016/j.exphem.2010.10.006

Linher-Melville, K., and Singh, G. (2017). The complex roles of STAT3 and STAT5 in maintaining redox balance: lessons from STAT-mediated xCT expression in cancer cells. *Mol. Cell. Endocrinol.* 451, 40–52. doi: 10.1016/j.mce.2017.02.014

Mairbäurl, H., and Weber, R. E. (2012). Oxygen transport by hemoglobin. *Compr. Physiol.* 2, 1463–1489. doi: 10.1002/cphy.c080113

Merino, C. F. (1950). Studies on blood formation and destruction in the polycythemia of high altitude. *Blood* 5, 1–31.

Mihov, D., Vogel, J., Gassmann, M., and Bogdanova, A. (2009). Erythropoietin activates nitric oxide synthase in murine erythrocytes. *Am. J. Physiol.* 297, C378–C388. doi: 10.1152/ajpcell.00543.2008

Milledge, J. S., and Bärtsch, P. (2014). "Blood and haemostasis," in *High Altitude: Human Adaptation to Hypoxia*, eds E.R. Swenson and P. Bärtsch (New York, NY: Springer), 203–216.

Nadarajan, V. S., Ooi, C. H., Sthaneshwar, P., and Thompson, M. W. (2010). The utility of immature reticulocyte fraction as an indicator of erythropoietic response to altitude training in elite cyclists. *Int. J. Lab. Hematol.* 32, 82–87. doi: 10.1111/j.1751-553X.2008.01132.x

Ohi, H., Tamano, M., Sudo, S., and Okada, N. (2003). Recombinant EPO therapy increases erythrocyte expression of complement regulatory proteins. *Am. J. Kidney Dis.* 41, 179–185. doi: 10.1053/ajkd.2003.50002

Pace, N., Meyer, L. B., and Vaughan, B. E. (1956). Erythrolysis on return of altitude acclimatized individuals to sea level. *J. Appl. Physiol.* 9, 141–144. doi: 10.1152/jappl.1956.9.2.141

Pak, O., Sydykov, A., Kosanovic, D., Schermuly, R. T., Dietrich, A., Schroder, K., et al. (2017). Lung ischaemia-reperfusion injury: the role of reactive oxygen species. *Adv. Exp. Med. Biol.* 967, 195–225. doi: 10.1007/978-3-319-63245-2_12

Paulson, R. F., Shi, L., and Wu, D. C. (2011). Stress erythropoiesis: new signals and new stress progenitor cells. *Curr. Opin. Hematol.* 18, 139–145. doi: 10.1097/MOH.0b013e32834521c8

Perry, J. M., Harandi, O. F., and Paulson, R. F. (2007). BMP4, SCF, and hypoxia cooperatively regulate the expansion of murine stress erythroid progenitors. *Blood* 109, 4494–4502. doi: 10.1182/blood-2006-04-016154

Prommer, N., Thoma, S., Quecke, L., Gutekunst, T., Volzke, C., Wachsmuth, N., et al. (2010). Total hemoglobin mass and blood volume of elite Kenyan runners. *Med. Sci. Sports Exerc.* 42, 791–797. doi: 10.1249/MSS.0b013e3181badd67

Rasmussen, P., Siebenmann, C., Diaz, V., and Lundby, C. (2013). Red cell volume expansion at altitude: a meta-analysis and Monte Carlo simulation. *Med. Sci. Sports Exerc.* 45, 1767–1772. doi: 10.1249/MSS.0b013e31829047e5

Reynafarje, C., Lozano, R., and Valdivieso, J. (1959). The polycythemia of high altitudes: iron metabolism and related aspects. *Blood* 14, 433–455.

Rhodes, M. M., Koury, S. T., Kopsombut, P., Alford, C. E., Price, J. O., and Koury, M. J. (2016). Stress reticulocytes lose transferrin receptors by an extrinsic process involving spleen and macrophages. *Am. J. Hematol.* 91, 875–882. doi: 10.1002/ajh.24421

Rice, L., Ruiz, W., Driscoll, T., Whitley, C. E., Tapia, R., Hachey, D. L., et al. (2001). Neocytolysis on descent from altitude: a newly recognized mechanism for the control of red cell mass. *Ann. Intern. Med.* 134, 652–656. doi: 10.7326/0003-4819-134-8-200104170-00010

Rifkind, R. A. (1966). Destruction of injured red cells *in vivo*. *Am. J. Med.* 41, 711–723. doi: 10.1016/0002-9343(66)90032-5

Risso, A., Ciana, A., Achilli, C., Antonutto, G., and Minetti, G. (2014). Neocytolysis: none, one or many? A reappraisal and future perspectives. *Front. Physiol.* 5:54. doi: 10.3389/fphys.2014.00054

Risso, A., Fabbro, D., Damante, G., and Antonutto, G. (2012). Expression of fetal hemoglobin in adult humans exposed to high altitude hypoxia. *Blood Cells Mol. Dis.* 48, 147–153. doi: 10.1016/j.bcmd.2011.12.004

Risso, A., Turello, M., Biffoni, F., and Antonutto, G. (2007). Red blood cell senescence and neocytolysis in humans after high altitude acclimatization. *Blood Cells Mol. Dis.* 38, 83–92. doi: 10.1016/j.bcmd.2006.10.161

Rivella, S. (2009). Ineffective erythropoiesis and thalassemias. *Curr. Opin. Hematol.* 16, 187–194. doi: 10.1097/MOH.0b013e32832990a4

Rogers, S. C., Said, A., Corcuera, D., McLaughlin, D., Kell, P., and Doctor, A. (2009). Hypoxia limits antioxidant capacity in red blood cells by altering glycolytic pathway dominance. *FASEB J.* 23, 3159–3170. doi: 10.1096/fj.09-130666

Ryan, B. J., Wachsmuth, N. B., Schmidt, W. F., Byrnes, W. C., Julian, C. G., Lovering, A. T., et al. (2014). AltitudeOmics: rapid hemoglobin mass alterations with early acclimatization to and de-acclimatization from 5,260 m in healthy humans. *PLoS ONE* 9:e108788. doi: 10.1371/journal.pone.0108788

Sánchez, C., Merino, C., and Figallo, M. (1970). Simultaneous measurement of plasma volume and cell mass in polycythemia of high altitude. *J. Appl. Physiol.* 28, 775–778. doi: 10.1152/jappl.1970.28.6.775

Sandoval, H., Thiagarajan, P., Dasgupta, S. K., Schumacher, A., Prchal, J. T., Chen, M., et al. (2008). Essential role for Nix in autophagic maturation of erythroid cells. *Nature* 454, 232–235. doi: 10.1038/nature07006

Sawka, M. N., Convertino, V. A., Eichner, E. R., Schnieder, S. M., and Young, A. J. (2000). Blood volume: importance and adaptations to exercise training, environmental stresses, and trauma/sickness. *Med. Sci. Sports Exerc.* 32, 332–348. doi: 10.1097/00005768-200002000-00012

Semenza, G. L. (2008). Mitochondrial autophagy: life and breath of the cell. *Autophagy.* 4, 534–536. doi: 10.4161/auto.5956

Siebenmann, C., Robach, P., and Lundby, C. (2017). Regulation of blood volume in lowlanders exposed to high altitude. *J. Appl. Physiol.* 123, 957–966. doi: 10.1152/japplphysiol.00118.2017

Siri, W. E., Van Dyke, D. C., Winchell, H. S., Pollycove, M., Parker, H. G., and Cleveland, A. S. (1966). Early erythropoietin, blood, and physiological responses to severe hypoxia in man. *J. Appl. Physiol.* 21, 73–80. doi: 10.1152/jappl.1966.21.1.73

Song, J., Sundar, K., Gangaraju, R., and Prchal, J. T. (2017). Regulation of erythropoiesis after normoxic return from chronic sustained and intermittent hypoxia. *J. Appl. Physiol.* 123, 1671–1675. doi: 10.1152/japplphysiol.00119.2017

Song, J., Yoon, D., Christensen, R. D., Horvathova, M., Thiagarajan, P., and Prchal, J. T. (2015). HIF-mediated increased ROS from reduced mitophagy and decreased catalase causes neocytolysis. *J. Mol. Med.* 93, 857–866. doi: 10.1007/s00109-015-1294-y

Stray-Gundersen, J., and Levine, B. D. (2008). Live high, train low at natural altitude. *Scand. J. Med. Sci. Sports* 18(Suppl. 1), 21–28. doi: 10.1111/j.1600-0838.2008.00829.x

Terrenato, L., Bertilaccio, C., Spinelli, P., and Colombo, B. (1981). The switch from haemoglobin F to A: the time course of qualitative and quantitative variations of haemoglobins after birth. *Br. J. Haematol.* 47, 31–41. doi: 10.1111/j.1365-2141.1981.tb02759.x

Trial, J., and Rice, L. (2004). Erythropoietin withdrawal leads to the destruction of young red cells at the endothelial-macrophage interface. *Curr. Pharm. Des.* 10, 183–190. doi: 10.2174/1381612043453423

Valtieri, M., Gabbianelli, M., Pelosi, E., Bassano, E., Petti, S., Russo, G., et al. (1989). Erythropoietin alone induces erythroid burst formation by human embryonic but not adult BFU-E in unicellular serum-free culture. *Blood* 74, 460–470.

Wachsmuth, N. B., Volzke, C., Prommer, N., Schmidt-Trucksass, A., Frese, F., Spahl, O., et al. (2013b). The effects of classic altitude training on hemoglobin mass in swimmers. *Eur. J. Appl. Physiol.* 113, 1199–1211. doi: 10.1007/s00421-012-2536-0

Wachsmuth, N., Kley, M., Spielvogel, H., Aughey, R. J., Gore, C. J., Bourdon, P. C., et al. (2013a). Changes in blood gas transport of altitude native soccer players near sea-level and sea-level native soccer players at altitude (ISA3600). *Br. J. Sports Med.* 47(Suppl. 1), i93–i99. doi: 10.1136/bjsports-2013-092761

Weber, R. E., Voelter, W., Fago, A., Echner, H., Campanella, E., and Low, P. S. (2004). Modulation of red cell glycolysis: interactions between vertebrate hemoglobins and cytoplasmic domains of band 3 red cell membrane proteins. *Am. J. Physiol.* 287, R454–R464. doi: 10.1152/ajpregu.00060.2004

Wenger, R. H., and Kurtz, A. (2011). Erythropoietin. *Compr. Physiol.* 1, 1759–1794. doi: 10.1002/cphy.c100075

Wojchowski, D. M., Menon, M. P., Sathyanarayana, P., Fang, J., Karur, V., Houde, E., et al. (2006). Erythropoietin-dependent erythropoiesis: new insights and questions. *Blood Cells Mol. Dis.* 36, 232–238. doi: 10.1016/j.bcmd.2006.01.007

Wu, D. C., and Paulson, R. F. (2010). Hypoxia regulates BMP4 expression in the murine spleen during the recovery from acute anemia. *PLoS ONE* 5:e11303. doi: 10.1371/journal.pone.0011303

Zhang, H., Bosch-Marce, M., Shimoda, L. A., Tan, Y. S., Baek, J. H., Wesley, J. B., et al. (2008). Mitochondrial autophagy is an HIF-1-dependent adaptive metabolic response to hypoxia. *J. Biol. Chem.* 283, 10892–10903. doi: 10.1074/jbc.M800102200

13

Is it Possible to Reverse the Storage-Induced Lesion of Red Blood Cells?

Gregory Barshtein[1]*, Dan Arbell[2], Leonid Livshits[1,3] and Alexander Gural[4]

[1] Faculty of Medicine, Biochemistry Department, Hebrew University of Jerusalem, Jerusalem, Israel, [2] Pediatric Surgery, Hadassah-Hebrew University Medical Center, Jerusalem, Israel, [3] Institute of Veterinary Physiology, University of Zurich, Zürich, Switzerland, [4] Blood Bank, Hadassah-Hebrew University Medical Center, Jerusalem, Israel

***Correspondence:**
Gregory Barshtein
gregoryba@ekmd.huji.ac.il

Cold-storage of packed red blood cells (PRBCs) in the blood bank is reportedly associated with alteration in a wide range of RBC features, which change cell storage each on its own timescale. Thus, some of the changes take place at an early stage of storage (during the first 7 days), while others occur later. We still do not have a clear understanding what happens to the damaged PRBC following their transfusion. We know that some portion (from a few to 10%) of transfused cells with a high degree of damage are removed from the bloodstream immediately or in the first hour(s) after the transfusion. The remaining cells partially restore their functionality and remain in the recipient's blood for a longer time. Thus, the ability of transfused cells to recover is a significant factor in PRBC transfusion effectiveness. In the present review, we discuss publications that examined RBC lesions induced by the cold storage, aiming to offer a better understanding of the time frame in which these lesions occur, with particular emphasis on the question of their reversibility. We argue that transfused RBCs are capable (in a matter of a few hours) of restoring their pre-storage levels of ATP and 2,3-DPG, with subsequent restoration of cell functionality, especially of those properties having a more pronounced ATP-dependence. The extent of reversal is inversely proportional to the extent of damage, and some of the changes cannot be reversed.

Keywords: red blood cells, rejuvenation, erythrocyte membrane, aging, blood banks, transfusion, deformability, fragility

INTRODUCTION

Red blood cell (RBC) transfusion is a life-saving procedure whose primary objective is to sustain tissue and organ oxygenation in patients with massive bleeding or acute anemia. Packed red blood cell (PRBC) donations for transfusion are routinely stored for up to 35 or 42 days, depending on the preservation solution. This time limit has been determined mainly by the recovery and the lifespan of the RBCs in the circulation of recipients.

During cold-storage, PRBCs undergo slow detrimental changes that are collectively termed storage lesion. Oxidative-stress and defective adenosine triphosphate (ATP) metabolism are the main driving forces in the development of PRBC lesion. Storage-related processes lead to significant metabolic and structural changes of erythrocytes that include global biochemical and biophysical alteration, remodeling of the cell membrane and cytoplasm composition (Hess, 2010; Obrador et al., 2015).

The most studied changes include: (ATP) and 2,3-bisphosphoglycerate (2.3-DPG) depletion (Hess, 2010), loss of cellular antioxidant capability (Racek et al., 1997; Dumaswala et al., 2000), changes in K^+ and Na^+ concentration (Olivieri et al., 1993; Cicha et al., 2000), loss of membrane' and skeleton proteins (Ciana et al., 2017; Orbach et al., 2017), loss of membrane lipids and changes in their in/out distribution, vesicle generation (Bosman et al., 2008, 2010), oxidation and remodeling of skeleton proteins (Wolfe et al., 1986), clustering of band 3 proteins (Pantaleo et al., 2008; Arashiki et al., 2013), alteration of nitric oxide signaling (Almac et al., 2014; Liu et al., 2014), decrease in antioxidant activity (Dumaswala et al., 1999; Dzik, 2008; Whillier et al., 2011) etc.

A number of these changes are interrelated and initiate a cascade of biochemical and structural changes which in turn lead to impairment in RBC functionality, specifically – alteration in the biophysical/mechanical properties of cells.

Each of the reported storage-induced alterations in PRBC properties occurs on its specific time-scale (d'Almeida et al., 2000; Bennett-Guerrero et al., 2007; D'Amici et al., 2007; Relevy et al., 2008; D'Alessandro et al., 2012; Gevi et al., 2012; Santacruz-Gomez et al., 2014; Kozlova et al., 2015; Bardyn et al., 2017). Some of these changes take place at an early stage of storage (during the first 7 days), while others occur later. Prudent et al. (2015) have extensively discussed this issue, distinguishing between the separate phases of PRBCs lesion development and providing a detailed scheme of the various changes on a time-scale. Different stages of cell aging are also reported by Nishino et al. (2009, 2013) and Gevi et al. (2012).

When a patient is being transfused with a PRBCs unit, cells with a specific set of features are administered into his bloodstream. Senescent transfused cells, with a high degree of damage, are removed from the bloodstream shortly following the transfusion (Hunsicker et al., 2018). Furthermore, we have recently demonstrated a dependence of transfusion-induced hemoglobin increment (determined upon completion of the transfusion) on the percentage of low-deformable cells in the population of the transfused RBCs (TRBCs) unit (Barshtein et al., 2017). We suggested that during the transfusion the relatively rigid cells in the TRBCs population (composing dozens of percentages) are immediately removed itself. This suggestion is in accord with previous reports indicating that the clearance of TRBCs starts directly with the administration of cells into the bloodstream (Luten et al., 2008; Bosman, 2013).

Rigid and fragile RBC are subject to facilitated removal from circulation within the first hours after transfusion, due to shear forces operating in the bloodstream (Nagababu et al., 2016). Thus, Luten et al. (2008) concluded that significant portion of the TRBCs that do not survive the first 24 h are removed from the circulation within the first few hours after transfusion.

Following removal of the extremely damaged cells, most of the TRBCs [in the range of 75% (Luten et al., 2008)] remain in the bloodstream of the recipient in an environment substantially different from the one in which they were stored. As a result, the remaining TRBCs can partially restore their functionality and to remain in the recipient's blood for a more extended period. The average lifespan of transfused RBCs is about 50–60 days, but it can be significantly shorter in the presence of factors reducing their survival (Liumbruno et al., 2009).

Accordingly, an assessment of reversibility of the cold-storage lesion is a critical issue in the field of RBCs storage and transfusion as the ability of transfused RBCs to restore their properties following transfusion. This ability largely determines TRBCs behavior in the bloodstream of the recipient.

In the present review, we discuss publications that examined RBC lesions induced by the cold-storage, aiming to offer a better understanding of the time frame in which these lesions occur, with particular emphasis on the question of their reversibility. Also, we propose an approach for assessing the potential for reversibility of the damage to specific properties of PRBCs.

POST-TRANSFUSION BEHAVIOR OF RBCs

Of all the properties of TRBCs, the ability to restore of ATP and 2,3-DPG levels is most extensively discussed in the literature. Since some physiological factors can modify the time course of the post-transfusion restoration, the reported time needed for full recovery varies widely from several hours to several days (Valtis, 1954; Beutler and Wood, 1969; Valeri and Hirsch, 1969; Enoki et al., 1986; Heaton et al., 1989). The ATP level in TRBCs rapidly increases in the recipient's bloodstream (Valeri and Hirsch, 1969; Heaton et al., 1989). Valeri and Hirsch (1969) suggested that this effect is associated with a rapid decrease in the donor cell Na^+ content during the 24 h post-transfusion period. In parallel, TRBC cellular K^+ content is gradually increased, with the rate of this increase being related to the increasing level of intracellular 2,3-DPG (Valeri and Hirsch, 1969).

Heaton et al. (1989) measured the levels of 2,3-DPG and ATP in transfused cells for 1 week following the transfusion. The authors demonstrated that an average of 95% of the recipients' pre-transfusion 2,3-DPG level was reached by 72 h, while ATP level in started increasing 1 h after transfusion (Heaton et al., 1989). D'Alessandro et al. (2010) have reported that the repairing of Na^+/K^+ pump activity occurred during 1 to 4 days.

In contrast to the data presented so far, some publications (Frank et al., 2013; Chadebech et al., 2016, 2017) have reported a deterioration in the TRBCs properties following their interaction with human plasma. Thus, Chadebech et al. (2016, 2017) demonstrated that an *ex vivo* incubation of PRBCs with the plasma of healthy subjects (Chadebech et al., 2016, 2017), patients with sepsis (Chadebech et al., 2017) and sickle anemia patients (Chadebech et al., 2016) induced alterations in the phosphatidylserine (PS) externalization and a decrease in the average cell size.

Frank et al. (2013) measured deformability of RBCs from post-surgery patients prior to and following a moderate ($\geq$five units) or a minimal ($\leq$four units) PRBC transfusion. They demonstrated that deformability of the patients' RBCs has decreased following transfusion as compared to pre-transfusion cells, and this abnormality was not reversed and even got worse during the subsequent 3 days.

WHAT LESION IS REVERSIBLE?

Which are the properties of the stored PRBCs that we can expect to be corrected, and which ones are not? This question is extensively discussed in the literature (Beutler et al., 1982; Luten et al., 2008; D'Alessandro et al., 2010; Prudent et al., 2015). For example, D'Alessandro et al. suggest that the reversibility of these changes is inversely proportional to the duration of storage (D'Alessandro et al., 2010). Prudent et al. takes a similar position (Prudent et al., 2015), with the authors concluding that an "early" lesion (i.e., one that occurs following first 2 weeks of storage) is reversible, while a "late" lesion (4 weeks and more) is not. This suggestion is supported by *in vivo* studies of TRBCs performed by Beutler et al. (1982) and Luten et al. (2008), who conclude that RBC storage is associated with irreversible damage that increases with storage duration.

DO ANY IRREVERSIBLE CHANGES OCCUR IN THE EARLY STAGES OF STORAGE?

During the first week of storage, RBC lesion is characterized by the formation of micro-defects in the RBC membrane and a decrease in the membrane roughness, as assessed by atomic force microscopy (Girasole et al., 2012; Pompeo et al., 2012; Kozlova et al., 2015; Acosta-Elias et al., 2017). For example, Kozlova et al. (2015) demonstrated that by days 9 to 12 topological defects in the form of "domains" appear on the membrane surface. These defects initially appear as grain-like structures ("grains") of up to 200 nm (on days 16–23), and later merge to form large defects, 400–1000 nm. This observation conforms with that of Girasole et al. (2012) and Pompeo et al. (2012), who used atomic force microscopy to examine storage-induced structural and metabolic changes in PRBCs. The authors demonstrated that the RBC roughness might be restored to the initial value only in samples stored for up to 4–5 days, whereas after the eighth day of storage the rejuvenation procedure appears to be inefficient. Girasole et al. (2010, 2012) concluded that some changes, localized on the membrane surface, appear when the ATP synthesis capacity declines to apparently sub-viable levels and the membrane-skeleton is permanently damaged (Pompeo et al., 2012).

Moreover, irreversible reduction in surface charge (Godin and Caprani, 1997; Silva et al., 2012; Erman et al., 2016) has been observed under different conditions of RBC *in vitro* aging. Specifically, Silva et al. (2012) examined the effect of cold-storage of human RBCs (collected into CPD-SAGM, leukodepleted and unleukodepleted) on the ξ-potential of the cell membrane, and demonstrated that the ξ-potential of cells decreases during the first week of storage. The same authors (Silva et al., 2012) have also demonstrated that ξ-potential decay (30%) of RBC samples (leukodepleted and not) was more pronounced during the first week of storage, suggesting that this decay is caused by oxidative damage generated by the production of reactive oxygen species.

The authors suggest that the decrease in RBC deformability observed during cell aging (*in vivo*) (Huang et al., 2014) and cold storage (Silva et al., 2012) could arise from a reduction of their ξ-potential.

Moreover, a release of microvesicles from RBC membrane starts at the second week of cold-storage. These vesicles are characterized by a significant fraction of lipid raft proteins [such as stomatin and flotillins (Salzer and Prohaska, 2001)] as well as oxidized or reactive signaling components commonly associated with senescent RBCs. Kriebardis et al. (2008) demonstrated that the vesicular protein content progressively increased over time, with a twofold increase in PRBCs stored for 17 days as compared to those stored for 7 days.

The formation of microvesicles leads to a decrease in the content of membrane proteins (Salzer and Prohaska, 2001; Wilkinson et al., 2008; D'Alessandro et al., 2012) and a change in the composition of the cytoskeleton. Thus, Ciana et al. (2017) suggested that part of the membrane skeleton is lost together with components of the lipid bilayer in a balanced way.

Song et al. (2017) demonstrated that during cold-storage the protein components of RBC skeleton are partially decomposed. The thickness of the cell membrane is reduced during storage and, specifically, shows a sharp decrease from the 6th to the 14th day of cold-storage.

Mechanism of vesiculation is discussed in detail in numerous publications (D'Alessandro et al., 2015; Antonelou and Seghatchian, 2016; Ciana et al., 2017). Nonetheless, the selective sorting of specific membrane components into microvesicles remains to be understood. In any case, regardless of the mechanism, the formation of vesicles leads to irreversible changes in the composition and structure of the membrane. Specifically, it induces a decrease in the area-volume ratio, which affects the cells' shape, their mechanical properties (Svetina, 2012) and survival in the bloodstream (Deplaine et al., 2011).

Thus, some basic cells properties are irreversibly altered during the first to third week of storage. These changes necessarily produce alterations in the functionality of the transfused erythrocytes, some of which cannot be fully reversed following transfusion (Barshtein et al., 2014).

POST-STORAGE REJUVENATION TREATMENT *IN VITRO*

One of the possible procedures proposed for the reversal of storage-induced damage is post-storage rejuvenation treatment, which consists of supplementing PRBC units with rejuvenation solution before their transfusion (Kiartivich et al., 1986; Lockwood et al., 2003; Verhoeven et al., 2006; Raat et al., 2009). A commercially available rejuvenation solution is produced under trademark Rejuvesol and consists of sodium pyruvate, inosine, adenine, and sodium phosphate. The FDA approves this solution and, although rarely applied in clinical blood banking, is widely used in research for restoring cellular ATP and 2,3-DPG levels (d'Almeida et al., 2000; Yoshida et al., 2008; Meyer et al., 2011). Of course, the research results should be interpreted with caution as an *in vitro* method with significant limitations for clinical interpretation.

The rejuvenation procedure can be carried out at 37°C ("warm") and 4°C ("cold"), with the "warm" type being more extensively studied than the cold one. Still, a comparison of the results reported by different authors (d'Almeida et al., 2000; Koshkaryev et al., 2009; Tchir et al., 2013; Barshtein et al., 2014; Kurach et al., 2014) leads to the conclusion that rejuvenation is more effective when performed at 37°C. In the following section, we will only consider results obtained with a warm treatment, which is consistent with the objective of the present review.

Indeed, during previous attempts to attenuate the impairment of PRBCs functionality caused by cold-storage, it was shown that rejuvenation treatment could restore intra-cellular ATP and 2,3-DPG levels and thus reverse a storage-induced alteration to various properties of cells (Dumaswala et al., 1992; Koshkaryev et al., 2009; Barshtein et al., 2014). Specifically, rejuvenation leads to repairing of PRBCs morphology (Usry et al., 1975) and mechanical properties: deformability (Barras et al., 1994; d'Almeida et al., 2000; Barshtein et al., 2014) and fragility (DeVenuto et al., 1974; Gelderman and Vostal, 2011; Barshtein et al., 2014), although, as could be expected, this positive effect decreases with an increasing storage duration (d'Almeida et al., 2000; Meyer et al., 2011).

Importantly, the effect of rejuvenation on stored PRBCs is not limited to the restoration of intracellular levels of ATP and 2,3-DPG: it was shown that treatment of stored cells by Rejuvesol had induced significant metabolic reprogramming, including reactivation of energy-generating and antioxidant pathways, and membrane lipid recycling (D'Alessandro et al., 2017).

REVERSIBILITY OF PRBC LESION *IN VITRO*

In this section, we will focus on the reversibility of specific functional properties of cells that determine their behavior after transfusion to the patient, especially – PS externalization and mechanical properties of their membrane.

The regulated plasma/membrane PS asymmetry is critical to many biological processes (Bratosin et al., 1998; Kuypers and de Jong, 2004; Lutz and Bogdanova, 2013; Dinkla et al., 2014). Thus, it has been shown that PRBCs storage initiates Ca^{2+} influx into cells with subsequent PS externalization and amplifies the susceptibility of TRBCs to eryptosis, the "suicidal" death (Lang et al., 2016). Furthermore, erythrocyte surface PS has been reported to activate coagulation and thus induce thrombosis (Chung et al., 2007; Shin et al., 2007; Gao et al., 2012).

PS externalization can be mediated by the decrease in the ATP level (Bitbol et al., 1987) and/or by activation of scramblase (Basse et al., 1996; Woon et al., 1999). Therefore, the storage-induced increase in intracellular $[Ca^{2+}]$ (Koshkaryev et al., 2009; Lang et al., 2016) may be sufficient to induce the observed elevation of PS-positive PRBCs via the activation of scramblase (Basse et al., 1996; Woon et al., 1999). Alternatively, Verhoeven et al. (2006) have reported that cold-storage did not activate scramblase (by Ca^{2+} influx), but rather inhibited flippase activity as a result of ATP depletion, which was subsequently reversed by the treatment with Rejuvesol (d'Almeida et al., 2000; Yoshida et al., 2008; Meyer et al., 2011). However, whatever the mechanism of action, since intracellular Ca^{2+} concentration is ATP dependent (Maher and Kuchel, 2003), the renewal of ATP content in PRBCs as a result of rejuvenation should lead to the restoring of phospholipids' asymmetry (Maher and Kuchel, 2003).

In agreement with this assumption, Koshkaryev et al. (2009) have recently shown that the storage-induced alterations in PRBCs (elevation of $[Ca^{2+}]$, and PS externalization) are almost completely rectified by post-storage rejuvenation treatment, which caused a decrease in RBC adhesion to endothelial cells.

In discrepancy to this observation, in our publication (Barshtein et al., 2014) we demonstrated that treatment with the Rejuvesol causes only partial restoration of the cells' mechanical properties (deformability and fragility).

To explain the difference in rejuvenation efficiency reported by different groups, we assumed that it is related to the degree of dependency of the specific property on the intracellular ATP concentration.

Indeed, it is well-known that various RBC functions and properties are mainly, if not solely, determined by the cell ATP level. Thus, it is plausible to expect the rejuvenation to be more effective in restoring cell properties that are strongly ATP-dependent.

To assess rejuvenation effectiveness (i.e., the degree of reversibility) we have formulated (Barshtein et al., 2014) rejuvenation effectiveness index (REI), describing the percentage of storage-induced damage to a specific RBC property that is restored by treatment.

In our publication (Barshtein et al., 2014) we summarized previously obtained results regarding reversibility of PRBC lesion and had shown that treatment of PRBCs with Rejuvesol had restored all tested properties. However, the extent of improvement varied considerably between the different measures, leading us to suggest that the REI is higher for features that are more ATP-dependent. Thus, for intracellular Ca^{2+} content and the level of PS externalization, REI is nearly 70%, with full recovery of RBC adhesion. In contrast, the rejuvenation efficacy in repairing the PRBC mechanical properties (deformability and fragility), was only 50%.

Of particular interest are the findings previously presented by us (Barshtein et al., 2014), showing that the efficacy of rejuvenation in the reversal of storage-induced impairment in the RBC mechanical properties depends on the extent of damage – thus, the higher the damage, the lesser the rejuvenation efficacy (Barshtein et al., 2014). Changes in RBC mechanical properties are often associated with irreversible structural alterations, such as changes in RBC surface-to-volume ratio due to vesiculation (Safeukui et al., 2012), or reduction in surface charge due to sialic acid degradation (Godin and Caprani, 1997; Huang et al., 2014), which are not expected to be affected by restoring the ATP content of RBC. These changes in the RBC membrane structure have been reported to increase with storage duration (Silva et al., 2012), thereby explaining why the rejuvenation efficacy is inversely related to the extent of storage-induced damage to PRBCs mechanical properties.

Thus, the ability of PRBCs to reverse (wholly or partially) their deformability and intracellular [2,3-DPG] content can explain the results obtained by Raat et al. (2009). The authors tested human PRBCs in an isovolemic transfusion model in rats after hemodilution. The cells were derived from units of PRBCs and transfused to animals with or without rejuvenation treatment before transfusion. It was demonstrated (Raat et al., 2009) that the rejuvenation of cells can completely reverse the reduced oxygenation capacity of long-stored human PRBCs in hemodiluted rats before transfusion.

LIMITATIONS

In presented mini-review, we discussed the reversibility of PRBC lesion induced by cold-storage. For this purpose, we reviewed different studies examining PRBC recovery under *in vivo, ex vivo,* and *in vitro* conditions. However, it is necessary to take into account the difference between the potential recoverability of a cell's specific feature(s), and the possibility of its restoration after a PRBC transfusion to the patient.

FUTURE DIRECTION

As demonstrated above, the reversibility of the RBC lesion *in vitro* (by incubation with Rejuvesol) has been extensively discussed in the cited literature. Unfortunately, this issue has been poorly studied under *in vivo* conditions, despite its theoretical and practical significance in assessing the role that storage lesion plays in transfusion outcome. Currently, PRBC units are supplied for transfusion on the first-in-first-out (FIFO) basis, assuming that their functionality is equal for all units with equal pre-transfusion storage duration. Thus, a number of large-scale clinical trials, both published (Hod et al., 2011; Steiner et al., 2015; Rapido et al., 2017; Stowell et al., 2017) and ongoing (Kekre et al., 2013), have focused their attention on the conditions of storage (specifically – on storage duration), and not on the properties of transfused RBCs and the reversibility of the storage lesion in the bloodstream. We believe that studying the PRBC lesion reversibility after transfusion should be the future direction of research on this subject, being of fundamental importance for assessing the survival of TRBCs in the bloodstream, and potentially leading to the improvement in the transfusion outcome.

CONCLUSION

It is well-documented that the cold-storage of PRBC units is associated with a change in a wide range of RBCs properties, each of them taking place on its own specific timescale. Thus, even at an early stage of storage (the first or second week), irreversible changes in the properties of the cells can already occur.

Despite the fact that the behavior of TRBCs in the recipient's bloodstream is still insufficiently studied, it can be argued at this stage that transfused cells are capable of restoring the pre-storage levels of ATP and 2,3-DPG, with subsequent restoration of cell functionality. This assumption is confirmed by the results of *in vitro* experiments demonstrating significant restoration of various PRBC features following incubation with a rejuvenation solution, especially those with a more pronounced ATP-dependence. The extent of reversal is inversely proportional to the extent of damage, and some of the changes cannot be fully reversed.

We hope that this review may stimulate further research into the field of cold storage and rejuvenation discussed here, and thus aid in the formulation of a new paradigm for PRBCs units inventory management.

AUTHOR CONTRIBUTIONS

GB, DA, LL, and AG have been involved in the analysis and discussion of studies relating to the subject and in the writing of the review.

REFERENCES

Acosta-Elias, M. A., Burgara-Estrella, A. J., Sarabia-Sainz, J. A., Silva-Campa, E., Angulo-Molina, A., Santacruz-Gomez, K. J., et al. (2017). Nano alterations of membrane structure on both gamma-irradiated and stored human erythrocytes. *Int. J. Radiat. Biol.* 93, 1306–1311. doi: 10.1080/09553002.2017.1393581

Almac, E., Bezemer, R., Hilarius-Stokman, P. M., Goedhart, P., de Korte, D., Verhoeven, A. J., et al. (2014). Red blood cell storage increases hypoxia-induced nitric oxide bioavailability and methemoglobin formation in vitro and in vivo. *Transfusion* 54, 3178–3185. doi: 10.1111/trf.12738

Antonelou, M. H., and Seghatchian, J. (2016). Update on extracellular vesicles inside red blood cell storage units: adjust the sails closer to the new wind. *Transfus. Apher. Sci.* 55, 92–104. doi: 10.1016/j.transci.2016.07.016

Arashiki, N., Kimata, N., Manno, S., Mohandas, N., and Takakuwa, Y. (2013). Membrane peroxidation and methemoglobin formation are both necessary for band 3 clustering: mechanistic insights into human erythrocyte senescence. *Biochemistry* 52, 5760–5769. doi: 10.1021/bi400405p

Bardyn, M., Rappaz, B., Jaferzadeh, K., Crettaz, D., Tissot, J. D., Moon, I., et al. (2017). Red blood cells ageing markers: a multi-parametric analysis. *Blood Transfus.* 15, 239–248. doi: 10.2450/2017.0318-16

Barras, J. P., Moldovanyi, A., Wagner, S., and Koerner, K. (1994). [Effect of rejuvenation on the rheologic properties of stored erythrocytes]. *Vasa* 23, 305–311.

Barshtein, G., Goldschmidt, N., Pries, A. R., Zelig, O., Arbell, D., and Yedgar, S. (2017). Deformability of transfused red blood cells is a potent effector of transfusion-induced hemoglobin increment: a study with beta-thalassemia major patients. *Am. J. Hematol.* 92, E559–E560. doi: 10.1002/ajh.24821

Barshtein, G., Gural, A., Manny, N., Zelig, O., Yedgar, S., and Arbell, D. (2014). Storage-induced damage to red blood cell mechanical properties can be only partially reversed by rejuvenation. *Transfus. Med. Hemother.* 41, 197–204. doi: 10.1159/000357986

Basse, F., Stout, J. G., Sims, P. J., and Wiedmer, T. (1996). Isolation of an erythrocyte membrane protein that mediates Ca^{2+}-dependent transbilayer movement of phospholipid. *J. Biol. Chem.* 271, 17205–17210. doi: 10.1074/jbc.271.29.17205

Bennett-Guerrero, E., Veldman, T. H., Doctor, A., Telen, M. J., Ortel, T. L., Reid, T. S., et al. (2007). Evolution of adverse changes in stored RBCs. *Proc. Natl. Acad. Sci. U.S.A.* 104, 17063–17068. doi: 10.1073/pnas.0708160104

Beutler, E., Kuhl, W., and West, C. (1982). The osmotic fragility of erythrocytes after prolonged liquid storage and after reinfusion. *Blood* 59, 1141–1147.

Beutler, E., and Wood, L. (1969). The in vivo regeneration of red cell 2,3 diphosphoglyceric acid (DPG) after transfusion of stored blood. *J. Lab. Clin. Med.* 74, 300–304.

Bitbol, M., Fellmann, P., Zachowski, A., and Devaux, P. F. (1987). Ion regulation of phosphatidylserine and phosphatidylethanolamine outside-inside translocation in human erythrocytes. *Biochim. Biophys. Acta* 904, 268–282. doi: 10.1016/0005-2736(87)90376-2

Bosman, G. J. (2013). Survival of red blood cells after transfusion: processes and consequences. *Front. Physiol.* 4:376. doi: 10.3389/fphys.2013.00376

Bosman, G. J., Stappers, M., and Novotny, V. M. (2010). Changes in band 3 structure as determinants of erythrocyte integrity during storage and survival after transfusion. *Blood Transfus.* 8, S48–S52. doi: 10.2450/2010.008s

Bosman, G. J., Werre, J. M., Willekens, F. L., and Novotny, V. M. (2008). Erythrocyte ageing in vivo and in vitro: structural aspects and implications for transfusion. *Transfus. Med.* 18, 335–347. doi: 10.1111/j.1365-3148.2008.00892.x

Bratosin, D., Mazurier, J., Tissier, J. P., Estaquier, J., Huart, J. J., Ameisen, J. C., et al. (1998). Cellular and molecular mechanisms of senescent erythrocyte phagocytosis by macrophages. A review. *Biochimie* 80, 173–195. doi: 10.1016/S0300-9084(98)80024-2

Chadebech, P., Bodivit, G., Razazi, K., de Vassoigne, C., Pelle, L., Burin-des-Roziers, N., et al. (2017). Red blood cells for transfusion in patients with sepsis: respective roles of unit age and exposure to recipient plasma. *Transfusion* 57, 1898–1904. doi: 10.1111/trf.14170

Chadebech, P., de Menorval, M. A., Bodivit, G., Mekontso-Dessap, A., Pakdaman, S., Jouard, A., et al. (2016). Evidence of benefits from using fresh and cryopreserved blood to transfuse patients with acute sickle cell disease. *Transfusion* 56, 1730–1738. doi: 10.1111/trf.13636

Chung, S. M., Bae, O. N., Lim, K. M., Noh, J. Y., Lee, M. Y., Jung, Y. S., et al. (2007). Lysophosphatidic acid induces thrombogenic activity through phosphatidylserine exposure and procoagulant microvesicle generation in human erythrocytes. *Arterioscler. Thromb. Vasc. Biol.* 27, 414–421. doi: 10.1161/01.ATV.0000252898.48084.6a

Ciana, A., Achilli, C., and Minetti, G. (2017). Spectrin and other membrane-skeletal components in human red blood cells of different age. *Cell. Physiol. Biochem.* 42, 1139–1152. doi: 10.1159/000478769

Cicha, I., Suzuki, Y., Tateishi, N., Shiba, M., Muraoka, M., Tadokoro, K., et al. (2000). Gamma-ray-irradiated red blood cells stored in mannitol-adenine-phosphate medium: rheological evaluation and susceptibility to oxidative stress. *Vox Sang.* 79, 75–82. doi: 10.1046/j.1423-0410.2000.7920075.x

D'Alessandro, A., D'Amici, G. M., Vaglio, S., and Zolla, L. (2012). Time-course investigation of SAGM-stored leukocyte-filtered red bood cell concentrates: from metabolism to proteomics. *Haematologica* 97, 107–115. doi: 10.3324/haematol.2011.051789

D'Alessandro, A., Gray, A. D., Szczepiorkowski, Z. M., Hansen, K., Herschel, L. H., and Dumont, L. J. (2017). Red blood cell metabolic responses to refrigerated storage, rejuvenation, and frozen storage. *Transfusion* 57, 1019–1030. doi: 10.1111/trf.14034

D'Alessandro, A., Kriebardis, A. G., Rinalducci, S., Antonelou, M. H., Hansen, K. C., Papassideri, I. S., et al. (2015). An update on red blood cell storage lesions, as gleaned through biochemistry and omics technologies. *Transfusion* 55, 205–219. doi: 10.1111/trf.12804

D'Alessandro, A., Liumbruno, G., Grazzini, G., and Zolla, L. (2010). Red blood cell storage: the story so far. *Blood Transfus.* 8, 82–88. doi: 10.2450/2009.0122-09

d'Almeida, M. S., Jagger, J., Duggan, M., White, M., Ellis, C., and Chin-Yee, I. H. (2000). A comparison of biochemical and functional alterations of rat and human erythrocytes stored in CPDA-1 for 29 days: implications for animal models of transfusion. *Transfus. Med.* 10, 291–303. doi: 10.1046/j.1365-3148.2000.00267.x

D'Amici, G. M., Rinalducci, S., and Zolla, L. (2007). Proteomic analysis of RBC membrane protein degradation during blood storage. *J. Proteome Res.* 6, 3242–3255. doi: 10.1021/pr070179d

Deplaine, G., Safeukui, I., Jeddi, F., Lacoste, F., Brousse, V., Perrot, S., et al. (2011). The sensing of poorly deformable red blood cells by the human spleen can be mimicked in vitro. *Blood* 117, e88–e95. doi: 10.1182/blood-2010-10-312801

DeVenuto, F., Brenneman, G., and Wilson, S. M. (1974). Rejuvenation of human red blood cells during liquid storage. *Transfusion* 14, 338–344. doi: 10.1111/j.1537-2995.1974.tb04542.x

Dinkla, S., Peppelman, M., van der Raadt, J., Atsma, F., Novotny, V. M., van Kraaij, M. G., et al. (2014). Phosphatidylserine exposure on stored red blood cells as a parameter for donor-dependent variation in product quality. *Blood Transfus.* 12, 204–209. doi: 10.2450/2013.0106-13

Dumaswala, U. J., Petrosky, T. L., and Greenwalt, T. J. (1992). Studies in red blood cell preservation. 6. Red cell membrane remodeling during rejuvenation. *Vox Sang.* 63, 12–15. doi: 10.1111/j.1423-0410.1992.tb01212.x

Dumaswala, U. J., Wilson, M. J., Wu, Y. L., Wykle, J., Zhuo, L., Douglass, L. M., et al. (2000). Glutathione loading prevents free radical injury in red blood cells after storage. *Free Radic. Res.* 33, 517–529. doi: 10.1080/10715760000301061

Dumaswala, U. J., Zhuo, L., Jacobsen, D. W., Jain, S. K., and Sukalski, K. A. (1999). Protein and lipid oxidation of banked human erythrocytes: role of glutathione. *Free Radic. Biol. Med.* 27, 1041–1049. doi: 10.1016/S0891-5849(99)00149-5

Dzik, W. (2008). Fresh blood for everyone? Balancing availability and quality of stored RBCs. *Transfus. Med.* 18, 260–265. doi: 10.1111/j.1365-3148.2008.00870.x

Enoki, Y., Watanabe, T., and Ohga, Y. (1986). Posttransfusional recovery of defective respiratory function of stored blood in dogs. *Jpn. J. Physiol.* 36, 1125–1139. doi: 10.2170/jjphysiol.36.1125

Erman, H., Aksu, U., Belce, A., Atukeren, P., Uzun, D., Cebe, T., et al. (2016). Gender and chronological age affect erythrocyte membrane oxidative indices in citrate phosphate dextrose adenine-formula 1 (CPDA-1) blood bank storage condition. *Gen. Physiol. Biophys.* 35, 343–351. doi: 10.4149/gpb_2016001

Frank, S. M., Abazyan, B., Ono, M., Hogue, C. W., Cohen, D. B., Berkowitz, D. E., et al. (2013). Decreased erythrocyte deformability after transfusion and the effects of erythrocyte storage duration. *Anesth. Analg.* 116, 975–981. doi: 10.1213/ANE.0b013e31828843e6

Gao, C., Xie, R., Yu, C., Wang, Q., Shi, F., Yao, C., et al. (2012). Procoagulant activity of erythrocytes and platelets through phosphatidylserine exposure and microparticles release in patients with nephrotic syndrome. *Thromb. Haemost.* 107, 681–689. doi: 10.1160/TH11-09-0673

Gelderman, M. P., and Vostal, J. G. (2011). Rejuvenation improves roller pump-induced physical stress resistance of fresh and stored red blood cells. *Transfusion* 51, 1096–1104. doi: 10.1111/j.1537-2995.2010.02972.x

Gevi, F., D'Alessandro, A., Rinalducci, S., and Zolla, L. (2012). Alterations of red blood cell metabolome during cold liquid storage of erythrocyte concentrates in CPD-SAGM. *J. Proteomics* 76, 168–180. doi: 10.1016/j.jprot.2012.03.012

Girasole, M., Pompeo, G., Cricenti, A., Longo, G., Boumis, G., Bellelli, A., et al. (2010). The how, when, and why of the aging signals appearing on the human erythrocyte membrane: an atomic force microscopy study of surface roughness. *Nanomedicine* 6, 760–768. doi: 10.1016/j.nano.2010.06.004

Girasole, M., Pompeo, G., Cricenti, A., Longo, G., Boumis, G., Bellelli, A., et al. (2012). The how, when, and why of the aging signals appearing on the human erythrocyte membrane: an atomic force microscopy study of surface roughness. *Nanomedicine* 6, 760–768. doi: 10.1016/j.nano.2010.06.004

Godin, C., and Caprani, A. (1997). Effect of blood storage on erythrocyte/wall interactions: implications for surface charge and rigidity. *Eur. Biophys. J.* 26, 175–182. doi: 10.1007/s002490050069

Heaton, A., Keegan, T., and Holme, S. (1989). In vivo regeneration of red cell 2,3-diphosphoglycerate following transfusion of DPG-depleted AS-1, AS-3 and CPDA-1 red cells. *Br. J. Haematol.* 71, 131–136. doi: 10.1111/j.1365-2141.1989.tb06286.x

Hess, J. R. (2010). Red cell storage. *J. Proteomics* 73, 368–373. doi: 10.1016/j.jprot.2009.11.005

Hod, E. A., Brittenham, G. M., Billote, G. B., Francis, R. O., Ginzburg, Y. Z., Hendrickson, J. E., et al. (2011). Transfusion of human volunteers with older, stored red blood cells produces extravascular hemolysis and circulating non-transferrin-bound iron. *Blood* 118, 6675–6682. doi: 10.1182/blood-2011-08-371849

Huang, Y. X., Wu, Z. J., Mehrishi, J., Huang, B. T., Chen, X. Y., Zheng, X. J., et al. (2014). Human red blood cell aging: correlative changes in surface charge and cell properties. *J. Cell. Mol. Med.* 15, 2634–2642. doi: 10.1111/j.1582-4934.2011.01310.x

Hunsicker, O., Hessler, K., Krannich, A., Boemke, W., Braicu, I., Sehouli, J., et al. (2018). Duration of storage influences the hemoglobin rising effect of red blood cells in patients undergoing major abdominal surgery. *Transfusion* doi: 10.1111/trf.14627

Kekre, N., Mallick, R., Allan, D., Tinmouth, A., and Tay, J. (2013). The impact of prolonged storage of red blood cells on cancer survival. *PLoS One* 8:e68820. doi: 10.1371/journal.pone.0068820

Kiartivich, S., Talalak, P., and Chandanayingyoung, D. (1986). The effect of rejuvenation on 2, 3-DPG level of preserved red blood cells. *J. Med. Assoc. Thai.* 69, 665–671.

Koshkaryev, A., Zelig, O., Manny, N., Yedgar, S., and Barshtein, G. (2009). Rejuvenation treatment of stored red blood cells reverses storage-induced adhesion to vascular endothelial cells. *Transfusion* 49, 2136–2143. doi: 10.1111/j.1537-2995.2009.02251.x

Kozlova, E., Chernysh, A., Moroz, V., Sergunova, V., Gudkova, O., and Kuzovlev, A. (2015). Nanodefects of membranes cause destruction of packed red blood cells during long-term storage. *Exp. Cell Res.* 337, 192–201. doi: 10.1016/j.yexcr.2015.07.009

Kriebardis, A. G., Antonelou, M. H., Stamoulis, K. E., Economou-Petersen, E., Margaritis, L. H., and Papassideri, I. S. (2008). RBC-derived vesicles during storage: ultrastructure, protein composition, oxidation, and signaling components. *Transfusion* 48, 1943–1953. doi: 10.1111/j.1537-2995.2008.01794.x

Kurach, J. D., Almizraq, R., Bicalho, B., Acker, J. P., and Holovati, J. L. (2014). The effects of rejuvenation during hypothermic storage on red blood cell membrane remodeling. *Transfusion* 54, 1595–1603. doi: 10.1111/trf.12490

Kuypers, F. A., and de Jong, K. (2004). The role of phosphatidylserine in recognition and removal of erythrocytes. *Cell. Mol. Biol.* 50, 147–158.

Lang, E., Pozdeev, V. I., Xu, H. C., Shinde, P. V., Behnke, K., Hamdam, J. M., et al. (2016). Storage of erythrocytes induces suicidal erythrocyte death. *Cell. Physiol. Biochem.* 39, 668–676. doi: 10.1159/000445657

Liu, C., Liu, X., Janes, J., Stapley, R., Patel, R. P., Gladwin, M. T., et al. (2014). Mechanism of faster NO scavenging by older stored red blood cells. *Redox Biol.* 2, 211–219. doi: 10.1016/j.redox.2013.12.014

Liumbruno, G., Bennardello, F., Lattanzio, A., Piccoli, P., and Rossetti, G. (2009). Recommendations for the transfusion of red blood cells. *Blood Transfus.* 7, 49–64. doi: 10.2450/2008.0020-08

Lockwood, W. B., Hudgens, R. W., Szymanski, I. O., Teno, R. A., and Gray, A. D. (2003). Effects of rejuvenation and frozen storage on 42-day-old AS-3 RBCs. *Transfusion* 43, 1527–1532. doi: 10.1046/j.1537-2995.2003.00551.x

Luten, M., Roerdinkholder-Stoelwinder, B., Schaap, N. P., de Grip, W. J., Bos, H. J., and Bosman, G. J. (2008). Survival of red blood cells after transfusion: a comparison between red cells concentrates of different storage periods. *Transfusion* 48, 1478–1485. doi: 10.1111/j.1537-2995.2008.01734.x

Lutz, H. U., and Bogdanova, A. (2013). Mechanisms tagging senescent red blood cells for clearance in healthy humans. *Front. Physiol.* 4:387. doi: 10.3389/fphys.2013.00387

Maher, A. D., and Kuchel, P. W. (2003). The Gardos channel: a review of the Ca^{2+}-activated K^+ channel in human erythrocytes. *Int. J. Biochem. Cell Biol.* 35, 1182–1197. doi: 10.1016/S1357-2725(02)00310-2

Meyer, E. K., Dumont, D. F., Baker, S., and Dumont, L. J. (2011). Rejuvenation capacity of red blood cells in additive solutions over long-term storage. *Transfusion* 51, 1574–1579. doi: 10.1111/j.1537-2995.2010.03021.x

Nagababu, E., Scott, A. V., Johnson, D. J., Goyal, A., Lipsitz, J. A., Barodka, V. M., et al. (2016). The impact of surgery and stored red blood cell transfusions on nitric oxide homeostasis. *Anesth. Analg.* 123, 274–282. doi: 10.1213/ANE.0000000000001392

Nishino, T., Yachie-Kinoshita, A., Hirayama, A., Soga, T., Suematsu, M., and Tomita, M. (2009). In silico modeling and metabolome analysis of long-stored erythrocytes to improve blood storage methods. *J. Biotechnol.* 144, 212–223. doi: 10.1016/j.jbiotec.2009.08.010

Nishino, T., Yachie-Kinoshita, A., Hirayama, A., Soga, T., Suematsu, M., and Tomita, M. (2013). Dynamic simulation and metabolome analysis of long-term erythrocyte storage in adenine-guanosine solution. *PLoS One* 8:e71060. doi: 10.1371/journal.pone.0071060

Obrador, R., Musulin, S., and Hansen, B. (2015). Red blood cell storage lesion. *J. Vet. Emerg. Crit. Care* 25, 187–199. doi: 10.1111/vec.12252

Olivieri, O., de Franceschi, L., de Gironcoli, M., Girelli, D., and Corrocher, R. (1993). Potassium loss and cellular dehydration of stored erythrocytes following incubation in autologous plasma: role of the KCl cotransport system. *Vox Sang.* 65, 95–102. doi: 10.1111/j.1423-0410.1993.tb02123.x

Orbach, A., Zelig, O., Yedgar, S., and Barshtein, G. (2017). Biophysical and biochemical markers of red blood cells fragility. *Transfus Med Hemother* 44, 183–187. doi: 10.1159/000452106

Pantaleo, A., Giribaldi, G., Mannu, F., Arese, P., and Turrini, F. (2008). Naturally occurring anti-band 3 antibodies and red blood cell removal under physiological and pathological conditions. *Autoimmun. Rev.* 7, 457–462. doi: 10.1016/j.autrev.2008.03.017

Pompeo, G., Girasole, M., Cricenti, A., Boumis, G., Bellelli, A., and Amiconi, S. (2012). Erythrocyte death in vitro induced by starvation in the absence of Ca^{2+}. *Biochim. Biophys. Acta* 1798, 1047–1055. doi: 10.1016/j.bbamem.2010.02.002

Prudent, M., Tissot, J. D., and Lion, N. (2015). In vitro assays and clinical trials in red blood cell aging: Lost in translation. *Transfus. Apher. Sci.* 52, 270–276. doi: 10.1016/j.transci.2015.04.006

Raat, N. J., Hilarius, P. M., Johannes, T., de Korte, D., Ince, C., and Verhoeven, A. J. (2009). Rejuvenation of stored human red blood cells reverses the renal microvascular oxygenation deficit in an isovolemic transfusion model in rats. *Transfusion* 49, 427–434. doi: 10.1111/j.1537-2995.2008.02002.x

Racek, J., Herynkova, R., Holecek, V., Jerabek, Z., and Slama, V. (1997). Influence of antioxidants on the quality of stored blood. *Vox Sang.* 72, 16–19. doi: 10.1159/000461951

Rapido, F., Brittenham, G. M., Bandyopadhyay, S., La Carpia, F., L'Acqua, C., McMahon, D. J., et al. (2017). Prolonged red cell storage before transfusion increases extravascular hemolysis. *J. Clin. Invest.* 127, 375–382. doi: 10.1172/JCI90837

Relevy, H., Koshkaryev, A., Manny, N., Yedgar, S., and Barshtein, G. (2008). Blood banking-induced alteration of red blood cell flow properties. *Transfusion* 48, 136–146. doi: 10.1111/j.1537-2995.2007.01491.x

Safeukui, I., Buffet, P. A., Deplaine, G., Perrot, S., Brousse, V., Ndour, A., et al. (2012). Quantitative assessment of sensing and sequestration of spherocytic erythrocytes by the human spleen. *Blood* 120, 424–430. doi: 10.1182/blood-2012-01-404103

Salzer, U., and Prohaska, R. (2001). Stomatin, flotillin-1, and flotillin-2 are major integral proteins of erythrocyte lipid rafts. *Blood* 97, 1141–1143. doi: 10.1182/blood.V97.4.1141

Santacruz-Gomez, K., Silva-Campa, E., Alvarez-Garcia, S., Mata-Haro, V., Soto-Puebla, D., and Pedroza-Montero, M. (2014). An AFM approach of RBC micro and nanoscale topographic features during storage. *World Acad. Sci. Eng. Technol. Int. J.* 8, 449–452.

Shin, J. H., Lim, K. M., Noh, J. Y., Bae, O. N., Chung, S. M., Lee, M. Y., et al. (2007). Lead-induced procoagulant activation of erythrocytes through phosphatidylserine exposure may lead to thrombotic diseases. *Chem. Res. Toxicol.* 20, 38–43. doi: 10.1021/tx060114

Silva, D. C., Jovino, C. N., Silva, C. A., Fernandes, H. P., Filho, M. M., Lucena, S. C., et al. (2012). Optical tweezers as a new biomedical tool to measure zeta potential of stored red blood cells. *PLoS One* 7:e31778. doi: 10.1371/journal.pone.0031778

Song, H., Liu, Y., Zhang, B., Tian, K., Zhu, P., Lu, H., et al. (2017). Study of in vitro RBCs membrane elasticity with AOD scanning optical tweezers. *Biomed. Opt. Express* 8, 384–394. doi: 10.1364/BOE.8.000384

Steiner, M. E., Ness, P. M., Assmann, S. F., Triulzi, D. J., Sloan, S. R., Delaney, M., et al. (2015). Effects of red-cell storage duration on patients undergoing cardiac surgery. *N. Engl. J. Med.* 372, 1419–1429. doi: 10.1056/NEJMoa1414219

Stowell, C. P., Whitman, G., Granger, S., Gomez, H., Assmann, S. F., Massey, M. J., et al. (2017). The impact of red blood cell storage duration on tissue oxygenation in cardiac surgery. *J. Thorac. Cardiovasc. Surg.* 153, 610–619e2. doi: 10.1016/j.jtcvs.2016.11.029

Svetina, S. (2012). Red blood cell shape and deformability in the context of the functional evolution of its membrane structure. *Cell. Mol. Biol. Lett.* 17, 171–181. doi: 10.2478/s11658-012-0001-z

Tchir, J. D., Acker, J. P., and Holovati, J. L. (2013). Rejuvenation of ATP during storage does not reverse effects of the hypothermic storage lesion. *Transfusion* 53, 3184–3191. doi: 10.1111/trf.12194

Usry, R. T., Moore, G. L., and Manalo, F. W. (1975). Morphology of stored, rejuvenated human erythrocytes. *Vox Sang.* 28, 176–183. doi: 10.1111/j.1423-0410.1975.tb02756.x

Valeri, C. R., and Hirsch, N. M. (1969). Restoration in vivo of erythrocyte adenosine triphosphate, 2,3-diphosphoglycerate, potassium ion, and sodium ion concentrations following the transfusion of acid-citrate-dextrose-stored human red blood cells. *J. Lab. Clin. Med.* 73, 722–733.

Valtis, D. J. (1954). Defective gas-transport function of stored red blood-cells. *Lancet* 266, 119–124. doi: 10.1016/S0140-6736(54)90978-2

Verhoeven, A. J., Hilarius, P. M., Dekkers, D. W., Lagerberg, J. W., and de Korte, D. (2006). Prolonged storage of red blood cells affects aminophospholipid translocase activity. *Vox Sang.* 91, 244–251. doi: 10.1111/j.1423-0410.2006.00822.x

Whillier, S., Raftos, J. E., Sparrow, R. L., and Kuchel, P. W. (2011). The effects of long-term storage of human red blood cells on the glutathione synthesis rate and steady-state concentration. *Transfusion* 51, 1450–1459. doi: 10.1111/j.1537-2995.2010.03026.x

Wilkinson, D. K., Turner, E. J., Parkin, E. T., Garner, A. E., Harrison, P. J., Crawford, M., et al. (2008). Membrane raft actin deficiency and altered Ca2+-induced vesiculation in stomatin-deficient overhydrated hereditary stomatocytosis. *Biochim. Biophys. Acta* 1778, 125–132. doi: 10.1016/j.bbamem.2007.09.016

Wolfe, L. C., Byrne, A. M., and Lux, S. E. (1986). Molecular defect in the membrane skeleton of blood bank-stored red cells. Abnormal spectrin-protein 4.1-actin complex formation. *J. Clin. Invest.* 78, 1681–1686. doi: 10.1172/JCI112762

Woon, L. A., Holland, J. W., Kable, E. P., and Roufogalis, B. D. (1999). Ca^{2+} sensitivity of phospholipid scrambling in human red cell ghosts. *Cell Calcium* 25, 313–320. doi: 10.1054/ceca.1999.0029

Yoshida, T., AuBuchon, J. P., Dumont, L. J., Gorham, J. D., Gifford, S. C., Foster, K. Y., et al. (2008). The effects of additive solution pH and metabolic rejuvenation on anaerobic storage of red cells. *Transfusion* 48, 2096–2105. doi: 10.1111/j.1537-2995.2008.01812.x

14

Proteomics of Stored Red Blood Cell Membrane and Storage-Induced Microvesicles Reveals the Association of Flotillin-2 With Band 3 Complexes

Michel Prudent[1,2], Julien Delobel[1], Aurélie Hübner[1], Corinne Benay[1], Niels Lion[1,2] and Jean-Daniel Tissot[1,2]*

[1] *Laboratoire de Recherche sur les Produits Sanguins, Recherche et Développement Produits, Transfusion Interrégionale CRS, Épalinges, Switzerland,* [2] *Faculté de Biologie et de Médecine, Université de Lausanne, Lausanne, Switzerland*

***Correspondence:**
Michel Prudent
Michel.prudent@itransfusion.ch

The storage of erythrocyte concentrates (ECs) induces lesions that notably affect metabolism, protein activity, deformability of red blood cells (RBCs), as well as the release of oxygen. Band 3 is one of the proteins affected during the *ex vivo* aging of RBCs. This membrane protein is an anion transporter, an anchor site for the cytoskeleton and other membrane proteins as well as a binding site for glycolytic enzymes and bears blood group antigens. In the present study, band 3 complexes were isolated from RBCs stored for 7 and 42 days in average ($n = 3$), as well as from microvesicles ($n = 3$). After extraction of membrane proteins with a deoxycholate containing buffer, band 3 complexes were co-immunoprecipitated on magnetic beads coated with two anti-band 3 antibodies. Both total membrane protein extracts and eluates (containing band 3 complexes) were separated on SDS-PAGE and analyzed by bottom-up proteomics. It revealed that three proteins were present or absent in band 3 complexes stemming from long-stored or short-stored ECs, respectively, whereas the membrane protein contents remained equivalent. These potential markers for storage-induced RBC aging are adenylosuccinate lyase (ADSL), α-adducin and flotillin-2, and were further analyzed using western blots. ADSL abundance tended to increase during storage in both total membrane protein and band 3 complexes, whereas α-adducin mainly tended to stay onto the membrane extract. Interestingly, flotillin-2 was equivalently present in total membrane proteins whereas it clearly co-immunoprecipitated with band 3 complexes during storage (1.6-fold-change, $p = 0.0024$). Moreover, flotillin-2 was enriched (almost threefold) in RBCs compared to microvesicles (MVs) ($p < 0.001$) and the amount found in MVs was associated to band 3 complexes. Different types of band 3 complexes are known to exist in RBCs and further studies will be required to better understand involvement of this protein in microvesiculation during the storage of RBCs.

Keywords: band 3, flotillin-2, immunoprecipitation, proteomics, red blood cells, storage, transfusion

---

Abbreviations: ACN, acetonitrile; Co-IP, co-immunoprecipitation; DC, deoxycholate; EC, erythrocyte concentrate; FA, formic acid; FT, flow through; LC, liquid chromatography; MS, mass spectrometry; MV, microvesicle; PBST, phosphate buffered saline tween; RBC, red blood cell; RT, room temperature; SAGM, saline-adenine-glucose-mannitol.

INTRODUCTION

The organization of the RBC membrane is tightly associated to band 3 macrocomplexes and cytoskeleton. Band 3 is the major protein in RBC membrane and is reported as three major complexes. The first one is the band 3 dimer-ankyrin complex attached to the spectrin chains, the second one is the junctional complex where the band 3 (as dimer) is attached to the cytoskeleton via a complex of adducins, protein 4.1 and actin and the last one is a free band 3 dimer (Kodippili et al., 2009; Burton and Bruce, 2011; Mankelow et al., 2012; Lux, 2016). The knowledge on the composition and organization of the multi-protein complexes in RBC membrane has evolved during the last decades, from the membrane skeleton (Byers and Branton, 1985) to the binding of Rh proteins (Bruce et al., 2003), the role of protein 4.1 (Salomao et al., 2008), protein 4.2 (Satchwell et al., 2009), adducins (Anong et al., 2009), dematin involved in actin binding (Khan et al., 2008) and in junctional complex integrity (Lu et al., 2016), and ankyrin in band 3 tetramer stability (Satchwell et al., 2016). The multiple role of these complexes encompasses the cell deformability required to fulfill the RBC function of O_2 delivery to tissue and organs (Mohandas and Gallagher, 2008; Kodippili et al., 2009; Burton and Bruce, 2011), in gas exchange process (Bruce et al., 2003) and in metabolism regulation (Chu et al., 2008).

These functions are altered during the storage of RBCs under blood banking conditions (i.e., stored at 4°C up to 42 or 56 days depending on the various additive solutions used). *In vitro* studies have shown an increase in hemolysis (depending on additive solution and manufacturing) and a leakage of potassium, an increase in volume and cell rigidity (Hess et al., 2000; Gov and Safran, 2005; Flatt et al., 2014; Sparrow et al., 2014), the cell shape changes (Blasi et al., 2012; Bardyn et al., 2017b; Roussel et al., 2017), an accumulation of MVs (Rubin et al., 2008; Sparrow et al., 2014), metabolic and antioxidant modulations (ATP and 2,3-DPG depletion), and pH lowering (Hess et al., 2000; Sparrow et al., 2014; Bordbar et al., 2016; Bardyn et al., 2017a), what is called storage lesions (Tinmouth and Chin-Yee, 2001; Hess and Greenwalt, 2002; D'Alessandro et al., 2015; Prudent et al., 2015b; Bardyn et al., 2017b). At the protein level, these storage lesions induce the aggregation and degradation of band 3, leading to the formation of neoantigens recognized by the macrophages for the cell clearance (Bosman et al., 2008), accumulation of hemoglobin, antioxidant and metabolic enzymes at the membrane such as peroxiredoxin-2 (Antonelou et al., 2010; Rinalducci et al., 2011), degradation of proteins and decrease in spectrins and ankyrin contents (D'Amici et al., 2007; Bosman et al., 2008), accumulation of oxidized proteins (in particular at the cytoskeleton) (Antonelou et al., 2010; Delobel et al., 2012; Delobel et al., 2016).

Vesiculation is another mechanism related to the aging of RBCs. *In vitro*, it serves to remove damaged materials [such as oxidized proteins (Delobel et al., 2012)] and senescence molecules (phospatidylserine exposed at the RBC surface, IgG, neoantigen on band 3), which postpones the cell removal and increases their survival upon transfusion (Bosman et al., 2008; Willekens et al., 2008). The number of MVs increases exponentially during storage (Rubin et al., 2008) and it has been shown that after an incubation of 1 h at 37°C, long-stored RBCs exposed even more phosphatidylserine, release more MVs and potassium (Burger et al., 2013), which could impact transfusion efficiency (Cognasse et al., 2015; Said et al., 2017). Moreover, MVs promote the generation of thrombin (Rubin et al., 2013), which may be viewed as representing a potential hemostatic agent [as shown by reduced bleeding time and blood loss in thrombocytopenic rabbits and in Plavix®-treated rats (Jy et al., 2013)], or maybe promoters of thrombotic events (Tissot et al., 2013). MVs are formed at cytoskeleton-free spaces within the membrane and microvesiculation is expected to be a lipid-raft-based process affected by the loss of ATP (Sens and Gov, 2007; Gov et al., 2009). Lipid-raft (Ciana et al., 2014) proteins like stomatin and flotillins were found to decrease in RBC membranes during storage (Kriebardis et al., 2007), and stomatin to be enriched in MVs (Salzer et al., 2002, 2008).

Band 3 complexes play a key role in membrane organization and could be affected by the storage. In the present article, band 3 complexes were isolated from RBCs stemming from short and long-stored ECs as well as storage-induced MVs, in order to better decipher the fate of band 3 complexes during storage.

MATERIALS AND METHODS

Chemicals

Acetonitrile, deoxycholic acid (DC), NaCl and ponceau S were from Sigma (Sigma-Aldrich, Steinheim, Germany), and bromophenol blue, Coomassie Bue Brilliant R-250 and FA from Fluka (Fluka Chemie, Buchs, Switzerland). Tween-20 was bought from Roche Diagnostics (Mannheim, Germany). DTE, glycerol and urea were purchased from MP Biomedicals (Illkirch, France), ammonium bicarbonate and iodoacetamide from ICN Biomedicals (Aurora, Ohio, United States), 0.9% NaCl from Baxter (Volketswil, Switzerland), 10x PBS (1x PBS eq. to 137 mM NaCl, 2.7 mM KCl, 8.1 mM Na_2HPO_4 and 1.8 mM KH_2PO_4) from Laboratorium Dr. G. Bichsel (Interlaken, Switzerland), EDTA from Merck (MSD Merck Sharp & Dohme, Luzern, Switzerland), Tris-HCl from BIO-RAD (Hercules, CA, United States), ethanol from Thommen-Furler AG (Rüti bei Büren, Switzerland), Top Block from Lubio Science (Luzern, Switzerland), benchMark Protein Ladder (prestained or not) from Invitrogen (Carlsbad, CA, United States), FITC mouse anti-Human CD47 antibody from BD Pharmingen (BD Biosciences, Franklin Lakes, NJ, United States), and Sequencing Grade Modified Trypsin (Trypsin) from Promega AG (Dübendorf, Switzerland). Deionized water (18.2 MΩ·cm) was prepared using a Purelab option Q-15 (Elga LabWater).

Blood Samples

Erythrocyte concentrates were prepared from whole blood donations. Briefly, 450 ± 50 mL of blood from healthy donors were mixed with 63 mL of citrate phosphate dextrose anticoagulant solution and left at 22°C overnight (NGR6428B, Fenwal, Lake Zurich, IL, United States). All blood components (i.e., RBCs, plasma and white blood cells- and platelets-containing buffy coat) were separated upon centrifugation at 3,500 *g* for 14 min. The separated components were then distributed among the sterile inter-connected blood bags by applying a semi-automated pressure (on an Optipress II, Fenwal, United States) on the centrifuged original blood donation bag. The RBCs were then transferred into a SAGM-containing bag to a total volume of 275 ± 75 mL and a hematocrit of 0.6 ± 0.1 *v/v*. A leukodepletion step was performed by gravity-based filtration. ECs were finally stored at 4°C. ECs that did not meet the quality criteria for blood transfusion, e.g., low hemoglobin content or a slightly too small volume, were used under the signed assent of blood donors.

No research on genetic material was carried out. Therefore, no specific ethical processing was required and these samples were used in agreement with the local legislation (Loi fédérale relative à la recherche sur l'être humain, LRH - RS 810.30" and "the "Ordonnance relative à la recherche sur l'être humain, ORH - RS 810.301").

Preparation of RBC Membranes

Four times 6 mL of ECs were collected from: three ECs (bags A, B, and C) after 5 days, 7 days, 6 days, and 41 days, 43 days, 42 days, respectively; and three others (bags D, E, and F) after 50, 38, and 42 days, respectively, for experiments on MVs. RBCs were washed twice in 0.9% NaCl (2 v) and spun down at 2,000 *g* during 10 min at 4°C. RBCs were lyzed by incubation 1 h at 4°C in a hypotonic 0.1x PBS solution under agitation (2 v of 0.1x PBS for 1 v of packed cells).

Membranes from bags A to F were separated by ultracentrifugation at 100,000 *g*, 30 min, 4°C, and washed twice with 0.9% NaCl before transferring to 1.5-mL tubes and washed 4 to 8 more times (centrifugation at 21,500 *g*, 30 min, 4°C) until to obtain pellets as white as possible. RBC membranes were stored at −70°C until protein extraction.

Microvesicles were harvested from the whole bags D, E, and F (approximately 4 to 6 times 40 mL plus one tube of 6 mL) after centrifugation at 2,000 *g* during 10 min at 4°C (the 6-mL tubes of RBCs were processed as before for membrane isolation). Cell-free supernatants were collected and ultracentrifuged at 100,000 *g*, 1 h, 4°C. MVs-containing pellets were washed two times with NaCl 0.9%. Then, the pellets were suspended in 1 mL of NaCl 0.9% and transferred to 1.5-mL tubes and stored at −28°C. MVs were quantified by flow cytometry as previously described by labeling 5 μL of samples with 5 μL of FITC mouse anti-human CD47 (Delobel et al., 2012).

Protein Extraction

Total membrane proteins were extracted fresh daily under native conditions from pelleted membranes with DC buffer: 1% DC in 50 mM Tris-HCl, 150 mM NaCl, pH 8.1. A final centrifugation was performed at 21,500 *g*, 30 min, 4°C. The supernatant, containing membrane proteins and cytoskeleton (Delobel et al., 2012), was saved at 4°C. Protein amounts were determined using the Bradford Protein Assay (BIO-RAD, United States), with a calibration curve composed of BSA dilutions.

Proteins from 80 million MVs were extracted with 400 μL of DC buffer (25 million for bag E) and were quantified using a nanodrop 2000c (Thermo scientific).

Isolation of Band 3 Complexes

Band 3 complexes were captured using Co-IP based on magnetic beads (Dynabeads M-270 Epoxy, Invitrogen, Oslo, Norway). Antibodies that target internal (extracellular) and N-terminal (intracellular) parts of band 3 sequence (BRIC 6 and BRIC 170, respectively, from NHS Blood and Transplant, Bristol, United Kingdom) were covalently bound to the beads using a standard protocol from the supplier (105 μg of antibodies in total on 7.5 mg of beads). For the experiments with the bags A to F, 2×6 sets of beads (containing 7.5 mg of beads each) were prepared, pooled and split in 2×6 equivalent tubes for homogeneity. Antibodies-coated beads were stored at 4°C before Co-IP.

Co-IPs were performed as shown in **Figure 1**. Beads were washed with 1x IP buffer (provided by the supplier). The tube was placed on a magnet which allows the beads to collect at the tube wall and remove the supernatant (to be saved or not). Two hundred μL of total membrane protein or MV extracts, that contained approximately 400 μg of proteins, were added on the beads and incubated 1 h at 4°C under agitation. The proteins that were not immunoprecipitated were collected in the FT and the beads containing the band 3 complexes were carefully washed 3× with 1× IP buffer followed by a final 5 min wash at RT under agitation in the last wash buffer (LWB, 0.5 M NH_4OAc, 0.5 mM $MgCl_2$, 0.1% Tween-20). Finally, the bead suspension was transferred to a clean tube for elution of band 3 complexes with 500 μL of elution buffer (EB, 0.5 M NH_4OH, 0.5 mM EDTA) by incubating 20 min at RT under agitation followed by a second elution with 500 μL of EB 10 min. Eluates were vacuum dried using a GeneVac EZ-2^{plus} (Genevac Ltd., Ipswich, United Kingdom).

SDS-PAGE and Western Blotting

Total membrane protein extracts, FTs and eluates were analyzed by SDS-PAGE. Ten μg of proteins from each sample and 3 μL of BenchMark Protein Ladder (or 10 μL of BenchMark Prestained Protein Ladder for western blot, WB) were loaded on gels (Mini-PROTEAN TGX gels, 4–15%, BIO-RAD, United States). The dried eluates were suspended in 20 μL of 1x Laëmmli buffer and loaded totally on the gel. Proteins were stained with Coomassie Brilliant Blue R250 and gels were destained so as to obtain the optimum contrast.

The WB analyses were performed on PVDF membranes (transfer 1 h at 100 V in Tris-Glycine buffer inside a Mini Trans-Blot Electrophoretic Transfer cell) against adenylosuccinate lyase (ADSL C-11 at 1/500), α-adducin (C-4, 1/1000) and flotillin-2 (B-6, 1/6000) from Santa Cruz Biotechnology, United States.

First Antibody

Membranes were rinsed with PBST (1× PBS + 0.05% Tween-20) and blocked 1 h at RT under agitation with Top Block buffer (4% in PBST). Then the membranes were rinsed and washed 2 × 5 min in PBST. The blot was incubated overnight at 4°C

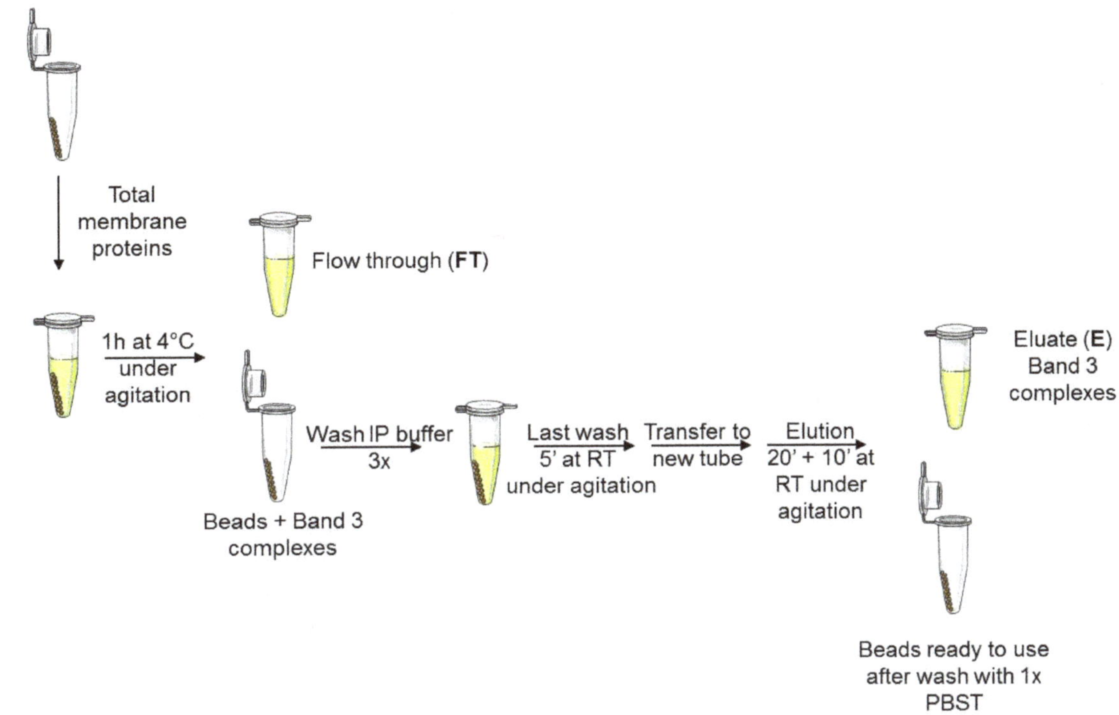

FIGURE 1 | Workflow for Co-IP of band 3 complexes. Magnetic beads were covalently coated with anti-band 3 antibodies (BRIC 6 and 170 specific to internal and N-ter band 3 sequence, respectively). Membrane proteins were extracted with 1% DC buffer. Beads were previously equilibrated with 1x IP buffer. Wash buffer: 1x IP buffer, Last wash buffer: 0.5 M NH_4OAc, 0.5 mM $MgCl_2$, 0.1% Tween-20. Elution buffer: 0.5 M NH_4OH, 0.5 mM EDTA. Beads were finally washed with 1x PBST and saved at 4°C for further co-IPs.

under agitation with the primary antibody (ADSL at 1/500 in Top block buffer). After a quick rinse and three washes of 5 min at RT in PBST, the membranes were re-incubated in Top Block buffer 20 min at RT under agitation, and were incubated 1 h at RT under agitation with the secondary antibody (Polyclonal goat anti-mouse immunoglobulins HRP, Dako, Denmark) diluted at 1/10,000 in Top Block buffer. The membranes were finally washed several times in PBST and were incubated at least twice 30 min at RT under agitation. The ECL reaction was achieved using the ECL western blotting detection reagents (GE Healthcare, Little Chalfont, Buckinghamshire, United Kingdom) 1 min in the dark and the images were acquired by means of ImageQuant LAS 500 (GE healthcare, Uppsala, Sweden).

Membranes Stripping

After the ECL reaction, the blots were rinsed and washed 3 × 5 min in PBST and then stripped 40 min at RT under agitation in 20 mL of Restore™ western blot stripping membrane (Thermo Scientific, Rockford, IL, United States). Then, the blots were rinsed and washed again 3 × 5 min in PBST before a new blocking 20 min at RT under agitation in Top Block buffer. Finally, they were rinsed, washed 2 × 5 min in PBST, and stored at 4°C for further immunodetection.

Second and Third Antibodies

After the membrane stripping, they were incubated with α-adducin diluted at 1/1,000 in Top Block buffer and the same procedure as before was applied. The last antibody tested was flotillin-2 diluted at 1/6,000 in Top Block buffer.

The WB membranes were finally stained with Ponceau red and scanned with a Personal Densitometer SI (GE Healthcare, United States).

Image Analyses and Statistic

Bands of interest were quantified by densitometry by means of the ImageQuant TL software (7.0, GE Healthcare, United States) and expressed as "volume." The data were then corrected by the total protein loading detected on Ponceau red by densitometry (see Supplementary Material). The relative volumes were calculated as follows:

$$\text{Relative Volume}_{\text{Protein}} = \text{Volume}_{\text{Protein, ECL}} / \text{Volume}_{\text{Whole proteins, Ponceau}}$$

where $\text{Volume}_{\text{Protein, ECL}}$ is the band volume of the protein of interest from WB and $\text{Volume}_{\text{Whole proteins, Ponceau}}$ is the amount of loaded proteins determined by the densitometry analyses of whole lane from Ponceau red-stained membrane. Then, abundances were expressed as relative to short-stored ECs (effect of storage) or RBCs (RBCs vs. MVs) conditions.

t-test analyses were performed between long- and short-stored ECs using the software GraphPad Prism version 6.07 (GraphPad Software Inc.). Two-way ANOVA was used for flotillin-2 data and multiple comparisons. *p*-values lower than 0.05 were considered as significant.

Proteomic Analysis

Each gel lane was cut in 8 bands (total membrane proteins and MVs experiments) and 8 or 13 bands (band 3 complexes in storage experiments) (**Supplementary Figure S4**), and proteins were in-gel digested (Delobel et al., 2012). Each excised band was treated and analyzed separately. Briefly, gel bands were washed with 50/50 ethanol/50 mM NH_4HCO_3. Proteins were reduced with 10 mM DTE in 50 mM NH_4HCO_3 1 h at 37°C under agitation, and alkylated with 55 mM iodoacetamide in 50 mM NH_4HCO_3 45 min at 37°C under agitation. Tryptic digestion was achieved by incubating gel bands in 12.5 ng/μL of trypsin (Sequencing Grade Modified Trypsin, Promega, Madison, WI, United States) in 50 mM NH_4HCO_3 and 10 mM $CaCl_2$ overnight at 37°C. Peptides were extracted sequentially in 50/45/5 ethanol/H_2O/FA then 70/25/5 ethanol/H_2O/FA. Peptide extracts were vacuum dried and resuspended, after washing, in 20 μL of 78/20/2 H_2O/FA/ACN for injection on LC coupled to mass spectrometry (LC-MS).

Ten microliter of peptide mixtures were analyzed onto an LC (UHPLC focused Thermo Scientific Dionex UltiMate 3000 Series from Thermo Scientific, Germering, Germany) coupled to an MS (amaZon ETD, Bruker Daltonik, Bremen, Germany) for protein identification. Peptide extract was loaded on a Dionex Acclaim PepMap RSLC column (300 μm × 15 cm, C18, 2 μm, 100 Å) at a 4 μL/min rate in a mixture of 95% eluent A (0.1% FA aqueous solution) and 5% of eluent B (H_2O/ACN 20/80 + 0.8% FA). Peptides were separated through a 40 min gradient, rising to 25% of eluent B in 30 min, then to 40% in 5 min, and finally to 90% in 10 min. Mass spectra of separated peptides were acquired in the positive scan mode from 300 to 1500 *m/z*. An automatic MS/MS fragmentation was performed on the three most intense precursor ions of each spectrum. Precursor ions were excluded from MS/MS fragmentation after appearance in one spectrum, and released after 0.15 min. Precursors presenting a 5% increase in intensity during their exclusion time were reconsidered for MS/MS fragmentation.

Protein identifications were performed through ProteinScape (Version 3.0, Bruker Daltonics, Bremen, Germany) and based on Mascot Server (version 2.4, Matrix Science Ltd., Boston, MA, United States). Spectra were submitted to database search with the following parameters: Database = SwissProt; Taxonomy = Homo sapiens (human); Enzyme = Trypsin, allow up to 1 missed cleavage; Modifications = Carbamidomethyl on cysteine (fixed) and methionine oxidation (variable); Peptide tolerance = ±0.35 Da; MS/MS tolerance = ±0.35 Da; Peptide charge = 2+, 3+, and 4+; peptide score threshold = 15 (35 for one peptide only), accepted proteins if Mascot score > 40 (25 when re-analyzed under Mascot) and accepted peptides if Mascot score > 20.

Protein lists from biological replicates (n = 3 for effect of aging and n = 3 for RBCs vs. MVs) were merged together for comparisons (see Supplementary Material and **Supplementary Tables S3–S6** for details).

RESULTS

Co-immunoprecipitation of Band 3 Complexes

Band 3 complexes were isolated from total membrane proteins from RBCs (**Figure 2a** and Supplementary Material). Membrane protein extracts showed a typical pattern including cytoskeleton proteins (e.g., α and β spectrins, protein 4.1), membrane proteins such as band 3 and proteins known to be localized to the membrane. FTs were similar to total membrane protein extracts because of the excess of incubated proteins regarding the binding capacity of the beads.

Six ECs were thus followed, total membrane proteins were extracted using DC-based buffer and band 3 complexes were isolated from RBCs at day 6 and day 42 (average), and from MVs using Co-IP. **Figure 2** shows the total membrane proteins (a and c) and protein contents after isolation of band 3 complexes (b and d). The protein distributions were quite similar between band 3 complexes and total membrane proteins. The main differences were the lower abundance of α and β spectrins relative to band 3, the lower abundance of low molecular weight proteins and the quasi absence of hemoglobin that was more important on bags D to F (IgG light chain was observed above 25 kDa). It emerges that hemoglobin derivatives do not bind to band 3 complexes but mainly to RBC membrane and that a large set of proteins is involved in these complexes, as expected. Protein 4.1 was less abundant in band 3 complexes than protein 4.2 even though their numbers of copies are equivalent (200,000 and 250,000 copies cell) (Burton and Bruce, 2011).

The MVs exhibit proteins mainly from the integral membrane, even though a few of them from the cytoskeleton, as the two spectrins and protein 4.1, and soluble proteins as hemoglobin (**Figure 2c**), were visible despite previous data (Lutz et al., 1977; Rubin et al., 2008; Salzer et al., 2008). As a consequence, the band 3 complexes isolated from MVs were free of spectrins which differs from RBCs-derived band 3 complexes (**Figure 2d**). The absence of proteins linking the skeleton to the membrane such as ankyrin, proteins 4.1 and 4.2 may suggest that mainly free complexes are expulsed through vesiculation.

Proteomic Analysis of Membrane Extracts and Band 3 Complexes

In the view of characterizing the protein content and pointing out the possible effect of storage, proteins were identified by a bottom-up proteomic approach. The whole gel lanes were cut in several pieces (**Supplementary Figure S4**), proteins were in-gel digested and analyzed by LC-MS/MS, and analyses were merged together in order to obtain a list of proteins per lane (see **Supplementary Tables**).

RBC Membrane Proteins

Forty-five proteins were identified in RBC total membrane proteins. Sixteen belonged exclusively to total membrane proteins, 2 were only found in band 3 complexes and 27 were common to both total membrane proteins and band 3 complexes (see **Supplementary Table S1**). In particular, 34

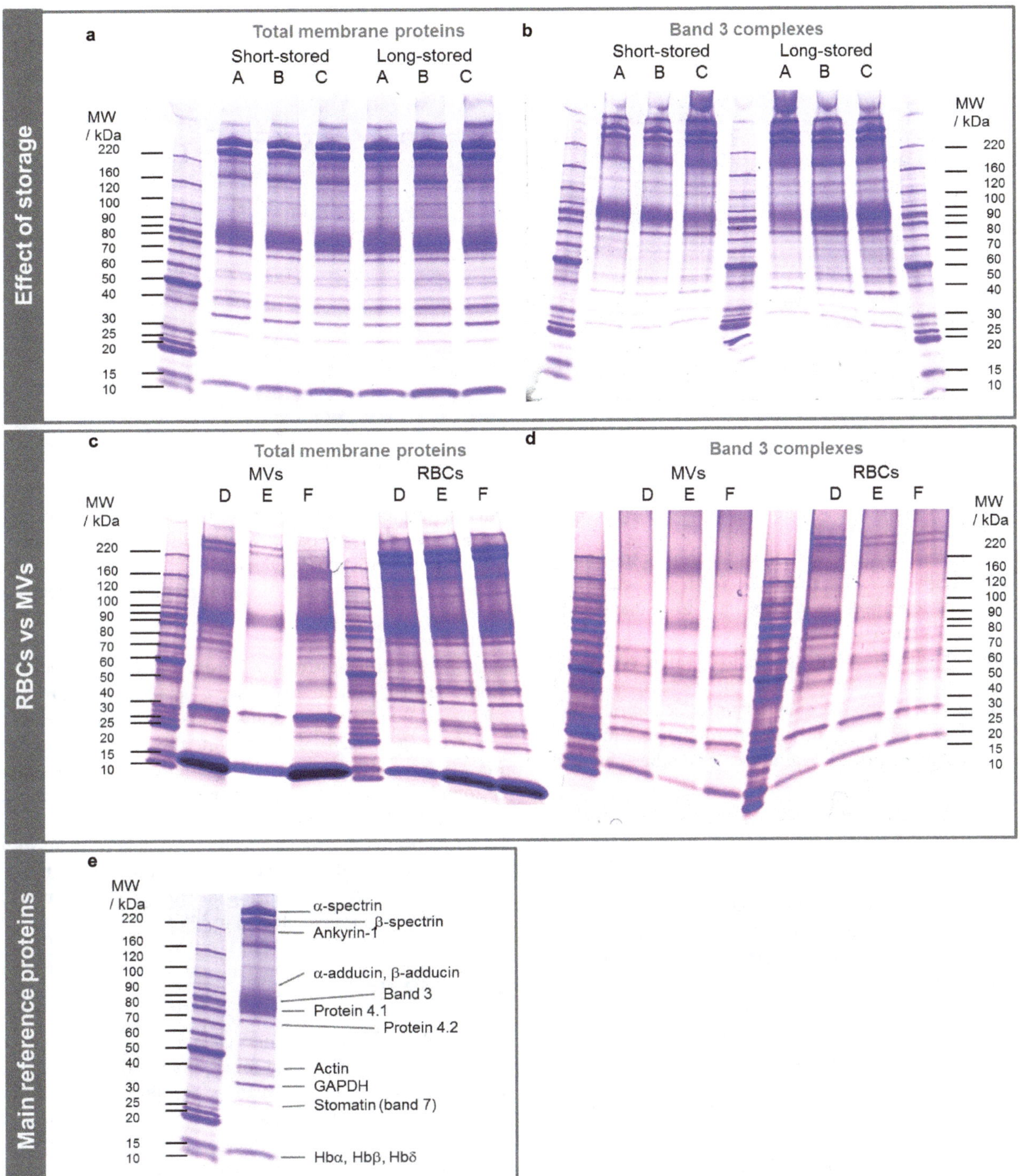

FIGURE 2 | SDS-PAGE of total membrane proteins and band 3 complexes from RBCs and MVs. **(a,c)** Total membrane proteins. **(b,d)** Co-IP of total membrane proteins, i.e., band 3 complexes. Proteins were extracted with 1% DC buffer. **(e)** Location of main proteins on a total membrane protein extract. A–F stand for bag numbers. Band 3 dimers are observed around 220 kDa, especially in **(d)**.

proteins were identified in both short- and long-stored total membrane proteins, 5 only in long-stored and 4 others only in short-stored ECs extracts; whereas 19 and 29 proteins were identified in band 3 complexes stemming from short- and long-stored ECs, respectively. These lists are limited because of the type of instrument used but the goal was to identify potential differences. The majority of those are known proteins of RBC membranes (Pasini et al., 2010; D'Alessandro et al., 2017)

TABLE 1 | Proteomic differences between band 3 complexes isolated from long- and short-stored erythrocyte concentrate (ECs).

Protein name	Accession number	Long-stored ECs			Short-stored ECs		
		L-A	L-B	L-C	S-A	S-B	S-C
Adenylosuccinate lyase	P30566	−	+	+*	−	−	−
Alpha-adducin	P35611	+	−	+	−	−	−
Flotillin-2	Q14254	+	+	+*	−	+*	−
ATP-citrate synthase	P53396	+	−	+*	−	−	+
Tropomodulin-1	P28289	−	+	−	−	+*	−
Ubiquitin-conjugating enzyme E2N	P61088	−	+	−	−	+*	−
Hemoglobin subunit delta	P02042	−	+	−	−	−	−
Phosphatidylinositol-5-phosphate 4-kinase	P48426	+	−	−	−	−	−
Ras-related protein Rap-1b	P61224	−	−	+	−	−	−
Ras-related protein Rap-2b	P61225	−	−	+	−	−	−

**Additional identification using Mascot search engine 2.4.1 (July 2013).*

and belong to the cytoskeleton: spectrins, actin, adducin; are glycoproteins: glycophorins A and C; and enzymes: GAPDH, aldolase, for instance.

Band 3 Complexes

Analyzing the effect of aging, it appears that only a few proteins co-immunoprecipitated with the band 3. In particular, three proteins were at least present in two long-stored bags and no more than one in short-stored bags (see **Table 1**). These latter proteins, namely adenylosuccinate lyase (ADSL), α-adducin and flotillin-2, were selected for WB analysis. Because of the MS instrument and the qualitative analysis, the selection of proteins was based on the presence or absence of proteins in samples and not on number of identified peptides or any other abundance scores.

Microvesicles

Thirty-two proteins were found in common between RBC membrane proteins and vesicles, 26 specific to RBCs and 25 to MVs (see **Supplementary Table S2**). Of interest, acetylcholinesterase was enriched in MVs as reported by Salzer et al. (2002). As for the band 3 complexes, the numbers are lower with 11 in common, 5 specific to RBCs and 7 to MVs. Complement C4 and galectin-7 were found exclusively on MVs-derived band 3 complexes and they are associated to complement and pro-apoptotic activities, respectively.

Quantification of ADSL, α-Adducin and Flotillin-2 by Western Blotting

Because of the sensitivity of WB, the segregation between the two groups was not as clear as reported by proteomics. The three proteins of interest were found in both short- and long-stored ECs (see **Figure 3**). No degradation was observed and the proteins were detected at their molecular weight (α-adducin is usually detected above the band 3, i.e., above 100 kDa). Their amounts tended to increase during storage without reaching statistical significances (**Figure 3b**). ADSL and α-adducin in band 3 complexes were preserved and tended to increase in the total membrane proteins; in particular α-adducin exhibited a fold change of 4.3 on membrane proteins extracted from long-stored EC ($p = 0.088$), specific to the membrane and not to band 3 complexes. The same tendency was observed in band 3 complexes, with marked effects for flotillin-2. It was clearly more abundant in long-stored ECs-derived band 3 complexes compared to short-stored ones with a fold change of 1.6 ($p = 0.0024$), but did not vary along storage in total membrane protein extracts ($p = 0.45$).

The quantity of flotillin-2 was clearly less important in total membrane proteins extracted from MVs compared to RBCs (more than threefold decrease, $p < 0.001$) (**Figure 4B**). As for band 3 complexes, a non-significant 1.3-fold decrease was observed ($p = 0.28$). In addition, the levels of flotillin-2 in MVs were equivalent in total membrane proteins and band 3 complexes, which suggest that the excreted flotillin-2 was associated to band 3 complexes.

These results show an association of these proteins to band 3 complexes during the storage of RBCs. In particular, the amount of flotillin-2 was constant during the storage, it associated to band 3 complexes and it was released in MVs.

DISCUSSION

The number of band 3 partners is important (28) onto this major RBC membrane protein and corresponds to the proteins reported in the literature. These partners are peripheral and integral membrane proteins and have different functions such as the cytoskeleton organization, energy metabolism, transmembrane transport and blood group antigen. The band 3 complexes isolation showed good specificity as confirmed by Co-IP on naked beads (no protein adsorption) and isotypic control (weak adsorption of band 3 and other unidentified proteins, and release of Ab) (see Supplementary Material and **Supplementary Figure S2**), which enable to study the effect of storage. It has to be noticed that band 3 complexes were isolated by Co-IP without any differentiation of the types of complexes (i.e., ankyrin, junctional or free complexes). The buffer used allows to extract both membrane and cytoskeleton proteins, as already described (Delobel et al., 2012). Moreover, the use of DC in the

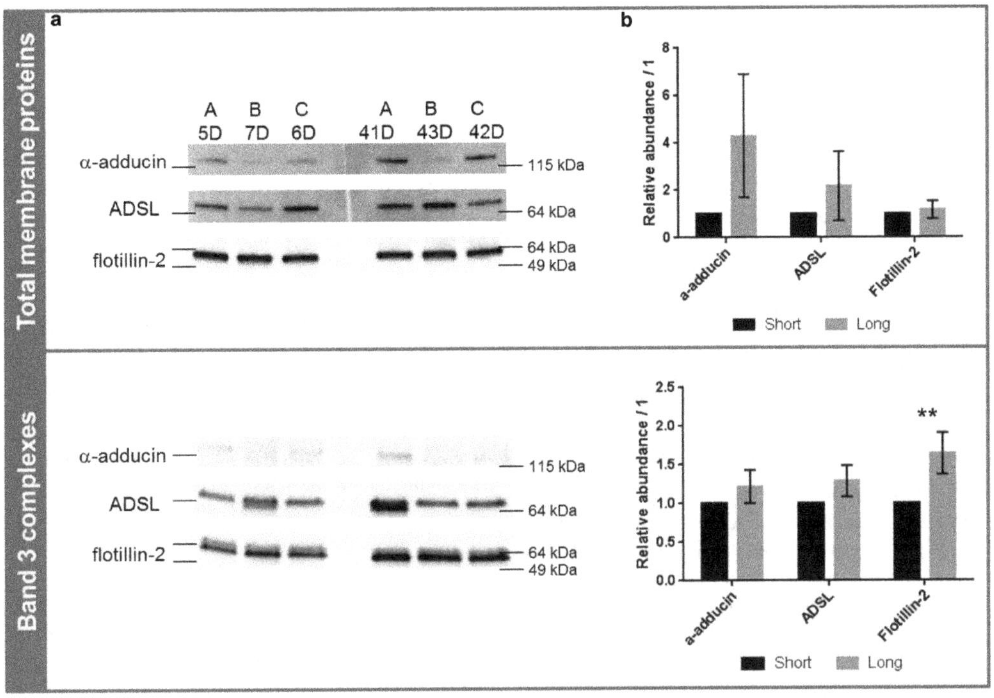

FIGURE 3 | Western blotting analysis of α-adducin, ADSL and flotillin-2 in total membrane proteins and band 3 complexes. **(a)** Western blot images in total membrane proteins (top) and band 3 complexes (bottom) in function of storage. **(b)** Corresponding densitometric analyses expressed as the mean of the band volume (n = 3) and relative to the protein loading. $^{**}p < 0.01$. Abundances were relative to short-stored ECs (see section "SDS-PAGE and Western Blotting" and Supplementary Material for details). A, B, and C stand for bag numbers; and D stands for days of storage.

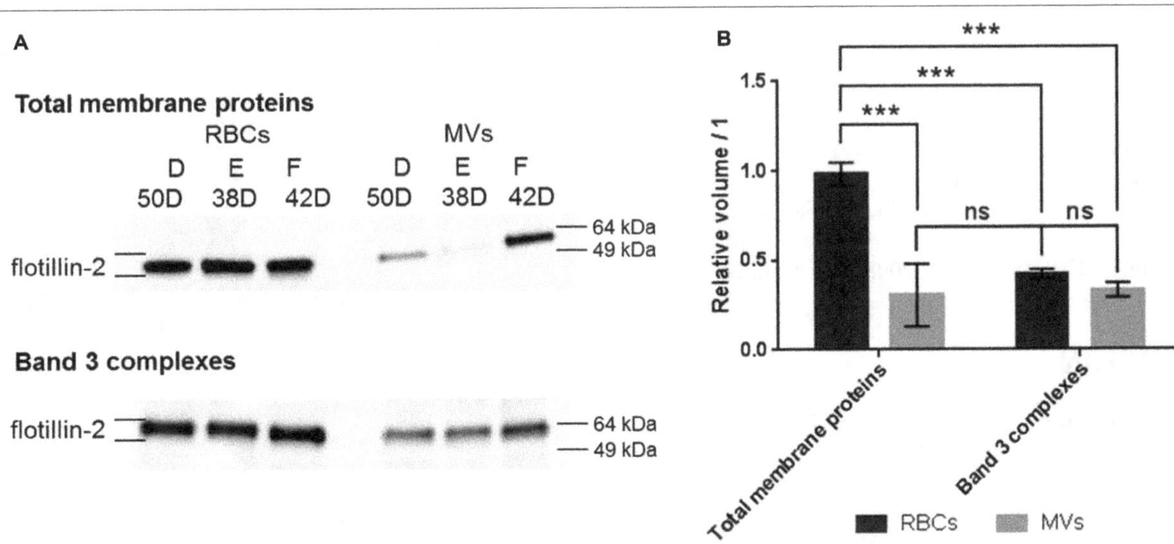

FIGURE 4 | Western blotting analysis of flotillin-2 in total membrane proteins and band 3 complexes from RBCs and MVs. **(A)** Western blot images in total membrane proteins (top) and band 3 complexes (bottom) stemming from RBCs and MVs. **(B)** Densitometric analyses of flotillin-2. Relative volumes were expressed as the mean of the band volume (n = 3) and relative to the protein loading (see section "SDS-PAGE and Western Blotting" and Supplementary Material for details). D, E, and F stand for bag numbers; and D stands for days of storage. $^{***}p < 0.001$.

extraction buffer may affect the association of a few proteins as protein 4.2. Indeed, washing of band 3 complexes-containing beads washed out protein 4.2 and spectrins (data not shown), as reported by Bruce et al. (2003).

The present study reveals the weak impact of *ex vivo* aging on band 3 complexes and 10 proteins were detected on long-stored EC-derived band 3 complexes. They play a role in metabolism activity, cytoskeleton organization and vesiculation such as Rap2

(Greco et al., 2006). A general accumulation trend of α-adducin on RBC membrane during the aging was observed, but it is not significant. α-adducin together with β subunit cap the fast-growing end of actin and recruit spectrins, and are involved in junction between band 3 and glucose transporter-1. It interacts also with dematin, a key protein in the organization of the junctional complex. It was reported (in mouse) that its absence induces the loss of adducin, actin and spectrin, and changes the RBC morphology (Lu et al., 2016). But the present data do not allow to conclude on this key protein (dematin was found both in short- and long-stored RBCs but was absent from MVs, see **Supplementary Tables S1, S2**).

The differences were significantly confirmed by WB for flotillin-2 that associates to band 3 complexes during the storage even though the data do not allow to specifically identify the proteins or the lipids driving the association. Flotillin-2 is a lipid raft-associated protein (Salzer and Prohaska, 2001) that is less abundant in MVs than in RBCs as previously reported (Salzer et al., 2002, 2008; Kriebardis et al., 2008). Since flotillin-2 was mainly found in MVs associated to band 3 complexes (**Figure 4**), it is speculated that flotillin-2 [known to be tightly associated with the cytoskeleton (Ciana et al., 2005)] could be specifically eliminated through the microvesiculation process at the end of the storage. In addition, stomatin, known to be enriched in MVs (Salzer et al., 2008), was also reported to be linked to flotillins and found in high molecular weight complexes (Rungaldier et al., 2013). These interactions may play a role in this process but the mechanism is unknown. This lipid raft-based process was also observed in calcium-induced microvesiculation (Salzer et al., 2002) though involving different sets of proteins (Prudent et al., 2015a). These observations are in agreement with the theory developed by Gov et al. (2009) where mobile components and breakage of the band 3-ankyrin anchors lead to vesiculation and morphology changes (Satchwell et al., 2016). Of course, other known mechanisms may be involved such as the loss of ATP-dependent aminophospholipid translocase (Salzer et al., 2008), the exposure of phosphatidyl serine or the accumulation of oxidized proteins (Kriebardis et al., 2008; Gov et al., 2009).

CONCLUSION

The isolation of band 3 complexes from RBCs revealed the high number of protein partners involving several functions. Moreover, it points out and confirms the association of flotillin-2 to band 3 complexes during the storage of RBCs and in storage-induced MVs. The role played in MVs remains unclear and the isolation of different types of complexes will be required to identify if a specific complex is involved in the binding of this protein during the storage. The stability of the protein complexes is influenced by protein-protein interactions and cell membrane organization. Post-translational modifications such as protein oxidation (Delobel et al., 2016; Reisz et al., 2016) or phosphorylation (Husain-Chishti et al., 1988; Harrison et al., 1991) impact the organization of the complexes. Therefore, these protein modifications could be further investigated during RBCs aging to provide more information on the storage lesions.

AUTHOR CONTRIBUTIONS

MP developed the co-IP, followed the EC bags, ran the proteomics, analyzed the data, and wrote the article. CB made the co-IP for the aging of ECs and in-gel digested the proteins. AH carried out the work on MVs. JD, NL, and J-DT reviewed the data and the manuscript. All authors read and approved the final version of the paper.

SUPPLEMENTARY MATERIAL

FIGURE S1 | Band 3 complexes captured using different antibodies against band 3. BRIC 6 (internal epitope), 155 (C-terminal) and 170 (N-terminal). NuPAGE Novex 4–12% gel from Invitrogen. Ten μg of proteins loaded and 5 μg of antibodies. FT, flow through (identical to protein extract); E, eluate; Ab, antibodies. BRIC 6 and 170 were chosen for co-IP.

FIGURE S2 | RBC total membrane proteins, adsorption on naked M-270 Epoxy beads and isotypic control. **Left**: NuPAGE Novex 4–12% gel from Invitrogen. Ten μg of proteins loaded. FT, flow through (identical to protein extract); E, eluate samples from co-IP on naked beads. M: molecular weight marker. **Right**: SDS-PAGE 4–15% gel from Bio-Rad. Ten μg of proteins loaded. E: eluate samples from co-IP on naked beads (1), on beads coated with an IgG against C23 (IgG, D-6, Santa-Cruz) (2), and on beads coated with BRIC 6 and BRIC 170 against band 3. No adsorption was observed on naked beads and only a few proteins were observed on the isotypic control (see text for details).

FIGURE S3 | SDS-PAGE analysis of co-IP band 3 complexes. In order to test the specificity of the beads and antibodies used, band 3 complexes were denatured with 1% SDS (+ or −) as is: before co-IP protein extract was incubated 5 min at RT under agitation in DC buffer containing 1% SDS. Red bars point to main differences. Green arrows are for the presence of released antibodies. FT, flow through (identical to protein extract); E, eluate samples. "+" and "−" signs stand for the presence or absence of SDS in the sample, respectively.

FIGURE S4 | Band excision of band 3 complexes for proteomics. **Top**: Effect of storage (bags A, B, and C). For bag B, additional bands were included as shown on the bottom right for numbering. **Bottom**: RBCs vs MVs (bags D, E, and F). Each red box represents a digested band. The same mapping was used for the total membrane proteins.

FIGURE S5 | Western blotting analyses of α-adducin, ADSL and flotillin-2 in total membrane extracts **(left)** and band 3 complexes **(right)** in function of RBC storage. Raw images. Acquisition times of 3 min for ADSL and flotillin-2, and 5 min for α-adducin. Green arrow: detection of released antibodies; blue arrow: remaining ADSL due to sequential detection. A, B, and C stand for the bags and D is for days of storage. Colored bands are for the MW markers (Pink band: 64 kDa).

FIGURE S6 | Western blotting analyses of flotillin-2 in total membrane extracts **(left)** and band 3 complexes **(right)** in function of their origin (RBCs or MVs). Raw images. Acquisition time of 3 min. Green arrow: detection of released antibodies. D, E, and F stand for the bags and D is for days of storage. Colored bands are for the MW markers (Pink band: 64 kDa).

FIGURE S7 | Example of image analyses by densitometry. **Left**: Western blotting of flotillin-2 on total membrane proteins. **Right**: Corresponding Ponceau red-stained membrane showing the total protein contents.

FIGURE S8 | Levels of protein expression in function of aging. Densitometric analyses of α-adducin, ADSL and flotillin-2 in total membrane proteins **(left)** and band 3 complexes **(right)**. Relative volumes were expressed as the mean of the band volume ($n = 3$) and relative to the protein loading. They were obtained for each protein and cannot be compared to another one (see section "SDS-PAGE and Western Blotting" and Supplementary Material for details). $^{**}p < 0.01$.

FIGURE S9 | Levels of flotillin-2 expression in RBCs and MVs. Densitometric analyses of flotillin-2 in total membrane proteins and band 3 complexes in function of the origin (RBCs or MVs). Relative volumes were expressed as the mean of the band volume ($n = 3$) and relative to the protein loading. Abundances were relative to RBCs (see "SDS-PAGE and Western Blotting" and Supplementary Material for details). $^{***}p < 0.001$; ns, non-significant.

TABLE S1 | Proteomic data. Effect of storage.

TABLE S2 | Proteomic data. RBCs vs. MVs.

TABLE S3 | Detailed proteomic data for **Figure 2a**.

TABLE S4 | Detailed proteomic data for **Figure 2b**.

TABLE S5 | Detailed proteomic data for **Figure 2c**.

TABLE S6 | Detailed proteomic data for **Figure 2d**.

REFERENCES

Anong, W. A., Franco, T., Chu, H. Y., Weis, T. L., Devlin, E. E., Bodine, D. M., et al. (2009). Adducin forms a bridge between the erythrocyte membrane and its cytoskeleton and regulates membrane cohesion. *Blood* 114, 1904–1912. doi: 10.1182/blood-2009-02-203216

Antonelou, M. H., Kriebardis, A. G., Stamoulis, K. E., Economou-Petersen, E., Margaritis, L. H., and Papassideri, I. S. (2010). Red blood cell aging markers during storage in citrate-phosphate-dextrose-saline-adenine-glucose-mannitol. *Transfusion* 50, 376–389. doi: 10.1111/j.1537-2995.2009.02449.x

Bardyn, M., Maye, S., Lesch, A., Delobel, J., Tissot, J.-D., Cortes-Salazar, F., et al. (2017a). The antioxidant capacity of erythrocyte concentrates is increased during the first week of storage and correlated with the uric acid level. *Vox Sang.* 112, 638–647. doi: 10.1111/vox.12563

Bardyn, M., Rappaz, B., Jaferzadeh, K., Crettaz, D., Tissot, J. D., Moon, I., et al. (2017b). Red blood cells ageing markers: a multi-parametric analysis. *Blood Transfus.* 15, 239–248. doi: 10.2450/2017.0318-16

Blasi, B., D'Alessandro, A., Ramundo, N., and Zolla, L. (2012). Red blood cell storage and cell morphology. *Transfus. Med.* 22, 90–96. doi: 10.1111/j.1365-3148.2012.01139.x

Bordbar, A., Johansson, P. I., Paglia, G., Harrison, S. J., Wichuk, K., Magnusdottir, M., et al. (2016). Identified metabolic signature for assessing red blood cell unit quality is associated with endothelial damage markers and clinical outcomes. *Transfusion* 56, 852–862. doi: 10.1111/trf.13460

Bosman, G., Lasonder, E., Luten, M., Roerdinkholder-Stoelwinder, B., Novotny, V. M. J., Bos, H., et al. (2008). The proteome of red cell membranes and vesicles during storage in blood bank conditions. *Transfusion* 48, 827–835. doi: 10.1111/j.1537-2995.2007.01630.x

Bruce, L. J., Beckmann, R., Ribeiro, M. L., Peters, L. L., Chasis, J. A., Delaunay, J., et al. (2003). A band 3-based macrocomplex of integral and peripheral proteins in the RBC membrane. *Blood* 101, 4180–4188. doi: 10.1182/blood-2002-09-2824

Burger, P., Kostova, E., Bloem, E., Hilarius-Stokman, P., Meijer, A. B., van den Berg, T. K., et al. (2013). Potassium leakage primes stored erythrocytes for phosphatidylserine exposure and shedding of pro-coagulant vesicles. *Br. J. Haematol.* 160, 377–386. doi: 10.1111/bjh.12133

Burton, N. M., and Bruce, L. J. (2011). Modelling the structure of the red cell membrane. *Biochem. Cell Biol.* 89, 200–215. doi: 10.1139/o10-154

Byers, T. J., and Branton, D. (1985). Visualization of the protein associations in the erythrocyte-membrane skeleton. *Proc. Natl. Acad. Sci. U.S.A.* 82, 6153–6157. doi: 10.1073/pnas.82.18.6153

Chu, H. Y., Breite, A., Ciraolo, P., Franco, R. S., and Low, P. S. (2008). Characterization of the deoxyhemoglobin binding site on human erythrocyte band 3: implications for O-2 regulation of erythrocyte properties. *Blood* 111, 932–938. doi: 10.1182/blood-2007-07-100180

Ciana, A., Achilli, C., and Minetti, G. (2014). Membrane rafts of the human red blood cell. *Mol. Membr. Biol.* 31, 47–57. doi: 10.3109/09687688.2014.896485

Ciana, A., Balduini, C., and Minetti, G. (2005). Detergent-resistant membranes in human erythrocytes and their connection to the membrane-skeleton. *J. Biosci.* 30, 317–328. doi: 10.1007/bf02703669

Cognasse, F., Hamzeh-Cognasse, H., Laradi, S., Chou, M.-L., Seghatchian, J., Burnouf, T., et al. (2015). The role of microparticles in inflammation and transfusion: a concise review. *Transfus. Apher. Sci.* 53, 159–167. doi: 10.1016/j.transci.2015.10.013

D'Alessandro, A., Dzieciatkowska, M., Nemkov, T., and Hansen, K. C. (2017). Red blood cell proteomics update: is there more to discover? *Blood Transfus.* 15, 182–187. doi: 10.2450/2017.0293-16

D'Alessandro, A., Kriebardis, A. G., Rinalducci, S., Antonelou, M. H., Hansen, K. C., Papassideri, I. S., et al. (2015). An update on red blood cell storage lesions, as gleaned through biochemistry and omics technologies. *Transfusion* 55, 205–219. doi: 10.1111/trf.12804

D'Amici, G. M., Rinalducci, S., and Zolla, L. (2007). Proteomic analysis of RBC membrane protein degradation during blood storage. *J. Proteome Res.* 6, 3242–3255. doi: 10.1021/pr070179d

Delobel, J., Prudent, M., Rubin, O., Crettaz, D., Tissot, J.-D., and Lion, N. (2012). Subcellular fractionation of stored red blood cells reveals a compartment-based protein carbonylation evolution. *J. Proteomics* 76, 181–193. doi: 10.1016/j.jprot.2012.05.004

Delobel, J., Prudent, M., Tissot, J. D., and Lion, N. (2016). Proteomics of the red blood cells carbonylome during blood banking of erythrocyte concentrates. *Proteomics Clin. Appl.* 10, 257–266. doi: 10.1002/prca.201500074

Flatt, J. F., Bawazir, W. M., and Bruce, L. J. (2014). The involvement of cation leaks in the storage lesion of red blood cells. *Front. Physiol.* 5:214. doi: 10.3389/fphys.2014.00214

Gov, N., Cluitmans, J., Sens, P., and Bosman, G. (2009). Cytoskeletal control of red blood cell shape: theory and practice of vesicle formation. *Adv. Planar Lipid Bilayers Liposomes* 10, 95–119. doi: 10.1016/s1554-4516(09)10004-2

Gov, N. S., and Safran, S. A. (2005). Red blood cell membrane fluctuations and shape controlled by ATP-induced cytoskeletal defects. *Biophys. J.* 88, 1859–1874. doi: 10.1529/biophysj.104.045328

Greco, F., Ciana, A., Pietra, D., Balduini, C., Minetti, G., and Torti, M. (2006). Rap2, but not Rap1 GTPase is expressed in human red blood cells and is involved in vesiculation. *Biochim. Biophys. Acta* 1763, 330–335. doi: 10.1016/j.bbamcr.2006.02.001

Harrison, M. L., Rathinavelu, P., Arese, P., Geahlen, R. L., and Low, P. S. (1991). Role of band-3 tyrosine phosphorylation in the regulation of erythrocyte glycolysis. *J. Biol. Chem.* 266, 4106–4111.

Hess, J. R., and Greenwalt, T. G. (2002). Storage of red blood cells: new approaches. *Transfus. Med. Rev.* 16, 283–295.

Hess, J. R., Lippert, L. E., Derse-Anthony, C. P., Hill, H. R., Oliver, C. K., Rugg, N., et al. (2000). The effects of phosphate, pH, and AS volume on RBCs stored in saline-adenine-glucose-mannitol solutions. *Transfusion* 40, 1000–1006. doi: 10.1046/j.1537-2995.2000.40081000.x

Husain-Chishti, A., Levin, A., and Branton, D. (1988). Abolition of actin-bundling by phosphorylation of human erythrocyte protein 4.9. *Nature* 334, 718–721. doi: 10.1038/334718a0

Jy, W., Johansen, M. E., Bidot, C., Horstman, L. L., and Ahn, Y. S. (2013). Red cell-derived microparticles (RMP) as haemostatic agent. *Thromb. Haemost.* 110, 751–760. doi: 10.1160/th12-12-0941

Khan, A. A., Hanada, T., Mohseni, M., Jeong, J. J., Zeng, L., Gaetani, M., et al. (2008). Dematin and adducin provide a novel link between the spectrin cytoskeleton and human erythrocyte membrane by directly interacting with glucose transporter-1. *J. Biol. Chem.* 283, 14600–14609. doi: 10.1074/jbc.M707818200

Kodippili, G. C., Spector, J., Sullivan, C., Kuypers, F. A., Labotka, R., Gallagher, P. G., et al. (2009). Imaging of the diffusion of single band 3 molecules on normal and mutant erythrocytes. *Blood* 113, 6237–6245. doi: 10.1182/blood-2009-02-205450

Kriebardis, A. G., Antonelou, M., Stamoulis, K., Economou-Petersen, E., Margaritis, L., and Papassideri, I. (2008). RBC-derived vesicles during storage-ultrastructure and lipid raft proteins participation. *Vox Sang.* 95, 190–190. doi: 10.1111/j.1537-2995.2008.01794.x

Kriebardis, A. G., Antonelou, M. H., Stamoulis, K. E., Economou-Petersen, E., Margaritis, L. H., and Papassideri, I. S. (2007). Storage-dependent remodeling of the red blood cell membrane is associated with increased immunoglobulin G binding, lipid raft rearrangement, and caspase activation. *Transfusion* 47, 1212–1220. doi: 10.1111/j.1537-2995.2007.01254.x

Lu, Y., Hanada, T., Fujiwara, Y., Nwankwo, J. O., Wieschhaus, A. J., Hartwig, J., et al. (2016). Gene disruption of dematin causes precipitous loss of erythrocyte membrane stability and severe hemolytic anemia. *Blood* 128, 93–103. doi: 10.1182/blood-2016-01-692251

Lutz, H. U., Liu, S. C., and Palek, J. (1977). Release of spectrin-free vesicles from human erythrocytes during ATP depletion.1. Characterization of spectrin-free vesicles. *J. Cell Biol.* 73, 548–560. doi: 10.1083/jcb.73.3.548

Lux, S. E. (2016). Anatomy of the red cell membrane skeleton: unanswered questions. *Blood* 127, 187–199. doi: 10.1182/blood-2014-12-512772

Mankelow, T. J., Satchwell, T. J., and Burton, N. M. (2012). Refined views of multi-protein complexes in the erythrocyte membrane. *Blood Cells Mol. Dis.* 49, 1–10. doi: 10.1016/j.bcmd.2012.03.001

Mohandas, N., and Gallagher, P. G. (2008). Red cell membrane: past, present, and future. *Blood* 112, 3939–3948. doi: 10.1182/blood-2008-07-161166

Pasini, E. M., Lutz, H. U., Mann, M., and Thomas, A. W. (2010). Red blood cell (RBC) membrane proteomics - Part I: proteomics and RBC physiology. *J. Proteomics* 73, 403–420. doi: 10.1016/j.jprot.2009.06.005

Prudent, M., Crettaz, D., Delobel, J., Seghatchian, J., Tissot, J. D., and Lion, N. (2015a). Differences between calcium-stimulated and storage-induced erythrocytes-derived microvesicles. *Transfus. Apher. Sci.* 53, 153–158. doi: 10.1016/j.transci.2015.10.012

Prudent, M., Tissot, J. D., and Lion, N. (2015b). In vitro assays and clinical trials in red blood cell aging: Lost in translation. *Transfus. Apher. Sci.* 52, 270–276. doi: 10.1016/j.transci.2015.04.006

Reisz, J. A., Wither, M. J., Dzieciatkowska, M., Nemkov, T., Issaian, A., Yoshida, T., et al. (2016). Oxidative modifications of glyceraldehyde 3-phosphate dehydrogenase regulate metabolic reprogramming of stored red blood cells. *Blood* 128, e32–e42. doi: 10.1182/blood-2016-05-714816

Rinalducci, S., D'Amici, G. M., Blasi, B., Vaglio, S., Grazzini, G., and Zolla, L. (2011). Peroxiredoxin-2 as a candidate biomarker to test oxidative stress levels of stored red blood cells under blood bank conditions. *Transfusion* 51, 1439–1449. doi: 10.1111/j.1537-2995.2010.03032.x

Roussel, C., Dussiot, M., Marin, M., Morel, A., Ndour, P. A., Duez, J., et al. (2017). Spherocytic shift of red blood cells during storage provides a quantitative whole cell-based marker of the storage lesion. *Transfusion* 57, 1007–1018. doi: 10.1111/trf.14015

Rubin, O., Crettaz, D., Canellini, G., Tissot, J. D., and Lion, N. (2008). Microparticles in stored red blood cells: an approach using flow cytometry and proteomic tools. *Vox Sang.* 95, 288–297. doi: 10.1111/j.1423-0410.2008.01101.x

Rubin, O., Delobel, J., Prudent, M., Lion, N., Kohl, K., Tucker, E. I., et al. (2013). Red blood cell-derived microparticles isolated from blood units initiate and propagate thrombin generation. *Transfusion* 53, 1744–1754. doi: 10.1111/trf.12008

Rungaldier, S., Oberwagner, W., Salzer, U., Csaszar, E., and Prohaska, R. (2013). Stomatin interacts with GLUT1/SLC2A1, band 3/SLC4A1, and aquaporin-1 in human erythrocyte membrane domains. *Biochim. Biophys. Acta* 1828, 956–966. doi: 10.1016/j.bbamem.2012.11.030

Said, A. S., Rogers, S. C., and Doctor, A. (2017). Physiologic Impact of circulating RBC microparticles upon blood-vascular interactions. *Front. Physiol.* 8:1120. doi: 10.3389/fphys.2017.01120

Salomao, M., Zhang, X. H., Yang, Y., Lee, S., Hartwig, J. H., Chasis, J. A., et al. (2008). Protein 4.1R-dependent multiprotein complex: new insights into the structural organization of the red blood cell membrane. *Proc. Natl. Acad. Sci. U.S.A.* 105, 8026–8031. doi: 10.1073/pnas.0803225105

Salzer, U., Hinterdorfer, P., Hunger, U., Borken, C., and Prohaska, R. (2002). Ca++-dependent vesicle release from erythrocytes involves stomatin-specific lipid rafts, synexin (annexin VII), and sorcin. *Blood* 99, 2569–2577. doi: 10.1182/blood.V99.7.2569

Salzer, U., and Prohaska, R. (2001). Stomatin, flotillin-1, and flotillin-2 are major integral proteins of erythrocyte lipid rafts. *Blood* 97, 1141–1143. doi: 10.1182/blood.V97.4.1141

Salzer, U., Zhu, R., Luten, M., Isobe, H., Pastushenko, V., Perkmann, T., et al. (2008). Vesicles generated during storage of red cells are rich in the lipid raft marker stomatin. *Transfusion* 48, 451–462. doi: 10.1111/j.1537-2995.2007.01549.x

Satchwell, T. J., Bell, A. J., Hawley, B. R., Pellegrin, S., Mordue, K. E., van Deursen, C. T., et al. (2016). Severe Ankyrin-R deficiency results in impaired surface retention and lysosomal degradation of RhAG in human erythroblasts. *Haematologica* 101, 1018–1027. doi: 10.3324/haematol.2016.146209

Satchwell, T. J., Shoemark, D. K., Sessions, R. B., and Toye, A. M. (2009). Protein 4.2: A complex linker. *Blood Cells Mol. Dis.* 42, 201–210. doi: 10.1016/j.bcmd.2009.01.005

Sens, P., and Gov, N. (2007). Force balance and membrane shedding at the red-blood-cell surface. *Phys. Rev. Lett.* 98:018102. doi: 10.1103/PhysRevLett.98.018102

Sparrow, R. L., Sran, A., Healey, G., Veale, M. F., and Norris, P. J. (2014). In vitro measures of membrane changes reveal differences between red blood cells stored in saline-adenine-glucose-mannitol and AS-1 additive solutions: a paired study. *Transfusion* 54, 560–568. doi: 10.1111/trf.12344

Tinmouth, A., and Chin-Yee, I. (2001). The clinical consequences of the red cell storage lesion. *Transfus. Med. Rev.* 15, 91–107. doi: 10.1053/tmrv.2001.22613

Tissot, J.-D., Canellini, G., Rubin, O., Angelillo-Scherrer, A., Delobel, J., Prudent, M., et al. (2013). Blood microvesicles: from proteomics to physiology. *Translat. Proteomics* 1, 38–52. doi: 10.1016/j.trprot.2013.04.004

Willekens, F. L. A., Werre, J. M., Groenen-Dop, Y. A. M., Roerdinkholder-Stoelwinder, B., de Pauw, B., and Bosman, G. (2008). Erythrocyte vesiculation: a self-protective mechanism? *Br. J. Haematol.* 141, 549–556. doi: 10.1111/j.1365-2141.2008.07055.x

15

From Erythroblasts to Mature Red Blood Cells: Organelle Clearance in Mammals

Martina Moras, Sophie D. Lefevre and Mariano A. Ostuni*

UMR-S1134 Integrated Biology of Red Blood Cell, INSERM, Université Paris Diderot, Sorbonne Paris Cité, Institut National de la Transfusion Sanguine, Laboratoire d'Excellence GR-Ex, Paris, France

***Correspondence:**
Mariano A. Ostuni
mariano.ostuni@inserm.fr

Erythropoiesis occurs mostly in bone marrow and ends in blood stream. Mature red blood cells are generated from multipotent hematopoietic stem cells, through a complex maturation process involving several morphological changes to produce a highly functional specialized cells. In mammals, terminal steps involved expulsion of the nucleus from erythroblasts that leads to the formation of reticulocytes. In order to produce mature biconcave red blood cells, organelles and ribosomes are selectively eliminated from reticulocytes as well as the plasma membrane undergoes remodeling. The mechanisms involved in these last maturation steps are still under investigation. Enucleation involves dramatic chromatin condensation and establishment of the nuclear polarity, which is driven by a rearrangement of actin cytoskeleton and the clathrin-dependent generation of vacuoles at the nuclear-cytoplasmic junction. This process is favored by interaction between the erythroblasts and macrophages at the erythroblastic island. Mitochondria are eliminated by mitophagy. This is a macroautophagy pathway consisting in the engulfment of mitochondria into a double-membrane structure called autophagosome before degradation. Several mice knock-out models were developed to identify mitophagy-involved proteins during erythropoiesis, but whole mechanisms are not completely determined. Less is known concerning the clearance of other organelles, such as smooth and rough ER, Golgi apparatus and ribosomes. Understanding the modulators of organelles clearance in erythropoiesis may elucidate the pathogenesis of different dyserythropoietic diseases such as myelodysplastic syndrome, leukemia and anemia.

Keywords: erythropoiesis, mitophagy, organelle clearance, reticulocytes, enucleation, erythroblast maturation

INTRODUCTION

Mature red blood cells (RBCs) result from a finely regulated process called erythropoiesis that produces 2 million RBCs every second in healthy human adults (Palis, 2014). The standard model of erythropoiesis starts with hematopoietic stem cells (HSCs) in the bone marrow (BM), giving rise to multipotent progenitors that go on to erythroid-committed precursors to mature RBC. This hierarchical relationship is, however, challenged, showing a greater plasticity for the cell's potential fates, with several studies in mice (Adolfsson et al., 2005) and recent new data in human (Notta et al., 2016).

Maturation from erythroid-committed precursors is called terminal erythropoiesis and occurs in the BM within erythroblastic islands, which consist of a central macrophage surrounded by erythroblasts, and ends in the blood stream where reticulocytes complete their maturation within 1–2 days. During this phase, proerythroblasts (Pro-E) undergo morphological changes, such as cell size reduction and chromatin condensation, produce specific proteins, such as hemoglobin, and exhibit a reduced proliferative capacity to give rise to basophilic (Baso-E), polychromatophilic (Poly-E) and orthochromatophilic (Ortho-E) erythroblasts, successively. Even though several growth factors are known to regulate erythropoiesis, Epo is the main regulator of erythropoiesis driving RBC precursor proliferation and differentiation, preventing erythroblast apoptosis (Koury and Bondurant, 1990; Ji et al., 2011). The macrophage-erythroblast interaction in the BM is essential since macrophages facilitate proliferation and differentiation and provide iron to the erythroblasts (de Back et al., 2014).

At the end of the terminal maturation, mammalian erythroblasts expel their nuclei and lose all their organelles, such as the Golgi apparatus, endoplasmic reticulum (ER), mitochondria and ribosomes. After expelling its nucleus, the reticulocyte maturation continues, losing 20–30% of the cell surface (Waugh et al., 1997; Da Costa et al., 2001) and eliminating any remaining membrane-bound cytosolic organelles through an autophagy/exosome-combined pathway (Blanc et al., 2005).

While extensive literature is done concerning the general mechanisms of erythropoiesis (Palis, 2014), this review focuses on the mechanisms and molecular actors involved during organelle clearance and membrane remodeling in order to produce fully functional biconcave mature RBCs. **Figure 1** summarizes the best characterized steps of organelle clearance throughout erythroblast terminal differentiation.

ENUCLEATION

The most spectacular aspect of mammalian erythropoiesis is the generation of enucleated cells. Enucleation occurs in orthochromatic erythroblasts producing two kinds of cells, the reticulocyte and the pyrenocyte [the nucleus surrounded by a tiny layer of cytoplasm and the plasma membrane (PM)]. Pyrenocytes are rapidly eliminated by the macrophages of the erythroblastic island, where phosphatidylserine exposure acts as an "eat me" signal (Yoshida et al., 2005).

Among the changes occurring during terminal differentiation, cell cycle arrest, chromatin and nuclear condensation and nuclear polarization are important for enucleation. In addition, nucleus expulsion is believed to be dependent on adhesion protein reorganization across the PM and macrophage interactions (Lee et al., 2004; Soni et al., 2006). The transcription factor KFL1 is required for enucleation (Parkins et al., 1995; Magor et al., 2015), regulating the expression of cell cycle proteins, deacetylases, caspases, and nuclear membrane proteins (Gnanapragasam et al., 2016; Gnanapragasam and Bieker, 2017).

Nuclear and chromatin condensation is essential for enucleation (Popova et al., 2009; Ji et al., 2010) and is dependent on the acetylation status of histones H3 and H4 under the control of histone acetyl transferases (HATs) and histone deacetylases (HDACs). Accordingly, Gcn5, an HAT protein, is down-regulated, and H3K9 and H4K5 histone acetylation decreases during mouse fetal erythropoiesis. In addition, Gcn5 is up regulated by c-Myc, which is known to decrease during the late phase of the erythropoiesis (Jayapal et al., 2010). With the same model, the role of HDAC2 protein was shown to be essential not only for chromatin condensation but also for the formation of the contractile actin ring (CAR), which is involved in nuclear pyknosis (Ji et al., 2010). Moreover, it was recently shown that major histones are released through a nuclear opening that is induced by caspase 3 activity-dependent lamin B cleavage and chromatin condensation (Gnanapragasam and Bieker, 2017).

Many studies demonstrate the cell cycle dependence of enucleation (Gnanapragasam and Bieker, 2017). Interestingly, the cyclin-induced E2F-2 transcription factor, which is a direct target of KLF1 during terminal erythropoiesis, appears to play a role in enucleation by inducing the expression of CRIK (Citron Rho-interacting kinase). Away from its regular targets related to microtubule organization and cytokinesis, CRIK participates in nuclear condensation (Swartz et al., 2017).

Cytoskeletal elements play an important role in erythroblast enucleation, acting in a similar manner to cytokinesis but in an asymmetric way. Specifically, as observed by electron and immunofluorescence microscopy, actin filaments (F-actin) condensate behind the extruding nucleus to form the CAR. The use of cytochalasin D, an F-actin inhibitor, causes the complete blockage of enucleation (Koury et al., 1989). Furthermore, the formation of the CAR is dependent on Rac1 GTPase and on mDia2, a Rho GTPase downstream effector, since down-regulating these two proteins disrupts the CAR formation and blocks erythroblast enucleation (Ji et al., 2008).

Regarding other cytoskeleton elements, the pharmacological inhibition of vimentin does not affect enucleation, which is in agreement with its decrease during human erythropoiesis (Dellagi et al., 1983). However, the deregulation of microtubules diminishes the enucleation rate. Microtubules form a basket around the nucleus (Koury et al., 1989), which is displaced near the PM at the late erythroblast stages, suggesting that this network must be essential for the polarization of the nucleus. Recently, the importance of the molecular motor dynein, which mediates unidirectional movement toward the minus end of the microtubules, was shown. Furthermore, PI3K activity is induced by microtubule polymers, improves the polarization efficiency and promotes nuclear movement. However, PI3K inhibition does not block, but only delays, mice enucleation (Wang et al., 2012).

In 2010, Crispino's group observed, by electron microscopy, the formation of vesicles close to the nuclear extrusion site in both primary murine and human erythroblasts, suggesting that another mechanism contributes to enucleation. Additionally, as shown by genetic invalidation, clathrin is needed for the vesicle formation (Keerthivasan et al., 2010). More recently, it was shown that survivin is required for erythroblast enucleation, but instead of acting on cytokinesis via the chromosome passenger complex, survivin contributes to enucleation through

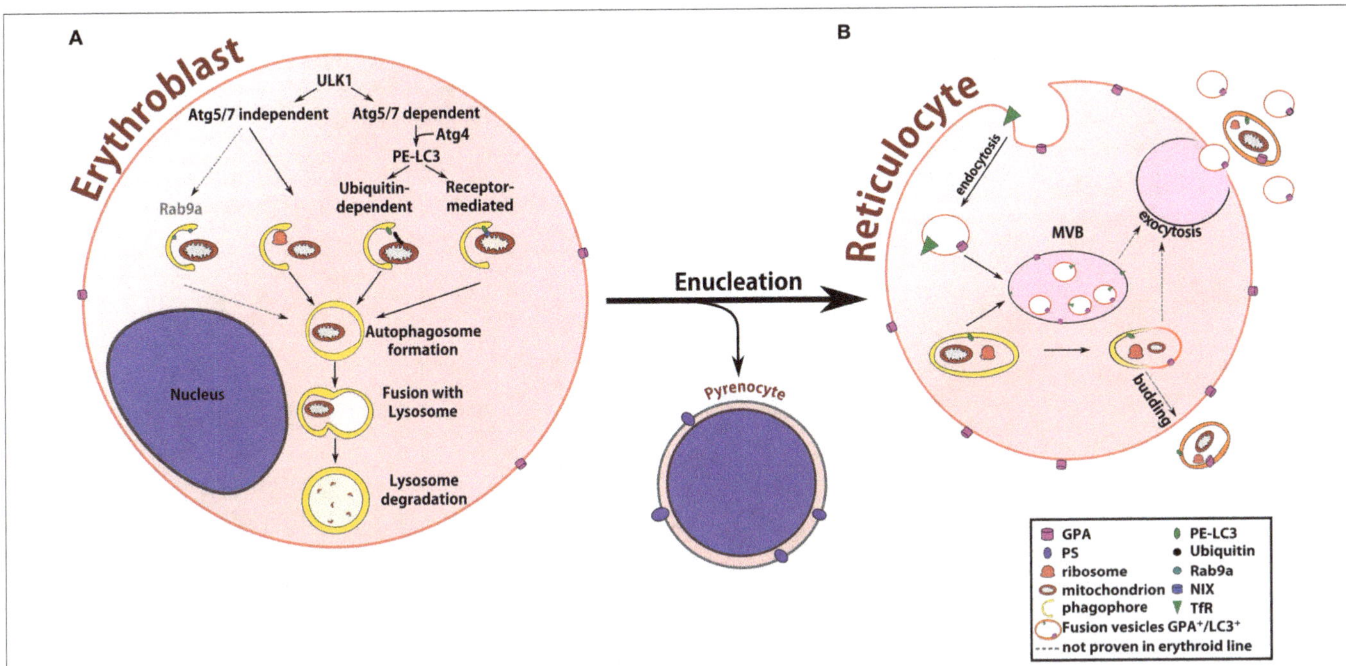

FIGURE 1 | Terminal maturation of erythroblasts. **(A)** At the erythroblast stage, two Ulk1-mediated autophagic pathways are activated to allow organelle clearance: the Atg5/7-dependent pathway with the proteolytic Atg4-dependent activation of MAPLC3, microtubule-associated protein 1 light channel 3 (LC3) and the Atg5/7-independent pathway, which is not related to the LC3 protein. LC3 activation allows its insertion into the phagophore membrane, starting the engulfment of organelles through the recognition of an ubiquitin signal or by the direct binding of specialized receptors at the organelle membrane. In non-erythroid cells, Rab9a is important for the formation of the phagophore during the Atg5/7-independent autophagic pathway. After the formation of the autophagosome, its fusion with the lysosome permits the degradation of organelles by hydrolytic enzymes. The enucleation process gives rise to the pyrenocyte and the reticulocyte, which still contains some organelles that must be eliminated for the final maturation into erythrocyte. **(B)** During this stage, unwanted membrane proteins, such as transferrin receptor (TfR), are internalized by endocytosis and expelled by exocytosis from multi-vesicular body structures. Glycophorin A (GPA)/LC3 double-positive vesicles containing organelle remnants are also found in reticulocytes, suggesting cooperation between the endocytosis (GPA$^+$) and autophagy (LC3$^+$) pathways to eliminate organelles. How autophagosomes interact with multivesicular bodies (MVBs) following the same pathway of membrane protein recycling or budding directly from the plasma membrane after fusion with endocytic vesicles, however, remains unknown.

an interaction with EPS15 and clathrin (Keerthivasan et al., 2012).

Clearly, we are still at the beginning of unraveling the molecular players involved in the enucleation process. Moreover, as shown in **Table 1**, most of the molecular players were identified in mice, and we are still lacking a demonstration that these players are also involved in human erythropoiesis.

Mitochondrial Clearance

The main mechanism for mitochondrial clearance is mitophagy, a selective type of autophagy that allows the degradation of damaged mitochondria. The importance of this process is highlighted by knowing that an impairment in mitochondrial function triggers an increase in reactive oxygen species production, which can in turn cause damage to cellular components (proteins, nucleic acid, and lipids) and trigger cell death (Lee et al., 2012).

During regular autophagy processes, stress or nutrient deprivation activates APM-activated protein kinase (AMPK), triggering two ubiquitin-dependent pathways (**Figure 1A**). One of these allows the assembly of the phagophore and involves several autophagy-related proteins (Atg), such as Atg5 and Atg7. The other aims to activate and lipidate LC3 (MAPLC3, microtubule-associated protein 1 light channel 3) by Atg4, a redox regulated protein. Atg4 and Atg7 cooperate to conjugate LC3 onto phosphatidylethanolamine in the lipid bilayer of the membrane originated from the ER-mitochondria contact site (Tooze and Yoshimori, 2010; Hamasaki et al., 2013). The elongated phagophore is then recruited to engulf targets via adaptor proteins, containing an LC3-interacting region (LIR) that forms a double-membrane autophagosome, which will fuse with a lysosome, initiating the degradation of the autophagosome components.

Upon mitochondria damage or depolarization, the mitochondrial membrane proteins are exposed and act as a beacon to recruit the phagophore membranes (Liu et al., 2014). An example is the PINK1 (P-TEN-induced kinase 1)-dependent recruitment of Parkin. Upon mitochondria depolarization, PINK1 accumulates at the OMM (outer mitochondrial membrane) and induces the mitochondrial translocation of Parkin, an RBR (ring-in-between)-type E3 ubiquitin ligase by direct phosphorylation (Kim et al., 2008; Narendra et al., 2010). The stabilization of Parkin at the OMM leads to the poly-ubiquitination of many proteins, inducing mitochondria fission and mobility stop and the phagophore recruitment by interacting with p62/SQSTM1, a LIR containing protein

TABLE 1 | Comparison between studies in human or mice erythroid cells or in other cell models.

	HUMAN erythroid cells	MICE erythroid cells	Other model or cell line
ENUCLEATION			
PS exposition in pyrenocytes		Yoshida et al., 2005	
Role of KFL1	Magor et al., 2015	Parkins et al., 1995	
Role of Gcn5		Jayapal et al., 2010	
Formation of CAR		Ji et al., 2010	
Role of F-actin		Koury et al., 1989	
Role of Rac1 and mDia2		Ji et al., 2008	
Role of E2F-2		Swartz et al., 2017	
Role of dynein	Kobayashi et al., 2016		
Role of PI3K		Wang et al., 2012	
Vesicular trafficking	Keerthivasan et al., 2010	Keerthivasan et al., 2010	
Role of survivin/EPS15/clathrin	Keerthivasan et al., 2012	Keerthivasan et al., 2012	
Apoptotic involvement		Krauss, 2005	Weil et al., 1999
MITOPHAGY			
PINK1 accumulation			Narendra et al., 2010
Role of Parkin			Kim et al., 2008; Geisler et al., 2010
LC3 Cleavage	Betin et al., 2013		
Lc3B binding through p62			Pankiv et al., 2007
Engulfment inside the autophagosome		Koury, 2005	
Role of NIX	Aerbajinai et al., 2003	Zhang et al., 2012; Sandoval et al., 2008 Schweers et al., 2007	Yuan et al., 2017
Atg7 independent pathway		Honda et al., 2014; Mortensen et al., 2010; Zhang et al., 2009	
Role of FUNDC1			Chen et al., 2017
Role of Bcl2-L-13			Murakawa et al., 2015
Role of optineurin			Wong and Holzbaur, 2014
Role of prohibitin 2			Wei et al., 2017
KRAB/KAP1-miRNA regulatory cascade	Barde et al., 2013	Barde et al., 2013	
Role of 15-LOX			Kühn et al., 1990; Grüllich et al., 2001 Vijayvergiya et al., 2004
Role of Rab		Wang et al., 2016	Hammerling et al., 2017a,b
Role of hemin regulation	Fader et al., 2016		
Role of NF-E2	Gothwal et al., 2016	Gothwal et al., 2016	
RIBOSOMES ELIMINATION			
Role of Ulk1		Kundu et al., 2008	
Atg7-Independent pathway		Mortensen et al., 2010	
PEROXISOME ELIMINATION			
Role of macroautophagy			Iwata, 2006
Role of 15-LOX			Yokota et al., 2001
Role of Lon proteases			Yokota et al., 2008
LYSOSOME ELIMINATION			
Role of p62			Hung et al., 2013
RNA ELIMINATION			
Role of pyrimidin nucleotidase	Valentine et al., 1974; Lee et al., 2014		
MEMBRANE REMODELING			
TfR removing			Johnstone et al., 1989; Killisch et al., 1992
AQP removing			Blanc et al., 2009
α4β1 integrin removing			Rieu et al., 2000
GLUT and AChE removing			Johnstone et al., 1987
GPA^+ exosomes	Griffiths et al., 2012		

(Geisler et al., 2010). Unlike regular mitophagy induction, targeted mitochondria, during erythroblast maturation, are fully functional. BNIP3L/NIX, a BH3-only integral OMM protein first identified in mouse reticulocytes, appears to be the major mitochondrial protein involved during terminal differentiation (Schweers et al., 2007; Sandoval et al., 2008). This protein is upregulated during erythropoiesis and induces mitochondrial membrane depolarization and membrane conjugated LC3 recruitment to the mitochondria (Aerbajinai et al., 2003; Novak et al., 2010). Nix action is not mediated by its BH3 domain but rather seems to be due to a cytoplasmic short linear motif, acting as a cellular signal to recruit other proteins (Zhang et al., 2012). However, whether Nix-induced mitochondrial depolarization activates the Parkin-dependent pathway is still unknown (Yuan et al., 2017).

Recently, other mitochondrial receptors were found to participate in mitophagy, such as FUNDC1, induced by MARCH5, an E3 ubiquitin ligase acting in hypoxic condition (Chen et al., 2017), Bcl2-L-13 (Murakawa et al., 2015), optineurin (Wong and Holzbaur, 2014), and Prohibitin 2 (Wei et al., 2017). It remains unknown whether they play a role in erythroid maturation.

Canonical Atg proteins also participate in terminal maturation. In human erythropoiesis, LC3 cleavage is under the control of the endopeptidase Atg4 and is needed for autophagosome maturation (Betin et al., 2013). In mice, Ulk1 (Atg1) expression correlates with terminal differentiation and participates in mitochondria and ribosome elimination (Chan et al., 2007; Kundu et al., 2008). The ubiquitination-dependent pathway also plays a role in reticulocyte maturation but is not essential. Indeed, in Atg7$^{-/-}$ reticulocytes, mitochondrial clearance is only partially affected (Zhang and Ney, 2009; Zhang et al., 2009). However, Nix and Ulk1 activation appears to be essential (Mortensen et al., 2010; Honda et al., 2014), suggesting the coexistence of both Atg5/Atg7-dependent and independent pathways during terminal differentiation.

Some studies suggest that the Atg5/7-independent degradation of mitochondria involves endosomal trafficking regulatory Rab proteins. Autophagosomes, formed in a Ulk1-dependent pathway, fuse with Golgi-derived vesicles and late endosomes in a Rab9a-dependent manner before they are targeted to the lysosomes (Wang et al., 2016). Interestingly, Rab proteins were also recently shown to be involved in mitochondria removal in a complete autophagy-independent pathway. Depolarized mitochondria appear to be engulfed in Rab5-positive endosomes that mature into Rab7-positive late endosomes and then fuse with lysosomes (Hammerling et al., 2017a,b). Unlike canonical autophagy, which involves the surrounding of a ubiquitin-decorated target by a double membrane structure, the entire mitochondria appears to be engulfed by an early endosome membrane invagination through the ESCRT machinery. Whether this might also occur in maturing erythroblasts is not known.

Mitophagy also appears to be transcriptionally regulated. Indeed, hemin-dependent differentiation of an erythroid cell line shows features of mitophagy (Fader et al., 2016). The NF-E2 transcription factor involved in globin gene expression also regulates mitophagy through the regulation of Nix and Ulk1 genes (Gothwal et al., 2016; Lupo et al., 2016). Another key regulator is the KRAB/KAP1-miRNA regulatory cascade, which acts as an indirect repressor of mitophagy genes in mice as well as in human cells, probably by the down and up regulation of a series of miRNAs, such as miR-351 that targets Nix (Barde et al., 2013).

In parallel to the autophagic pathway, cytosolic degradation seems to occur during reticulocyte maturation. 15-lipoxygenase (15-LOX), an enzyme that catalyzes the dioxygenation of polyunsaturated fatty acids, is translationally inhibited until the reticulocyte stage and acts to permeabilize organelle membranes, allowing proteasome access and degradation. Interestingly, only mitochondria elimination is affected, while ribosome clearance remains efficient when using a lipoxygenase inhibitor (Grüllich et al., 2001). This mechanism is still controversial, as 15-LOX might also act in the autophagy pathway as an OMM pH gradient disruptor that can induce mitophagy (Vijayvergiya et al., 2004), and on the oxidation of phospholipids conjugating with LC3 during the autophagosome formation; even so, these features, as shown in **Table 1** were not demonstrated in erythroid cells yet (Morgan et al., 2015).

Ribosomes and Other Organelles

In general, autophagy plays an essential role in the elimination of other organelles, such as lysosomes, peroxisomes and ER. However, the literature presents only very few studies in erythroid cells (**Table 1**).

While Nix is required for mitochondria removal, Ulk1 is involved in ribosome and mitochondria degradation (Schweers et al., 2007; Kundu et al., 2008; Sandoval et al., 2008). Similarly, an efficient clearance of ribosomes and ER and the inhibition of mitophagy was observed in Atg7$^{-/-}$ mice (Mortensen et al., 2010). These data suggest that non-autophagic or Atg7-independent autophagic pathways might exist for the elimination of other organelles (**Figure 1A**).

In non-erythroid cells from mammals, it was proposed that peroxisomes are eliminated by three different pathways: macroautophagy (Iwata, 2006), 15-LOX mediated (Yokota et al., 2001) and the peroxisomal Lon proteases (Yokota et al., 2008). Furthermore, the autophagic degradation of lysosomes (lysophagy) was recently identified in HeLa cells where it is mediated by ubiquitination and involves p62 protein (Hung et al., 2013). The similarities between pexophagy/lysophagy and mitophagy in non-erythroid cells suggest that autophagy pathways might also be involved in erythroblast terminal maturation.

After enucleation, reticulocytes mature in the bone marrow (R1) and then exit in the blood stream (R2) to complete the process. While the degradation of organelles starts at the time of enucleation, the elimination of mRNA occurs in the blood stream and is mediated by ribonucleases, generating nucleotides that are degraded by the erythroid pyrimidine nucleotidase. This elimination is crucial, as the deficiency in this enzyme causes hemolytic anemia (Valentine et al., 1974). mRNAs in R2 reticulocytes mainly belong to three overlapping categories: transport, metabolic and signal transduction (Lee et al., 2014), and their presence is essential to reach the mature RBC stage. This supports the importance of the exosome pathway for the final maturation into RBCs with an active elimination of other subcellular components.

Exocytosis and Membrane Remodeling

Exosomes are small vesicles that are secreted into the extracellular medium from various kind of cells. PM invaginations form early endosomes that engulf various targets forming multivesicular bodies (MVB, late endosomes) that eventually fuse with the PM and release exosomes. In reticulocytes, this pathway is thought to be involved in cell volume and membrane remodeling to reduce volume and remove unwanted membrane proteins. This was first discovered in sheep reticulocytes where transferrin receptor (TfR) is first internalized into small vesicles of 100–200 nm before being engulfed into the MVBs (Pan et al., 1985; Johnstone et al., 1989). The internalization step is clathrin-dependent, and the degradation is lysosome-independent and occurs by exocytosis after the fusion of the MVBs with the PM as shown in **Figure 1B** (Killisch et al., 1992). This process is required for the final elimination of other membrane proteins that are essential for the reticulocyte but are absent in the mature cell. Proteins such as aquaporin-1 (AQP1) (Blanc et al., 2009), α4β1 integrin (Rieu et al., 2000), glucose transporter and acetylcholinestarase (Johnstone et al., 1987) are found in glycophorine-A (GPA) positive endosomes while cytoskeletal proteins, such as actin or spectrin have never been found in these endosomes (Liu et al., 2010).

While plenty of evidence notes the role of autophagy in removing organelles during terminal maturation, the degradation step itself shows discrepancies with canonical proteolysis involving lysosomal proteins because of the disappearance of the lysosomal compartment during the maturation and removal of LAMP2 by exocytosis (Barres et al., 2010). Recently, GPA-positive endosomes were found to express LC3 at the endosome membrane, suggesting the cooperation of both autophagy and exocytosis in the removal of remnant organelles in R2 reticulocytes. These hybrid vesicles contain mitochondria, Golgi and lysosomes might be formed by the fusion of the outer-membrane of the autophagosome and the PM derived endosome (Griffiths et al., 2012). The exocytosis of this vesicle might be favored by the spleen, as splenectomized patients present large vacuoles inside reticulocytes (Holroyde and Gardner, 1970).

It should be pointed out the importance of lipids domain such as cholesterol and sphingomyelin-enriched domains in the PM remodeling, as they were find both in membrane vesiculation specific sites (Leonard et al., 2017).

CONCLUSION

Even if all the animal models used to identify the molecular players involved during terminal differentiation exhibit maturation defects and anemia, links between organelle clearance and human hematological diseases are still mostly unknown. Erythroid disorders, such as β-thalassemia and myelodysplastic syndrome (MDS), are characterized by ineffective hematopoiesis, anemia, dissociation between proliferation and differentiation of progenitor cells and the inefficient elimination of aggregated protein (Arber et al., 2016; Taher et al., 2017). Indeed, defects in reticulocyte maturation and autophagy are identified in HbE/β-thalassemia patients (Lithanatudom et al., 2011; Khandros et al., 2012; Butthep et al., 2015), and enucleation defects are found in MDS patients (Garderet et al., 2010; Park et al., 2016). Impaired autophagy is involved in cytosolic toxic Lyn accumulation and mitochondria and lysosome degradation delay in chorea-acanthocytosis (Lupo et al., 2016). The use of autophagy modulators is beneficial in the case of SCD or β-thalassemia (Franco et al., 2014; Jagadeeswaran et al., 2017). Moreover, anemia in Pearson's syndrome was recently linked to incomplete mitochondrial clearance from reticulocytes (Palis, 2014) and an asynchronization of iron loading (Ahlqvist et al., 2015), while sickle cells patients showed an accumulation of proteins in their erythrocytes suggesting a defect in exosomal pathway (De Franceschi, 2009; Carayon et al., 2011).

Unraveling the molecular mechanisms and interplays ruling erythroblast terminal maturation would be priceless in hematological disease therapy. However, much of our knowledge regarding human erythropoiesis is based on animal models and/or *ex vivo* cultured human progenitor cells (**Table 1**). Great care should be applied when interpreting results, considering the important differences between mouse and human erythropoiesis as well as the *in vivo* and *in vitro* environments, as highlighted in the extensive transcriptome analysis across a terminal erythroid differentiation study (An et al., 2014).

AUTHOR CONTRIBUTIONS

All authors listed have made a substantial, direct and intellectual contribution to the work, and approved it for publication.

ACKNOWLEDGMENTS

MM is funded by the European Union's Horizon 2020 research and innovation programme under the Marie Skłodowska-Curie grant agreement No. 665850. We thank I. Marginedas-Freixa and C. Hattab for helpful discussions.

REFERENCES

Adolfsson, J., Månsson, R., Buza-Vidas, N., Hultquist, A., Liuba, K., Jensen, C. T., et al. (2005). Identification of Flt3+ lympho-myeloid stem cells lacking erythro-megakaryocytic potential. *Cell* 121, 295–306. doi: 10.1016/j.cell.2005.02.013

Aerbajinai, W., Giattina, M., Lee, T. Y., Raffield, M., and Miller, J. L. (2003). The proapoptotic factor Nix is coexpressed with Bcl-xL during terminal erythroid differentiation. *Blood* 102, 712–717. doi: 10.1182/blood-2002-11-3324

Ahlqvist, K. J., Leoncini, S., Pecorelli, A., Wortmann, S. B., Ahola, S., Forsström, S., et al. (2015). MtDNA mutagenesis impairs elimination of mitochondria during erythroid maturation leading to enhanced erythrocyte destruction. *Nat. Commun.* 6:6494. doi: 10.1038/ncomms7494

An, X., Schulz, V. P., Li, J., Wu, K., Liu, J., Xue, F., et al. (2014). Global transcriptome analyses of human and murine terminal erythroid differentiation. *Blood* 123, 3466–3477. doi: 10.1182/blood-2014-01-548305

Arber, D. A., Orazi, A., Hasserjian, R., Thiele, J., Borowitz, M. J., Le Beau, M. M., et al. (2016). The 2016 revision to the World Health Organization classification of myeloid neoplasms and acute leukemia. *Blood* 127, 2391–2405. doi: 10.1182/blood-2016-03-643544

Barde, I., Rauwel, B., Marin-Florez, R. M., Corsinotti, A., Laurenti, E., Verp, S., et al. (2013). A KRAB/KAP1-miRNA cascade regulates erythropoiesis through stage-specific control of mitophagy. *Science* 340, 350–353. doi: 10.1126/science.1232398

Barres, C., Blanc, L., Bette-Bobillo, P., Andre, S., Mamoun, R., Gabius, H.-J., et al. (2010). Galectin-5 is bound onto the surface of rat reticulocyte exosomes and modulates vesicle uptake by macrophages. *Blood* 115, 696–705. doi: 10.1182/blood-2009-07-231449

Betin, V. M. S., Singleton, B. K., Parsons, S. F., Anstee, D. J., and Lane, J. D. (2013). Autophagy facilitates organelle clearance during differentiation of human erythroblasts: evidence for a role for ATG4 paralogs during autophagosome maturation. *Autophagy* 9, 881–893. doi: 10.4161/auto.24172

Blanc, L., De Gassart, A., Géminard, C., Bette-Bobillo, P., and Vidal, M. (2005). Exosome release by reticulocytes—an integral part of the red blood cell differentiation system. *Blood Cells. Mol. Dis.* 35, 21–26. doi: 10.1016/j.bcmd.2005.04.008

Blanc, L., Liu, J., Vidal, M., Chasis, J. A., An, X., and Mohandas, N. (2009). The water channel aquaporin-1 partitions into exosomes during reticulocyte maturation: implication for the regulation of cell volume. *Blood* 114, 3928–3934. doi: 10.1182/blood-2009-06-230086

Butthep, P., Wisedpanichkij, R., Jindadamrongwech, S., and Fucharoen, S. (2015). Elevated erythropoietin and cytokines levels are related to impaired reticulocyte maturation in thalassemic patients. *Blood Cells. Mol. Dis.* 54, 170–176. doi: 10.1016/j.bcmd.2014.11.007

Carayon, K., Chaoui, K., Ronzier, E., Lazar, I., Bertrand-Michel, J., Roques, V., et al. (2011). Proteolipidic composition of exosomes changes during reticulocyte maturation. *J. Biol. Chem.* 286, 34426–34439. doi: 10.1074/jbc.M111.257444

Chan, E. Y. W., Kir, S., and Tooze, S. A. (2007). siRNA screening of the kinome identifies ULK1 as a multidomain modulator of autophagy. *J. Biol. Chem.* 282, 25464–25474. doi: 10.1074/jbc.M703663200

Chen, Z., Siraj, S., Liu, L., and Chen, Q. (2017). MARCH5-FUNDC1 axis fine-tunes hypoxia induced mitophagy. *Autophagy* 13, 1244–1245. doi: 10.1080/15548627.2017.1310789

Da Costa, L., Mohandas, N., Sorette, M., Grange, M.-J., Tchernia, G., and Cynober, T. (2001). Temporal differences in membrane loss lead to distinct reticulocyte features in hereditary spherocytosis and in immune hemolytic anemia. *Blood* 98, 2894–2899. doi: 10.1182/blood.V98.10.2894

de Back, D. Z., Kostova, E. B., van Kraaij, M., van den Berg, T. K., and van Bruggen, R. (2014). Of macrophages and red blood cells; a complex love story. *Front. Physiol.* 5:9. doi: 10.3389/fphys.2014.00009

De Franceschi, L. (2009). Pathophisiology of sickle cell disease and new drugs for the treatment. *Mediterr. J. Hematol. Infect. Dis.* 1:e2009024. doi: 10.4084/MJHID.2009.024

Dellagi, K., Vainchenker, W., Vinci, G., Paulin, D., and Brouet, J. C. (1983). Alteration of vimentin intermediate filament expression during differentiation of human hemopoietic cells. *EMBO J.* 2, 1509–1514.

Fader, C. M., Salassa, B. N., Grosso, R. A., Vergara, A. N., and Colombo, M. I. (2016). Hemin induces mitophagy in a leukemic erythroblast cell line: hemin induces mitophagy in K562 cells. *Biol. Cell* 108, 77–95. doi: 10.1111/boc.201500058

Franco, S. S., De Falco, L., Ghaffari, S., Brugnara, C., Sinclair, D. A., Matté, A., et al. (2014). Resveratrol accelerates erythroid maturation by activation of FoxO3 and ameliorates anemia in beta-thalassemic mice. *Haematologica* 99, 267–275. doi: 10.3324/haematol.2013.090076

Garderet, L., Kobari, L., Mazurier, C., De Witte, C., Giarratana, M.-C., Perot, C., et al. (2010). Unimpaired terminal erythroid differentiation and preserved enucleation capacity in myelodysplastic 5q(del) clones: a single cell study. *Haematologica* 95, 398–405. doi: 10.3324/haematol.2009.012773

Geisler, S., Holmström, K. M., Skujat, D., Fiesel, F. C., Rothfuss, O. C., Kahle, P. J., et al. (2010). PINK1/Parkin-mediated mitophagy is dependent on VDAC1 and p62/SQSTM1. *Nat. Cell Biol.* 12, 119–131. doi: 10.1038/ncb2012

Gnanapragasam, M. N., and Bieker, J. J. (2017). Orchestration of late events in erythropoiesis by KLF1/EKLF. *Curr. Opin. Hematol.* 24, 183–190. doi: 10.1097/MOH.0000000000000327

Gnanapragasam, M. N., McGrath, K. E., Catherman, S., Xue, L., Palis, J., and Bieker, J. J. (2016). EKLF/KLF1-regulated cell cycle exit is essential for erythroblast enucleation. *Blood* 128, 1631–1641. doi: 10.1182/blood-2016-03-706671

Gothwal, M., Wehrle, J., Aumann, K., Zimmermann, V., Grunder, A., and Pahl, H. L. (2016). A novel role for nuclear factor-erythroid 2 in erythroid maturation by modulation of mitochondrial autophagy. *Haematologica* 101, 1054–1064. doi: 10.3324/haematol.2015.132589

Griffiths, R. E., Kupzig, S., Cogan, N., Mankelow, T. J., Betin, V. M. S., Trakarnsanga, K., et al. (2012). Maturing reticulocytes internalize plasma membrane in glycophorin A-containing vesicles that fuse with autophagosomes before exocytosis. *Blood* 119, 6296–6306. doi: 10.1182/blood-2011-09-376475

Grüllich, C., Duvoisin, R. M., Wiedmann, M., and Van Leyen, K. (2001). Inhibition of 15-lipoxygenase leads to delayed organelle degradation in the reticulocyte. *FEBS Lett.* 489, 51–54. doi: 10.1016/S0014-5793(01)02080-4

Hamasaki, M., Furuta, N., Matsuda, A., Nezu, A., Yamamoto, A., Fujita, N., et al. (2013). Autophagosomes form at ER-mitochondria contact sites. *Nature* 495, 389–393. doi: 10.1038/nature11910

Hammerling, B. C., Najor, R. H., Cortez, M. Q., Shires, S. E., Leon, L. J., Gonzalez, E. R., et al. (2017a). A Rab5 endosomal pathway mediates Parkin-dependent mitochondrial clearance. *Nat. Commun.* 8:14050. doi: 10.1038/ncomms14050

Hammerling, B. C., Shires, S. E., Leon, L. J., Cortez, M. Q., and Gustafsson, Å. B. (2017b). Isolation of Rab5-positive endosomes reveals a new mitochondrial degradation pathway utilized by BNIP3 and Parkin. *Small GTPases* 11, 1–8. doi: 10.1080/21541248.2017.1342749

Holroyde, C. P., and Gardner, F. H. (1970). Acquisition of autophagic vacuoles by human erythrocytes physiological role of the spleen. *Blood* 36, 566–575.

Honda, S., Arakawa, S., Nishida, Y., Yamaguchi, H., Ishii, E., and Shimizu, S. (2014). Ulk1-mediated Atg5-independent macroautophagy mediates elimination of mitochondria from embryonic reticulocytes. *Nat. Commun.* 5:4004. doi: 10.1038/ncomms5004

Hung, Y.-H., Chen, L. M.-W., Yang, J.-Y., and Yuan Yang, W. (2013). Spatiotemporally controlled induction of autophagy-mediated lysosome turnover. *Nat. Commun.* 4:2111. doi: 10.1038/ncomms3111

Iwata, J. (2006). Excess peroxisomes are degraded by autophagic machinery in mammals. *J. Biol. Chem.* 281, 4035–4041. doi: 10.1074/jbc.M512283200

Jagadeeswaran, R., Vazquez, B. A., Thiruppathi, M., Ganesh, B. B., Ibanez, V., Cui, S., et al. (2017). Pharmacological inhibition of LSD1 and mTOR reduces mitochondrial retention and associated ROS levels in the red blood cells of sickle cell disease. *Exp. Hematol.* 50, 46–52. doi: 10.1016/j.exphem.2017.02.003

Jayapal, S. R., Lee, K. L., Ji, P., Kaldis, P., Lim, B., and Lodish, H. F. (2010). Down-regulation of Myc is essential for terminal erythroid maturation. *J. Biol. Chem.* 285, 40252–40265. doi: 10.1074/jbc.M110.181073

Ji, P., Jayapal, S. R., and Lodish, H. F. (2008). Enucleation of cultured mouse fetal erythroblasts requires Rac GTPases and mDia2. *Nat. Cell Biol.* 10, 314–321. doi: 10.1038/ncb1693

Ji, P., Yeh, V., Ramirez, T., Murata-Hori, M., and Lodish, H. F. (2010). Histone deacetylase 2 is required for chromatin condensation and subsequent enucleation of cultured mouse fetal erythroblasts. *Haematologica* 95, 2013–2021. doi: 10.3324/haematol.2010.029827

Ji, Y. Q., Zhang, Y. Q., Li, M. Q., Du, M. R., Wei, W. W., and Li, D. J. (2011). EPO improves the proliferation and inhibits apoptosis of trophoblast and decidual stromal cells through activating STAT-5 and inactivating p38 signal in human early pregnancy. *Int. J. Clin. Exp. Pathol.* 4, 765–774.

Johnstone, R. M., Adam, M., Hammond, J. R., Orr, L., and Turbide, C. (1987). Vesicle formation during reticulocyte maturation. Association of plasma membrane activities with released vesicles (exosomes). *J. Biol. Chem.* 262, 9412–9420.

Johnstone, R. M., Bianchini, A., and Teng, K. (1989). Reticulocyte maturation and exosome release: transferrin receptor containing exosomes shows multiple plasma membrane functions. *Blood* 19, 1844–1851.

Keerthivasan, G., Liu, H., Gump, J. M., Dowdy, S. F., Wickrema, A., and Crispino, J. D. (2012). A novel role for survivin in erythroblast enucleation. *Haematologica* 97, 1471–1479. doi: 10.3324/haematol.2011.061093

Keerthivasan, G., Small, S., Liu, H., Wickrema, A., and Crispino, J. D. (2010). Vesicle trafficking plays a novel role in erythroblast enucleation. *Blood* 116, 3331–3340. doi: 10.1182/blood-2010-03-277426

Khandros, E., Thom, C. S., D'Souza, J., and Weiss, M. J. (2012). Integrated protein quality-control pathways regulate free α-globin in murine β-thalassemia. *Blood* 119, 5265–5275. doi: 10.1182/blood-2011-12-397729

Killisch, I., Steinlein, P., Romisch, K., Hollinshead, R., Beug, H., and Griffiths, G. (1992). Characterization of early and late endocytic compartments of the transferrin cycle. Transferrin receptor antibody blocks erythroid differentiation by trapping the receptor in the early endosome. *J. Cell Sci.* 103, 211–232.

Kim, Y., Park, J., Kim, S., Song, S., Kwon, S.-K., Lee, S.-H., et al. (2008). PINK1 controls mitochondrial localization of Parkin through direct phosphorylation. *Biochem. Biophys. Res. Commun.* 377, 975–980. doi: 10.1016/j.bbrc.2008.10.104

Kobayashi, I., Ubukawa, K., Sugawara, K., Asanuma, K., Guo, Y.-M., Yamashita, J., et al. (2016). Erythroblast enucleation is a dynein-dependent process. *Exp. Hematol.* 44, 247–256.e12. doi: 10.1016/j.exphem.2015.12.003

Koury, S. T., Koury, M. J., and Bondurant, M. C. (1989). Cytoskeletal distribution and function during the maturation and enucleation of 13 mammalian erythroblasts. *J. Cell Biol.* 109, 3005–3013.

Koury, M. J. (2005). *In vitro* maturation of nascent reticulocytes to erythrocytes. *Blood* 105, 2168–2174. doi: 10.1182/blood-2004-02-0616

Koury, M. J., and Bondurant, M. C. (1990). Control of red cell production: the roles of programmed cell death (apoptosis) and erythropoietin. *Transfusion* 30, 673–674. doi: 10.1046/j.1537-2995.1990.30891020321.x

Krauss, S. W. (2005). Nuclear substructure reorganization during late-stage erythropoiesis is selective and does not involve caspase cleavage of major nuclear substructural proteins. *Blood* 106, 2200–2205. doi: 10.1182/blood-2005-04-1357

Kühn, H., Belkner, J., and Wiesner, R. (1990). Subcellular distribution of lipoxygenase products in rabbit reticulocyte membranes. *FEBS J.* 191, 221–227. doi: 10.1111/j.1432-1033.1990.tb19113.x

Kundu, M., Lindsten, T., Yang, C.-Y., Wu, J., Zhao, F., Zhang, J., et al. (2008). Ulk1 plays a critical role in the autophagic clearance of mitochondria and ribosomes during reticulocyte maturation. *Blood* 112, 1493–1502. doi: 10.1182/blood-2008-02-137398

Lee, E., Choi, H. S., Hwang, J. H., Hoh, J. K., Cho, Y.-H., and Baek, E. J. (2014). The RNA in reticulocytes is not just debris: it is necessary for the final stages of erythrocyte formation. *Blood Cells. Mol. Dis.* 53, 1–10. doi: 10.1016/j.bcmd.2014.02.009

Lee, J. C.-M., Gimm, J. A., Lo, A. J., Koury, M. J., Krauss, S. W., Mohandas, N., et al. (2004). Mechanism of protein sorting during erythroblast enucleation: role of cytoskeletal connectivity. *Blood* 103, 1912–1919. doi: 10.1182/blood-2003-03-0928

Lee, J., Giordano, S., and Zhang, J. (2012). Autophagy, mitochondria and oxidative stress: cross-talk and redox signalling. *Biochem. J.* 441, 523–540. doi: 10.1042/BJ20111451

Leonard, C., Conrard, L., Guthmann, M., Pollet, H., Carquin, M., Vermylen, C., et al. (2017). Contribution of plasma membrane lipid domains to red blood cell (re)shaping. *Sci. Rep.* 7:4264. doi: 10.1038/s41598-017-04388-z

Lithanatudom, P., Wannatung, T., Leecharoenkiat, A., Svasti, S., Fucharoen, S., and Smith, D. R. (2011). Enhanced activation of autophagy in β-thalassemia/Hb E erythroblasts during erythropoiesis. *Ann. Hematol.* 90, 747–758. doi: 10.1007/s00277-010-1152-5

Liu, J., Guo, X., Mohandas, N., Chasis, J. A., and An, X. (2010). Membrane remodeling during reticulocyte maturation. *Blood* 115, 2021–2027. doi: 10.1182/blood-2009-08-241182

Liu, L., Sakakibara, K., Chen, Q., and Okamoto, K. (2014). Receptor-mediated mitophagy in yeast and mammalian systems. *Cell Res.* 24, 787–795. doi: 10.1038/cr.2014.75

Lupo, F., Tibaldi, E., Matte, A., Sharma, A. K., Brunati, A. M., Alper, S. L., et al. (2016). A new molecular link between defective autophagy and erythroid abnormalities in chorea-acanthocytosis. *Blood* 128, 2976–2987. doi: 10.1182/blood-2016-07-727321

Magor, G. W., Tallack, M. R., Gillinder, K. R., Bell, C. C., McCallum, N., Williams, B., et al. (2015). KLF1-null neonates display hydrops fetalis and a deranged erythroid transcriptome. *Blood* 125, 2405–2417. doi: 10.1182/blood-2014-08-590968

Morgan, A. H., Hammond, V. J., Sakoh-Nakatogawa, M., Ohsumi, Y., Thomas, C. P., Blanchet, F., et al. (2015). A novel role for 12/15-lipoxygenase in regulating autophagy. *Redox Biol.* 4, 40–47. doi: 10.1016/j.redox.2014.11.005

Mortensen, M., Ferguson, D. J. P., Edelmann, M., Kessler, B., Morten, K. J., Komatsu, M., et al. (2010). Loss of autophagy in erythroid cells leads to defective removal of mitochondria and severe anemia *in vivo*. *Proc. Natl. Acad. Sci. U.S.A.* 107, 832–837. doi: 10.1073/pnas.0913170107

Murakawa, T., Yamaguchi, O., Hashimoto, A., Hikoso, S., Takeda, T., Oka, T., et al. (2015). Bcl-2-like protein 13 is a mammalian Atg32 homologue that mediates mitophagy and mitochondrial fragmentation. *Nat. Commun.* 6:7527. doi: 10.1038/ncomms8527

Narendra, D. P., Jin, S. M., Tanaka, A., Suen, D.-F., Gautier, C. A., Shen, J., et al. (2010). PINK1 is selectively stabilized on impaired mitochondria to activate Parkin. *PLoS Biol.* 8:e1000298. doi: 10.1371/journal.pbio.1000298

Notta, F., Zandi, S., Takayama, N., Dobson, S., Gan, O. I., Wilson, G., et al. (2016). Distinct routes of lineage development reshape the human blood hierarchy across ontogeny. *Science* 351:aab2116. doi: 10.1126/science.aab2116

Novak, I., Kirkin, V., McEwan, D. G., Zhang, J., Wild, P., Rozenknop, A., et al. (2010). Nix is a selective autophagy receptor for mitochondrial clearance. *EMBO Rep.* 11, 45–51. doi: 10.1038/embor.2009.256

Palis, J. (2014). Primitive and definitive erythropoiesis in mammals. *Front. Physiol.* 5:3. doi: 10.3389/fphys.2014.00003

Pan, B.-T., Teng, K., Wu, C., Adam, M., and Johnstone, R. M. (1985). Electron microscopic evidence for externalization of the transferrin receptor in vesicular form in sheep reticulocytes. *J. Cell Biol.* 101, 942–948. doi: 10.1083/jcb.101.3.942

Pankiv, S., Clausen, T. H., Lamark, T., Brech, A., Bruun, J.-A., Outzen, H., et al. (2007). p62/SQSTM1 binds directly to Atg8/LC3 to facilitate degradation of ubiquitinated protein aggregates by autophagy. *J. Biol. Chem.* 282, 24131–24145. doi: 10.1074/jbc.M702824200

Park, S. M., Ou, J., Chamberlain, L., Simone, T. M., Yang, H., Virbasius, C.-M., et al. (2016). U2AF35(S34F) promotes transformation by directing aberrant aTG7 pre-mRNA 3′ end formation. *Mol. Cell* 62, 479–490. doi: 10.1016/j.molcel.2016.04.011

Parkins, A. C., Sharpe, A. H., and Orkin, S. H. (1995). Lethal β-thalassaemia in mice lacking the erythroid CACCC-transcription factor EKLF. *Nature* 375, 318–322. doi: 10.1038/375318a0

Popova, E. Y., Krauss, S. W., Short, S. A., Lee, G., Villalobos, J., Etzell, J., et al. (2009). Chromatin condensation in terminally differentiating mouse erythroblasts does not involve special architectural proteins but depends on histone deacetylation. *Chromosome Res.* 17, 47–64. doi: 10.1007/s10577-008-9005-y

Rieu, S., Géminard, C., Rabesandratana, H., Sainte-Marie, J., and Vidal, M. (2000). Exosomes released during reticulocyte maturation bind to fibronectin via integrin α4β1. *Eur. J. Biochem.* 267, 583–590. doi: 10.1046/j.1432-1327.2000.01036.x

Sandoval, H., Thiagarajan, P., Dasgupta, S. K., Schumacher, A., Prchal, J. T., Chen, M., et al. (2008). Essential role for Nix in autophagic maturation of erythroid cells. *Nature* 454, 232–235. doi: 10.1038/nature07006

Schweers, R. L., Zhang, J., Randall, M. S., Loyd, M. R., Li, W., Dorsey, F. C., et al. (2007). NIX is required for programmed mitochondrial clearance during reticulocyte maturation. *Proc. Natl. Acad. Sci. U.S.A.* 104, 19500–19505. doi: 10.1073/pnas.0708818104

Soni, S., Bala, S., Gwynn, B., Sahr, K. E., Peters, L. L., and Hanspal, M. (2006). Absence of erythroblast macrophage protein (Emp) leads to failure of erythroblast nuclear extrusion. *J. Biol. Chem.* 281, 20181–20189. doi: 10.1074/jbc.M603226200

Swartz, K. L., Wood, S. N., Murthy, T., Ramirez, O., Qin, G., Pillai, M. M., et al. (2017). E2F-2 promotes nuclear condensation and enucleation of terminally differentiated erythroblasts. *Mol. Cell. Biol.* 37:e00274–e00216. doi: 10.1128/MCB.00274-16

Taher, A. T., Weatherall, D. J., and Cappellini, M. D. (2017). Thalassaemia. *Lancet.* doi: 10.1016/S0140-6736(17)31822-6. [Epub ahead of print].

Tooze, S. A., and Yoshimori, T. (2010). The origin of the autophagosomal membrane. *Nat. Cell Biol.* 12, 831–835. doi: 10.1038/ncb0910-831

Valentine, W. N., Fink, K., Paglia, D. E., Harris, S. R., and Adams, W. S. (1974). Hereditary hemolytic anemia with human erythrocyte pyrimidine 5′-nucleotidase deficiency. *J. Clin. Invest.* 54, 866–879. doi: 10.1172/JCI107826

Vijayvergiya, C., De Angelis, D., Walther, M., Kühn, H., Duvoisin, R. M., Smith, D. H., et al. (2004). High-level expression of rabbit 15-lipoxygenase induces collapse of the mitochondrial pH gradient in cell culture. *Biochemistry* 43, 15296–15302. doi: 10.1021/bi048745v

Wang, J., Fang, Y., Yan, L., Yuan, N., Zhang, S., Xu, L., et al. (2016). Erythroleukemia cells acquire an alternative mitophagy capability. *Sci. Rep.* 6:24641. doi: 10.1038/srep24641

Wang, J., Ramirez, T., Ji, P., Jayapal, S. R., Lodish, H. F., and Murata-Hori, M. (2012). Mammalian erythroblast enucleation requires PI3K-dependent cell polarization. *J. Cell Sci.* 125, 340–349. doi: 10.1242/jcs.088286

Waugh, R. E., McKenney, J. B., Bauserman, R. G., Brooks, D. M., Valeri, C. R., and Snyder, L. M. (1997). Surface area and volume changes during maturation of reticulocytes in the circulation of the baboon. *J. Lab. Clin. Med.* 129, 527–535. doi: 10.1016/S0022-2143(97)90007-X

Wei, Y., Chiang, W.-C., Sumpter, R., Mishra, P., and Levine, B. (2017). Prohibitin 2 is an inner mitochondrial membrane mitophagy receptor. *Cell* 168, 224–238.e10. doi: 10.1016/j.cell.2016.11.042

Weil, M., Raff, M. C., and Braga, V. M. (1999). Caspase activation in the terminal differentiation of human epidermal keratinocytes. *Curr. Biol.* 9, 361–365. doi: 10.1016/S0960-9822(99)80162-6

Wong, Y. C., and Holzbaur, E. L. (2014). Optineurin is an autophagy receptor for damaged mitochondria in parkin-mediated mitophagy that is disrupted by an ALS-linked mutation. *Proc. Natl. Acad. Sci. U.S.A.* 111, E4439–E4448. doi: 10.1073/pnas.1405752111

Yokota, S., Haraguchi, C. M., and Oda, T. (2008). Induction of peroxisomal lon protease in rat liver after di-(2-ethylhexyl)phthalate treatment. *Histochem. Cell Biol.* 129, 73–83. doi: 10.1007/s00418-007-0328-0

Yokota, S., Oda, T., and Fahimi, H. D. (2001). The role of 15-lipoxygenase in disruption of the peroxisomal membrane and in programmed degradation of peroxisomes in normal rat liver. *J. Histochem. Cytochem.* 49, 613–621. doi: 10.1177/002215540104900508

Yoshida, H., Kawane, K., Koike, M., Mori, Y., Uchiyama, Y., and Nagata, S. (2005). Phosphatidylserine-dependent engulfment by macrophages of nuclei from erythroid precursor cells. *Nature* 437, 754–758. doi: 10.1038/nature03964

Yuan, Y., Zheng, Y., Zhang, X., Chen, Y., Wu, X., Wu, J., et al. (2017). BNIP3L/NIX-mediated mitophagy protects against ischemic brain injury independent of PARK2. *Autophagy* 13, 1754–1766. doi: 10.1080/15548627.2017.1357792

Zhang, J., Loyd, M. R., Randall, M. S., Waddell, M. B., Kriwacki, R. W., and Ney, P. A. (2012). A short linear motif in BNIP3L (NIX) mediates mitochondrial clearance in reticulocytes. *Autophagy* 8, 1325–1332. doi: 10.4161/auto.20764

Zhang, J., and Ney, P. (2009). Autophagy-dependent and-independent mechanisms of mitochondrial clearance during reticulocyte maturation. *Autophagy* 5, 1064–1065. doi: 10.4161/auto.5.7.9749

Zhang, J., Randall, M. S., Loyd, M. R., Dorsey, F. C., Kundu, M., Cleveland, J. L., et al. (2009). Mitochondrial clearance is regulated by Atg7-dependent and independent mechanisms during reticulocyte maturation. *Blood* 114, 157–164. doi: 10.1182/blood-2008-04-151639

16

The Shape Shifting Story of Reticulocyte Maturation

Elina Ovchynnikova[1,2†], Francesca Aglialoro[1,2†], Marieke von Lindern[1,2] and Emile van den Akker[1,2]*

[1] *Department of Hematopoiesis, Sanquin Research, Amsterdam, Netherlands,* [2] *Landsteiner Laboratory, Academic Medical Center, University of Amsterdam, Amsterdam, Netherlands*

***Correspondence:**
Emile van den Akker
e.vandenakker@sanquin.nl

† *These authors have contributed equally to this work.*

The final steps of erythropoiesis involve unique cellular processes including enucleation and reorganization of membrane proteins and the cytoskeleton to produce biconcave erythrocytes. Surprisingly this process is still poorly understood. *In vitro* erythropoiesis protocols currently produce reticulocytes rather than biconcave erythrocytes. In addition, immortalized lines and iPSC-derived erythroid cell suffer from low enucleation and suboptimal final maturation potential. In light of the increasing prospect to use *in vitro* produced erythrocytes as (personalized) transfusion products or as therapeutic delivery agents, the mechanisms driving this last step of erythropoiesis are in dire need of resolving. Here we review the elusive last steps of reticulocyte maturation with an emphasis on protein sorting during the defining steps of reticulocyte formation during enucleation and maturation.

Keywords: reticulocytes, erythropoiesis, differentiation, protein sorting, enucleation, maturation

INTRODUCTION

Production of red blood cells for transfusion can have several distinct benefits for healthcare and patient wellbeing (Douay and Andreu, 2007; Goodnough and Murphy, 2014; Shah et al., 2014; Benedetto et al., 2015). Alloimmunization is one of the major complications of blood transfusion and particularly affects patients who are frequently transfused. Observational studies conducted on random patients who received incidental transfusions demonstrated 1–3% alloimmunization. However, in patients with sickle cell disease (SCD) who receive chronic transfusions this can increase to 8% or even as high as 76% (Campbell-Lee and Kittles, 2014; Alkindi et al., 2017). In severe cases the only option available for the patient is a stem cell transplantation, which carries significant risk on its own. *In vitro* production of transfusable red blood cells can ensure better availability of matched blood, helping in the reduction of alloimmunization and contributing to more efficient treatment of such diseases as hemoglobinopathies and MDS. Apart from possible immune reactions, donor blood can be a source of blood borne diseases such as Hepatitis B and HIV. Produced *in vitro* red blood cells will be safe in terms of infections spreading. Another application for *in vitro* cultured red cells may be as vehicle for therapeutic agents, delivering cargo to specific parts in the body (Muzykantov, 2010; Crossan et al., 2011). Production of cultured red blood cells, however, faces a couple of challenges. First is quantity of production. One unit of blood transfused to the patient contains about 2 trillion red blood cells and annual transfusion need counts up to 90 million units in the world annually (World Health Organisation [WHO], 2017). Currently existing laboratory culture systems of red blood cells are not able to generate satisfactory number of red blood cells in efficient and cost-effective fashion, which need to be improved. Second challenge of red blood cells production is the quality of product. Existing laboratory culture systems give rise to reticulocytes of different stages of maturity using various culture systems and starting material depending or not depending on co-culture with specific stromal cells (Migliaccio et al., 2002, 2010; Giarratana et al., 2005; Leberbauer et al., 2005; Miharada et al., 2006; van den Akker et al., 2010a; Shah et al., 2016; Trakarnsanga et al., 2017). Reticulocytes are immature red blood cells that lost their nucleus but still retain residual RNA. Reticulocytes can perform the main function of red blood cells-oxygen transport. However, they have not yet adopted the unique biconcave shape of mature red blood cells that ensures their stability and flexibility to withstand blood flow shear stress. Luc Douay and coworkers published unique research in which they performed autologous transfusion of ^{51}Cr labeled *in vitro* cultured red blood cells to a human volunteer (Giarratana et al., 2011), reporting a reticulocyte half-life of approximately 26 days post injection. The life span of red blood cell is 120 days, which suggests that the *in vitro* cultured reticulocytes exhibit high clearance, possibly due to their low stability and immaturity. Effective use of cultured red blood cells for transfusion purposes may benefit from maturation of reticulocytes to mature erythrocytes, a process that is ill-defined and poorly understood. It is known that after the enucleation process, reticulocytes enter the bloodstream where they complete their maturation into fully functional erythrocytes within 3 days (Chasis et al., 1989). The reticulocyte stage of erythroid differentiation is brief, however, involves an extensive array of changes. During maturation reticulocytes undergo membrane remodeling, lose up to 20% of membrane, eliminate residual organelles and RNA and gain bi-concaveness (Gronowicz et al., 1984). Understanding the processes and factors involved in maturation of reticulocytes is an important step toward development of culture system producing transfusion-ready red blood cells. This review covers recent findings in the process of reticulocyte maturation with an implication in red blood cell production. **Table 1** indicates commonly used abbreviations throughout the review.

TABLE 1 | Abbreviations and function.

Acronym	Full name
MDS	Myelodysplastic syndrom
HIV	Human Immunodeficiency Virus
BMP-4	Bone Morphogenetic Protein 4
IL-6	Interleukin 6
TNF-alpha	Tumor Necrosis Factor alpha
INF-gamma	Interferon gamma
VCAM-1	Vascular Cell Adhesion Molecule 1
ICAM-4	Intracellular Adhesion Molecule 4
Gas6	Growth arrest-specific 6
Epo	Erythropoietin
PI3K	Phosphatidylinositol-4,5-bisphosphate 3-kinase
PKB	Protein Kinase B
TAM-receptor	Tyrosine Activation Motif receptor
CAR	Contractile Actomyosine Ring
CRIK	Citron Rho-interacting Kinase
Rho-GTPase	Rho-Guanosine TriPhosphate
MLC2	Myosin regulatory Light Chain 2
HAT	Histone Acetyl Transferase
HDAC	Histone Deacetylase
Gnc5	General control non-derepressible 5
MERTK	Proto-oncogene tyrosine-protein kinase MER
CD34	Cluster of differentiation; transmembrane phosphoglycoprotein
RhAG	Rh-Associated Glycoprotein
GPC	Glycophorin C
EMP	Erythroblast Macrophage Protein
CD147	Basignin
Xk	Kell blood group precursor
Rh	Rhesus
CD47	Integrin Associated Protein
CD49d	Integrin alpha subunit
CD71	Transferrin Receptor 1 (Trf1)
TO	Thiazole Orange
KCC	Potassium Chloride Cotransporter
LPA	Lysophosphatidic Acid
SCD	Sickle Cell Disease
Lu	Lutheran
BCAM	Basal Cell Adhesion Molecule
PKA	Protein Kinase A
GLUT4	Glucose transporter type 4
GPA	Glycophorin A
MVEs	Multivesicular Endosomes
ESCRT	Endosomal sorting complexes required for transport
AQP1	Aquaporin 1
MVB	Multivesicular Body
LC3	Light chain 3b
Rab11	Ras-related protein
LW	Landsteiner-Wiener
CD44	Cell surface glycoprotein

THE ELUSIVE AND ILL-DEFINED ROLE OF MACROPHAGES WITHIN ERYTHROBLASTIC ISLANDS

Terminal erythroid differentiation within bone marrow as well as during ontogeny takes place at specialized multicellular structures called erythroblastic islands (Bessis, 1958; Mohandas and Prenant, 1978) (**Figure 1**). Erythroblastic islands are composed of a central macrophage surrounded by differentiating erythroblasts and reticulocytes. It is unknown whether the primary function of the central macrophage is mainly to engulf and digest the expulsed nuclei, or whether the mutual interaction between the macrophage and the maturing erythroblasts contribute to the erythroid differentiation program and/or macrophage function. Adding to this confusion are the numerous knockouts that interfere with putative interaction partners facilitating the association between erythroid and macrophages that may or may not result in anemia (Sadahira et al., 1995; Hanspal et al., 1998b; Lee et al., 2006; Soni et al., 2006; Heideveld and van den Akker, 2017). Equally confusing is the observation that specific ablation of CD163+ macrophages in mice, although somewhat attenuating erythropoiesis, does not result in anemia (Chow et al., 2011). Differentiating erythroblasts follow distinct morphological changes that define the nomenclature. The early erythroblast stage is characterized

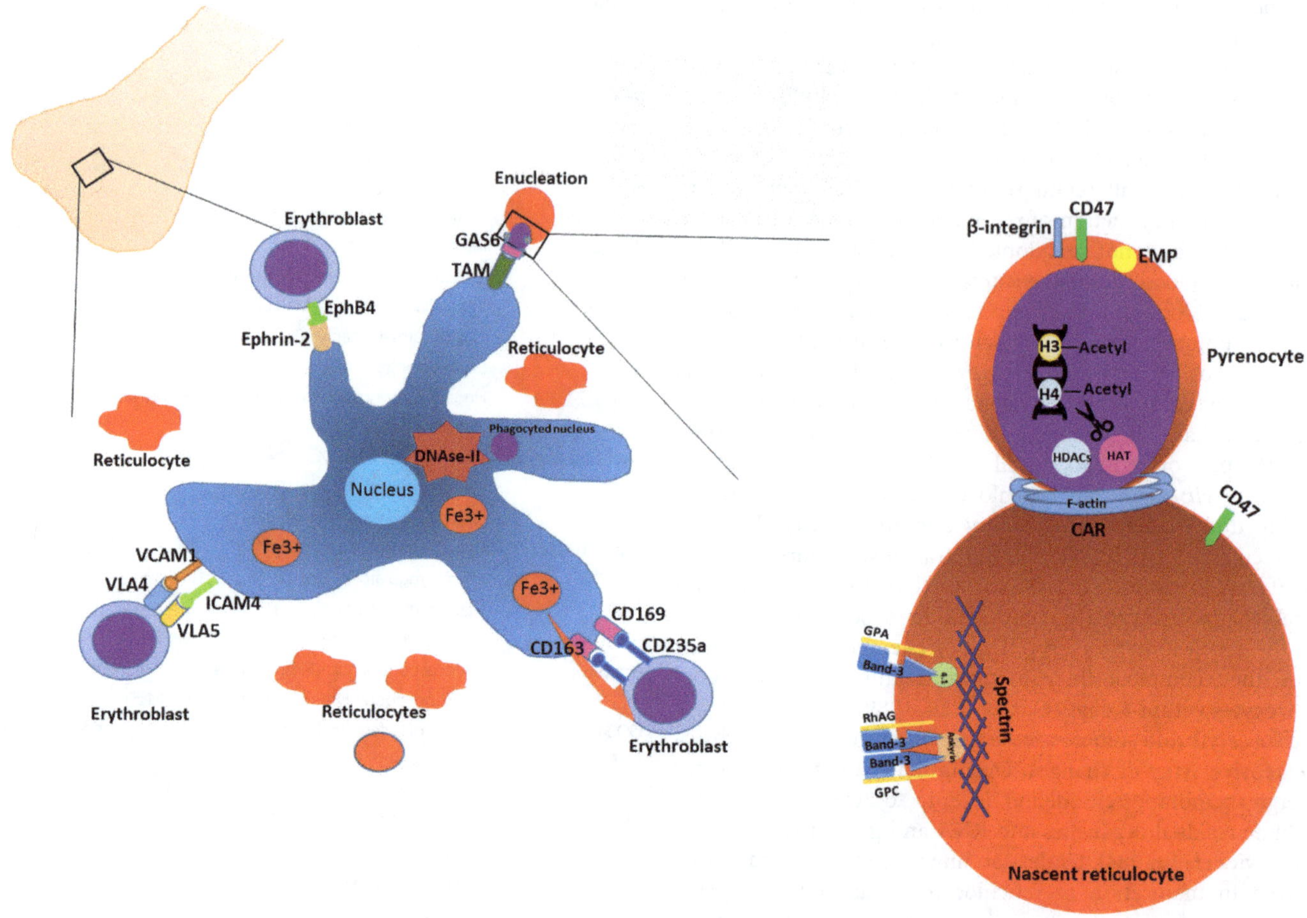

FIGURE 1 | Enucleation and reticulocyte formation in the bone marrow. Erythropoiesis in the bone marrow occurs in structures termed macrophage islands consisting of a central macrophage, surrounded by erythroid cells at different maturation stages and reticulocytes. In order to facilitate the interaction with erythroblasts, macrophage expresses various adhesion molecules such as VCAM1, ICAM4, CD169, CD163. In the erythroid niche, central macrophages play a nursing role for developing erythroblasts. Moreover, macrophage facilitates the enucleation process by phagocytosing and degrading of extruded nuclei through, e.g., interacting with erythroblast via, e.g., GAS6-TAM ligand-receptor tandem. Enucleation of erythroblasts is a complex process which includes condensation of chromatin, deacetylation of histones, formation of CAR and further abscission. Enucleation is coupled to the sorting of unwanted proteins to the pyrenocyte and retention of essential proteins. Generally, cytoskeleton-associated proteins and integral membrane proteins remain in the reticulocytes. Adhesion molecules such as β-integrin, are predominantly sorted to the pyrenocytes (see text).

by a large cell size, 12–20 μm in diameter, with a nucleus that occupies up to 80% of the cell volume. Nuclei of erythroblasts contain a large number of nucleoli. Basophilic erythroblasts are smaller and characterized by increased condensation of chromatin, combined with basophilic cytoplasm. Polychromatic erythroblasts are characterized by emerging hemoglobinization of the cytoplasm and irregularly condensed nuclei. In orthochromatic erythroblasts hemoglobinization is nearly completed, and nuclei are pyknotic. In this stage the cells do not expel several nuclei expulsion and differentiation to reticulocytes. The concept of erythroblastic islands was introduced by Bessis (1958) who analyzed transmission electron micrographs of bone marrow sections (Bessis, 1958). Bessis hypothesized that central macrophages play a supporting role during erythropoiesis by providing ferritin to the cells and by phagocytosis of expelled nuclei (Bessis and Breton-Gorius, 1962). The hypothesis of Bessis was reinforced by the study of Mohandas on hyper transfused rats (Mohandas and Prenant, 1978) in which erythropoiesis and the number of erythroblast-macrophage clusters is suppressed. Single stimulation of these rats with erythropoietin induced synchronous differentiation of resting erythroblast precursor cells. These experiments allowed to detect the individual clusters of erythroblasts within the bone marrow and link the formation of these multicellular structures to erythropoiesis. Quantitative light and electron microscopy of rat bone marrow sections demonstrated that islands form far from the sinuses accommodate mostly pro-erythroblasts, while the islands situated in the proximity to bone marrow sinuses contained more of differentiating erythroblasts and reticulocytes (Mohandas and Prenant, 1978; Yokoyama et al., 2003). It was proposed by Yokoyama et al. (2003) that erythroblastic islands can migrate toward the sinuses as differentiation of erythroid cells progresses, albeit through unknown mechanisms. This hypothesis, however, requires experimental reinforcement as it is unknown what signals, intrinsic or extrinsic, drive this apparent dynamic process. Co-culture of CD34+ cells with stromal cells or macrophages results in nearly complete enucleation, compared to feeder-free cultures (Giarratana et al., 2005 #729; Fujimi et al., 2008; Lu et al., 2008 #1723). Importantly, other studies have shown that erythroid terminal differentiation to complete enucleation can occur independent of central macrophages and that resulting reticulocytes can mature to biconcave erythrocytes upon injection into the bloodstream (Leberbauer et al., 2005; Ji et al., 2010; van den Akker et al., 2010a; Giarratana et al., 2011). So, although for enucleation and reticulocyte formation macrophages appear to be dispensable, macrophages may provide signals that optimize specific but ill-defined erythroid maturation processes that may be crucial for the eventual reticulocyte stability and function. In addition, specific culture systems/protocols may be more suitable to investigate specific signal transduction and transcriptional programs induced by the interplay between macrophages and erythroid cells and may for instance only manifest upon suboptimal culture conditions. For instance, macrophages within the erythroblastic island regulate erythropoiesis by multiple mechanisms including secretion of soluble factors and cell–cell contact. Macrophages have been shown to secrete BMP4, which can stimulate proliferation of erythroblasts (Millot et al., 2010; Heideveld et al., 2015). Macrophages also support erythropoiesis by secreting ferritin which is later taken up by erythroblasts via transferrin receptor or endocytosis (Meyron-Holtz et al., 1999; Leimberg et al., 2008; Kim et al., 2015). Secretion of IL-6, TNF-α, and INF-γ by macrophages down-regulates erythroid differentiation, while TGF-β suppresses proliferation of early erythroblasts, and enhances differentiation (Zermati et al., 2000; Bohmer, 2004). Direct cell-cell interactions also regulate erythropoiesis within the islands. Several adhesion molecules have been identified that direct contact of erythroblasts with the central macrophage. Emp knockout mice die perinatal due to severe defects in hematopoiesis and have a complete lack of F4/80 erythroblastic island macrophages, whilst erythroid cells display defects in enucleation and undergo increased apoptosis (Hanspal et al., 1998b). Another protein described to mediate erythroid-macrophage interaction and which can be used as a marker of central macrophages is VCAM-1 (Chow et al., 2011). Erythroblasts utilize α4β1 integrin and ICAM4 to bind to VCAM-1 and establish a tight contact with the macrophage and neighboring erythroblasts (Palis, 2016; Seu et al., 2017). Blocking of α4β1integrin with antibodies decreased cell proliferation and increased apoptosis *in vitro* and arrests erythropoiesis at E12 in α4 deficient mice (Sadahira et al., 1995; Lee et al., 2006). Interestingly though VCAM knockout mice do not display any phenotype regarding erythropoiesis, shedding doubt on whether VCAM is the interaction partner of α4β1 integrin (Ulyanova et al., 2016). Erythroblasts themselves can modulate inhibitory signaling from macrophages. Erythropoietin induces the secretion of Gas6 by erythroblasts which enhances the survival response to Epo-receptor signaling through PI3K and PKB-kinase signaling (Angelillo-Scherrer et al., 2008) and may function to facilitate phagocytosis of extruded nuclei through GAS6-dependent TAM-receptor present on central macrophages, which are expressed on human bone marrow and fetal liver macrophages (Toda et al., 2014; Heideveld and van den Akker, 2017). So although specific partners that facilitate the interaction between erythroid cells and macrophages as well as paracrine signaling has been found, the precise role of the central macrophage to the differentiation process of erythroid cells remains ill-defined. Recent phenotypic analysis of central macrophage populations in human bone marrow and fetal liver, together with the development of *in vitro* models now allows for *in vitro* experiments that could shed further light onto this elusive macrostructure (Hom et al., 2015; Belay et al., 2017; Heideveld and van den Akker, 2017; Seu et al., 2017).

ENUCLEATION

Enucleation of late stage erythroblasts or orthochromatic normoblasts is a unique cellular process that gives rise to reticulocytes [also reviewed in (Migliaccio, 2010)]. The only other cells in the body that undergo enucleation are the cells in the lens of our eyes. Before enucleation occurs, erythroblasts undergo cell cycle arrest, the chromatin condenses and the nucleus locates to the edge of the cell (Keerthivasan et al., 2011). Initially, enucleation was thought to be a specific form of apoptosis, which was based on microscopic detection of karyolysis and partial leakage of nuclear content into the cytoplasm (Simpson and Kling, 1967). In addition, the enucleation process in keratinocytes and fiber lens cells has also been described as a specific mechanism of programmed cell death (Bassnett, 1997; Yamamoto-Tanaka et al., 2014). However, reduction of caspase expression or inhibition of caspase activity demonstrated little to no involvement of caspases in erythroid enucleation (Carlile et al., 2004; Yoshida et al., 2005). Instead, recent evidence supports a model of asymmetric cytokinesis to separate the nucleus from the cell. This implies that the enucleating cell should display a cleavage furrow, the contractile actomyosine ring (CAR) and a stage of completion with abscission (Barr and Gruneberg, 2007) (**Figure 1**).

The Mechanism of Enucleation

A few players in cytokinesis were shown to play a role in enucleation. Citron Rho-interacting kinase (CRIK), a mitotic kinase known to interact with Rho-GTPases (Magor et al., 2015), regulates the length of astral microtubules and the orientation of the spindle in dividing cells. During enucleation, CRIK participates in the nuclear condensation and is involved in the formation of the CAR, possibly via interaction with MLC2 (Swartz et al., 2017). Another essential factor involved in enucleation is deacetylation of histones H3 and H4. Regulation of the acetylation status of those histones is carried out by enzymes histone acetyl transferase (HAT) and histone deacetylase (HDACs) (Ji et al., 2010). It has been shown that during late stage fetal erythropoiesis in mice Gcn5 and c-Myc are downregulated and histone deacetylase 2 is upregulated, which results in the chromatin condensation and CAR formation (Jayapal et al., 2010). Konstantidinis described the formation of an actin-myosine ring upon initiation of enucleation. Actin-myosin ring contracts and the condensed nucleus is expelled out of the cell together with the thin rim of cytoplasm and plasma membrane to form the pyrenocyte (Konstantinidis et al., 2012). As well as in cytokinesis, the cytoskeleton plays an important role in erythroblast enucleation. Immunofluorescent and microscopic studies demonstrated the condensation of F-actin filaments and formation of CAR can be disrupted by cytochalasin and depends on Rho-GTPase activity and downstream mDia activation (Sawada et al., 1989; Ji et al., 2008). Formation of microtubules plays an essential role in nucleus polarization and extrusion. It has been shown that inhibition of PI3K decreases nuclear polarization efficiency and delays the enucleation in mice (Wang et al., 2012). The mechanism of asymmetric cytokinesis is sustained by a second process that may act concurrently: the formation and trafficking of vesicles during abscission. During this final stage of cytokinesis, vesicles move toward the midbody region, fuse and promote the separation of the daughter cell (Gromley et al., 2005). Vesicles mainly contribute to enucleation by supplying membranes to the progressing tip of the cleavage furrow and thus facilitating the separation of pyrenocyte from reticulocyte. Disruption of vesicle trafficking and inhibition of clathrin expression blocked the enucleation of erythroblasts, suggesting that vesicle trafficking has an essential role in nuclear extrusion process (Keerthivasan et al., 2010). Of note, the eventual phagocytosis of the extruded nuclei occurs via protein-S dependent and MERTK dependent processes (Toda et al., 2014). High enucleation rates have been described for *in vitro* culture systems that initiate from cord blood, fetal or adult CD34+ hematopoietic stem and progenitor cells (Leberbauer et al., 2005; van den Akker et al., 2010a; Giarratana et al., 2011). In contrast, enucleation is generally poor in immortalized cell lines and erythroid cells derived from induced pluripotent stem cells (Lapillonne et al., 2010; Kurita et al., 2013; Trakarnsanga et al., 2017) [reviewed by (Focosi and Amabile, 2017)]. Resolving the fine details of the enucleation process and events leading up to enucleation may facilitate and improve the production of erythrocytes from these immortal sources. This is important as immortalized lines provide a considerable simplification of the *in vitro* erythrocyte production method, can be genetically altered to express specific blood groups or therapeutic cargo and can be standardized.

Protein Sorting During Enucleation

During erythroblast enucleation, plasma membrane and cytoskeletal proteins undergo reorganization while the nucleus, surrounded by plasma membrane, separates from the reticulocyte. A key aspect of this process is the distribution of (membrane) proteins to the pyrenocyte and/or reticulocytes, which may be through active sorting of specific proteins or through non-specific simple redistribution. By consequence, protein sorting during enucleation determines the protein content of reticulocyte membranes and possibly also intracellular proteins. Cytoskeletal proteins important for erythrocyte function, such as the erythrocyte Spectrins, Ankyrin, and protein 4.1, remain within the nascent reticulocyte (Sawada et al., 1989; Wickrema et al., 1994). Integral membrane proteins that are associated with the cytoskeleton, such as Glycophorin A (Lee et al., 2004), Band 3, RhAG, GPC; (Salomao et al., 2010) are thus predominantly found on the reticulocyte. Some proteins are specifically sorted to the pyrenocyte, such as the erythroblast macrophage protein (EMP), β1 integrin, Basignin (or CD147) and other adhesion molecules (Lee et al., 2004; Soni et al., 2006; Griffiths et al., 2012; Gautier et al., 2016). Distinct differences in the membrane composition of pyrenocytes and reticulocytes is likely to direct macrophages to phagocytose extruded nuclei. The mechanism of selective retention or exclusion of specific proteins within newly generated reticulocytes is still largely unknown but involve association with the erythroid specific Spectrin/Ankyrin cytoskeleton (Lee et al., 2004; Keerthivasan et al., 2011; Satchwell et al., 2016). During erythropoiesis the cytoskeleton is rearranged to facilitate large protein membrane networks that control the structural integrity of erythrocytes in the circulation through regulation of morphology by modulation of protein-cytoskeleton interactions or ion-transport (Bruce et al., 2009; van den Akker et al., 2010b; Satchwell et al., 2011). These networks can be roughly divided into an Ankyrin network and a junctional network [for review see (Bruce, 2008; van den Akker et al., 2010c)]. Mutations within proteins that comprise these complexes results in an array of erythrocyte specific diseases like hereditary spherocytosis and elliptocytosis [reviewed in (Da Costa et al., 2013; Gallagher, 2013)]. It has been proposed that inclusion of proteins within such networks facilitates reticulocyte retention during enucleation and vice versa localization to the nuclei upon non-inclusion (Satchwell et al., 2016). For instance GPC is located to the pyrenocyte in 4.1 deficient erythroblasts while this protein normally is sorted to reticulocytes, and GPA and Rh-associated antigens are misdirected to the pyrenocyte in ankyrin deficient erythroblasts (Chasis et al., 1993; Satchwell et al., 2016). Aberrant sorting of proteins during enucleation may lay fundament to the development of pathologies like Hereditary spherocytosis and elliptocytosis. Mutations within membrane proteins or cytoskeleton proteins resulting in disturbed/weakened association between specific membrane proteins with the cytoskeleton lead to aberrant distribution to pyrenocytes (Salomao et al., 2010; Satchwell et al., 2016). A strict hierarchy is present that results from inter-dependency of specific membrane protein expression. For instance, loss of RhAG will lead to a complete loss of Rh proteins, a loss of Kell means a loss of Xk, and loss of RhCE or protein 4.2 leads to a significantly reduced level of CD47 (Cherif-Zahar et al., 1996; Rivera et al., 2013; Mordue et al., 2017). Thus mutations within such "master" proteins may have significant domino effects on other proteins and thus the constitution and functionality of these large membrane complexes affecting erythrocyte stability. However, for proteins that are not part of these cytoskeleton-membrane protein hubs it is unknown if underlying mechanisms are specific or not. More work is required in order to determine the exact mechanism of protein sorting during enucleation. Understanding the nature of the sorting process can shed some light on the protein loss combined to the mutation in membrane-cytoskeleton complexes. This knowledge can aid in development of possible prevention and treatment of Hereditary spherocytosis and Elliptocytosis. In addition, direction of specific membrane proteins to these large membrane complexes may facilitate specific incorporation of therapeutic proteins to be used as delivery tools. A role for lipid composition to the sorting of proteins cannot be ruled out as it has been shown that lipid modifications and alterations during pathology associate with increased adhesion capabilities of erythrocytes (Hillery et al., 1996; Connor et al., 1997; Kuypers et al., 2007).

MATURATION OF RETICULOCYTES IN THE CIRCULATION

Although the term reticulocytes generally refers to enucleated erythroid cells that are not yet fully biconcave, one must appreciate these reticulocytes are a heterogeneous population of all stages in between enucleated reticulocytes and erythrocytes (Malleret et al., 2013; Ovchynnikova et al., 2017). These stages are characterized by progressive loss of RNA and membrane proteins that are cleared during maturation, such as CD71 or CD49d. In addition, reticulocyte maturation can be defined by size, morphology, biomechanical properties and metabolic state (Malleret et al., 2013). Diversity within the reticulocyte population was first described in early 1930's (Heilmeyer and Westhäuser, 1932). Based on brilliant Cresyl blue staining patterns, four stages were identified in the circulation: group I, group II, group III, and group IV (Heilmeyer and Westhäuser, 1932). Implementation of flow cytometry methods and use of Thiazole Orange (TO) to visualize RNA provided a more advanced reticulocyte maturity index classification system (Davis et al., 1995; Choi and Pai, 2001; Wollmann et al., 2014). This system, however, is proven to be inaccurate in certain conditions. Presence of hemoparasites and pathological erythrocyte inclusions such as Howell–Jolly bodies may result in false positive staining. Gradual loss of the transferrin receptor makes it an informative marker for reticulocyte maturation (Malleret et al., 2013). Based on CD71 staining of cord blood derived reticulocytes Malleret et al. (2013) described four stages of reticulocyte maturity namely CD71high, CD71medium, CD71low and CD71negative. Utilization of TO staining together with CD71 provides a more accurate distinction of various stages of reticulocyte maturation, mostly due to the fact that CD71 loss occurs prior to the loss of RNA. Based on CD71/TO dual staining it is possible to differentiate four stages of reticulocyte maturation from early reticulocytes R1 to late reticulocytes R4 (Malleret et al., 2013; Ovchynnikova et al., 2017). Upon release from the erythroblastic island, reticulocytes are irregularly shaped, multilobular cells that are far from being flexible compared to mature red blood cell (Mel et al., 1977; Malleret et al., 2013). To adopt a bi-concave morphology, stability, and the ability to deform these cells have to undergo a maturation process. Membrane-cytoskeleton rearrangement may be an important step allowing the transition from an unstructured reticulocyte to a morphologically biconcave and functional erythrocyte (Waugh et al., 1997, 2001). It takes 1–2 days in the circulation for the reticulocyte to obtain bi-concaveness and mature into fully functional erythrocytes (Chasis et al., 1989). Surprisingly, mature reticulocytes are stable and deformable as mature erythrocytes, while in young reticulocytes mechanical stability and membrane deformability are decreased (Chasis et al., 1989; Waugh et al., 1997). In addition, extracellular epitope exposure of specific membrane proteins is changing during reticulocyte maturation (Malleret et al., 2013; Ovchynnikova et al., 2017). This most likely involves specific protein reorganization into large protein complexes masking specific epitopes but could also suggest structural protein remodeling due through specific interactions or through lipid content remodeling (Sailaja et al., 2004; Ovchynnikova et al., 2017). Unfortunately, not much is known about how volume loss and discoid shaping are manifesting during differentiation, and what is known is mainly obtained from animals with reticulocytosis caused by stress erythropoiesis. Generalizing, there are three major events occurring in this time window: volume control, membrane remodeling and vesicularization (**Figure 2**).

Reticulocyte Volume Control

It has been calculated that the average cell volume of a reticulocyte once egressed from the bone marrow is 115 fL and decreases to

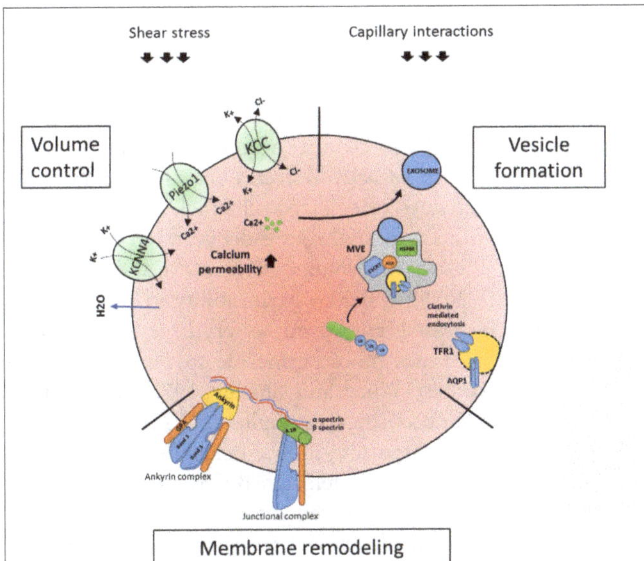

FIGURE 2 | Processes occurring within the maturing circulating reticulocyte. Once enucleated, the newly formed reticulocyte migrates to the peripheral blood where it completes its maturation in a surrounding eliciting external forces, shear stress and capillary/splenic interactions. Three major events occurring are volume control, membrane remodeling and vesicularization. As for volume control, a key role is played by ion channels KCNN4 (or Gardos), Piezo1 and KCC1 (see text). During reticulocyte maturation an active membrane remodeling is also occurring, in which the two main red blood cells complexes, the ankyrin and the junctional complexes (linked through a cytoskeleton network) are involved (see text). Lastly, the reticulocyte makes use of the ESCRT- mediated multi vesicular body (MVB) machinery to expel unwanted proteins. Proteins, e.g., TFR1 and Aquaporin1 are ubiquitinated and routed to the MVB where the ESCRT complex (in particular its associated protein Alix and Hsp60) contributes in assembling the MVB; this process will result in exosome releasing, which is also described to be triggered by calcium influx (see text). All three processes are mechanistically linked (see text) and need to occur in order for a reticulocyte to mature to an erythrocyte.

85 fL in mature erythrocytes, while the hemoglobin concentration (CHC) is increasing from 27 to 33 g/dL (Gallagher, 2017). Reticulocyte volume loss can be attributed to two processes, (i) through loss of membranes and intracellular remnants due to exosome/vesicle formation/shedding and (ii) through actions of transporters that regulate the cation/anion and water content and thereby cell volume. The contribution of each process to the eventual 20% loss of cell volume is not known. The potassium chloride cotransporter (KCC) is important in these processes. When KCC is activated, the cell loses potassium, chloride and water leading to cell volume loss. It was demonstrated that KCC activity decreases during reticulocyte maturation (Canessa et al., 1987; Bize et al., 2003; Quarmyne et al., 2011). It was also proven that Sickle Cell reticulocytes have an altered regulation of KCC activity, possibly being the cause of Sickle Cells dehydration. In conjunction with KCC, the mechanosensitive channel Piezo1 plays a role in volume regulation (Bagriantsev et al., 2014). When activated, Piezo1 causes Ca^{2+} to enter the cell, leading to the activation of the Gardos-channel associated with a change on K+ and Cl− influx and water loss, essential events that allow the red blood cell to narrow through the blood capillaries (Fermo et al., 2017). Presently, numerous gain of function mutations in the mechanosensor Piezo1 have been found that cause the most common form of hereditary stomatocytosis namely hereditary xerocytosis (Zarychanski et al., 2012; Albuisson et al., 2013; Andolfo et al., 2013; Da Costa et al., 2013; Archer et al., 2014; Beneteau et al., 2014; Sandberg et al., 2014). Interestingly, a Piezo channel agonist independent of the mechanosensitive mode of activation has been found, YODA1, that selectively activates the Piezo channel function. This induces calcium influx and erythrocyte dehydration confirming its the role of Piezo-1 in volume control (Cahalan et al., 2015; Syeda et al., 2015). Calcium permeability in reticulocytes is significantly increased compared to erythrocytes. Healthy reticulocytes are 43 times more permeable to Ca^{2+} compared to mature erythrocytes (Wiley and Shaller, 1977), which may be linked to mechanosensing, through, e.g., Piezo1. Indeed, inhibiting *N*-methyl-D-aspartate-induced calcium influx during erythroid maturation results in defective differentiation (Makhro et al., 2013). In addition, increased intracellular calcium levels due to secondary calcium-dependent phosphorylation processes have been observed in reticulocytes and may possibly link to specific phosphorylation of junctional and ankyrin complex proteins necessary for erythrocyte structural integrity (de Haro et al., 1985; Liu et al., 2010). Not all signal transduction that results in calcium influx in erythrocytes is functional in reticulocytes indicating an interesting signal specificity. For instance, lysophosphatidic acid (LPA) stimulation of RBCs is known to increase Ca^{2+} influx in erythrocytes (Yang et al., 2000), however, reticulocytes lack a Ca^{2+} response to LPA stimulation (Wang et al., 2013). Interestingly, Ca^{2+} ionophore-induced laminin association in SCD erythrocytes was not observed in reticulocytes (Burnett et al., 2004). It is known that increased Ca^{2+} flux induces release of vesicles in erythrocytes, which can contribute to the vast membrane loss during reticulocyte maturation (Kostova et al., 2015). How calcium signaling contributes to reticulocyte maturation will need to be further investigated, but reticulocytes express several surface molecules that induce Ca^{2+} fluxes.

Extracellular Factors Involved in Reticulocyte Maturation

Exiting the bone marrow, reticulocytes end up in a complex environment where their fate and development may be determined by a plethora of factors such as interactions with other blood components, endothelial cells, red pulp macrophages of the spleen, macrophages in liver and physical forces such as shear stress and osmolarity changes. Whilst the role of splenic and liver interactions in the development of reticulocyte was extensively studied (Yuditskaya et al., 2010; Klei et al., 2017), the influence of the shear stress forces and capillary interactions remains to date unclear. Reticulocytes share characteristics with erythrocytes of sickle cell disease (SCD) patients. Therefore, the physiology of sickle cells and their interaction with endothelium can shed some light on the fate of healthy reticulocytes in the blood stream. Patients with SCD are prone to develop painful vaso-occlusive crisis, which is characterized by abnormal interaction between red cells, leukocytes and endothelium and can lead to aggregate formation (Manodori et al., 1998). Reticulocyte-specific maintenance expression of adhesion proteins that may facilitate interaction with the endothelium. Among those proteins are $\alpha_4\beta_1$ integrin which is widely expressed on reticulocytes and interacts with VCAM-1, CD47 which binds to thrombospondin and Lu/BCAM which interacts with laminin (Gee and Platt, 1995; Udani et al., 1998). Hillery et al. (1996) showed that during reticulocytosis an increase, albeit modest, in thrombospondin association was observed, which may indicate increased endothelial interaction of reticulocytes. Although interactions with the endothelium would generally be considered as unwanted, it is unknown why reticulocytes still express specific receptors that could facilitate these interactions and if a so whether biological relevance can be found concerning endothelial interactions. Sickle cells display a higher activation status of Lutheran while healthy reticulocytes display higher expression of Lu/BCAM compared to erythrocytes, while the activation status of Lutheran in reticulocytes is less clear (Malleret et al., 2013). Binding of sickle cells to laminin is mediated via stimulation of β-adrenergic receptor and subsequent activation of $G_{\alpha s}$, which stimulates adenylyl cyclase. This enzyme induces conversion of ATP to cAMP, which activates PKA. This kinase mediates Lu/BCAM adhesion to laminin via yet unknown targets (Hines et al., 2003). Another molecule which is upregulated on sickle cells as well as on healthy reticulocytes is CD47, which binds to soluble and surface associated thrombospondin. Brittain et al. (2001) demonstrated increased affinity of sickle cells to thrombospondin upon shear stress application via activation of G_1 tyrosine kinase pathway. The relations between maturing red blood cells and macrophages of spleen and liver is important. It is proposed that macrophages of red pulp take part in "polishing" of the red cell membrane by removing excessive membranes and exosomes [reviewed by (Klei et al., 2017)]. Indicative of this "polishing" role is the presence of exosomes and inclusions such as Howell–Jolly bodies in splenectomized patients, whereas in healthy patients less than 2% of red blood cells have visible inclusions. Splenectomized patients show an increase in reticulocyte numbers. It has been speculated that this is due to delayed maturation and not by increased erythroid flux (De Haan et al., 1988). General reticulocyte parameters like morphological changes or volume loss are, however, not affected upon splenectomy indicating that spleen macrophages are not essential for these maturation parameters. Despite the specific quality control functions by splenic macrophages, reticulocyte maturation proceeds as normal in splenectomized patient indicating that reticulocyte maturation is partly intrinsic, or dependent on passage through other erythroid-regulating organs such as the liver, and may be promoted by other processes such as shear stress-induced signaling or endothelial interactions.

Membrane and Cytoskeleton Remodeling During Reticulocyte Maturation

Reticulocyte maturation is accompanied not only by a loss of cytosolic organelles, but also by an intense membrane remodeling. In red blood cells, two major membrane complexes are found: the ankyrin complex and the junctional (or 4.1 based) complex. These complexes are linked through a fine cytoskeletal network which involves spectrin as the main constituent. The anion transporter protein Band 3 (Anion Exchanger 1) plays a key role, as it is the main component of both complexes and anchors them to the cytoskeleton (Mohandas and Gallagher, 2008; van den Akker et al., 2010c). The cytoskeletal network comprises proteins like α-spectrin, β-spectrin, actin, protein 4.1R, ankyrin R, protein 4.2, p55, adducin, dematin, tropomyosin, and tropomodulin (Liu et al., 2011). Ankyrin deficiency causes a disruption of the membrane network, including the incapacity of Band 3 to form tetrameric complex and degradation of protein 4.2, together with loss of reticulocytes protein due to increased sorting of these proteins in the pyrenocyte (Satchwell et al., 2016). Some of these proteins are also lost during normal reticulocyte maturation, such as cytosolic actin and tubulin while some non-cytoskeletal proteins including GLUT4, $Na^{+}K^{+}$ ATPase, GPA and CD47 are only reduced (Liu et al., 2010). The reduction involves also the membrane protein Glycophorin A (GPA), although in our recent study we showed that during reticulocyte maturation GPA expression is only changing slightly compared to mature erythrocytes (Ovchynnikova et al., 2017). Band 3, Rh, RhAG, GPC, and XK are increased, most probably due to a loss of the membrane surface (Liu et al., 2010). The mechanisms behind the differential change in expression of the membrane proteins are nowadays still unknown. The loss of tubulin and actin has been proved to be mediated by the ubiquitin-proteasome system (Liu et al., 2010). Phosphorylation of certain proteins could play a role. Indeed, phosphorylation of 4.1 protein is significantly higher in reticulocytes compared to erythrocytes (Liu et al., 2010). Phosphorylation of protein 4.1 regulates the strength of the spectrin-p55-4.1R ternary complex, and increased phosphorylation in reticulocytes weakens the association of these proteins in reticulocytes compared to erythrocytes (Manno et al., 2005). Decreasing 4.1 phosphorylation during reticulocyte maturation will strengthen the junctional complex and regulates the mechanical stress mature erythrocytes can endure. Interestingly, a spectrin fragment mimicking a β spectrin region involved in the ternary complex formation is incorporated more easily in reticulocytes than erythrocytes, resulting in a more unstable junctional complex in reticulocytes (Manno et al., 2005). Interestingly other proteins comprising the junctional complex, GPC, XK, and Kell, are more extractable upon detergent treatment underscoring the weakened link of these membrane proteins to the underlying spectrin cytoskeleton. In contrast, proteins within the ankyrin complex remain bound to cytoskeleton (band 3, Rh, RhAG, and GPA), suggesting that during reticulocyte maturation the latter complex is already formed, while the former is still remodeling, eventually contributing to a more stable cell with an higher tolerance toward shear stress. Presently little is known about the regulation of these complexes through phosphorylation in reticulocytes. The assembly of these complexes during erythropoiesis is critical to the eventual stability of *in vitro* produced erythrocytes. Indeed, due to the optimization of *in vitro* human and mouse erythroblast culture systems, we are beginning to understand the assembly of these large protein complexes during erythropoiesis (Tchernia et al., 1981; Hanspal et al., 1992, 1998a; van den Akker et al., 2010b; Satchwell et al., 2011; Trakarnsanga et al., 2017).

Protein Removal During Reticulocyte Maturation Through Exosome Shedding

Another example of membrane remodeling involves the transferrin receptor TFR1 (also referred as CD71). In general, iron-loaded transferrin binds to TFR1 and internalizes via clathrin-mediated endocytosis. In the endosome the transferrin-receptor is stripped of the iron and transferrin-receptor complex returns to the membrane, where TFR1 release apo-transferrin and with that finishes the cycle (Hentze et al., 2010). But how is TFR1 lost in reticulocytes? As heme production and transcription of globins is shut down due to mitochondrial loss and enucleation, respectively, there is no need to import the oxidative-damage-inducing iron anymore. Thus, the nascent reticulocyte has incorporated all the iron needed, and the transferrin receptor must be removed, in order to prevent overloading of iron. This involves the switching from recycling of the receptor to the encapsulation into vesicles that will be removed. It is known since 1983 that the transferrin receptor sheds into vesicles. In fact, the term exosome or vesicle release has been shown for the first time in reticulocytes (Johnstone et al., 1987), but it was only later that these vesicles were defined as exosomes. This receptor is sorted through the multivesicular endosomes (MVEs) pathway, that terminates with the incorporation of TFR1 in a new formed vesicle that is subsequently fused with plasma membrane in order for the content to be released into the extracellular medium (Pan et al., 1985). About the molecular players involved in this process, it has been shown that hsp60 and the ESCRT associated protein Alix co-localize with TFR1 in reticulocytes exosomes, confirming the involvement of the endosomal – vesicular pathway in exosomes formation (Geminard et al., 2004). Interestingly, CD71 shedding can also be regulated in Ca^{2+} dependent manner and activated by extracellular transferrin (Savina et al., 2003). Among proteins that are cleared from reticulocytes through formation of vesicles is Aquaporin 1 (AQP1). This water channel is responsible for keeping a proper plasma membrane tonicity, in response to different osmotic perturbations. It co-localizes with TFR1 in the plasma membrane and in reticulocytes endosomal compartments (Blanc et al., 2009). Together with the knowledge that the loss of aquaporin-1 has been described as a prototype example of degradation through exosomes, recent data show that AQP1 is expressed at higher levels in adult red blood cell compared to cord blood cells, as well as in adult reticulocytes compared to cord reticulocytes. Such a difference possibly reflects a different gas exchange regulation in adult and neonatal red blood cells, although this remains to be confirmed (Schutte et al., 2016). Together with TFR1 and aquaporin 1, multiple proteins need to be disposed from the plasma membrane or the cytosol during reticulocyte maturation, presumably and sensibly from an evolutionary point of view via the same mechanism. The major process involves different routes of targeting proteins to multivesicular bodies (MVB), including the lipid domain inclusion, cytosolic inclusion and lectin mediated inclusion, targeting ubiquitinated, HSC/HSP bounds proteins and glycosylated proteins to MVBs (Guinez et al., 2007; Carayon et al., 2011). The ESCRT (Endosomal Sorting Complex Required for Transport) machinery comprises four complexes: ESCRT 0, I, II, III that are involved in MVB formation. Briefly, in the endosomal lumen, ESCRT 0, which has multiple ubiquitin binding domains, binds the ubiquitinated cargo (i.e., proteins destined to be included in the vesicles) and engages the other ESCRT subunits, while facilitating interactions with clathrin domains. ESCRT I and II are recruited and cause the deforming and involution of the membrane. The process is terminated by recruitment of ESCRT III by simultaneously pulling the cargo into the invagination and generating the MVB. It is generally believed that ESCRT complexes recognize ubiquitinated membrane proteins that need to be sorted into MVB (Odorizzi et al., 1998; Raiborg and Stenmark, 2009; Hislop and von Zastrow, 2011). In contrast, intracellular proteins may be routed to MVB via HSP70/HSC70 via ill-defined mechanisms. These mechanisms include, (i) HSC70 interacting with the endosomal membrane via electrostatic associations using its C-terminal basic region (Sahu et al., 2011), (ii) interactions with the ESCRT complex again via ubiquitin-modified targets (Dajani et al., 2001) or (iii) through ubiquitination of hsc70 itself (Pridgeon et al., 2009). Hsc70-dependent microautophagic processes are thus probably linked to MVB targeting and removal of unwanted proteins. Recently, UBE2O, an E2-E3 hybrid enzyme, which acts both as ubiquitin-conjugating enzyme and ubiquitin ligase has been found to play a key role in erythroid proteome remodeling among which ribosome elimination (Nguyen et al., 2017). A further link between autophagy and plasma-membrane vesicles was found with the co-localization of glycophorin A and the autophagy protein LC3 on intracellular reticulocyte vesicles (Griffiths et al., 2012). Griffiths et al propose that the final remnants of the plasma membrane are removed via an autophagosome/endosome hybrid compartment. Exosome composition indeed changes in protein composition during maturation (Carayon et al., 2011). Whether these vesicles are different entities or similar remains to be investigated as in other cell types the autophagosome can fuse with endocytic structures such as MVBs to generate an amphisome (Berg et al., 1998). Furthermore, efficient autophagic degradation requires functional MVBs and their fusion is again calcium dependent (Fader and Colombo, 2009). Normally, besides exosome release, these vesicle bodies are destined to fuse with the lysosome, causing the degradation of specific proteins (Saksena et al., 2007). However, in maturing reticulocytes these vesicles are exclusively re-routed to a secretory pathway (Pan et al., 1985; Blanc et al., 2009). The mechanisms and in particular the pathways involved in the formation and fusion of the vesicles with the membrane and consequential secretion are not yet fully understood. In the erythroleukemia cell line K562, exosome secretion is caused by an intracellular Ca^{2+} influx (Savina et al., 2003). Indeed, significant vesicle formation can be induced upon treatment of erythrocytes with the calcium ionophore ionomycin or through PKC activation (Kostova et al., 2015; Nguyen et al., 2016). Moreover, docking and fusion of MVB to the plasma membrane is regulated by calcium dependent small GTPase Rab11 (Savina et al., 2005). Of note, Rab11 has been shown to associate with the pericentriolar recycling endosome, as well as being involved in the regulation of transferrin recycling in the endosome (Ullrich et al., 1996). It is tempting to speculate that during reticulocyte maturation, routing of non-wanted proteins utilizes the same mechanism through which TFR1 is removed. The role of calcium signaling in MVB formation and fusion as well as the increased permeability of reticulocyte to calcium suggest a prominent but ill-characterized role for calcium signaling during reticulocyte formation. The formation, regulation and contents of MVB during reticulocyte maturation requires more attention as (i) it may provide key improvement to the *in vitro* culture of mature erythrocytes rather than the reticulocytes that are currently the end-stage of most culture protocols and (ii) specific pathologies may already manifest and initiate in the reticulocyte stage due to malfunctions within the sorting/secretory machinery. For instance, in dominant inherited beta-thalassemia's, a heterozygous mutation in the beta globin chain results in unstable hemoglobins and rapid degradation of the beta chains, which may overload the available chaperone/sorting system resulting in additional secondary defects. In addition, an array of erythrocyte diseases is characterized by aberrant expression of membrane proteins that are normally completely or partially removed during erythropoiesis (e.g., BCAM, LW or CD44). However, specificity for over-expression of a small selection of membrane proteins is not easy to explain via the general mechanism of MVB-mediated protein removal. Although lists of proteins identified in reticulocyte exosomes have been published (Carayon et al., 2011), more in-depth research into the extruded but also the intracellular vesicles bodies may uncover much needed insight into the cargo and may identify crucial proteins that play a role in the formation and secretion machinery. The fate of exosomes is interesting from a signaling and immunogenic point of view. The membrane of reticulocyte exosomes contains 20%

exposed Phosphatidylserine (PS) on the outer leaflet, which is a potent phagocytic trigger for many cells including cells that are in close contact with reticulocytes, e.g., endothelial cells, macrophages and neutrophils (Vidal et al., 1989). This provides a safe clearance mechanism; however, these vesicles may also function as conveyors of specific signals upon uptake by target cells. Research on this topic and specifically concerning reticulocyte exosomes is lacking.

CONCLUSION

In the bone marrow erythropoiesis progresses until the enucleated reticulocyte stage, after which the reticulocytes are released into the circulation where final maturation occurs. Is there an evolutionary benefit for this maturation to occur in the circulation and not within the bone marrow? Early reticulocytes seem non-optimally adapted to the shear stress within the circulation and display lower deformability. Despite this, it also becomes increasingly clear that reticulocyte maturation is an interplay between intrinsic processes and extrinsic processes, including exosome formation, interactions with splenic and liver cells (e.g., macrophages) and circulation-induced shear forces. Interestingly, erythroid culture protocols are mainly driven by the intrinsic ability of erythroblasts to differentiate into reticulocytes but fail to produce fully biconcave erythrocytes, stressing that specific maturation cues are missing. Although, these missing signals may partly originate from the bone marrow niche, it is surprising that pure >95% enucleated reticulocytes can be cultured without this support (Miharada et al., 2006; van den Akker et al., 2010a; Giarratana et al., 2011). Failure to progress from reticulocytes to fully biconcave erythrocytes thus suggests a lack of signals that may be partly independent and dependent of the bone marrow niche. Of note, also stromal co-cultures (MS5 or OP9) do not completely result in reticulocyte maturation to erythrocytes (Giarratana et al., 2005; Lu et al., 2008). Indeed, a recent study published a characterization of the secretory proteins from OP9, and such studies may eventually point to specific factors to will further facilitating erythropoiesis and possibly reticulocyte maturation (Trakarnsanga et al., 2018). One such extrinsic signal may be transport/exchange regulation of volume control upon circulation-induced shear stress to facilitate reticulocyte maturation. However, more research must be performed dissecting the contribution and connections between intrinsic processes and extrinsic factors to this maturation. Even prior to this, the field is currently still assessing the identity/nature of these external factors and their concomitant erythrocyte "signal transducer" counterparts before characterization and optimization can begin. For instance, the connection between exosome formation, cargo selection (e.g., ubiquitination) and cation/anion permeability/conductance is interesting to pursue. With the aid of novel techniques to separate and discriminate the various reticulocyte maturation stages and the progressive use of lower cell numbers in -omic approaches will facilitate this research. Future erythroid culture protocols will need to incorporate the regulation (activation) of these processes to ensure complete differentiation to fully biconcave erythrocytes. The promise of *in vitro* cultured patient catered personalized transfusion products as well as erythrocytes carrying specific cargo for therapeutic purposes are potent drivers that justify research into this last elusive step of erythropoiesis.

AUTHOR CONTRIBUTIONS

EO, FA, MvL, and EA wrote the manuscript. The manuscript was critically revised by all authors.

REFERENCES

Albuisson, J., Murthy, S. E., Bandell, M., Coste, B., Louis-Dit-Picard, H., and Mathur, J. (2013). Dehydrated hereditary stomatocytosis linked to gain-of-function mutations in mechanically activated PIEZO1 ion channels. *Nat. Commun.* 4:1884. doi: 10.1038/ncomms2899

Alkindi, S., AlMahrooqi, S., AlHinai, S., AlMarhoobi, A., Al-Hosni, S., Daar, S., et al. (2017). Alloimmunization in patients with sickle cell disease and thalassemia: experience of a single centre in oman. *Mediterr. J. Hematol. Infect. Dis.* 9:e2017013. doi: 10.4084/MJHID.2017.013

Andolfo, I., Alper, S. L., Delaunay, J., Auriemma, C., Russo, R., and Asci, R. (2013). Missense mutations in the ABCB6 transporter cause dominant familial pseudohyperkalemia. *Am. J. Hematol.* 88, 66–72. doi: 10.1002/ajh.23357

Angelillo-Scherrer, A., Burnier, L., Lambrechts, D., Fish, R. J., Tjwa, M., and Plaisance, S. (2008). Role of Gas6 in erythropoiesis and anemia in mice. *J. Clin. Invest.* 118, 583–596. doi: 10.1172/JCI30375

Archer, N. M., Shmukler, B. E., Andolfo, I., Vandorpe, D. H., Gnanasambandam, R., and Higgins, J. M. (2014). Hereditary xerocytosis revisited. *Am. J. Hematol.* 89, 1142–1146. doi: 10.1002/ajh.23799

Bagriantsev, S. N., Gracheva, E. O., and Gallagher, P. G. (2014). Piezo proteins: regulators of mechanosensation and other cellular processes. *J. Biol. Chem.* 289, 31673–31681. doi: 10.1074/jbc.R114.612697

Barr, F. A., and Gruneberg, U. (2007). Cytokinesis: placing and making the final cut. *Cell* 131, 847–860. doi: 10.1016/j.cell.2007.11.011

Bassnett, S. (1997). Fiber cell denucleation in the primate lens. *Invest. Ophthalmol. Vis. Sci.* 38, 1678–1687.

Belay, E., Hayes, B. J., Blau, C. A., and Torok-Storb, B. (2017). Human cord blood and bone marrow CD34+ cells generate macrophages that support erythroid islands. *PLoS One* 12:e0171096. doi: 10.1371/journal.pone.0171096

Benedetto, D., Rao, C. M., Cefalu, C., Aguglia, D. O., Cattadori, G., and D'Ascola, D. G. (2015). Effects of blood transfusion on exercise capacity in thalassemia major patients. *PLoS One* 10:e0127553. doi: 10.1371/journal.pone.0127553

Beneteau, C., Thierry, G., Blesson, S., Le Vaillant, C., Picard, V., and Bene, M. C. (2014). Recurrent mutation in the PIEZO1 gene in two families of hereditary xerocytosis with fetal hydrops. *Clin. Genet.* 85, 293–295. doi: 10.1111/cge.12147

Berg, T. O., Fengsrud, M., Stromhaug, P. E., Berg, T., and Seglen, P. O. (1998). Isolation and characterization of rat liver amphisomes. Evidence for fusion of autophagosomes with both early and late endosomes. *J. Biol. Chem.* 273, 21883–21892. doi: 10.1074/jbc.273.34.21883

Bessis, M. (1958). Erythroblastic island, functional unity of bone marrow. *Rev. Hematol.* 13, 8–11.

Bessis, M. C., and Breton-Gorius, J. (1962). Iron metabolism in the bone marrow as seen by electron microscopy: a critical review. *Blood* 19, 635–663.

Bize, I., Taher, S., and Brugnara, C. (2003). Regulation of K-Cl cotransport during reticulocyte maturation and erythrocyte aging in normal and sickle erythrocytes. *Am. J. Physiol. Cell Physiol.* 285, C31–C38. doi: 10.1152/ajpcell.00447.2002

Blanc, L., Liu, J., Vidal, M., Chasis, J. A., An, X., and Mohandas, N. (2009). The water channel aquaporin-1 partitions into exosomes during reticulocyte maturation: implication for the regulation of cell volume. *Blood* 114, 3928–3934. doi: 10.1182/blood-2009-06-230086

Bohmer, R. M. (2004). IL-3-dependent early erythropoiesis is stimulated by autocrine transforming growth factor beta. *Stem Cells* 22, 216–224. doi: 10.1634/stemcells.22-2-216

Brittain, J. E., Mlinar, K. J., Anderson, C. S., Orringer, E. P., and Parise, L. V. (2001). Integrin-associated protein is an adhesion receptor on sickle red blood cells for immobilized thrombospondin. *Blood* 97, 2159–2164. doi: 10.1182/blood.V97.7.2159

Bruce, L. J. (2008). Red cell membrane transport abnormalities. *Curr. Opin. Hematol.* 15, 184–190. doi: 10.1097/MOH.0b013e3282f97b0a

Bruce, L. J., Guizouarn, H., Burton, N. M., Gabillat, N., Poole, J., and Flatt, J. F. (2009). The monovalent cation leak in overhydrated stomatocytic red blood cells results from amino acid substitutions in the Rh-associated glycoprotein. *Blood* 113, 1350–1357. doi: 10.1182/blood-2008-07-171140

Burnett, S. H., Kershen, E. J., Zhang, J., Zeng, L., Straley, S. C., and Kaplan, A. M. (2004). Conditional macrophage ablation in transgenic mice expressing a Fas-based suicide gene. *J. Leukoc. Biol.* 75, 612–623. doi: 10.1189/jlb.0903442

Cahalan, S. M., Lukacs, V., Ranade, S. S., Chien, S., Bandell, M., and Patapoutian, A. (2015). Piezo1 links mechanical forces to red blood cell volume. *eLife* 4:e07370. doi: 10.7554/eLife.07370

Campbell-Lee, S. A., and Kittles, R. A. (2014). Red blood cell alloimmunization in sickle cell disease: listen to your ancestors. *Transfus. Med. Hemother.* 41, 431–435. doi: 10.1159/000369513

Canessa, M., Fabry, M. E., Blumenfeld, N., and Nagel, R. L. (1987). Volume-stimulated, Cl-dependent K+ efflux is highly expressed in young human red cells containing normal hemoglobin or HbS. *J. Membr. Biol.* 97, 97–105. doi: 10.1007/BF01869416

Carayon, K., Chaoui, K., Ronzier, E., Lazar, I., Bertrand-Michel, J., and Roques, V. (2011). Proteolipidic composition of exosomes changes during reticulocyte maturation. *J. Biol. Chem.* 286, 34426–34439. doi: 10.1074/jbc.M111.257444

Carlile, G. W., Smith, D. H., and Wiedmann, M. (2004). Caspase-3 has a nonapoptotic function in erythroid maturation. *Blood* 103, 4310–4316. doi: 10.1182/blood-2003-09-3362

Chasis, J. A., Coulombel, L., Conboy, J., McGee, S., Andrews, K., and Kan, Y. W. (1993). Differentiation-associated switches in protein 4.1 expression. Synthesis of multiple structural isoforms during normal human erythropoiesis. *J. Clin. Invest.* 91, 329–338. doi: 10.1172/JCI116189

Chasis, J. A., Prenant, M., Leung, A., and Mohandas, N. (1989). Membrane assembly and remodeling during reticulocyte maturation. *Blood* 74, 1112–1120.

Cherif-Zahar, B., Raynal, V., Gane, P., Mattei, M. G., Bailly, P., and Gibbs, B. (1996). Candidate gene acting as a suppressor of the RH locus in most cases of Rh-deficiency. *Nat. Genet.* 12, 168–173. doi: 10.1038/ng0296-168

Choi, J. W., and Pai, S. H. (2001). Reticulocyte subpopulations and reticulocyte maturity index (RMI) rise as body iron status falls. *Am. J. Hematol.* 67, 130–135. doi: 10.1002/ajh.1091

Chow, A., Lucas, D., Hidalgo, A., Mendez-Ferrer, S., Hashimoto, D., and Scheiermann, C. (2011). Bone marrow $CD169^{+}$ macrophages promote the retention of hematopoietic stem and progenitor cells in the mesenchymal stem cell niche. *J. Exp. Med.* 208, 261–271. doi: 10.1084/jem.20101688

Connor, W. E., Lin, D. S., Thomas, G., Ey, F., DeLoughery, T., and Zhu, N. (1997). Abnormal phospholipid molecular species of erythrocytes in sickle cell anemia. *J. Lipid Res.* 38, 2516–2528.

Crossan, G. P., van der Weyden, L., Rosado, I. V., Langevin, F., Gaillard, P. H., and McIntyre, R. E. (2011). Disruption of mouse Slx4, a regulator of structure-specific nucleases, phenocopies Fanconi Anemia. *Nat. Genet.* 43, 147–152. doi: 10.1038/ng.752

Da Costa, L., Galimand, J., Fenneteau, O., and Mohandas, N. (2013). Hereditary spherocytosis, elliptocytosis, and other red cell membrane disorders. *Blood Rev.* 27, 167–178. doi: 10.1016/j.blre.2013.04.003

Dajani, R., Fraser, E., Roe, S. M., Young, N., Good, V., and Dale, T. C. (2001). Crystal structure of glycogen synthase kinase 3 beta: structural basis for phosphate-primed substrate specificity and autoinhibition. *Cell* 105, 721–732. doi: 10.1016/S0092-8674(01)00374-9

Davis, B. H., Ornvold, K., and Bigelow, N. C. (1995). Flow cytometric reticulocyte maturity index: a useful laboratory parameter of erythropoietic activity in anemia. *Cytometry* 22, 35–39. doi: 10.1002/cyto.990220107

De Haan, L. D., Werre, J. M., Ruben, A. M., Huls, A. H., de Gier, J., and Staal, G. E. (1988). Reticulocyte crisis after splenectomy: evidence for delayed red cell maturation? *Eur. J. Haematol.* 41, 74–79. doi: 10.1111/j.1600-0609.1988.tb00872.x

de Haro, C., de Herreros, A. G., and Ochoa, S. (1985). Protein phosphorylation and translational control in reticulocytes: activation of the heme-controlled translational inhibitor by calcium ions and phospholipid. *Curr. Top. Cell. Regul.* 27, 63–81. doi: 10.1016/B978-0-12-152827-0.50013-X

Douay, L., and Andreu, G. (2007). Ex vivo production of human red blood cells from hematopoietic stem cells: what is the future in transfusion? *Transfus. Med. Rev.* 21, 91–100. doi: 10.1016/j.tmrv.2006.11.004

Fader, C. M., and Colombo, M. I. (2009). Autophagy and multivesicular bodies: two closely related partners. *Cell Death Differ.* 16, 70–78. doi: 10.1038/cdd.2008.168

Fermo, E., Bogdanova, A., Petkova-Kirova, P., Zaninoni, A., Marcello, A. P., and Makhro, A. (2017). 'Gardos Channelopathy': a variant of hereditary Stomatocytosis with complex molecular regulation. *Sci. Rep.* 7:1744. doi: 10.1038/s41598-017-01591-w

Focosi, D., and Amabile, G. (2017). Induced pluripotent stem cell-derived red blood cells and platelet concentrates: from bench to bedside. *Cells* 7:E2. doi: 10.3390/cells7010002

Fujimi, A., Matsunaga, T., Kobune, M., Kawano, Y., Nagaya, T., Tanaka, I., et al. (2008). Ex vivo large-scale generation of human red blood cells from cord blood CD_{34}^{+} cells by co-culturing with macrophages. *Int. J. Hematol.* 87, 339–350. doi: 10.1007/s12185-008-0062-y

Gallagher, P. G. (2013). Abnormalities of the erythrocyte membrane. *Pediatr. Clin. North Am.* 60, 1349–1362. doi: 10.1016/j.pcl.2013.09.001

Gallagher, P. G. (2017). Disorders of erythrocyte hydration. *Blood* 130, 2699–2708. doi: 10.1182/blood-2017-04-590810

Gautier, E. F., Ducamp, S., Leduc, M., Salnot, V., Guillonneau, F., and Dussiot, M. (2016). Comprehensive proteomic analysis of human erythropoiesis. *Cell Rep.* 16, 1470–1484. doi: 10.1016/j.celrep.2016.06.085

Gee, B. E., and Platt, O. S. (1995). Sickle reticulocytes adhere to VCAM-1. *Blood* 85, 268–274.

Geminard, C., De Gassart, A., Blanc, L., and Vidal, M. (2004). Degradation of AP2 during reticulocyte maturation enhances binding of hsc70 and Alix to a common site on TFR for sorting into exosomes. *Traffic* 5, 181–193. doi: 10.1111/j.1600-0854.2004.0167.x

Giarratana, M. C., Kobari, L., Lapillonne, H., Chalmers, D., Kiger, L., and Cynober, T. (2005). Ex vivo generation of fully mature human red blood cells from hematopoietic stem cells. *Nat. Biotechnol.* 23, 69–74. doi: 10.1038/nbt1047

Giarratana, M. C., Rouard, H., Dumont, A., Kiger, L., Safeukui, I., and Le Pennec, P. Y. (2011). Proof of principle for transfusion of in vitro-generated red blood cells. *Blood* 118, 5071–5079. doi: 10.1182/blood-2011-06-362038

Goodnough, L. T., and Murphy, M. F. (2014). Do liberal blood transfusions cause more harm than good? *BMJ* 349:g6897. doi: 10.1136/bmj.g6897

Griffiths, R. E., Kupzig, S., Cogan, N., Mankelow, T. J., Betin, V. M., and Trakarnsanga, K. (2012). Maturing reticulocytes internalize plasma membrane in glycophorin A-containing vesicles that fuse with autophagosomes before exocytosis. *Blood* 119, 6296–6306. doi: 10.1182/blood-2011-09-376475

Gromley, A., Yeaman, C., Rosa, J., Redick, S., Chen, C. T., and Mirabelle, S. (2005). Centriolin anchoring of exocyst and SNARE complexes at the midbody is required for secretory-vesicle-mediated abscission. *Cell* 123, 75–87. doi: 10.1016/j.cell.2005.07.027

Gronowicz, G., Swift, H., and Steck, T. L. (1984). Maturation of the reticulocyte in vitro. *J. Cell Sci.* 71, 177–197.

Guinez, C., Mir, A. M., Leroy, Y., Cacan, R., Michalski, J. C., and Lefebvre, T. (2007). Hsp70-GlcNAc-binding activity is released by stress, proteasome inhibition, and protein misfolding. *Biochem. Biophys. Res. Commun.* 361, 414–420. doi: 10.1016/j.bbrc.2007.07.020

Hanspal, M., Golan, D. E., Smockova, Y., Yi, S. J., Cho, M. R., and Liu, S. C. (1998a). Temporal synthesis of band 3 oligomers during terminal maturation of mouse erythroblasts. Dimers and tetramers exist in the membrane as preformed stable species. *Blood* 92, 329–338.

Hanspal, M., Hanspal, J. S., Kalraiya, R., Liu, S. C., Sahr, K. E., and Howard, D. (1992). Asynchronous synthesis of membrane skeletal proteins during terminal maturation of murine erythroblasts. *Blood* 80, 530–539.

Hanspal, M., Smockova, Y., and Uong, Q. (1998b). Molecular identification and functional characterization of a novel protein that mediates the attachment of erythroblasts to macrophages. *Blood* 92, 2940–2950.

Heideveld, E., Masiello, F., Marra, M., Esteghamat, F., Yagci, N., and von Lindern, M. (2015). $CD14^+$ cells from peripheral blood positively regulate hematopoietic stem and progenitor cell survival resulting in increased erythroid yield. *Haematologica* 100, 1396–1406. doi: 10.3324/haematol.2015.125492

Heideveld, E., and van den Akker, E. (2017). Digesting the role of bone marrow macrophages on hematopoiesis. *Immunobiology* 222, 814–822. doi: 10.1016/j.imbio.2016.11.007

Heilmeyer, L., and Westhäuser, R. (1932). Reifungsstadien an überlebenden reticulozyten in vitro und ihre bedeutung für die schaetzung der täglichen haemoglobin-produktion in vivo. *Ztschr. Klin. Med.* 121, 361–379.

Hentze, M. W., Muckenthaler, M. U., Galy, B., and Camaschella, C. (2010). Two to tango: regulation of Mammalian iron metabolism. *Cell* 142, 24–38. doi: 10.1016/j.cell.2010.06.028

Hillery, C. A., Du, M. C., Montgomery, R. R., and Scott, J. P. (1996). Increased adhesion of erythrocytes to components of the extracellular matrix: isolation and characterization of a red blood cell lipid that binds thrombospondin and laminin. *Blood* 87, 4879–4886.

Hines, P. C., Zen, Q., Burney, S. N., Shea, D. A., Ataga, K. I., and Orringer, E. P. (2003). Novel epinephrine and cyclic AMP-mediated activation of BCAM/Lu-dependent sickle (SS) RBC adhesion. *Blood* 101, 3281–3287. doi: 10.1182/blood-2001-12-0289

Hislop, J. N., and von Zastrow, M. (2011). Role of ubiquitination in endocytic trafficking of G-protein-coupled receptors. *Traffic* 12, 137–148. doi: 10.1111/j.1600-0854.2010.01121.x

Hom, J., Dulmovits, B. M., Mohandas, N., and Blanc, L. (2015). The erythroblastic island as an emerging paradigm in the anemia of inflammation. *Immunol. Res.* 63, 75–89. doi: 10.1007/s12026-015-8697-2

Jayapal, S. R., Lee, K. L., Ji, P., Kaldis, P., Lim, B., and Lodish, H. F. (2010). Down-regulation of Myc is essential for terminal erythroid maturation. *J. Biol. Chem.* 285, 40252–40265. doi: 10.1074/jbc.M110.181073

Ji, P., Jayapal, S. R., and Lodish, H. F. (2008). Enucleation of cultured mouse fetal erythroblasts requires Rac GTPases and mDia2. *Nat. Cell Biol.* 10, 314–321. doi: 10.1038/ncb1693

Ji, P., Yeh, V., Ramirez, T., Murata-Hori, M., and Lodish, H. F. (2010). Histone deacetylase 2 is required for chromatin condensation and subsequent enucleation of cultured mouse fetal erythroblasts. *Haematologica* 95, 2013–2021. doi: 10.3324/haematol.2010.029827

Johnstone, R. M., Adam, M., Hammond, J. R., Orr, L., and Turbide, C. (1987). Vesicle formation during reticulocyte maturation. Association of plasma membrane activities with released vesicles (exosomes). *J. Biol. Chem.* 262, 9412–9420.

Keerthivasan, G., Small, S., Liu, H., Wickrema, A., and Crispino, J. D. (2010). Vesicle trafficking plays a novel role in erythroblast enucleation. *Blood* 116, 3331–3340. doi: 10.1182/blood-2010-03-277426

Keerthivasan, G., Wickrema, A., and Crispino, J. D. (2011). Erythroblast enucleation. *Stem Cells Int.* 2011:139851. doi: 10.4061/2011/139851

Kim, P. G., Nakano, H., Das, P. P., Chen, M. J., Rowe, R. G., and Chou, S. S. (2015). Flow-induced protein kinase A-CREB pathway acts via BMP signaling to promote HSC emergence. *J. Exp. Med.* 212, 633–648. doi: 10.1084/jem.20141514

Klei, T. R., Meinderts, S. M., van den Berg, T. K., and van Bruggen, R. (2017). From the cradle to the grave: the role of macrophages in erythropoiesis and erythrophagocytosis. *Front. Immunol.* 8:73. doi: 10.3389/fimmu.2017.00073

Konstantinidis, D. G., Pushkaran, S., Johnson, J. F., Cancelas, J. A., Manganaris, S., and Harris, C. E. (2012). Signaling and cytoskeletal requirements in erythroblast enucleation. *Blood* 119, 6118–6127. doi: 10.1182/blood-2011-09-379263

Kostova, E. B., Beuger, B. M., Klei, T. R., Halonen, P., Lieftink, C., and Beijersbergen, R. (2015). Identification of signalling cascades involved in red blood cell shrinkage and vesiculation. *Biosci. Rep.* 35:e00187. doi: 10.1042/BSR20150019

Kurita, R., Suda, N., Sudo, K., Miharada, K., Hiroyama, T., and Miyoshi, H. (2013). Establishment of immortalized human erythroid progenitor cell lines able to produce enucleated red blood cells. *PLoS One* 8:e59890. doi: 10.1371/journal.pone.0059890

Kuypers, F. A., Larkin, S. K., Emeis, J. J., and Allison, A. C. (2007). Interaction of an annexin V homodimer (Diannexin) with phosphatidylserine on cell surfaces and consequent antithrombotic activity. *Thromb. Haemost.* 97, 478–486. doi: 10.1160/TH06-08-0436

Lapillonne, H., Kobari, L., Mazurier, C., Tropel, P., Giarratana, M. C., and Zanella-Cleon, I. (2010). Red blood cell generation from human induced pluripotent stem cells: perspectives for transfusion medicine. *Haematologica* 95, 1651–1659. doi: 10.3324/haematol.2010.023556

Leberbauer, C., Boulme, F., Unfried, G., Huber, J., Beug, H., and Mullner, E. W. (2005). Different steroids co-regulate long-term expansion versus terminal differentiation in primary human erythroid progenitors. *Blood* 105, 85–94. doi: 10.1182/blood-2004-03-1002

Lee, G., Lo, A., Short, S. A., Mankelow, T. J., Spring, F., and Parsons, S. F. (2006). Targeted gene deletion demonstrates that the cell adhesion molecule ICAM-4 is critical for erythroblastic island formation. *Blood* 108, 2064–2071. doi: 10.1182/blood-2006-03-006759

Lee, J. C., Gimm, J. A., Lo, A. J., Koury, M. J., Krauss, S. W., and Mohandas, N. (2004). Mechanism of protein sorting during erythroblast enucleation: role of cytoskeletal connectivity. *Blood* 103, 1912–1919. doi: 10.1182/blood-2003-03-0928

Leimberg, M. J., Prus, E., Konijn, A. M., and Fibach, E. (2008). Macrophages function as a ferritin iron source for cultured human erythroid precursors. *J. Cell. Biochem.* 103, 1211–1218. doi: 10.1002/jcb.21499

Liu, J., Guo, X., Mohandas, N., Chasis, J. A., and An, X. (2010). Membrane remodeling during reticulocyte maturation. *Blood* 115, 2021–2027. doi: 10.1182/blood-2009-08-241182

Liu, J., Mohandas, N., and An, X. (2011). Membrane assembly during erythropoiesis. *Curr. Opin. Hematol.* 18, 133–138. doi: 10.1097/MOH.0b013e32834521f3

Lu, S. J., Feng, Q., Park, J. S., Vida, L., Lee, B. S., and Strausbauch, M. (2008). Biologic properties and enucleation of red blood cells from human embryonic stem cells. *Blood* 112, 4475–4484. doi: 10.1182/blood-2008-05-157198

Magor, G. W., Tallack, M. R., Gillinder, K. R., Bell, C. C., McCallum, N., and Williams, B. (2015). KLF1-null neonates display hydrops fetalis and a deranged erythroid transcriptome. *Blood* 125, 2405–2417. doi: 10.1182/blood-2014-08-590968

Makhro, A., Hanggi, P., Goede, J. S., Wang, J., Bruggemann, A., and Gassmann, M. (2013). N-methyl-D-aspartate receptors in human erythroid precursor cells and in circulating red blood cells contribute to the intracellular calcium regulation. *Am. J. Physiol. Cell Physiol.* 305, C1123–C1138. doi: 10.1152/ajpcell.00031.2013

Malleret, B., Xu, F., Mohandas, N., Suwanarusk, R., Chu, C., and Leite, J. A. (2013). Significant biochemical, biophysical and metabolic diversity in circulating human cord blood reticulocytes. *PLoS One* 8:e76062. doi: 10.1371/journal.pone.0076062

Manno, S., Takakuwa, Y., and Mohandas, N. (2005). Modulation of erythrocyte membrane mechanical function by protein 4.1 phosphorylation. *J. Biol. Chem.* 280, 7581–7587. doi: 10.1074/jbc.M410650200

Manodori, A. B., Matsui, N. M., Chen, J. Y., and Embury, S. H. (1998). Enhanced adherence of sickle erythrocytes to thrombin-treated endothelial cells involves interendothelial cell gap formation. *Blood* 92, 3445–3454.

Mel, H. C., Prenant, M., and Mohandas, N. (1977). Reticulocyte motility and form: studies on maturation and classification. *Blood* 49, 1001–1009.

Meyron-Holtz, E. G., Vaisman, B., Cabantchik, Z. I., Fibach, E., Rouault, T. A., and Hershko, C. (1999). Regulation of intracellular iron metabolism in human erythroid precursors by internalized extracellular ferritin. *Blood* 94, 3205–3211.

Migliaccio, A. R. (2010). Erythroblast enucleation. *Haematologica* 95, 1985–1988. doi: 10.3324/haematol.2010.033225

Migliaccio, G., Di Pietro, R., di Giacomo, V., Di Baldassarre, A., Migliaccio, A. R., and Maccioni, L. (2002). In vitro mass production of human erythroid cells from the blood of normal donors and of thalassemic patients. *Blood Cells Mol. Dis.* 28, 169–180. doi: 10.1006/bcmd.2002.0502

Migliaccio, G., Sanchez, M., Masiello, F., Tirelli, V., Varricchio, L., and Whitsett, C. (2010). Humanized culture medium for clinical expansion of human erythroblasts. *Cell Transplant.* 19, 453–469. doi: 10.3727/096368909X485049

Miharada, K., Hiroyama, T., Sudo, K., Nagasawa, T., and Nakamura, Y. (2006). Efficient enucleation of erythroblasts differentiated in vitro from hematopoietic stem and progenitor cells. *Nat. Biotechnol.* 24, 1255–1256. doi: 10.1038/nbt1245

Millot, S., Andrieu, V., Letteron, P., Lyoumi, S., and Hurtado-Nedelec, M. (2010). Erythropoietin stimulates spleen BMP4-dependent stress erythropoiesis and partially corrects anemia in a mouse model of generalized inflammation. *Blood* 116, 6072–6081. doi: 10.1182/blood-2010-04-281840

Mohandas, N., and Gallagher, P. G. (2008). Red cell membrane: past, present, and future. *Blood* 112, 3939–3948. doi: 10.1182/blood-2008-07-161166

Mohandas, N., and Prenant, M. (1978). Three-dimensional model of bone marrow. *Blood* 51, 633–643.

Mordue, K. E., Hawley, B. R., Satchwell, T. J., and Toye, A. M. (2017). CD47 surface stability is sensitive to actin disruption prior to inclusion within the band 3 macrocomplex. *Sci. Rep.* 7:2246. doi: 10.1038/s41598-017-02356-1

Muzykantov, V. R. (2010). Drug delivery by red blood cells: vascular carriers designed by mother nature. *Expert Opin. Drug Deliv.* 7, 403–427. doi: 10.1517/17425241003610633

Nguyen, A. T., Prado, M. A., Schmidt, P. J., Sendamarai, A. K., Wilson-Grady, J. T., and Min, M. (2017). UBE2O remodels the proteome during terminal erythroid differentiation. *Science* 357:eaan0218. doi: 10.1126/science.aan0218

Nguyen, D. B., Ly, T. B., Wesseling, M. C., Hittinger, M., Torge, A., and Devitt, A. (2016). Characterization of microvesicles released from human red blood cells. *Cell. Physiol. Biochem.* 38, 1085–1099. doi: 10.1159/000443059

Odorizzi, G., Babst, M., and Emr, S. D. (1998). Fab1p PtdIns(3)P 5-kinase function essential for protein sorting in the multivesicular body. *Cell* 95, 847–858. doi: 10.1016/S0092-8674(00)81707-9

Ovchynnikova, E., Aglialoro, F., Bentlage, A. E. H., Vidarsson, G., Salinas, N. D., and von Lindern, M. (2017). DARC extracellular domain remodeling in maturating reticulocytes explains *Plasmodium vivax* tropism. *Blood* 130, 1441–1444. doi: 10.1182/blood-2017-03-774364

Palis, J. (2016). Interaction of the macrophage and primitive erythroid lineages in the Mammalian embryo. *Front. Immunol.* 7:669. doi: 10.3389/fimmu.2016.00669

Pan, B. T., Teng, K., Wu, C., Adam, M., and Johnstone, R. M. (1985). Electron microscopic evidence for externalization of the transferrin receptor in vesicular form in sheep reticulocytes. *J. Cell Biol.* 101, 942–948. doi: 10.1083/jcb.101.3.942

Pridgeon, J. W., Webber, E. A., Sha, D., Li, L., and Chin, L. S. (2009). Proteomic analysis reveals Hrs ubiquitin-interacting motif-mediated ubiquitin signaling in multiple cellular processes. *FEBS J.* 276, 118–131. doi: 10.1111/j.1742-4658.2008.06760.x

Quarmyne, M. O., Risinger, M., Linkugel, A., Frazier, A., and Joiner, C. (2011). Volume regulation and KCl cotransport in reticulocyte populations of sickle and normal red blood cells. *Blood Cells Mol. Dis.* 47, 95–99. doi: 10.1016/j.bcmd.2011.04.007

Raiborg, C., and Stenmark, H. (2009). The ESCRT machinery in endosomal sorting of ubiquitylated membrane proteins. *Nature* 458, 445–452. doi: 10.1038/nature07961

Rivera, A., Kam, S. Y., Ho, M., Romero, J. R., and Lee, S. (2013). Ablation of the Kell/Xk complex alters erythrocyte divalent cation homeostasis. *Blood Cells Mol. Dis.* 50, 80–85. doi: 10.1016/j.bcmd.2012.10.002

Sadahira, Y., Yoshino, T., and Monobe, Y. (1995). Very late activation antigen 4-vascular cell adhesion molecule 1 interaction is involved in the formation of erythroblastic islands. *J. Exp. Med.* 181, 411–415. doi: 10.1084/jem.181.1.411

Sahu, R., Kaushik, S., Clement, C. C., Cannizzo, E. S., Scharf, B., and Follenzi, A. (2011). Microautophagy of cytosolic proteins by late endosomes. *Dev. Cell* 20, 131–139. doi: 10.1016/j.devcel.2010.12.003

Sailaja, Y. R., Baskar, R., Srinivas Rao, C. S., and Saralakumari, D. (2004). Membrane lipids and protein-bound carbohydrates status during the maturation of reticulocytes to erythrocytes in type 2 diabetics. *Clin. Chim. Acta* 341, 185–192. doi: 10.1016/j.cccn.2003.12.003

Saksena, S., Sun, J., Chu, T., and Emr, S. D. (2007). ESCRTing proteins in the endocytic pathway. *Trends Biochem. Sci.* 32, 561–573. doi: 10.1016/j.tibs.2007.09.010

Salomao, M., Chen, K., Villalobos, J., Mohandas, N., An, X., and Chasis, J. A. (2010). Hereditary spherocytosis and hereditary elliptocytosis: aberrant protein sorting during erythroblast enucleation. *Blood* 116, 267–269. doi: 10.1182/blood-2010-02-264127

Sandberg, M. B., Nybo, M., Birgens, H., and Frederiksen, H. (2014). Hereditary xerocytosis and familial haemolysis due to mutation in the PIEZO1 gene: a simple diagnostic approach. *Int. J. Lab. Hematol.* 36, e62–e65. doi: 10.1111/ijlh.12172

Satchwell, T. J., Bell, A. J., Hawley, B. R., Pellegrin, S., Mordue, K. E., and van Deursen, C. T. (2016). Severe Ankyrin-R deficiency results in impaired surface retention and lysosomal degradation of RhAG in human erythroblasts. *Haematologica* 101, 1018–1027. doi: 10.3324/haematol.2016.146209

Satchwell, T. J., Bell, A. J., Pellegrin, S., Kupzig, S., Daniels, G., Ridgwell, K., et al. (2011). Critical band 3 multiprotein complex interactions establish early during human erythropoiesis. *Blood* 118, 182–191. doi: 10.1182/blood-2010-10-314187

Savina, A., Fader, C. M., Damiani, M. T., and Colombo, M. I. (2005). Rab11 promotes docking and fusion of multivesicular bodies in a calcium-dependent manner. *Traffic* 6, 131–143. doi: 10.1111/j.1600-0854.2004.00257.x

Savina, A., Furlan, M., Vidal, M., and Colombo, M. I. (2003). Exosome release is regulated by a calcium-dependent mechanism in K562 cells. *J. Biol. Chem.* 278, 20083–20090. doi: 10.1074/jbc.M301642200

Sawada, K., Krantz, S. B., Dessypris, E. N., Koury, S. T., and Sawyer, S. T. (1989). Human colony-forming units-erythroid do not require accessory cells, but do require direct interaction with insulin-like growth factor I and/or insulin for erythroid development. *J. Clin. Invest.* 83, 1701–1709. doi: 10.1172/JCI114070

Schutte, J., Wang, H., Antoniou, S., Jarratt, A., Wilson, N. K., and Riepsaame, J. (2016). An experimentally validated network of nine haematopoietic transcription factors reveals mechanisms of cell state stability. *eLife* 5:e11469. doi: 10.7554/eLife.11469

Seu, K. G., Papoin, J., Fessler, R., Hom, J., Huang, G., and Mohandas, N. (2017). Unraveling macrophage heterogeneity in erythroblastic islands. *Front. Immunol.* 8:1140. doi: 10.3389/fimmu.2017.01140

Shah, S., Huang, X., and Cheng, L. (2014). Concise review: stem cell-based approaches to red blood cell production for transfusion. *Stem Cells Transl. Med.* 3, 346–355. doi: 10.5966/sctm.2013-0054

Shah, S. N., Gelderman, M. P., Lewis, E. M., Farrel, J., Wood, F., and Strader, M. B. (2016). Evaluation of stem cell-derived red blood cells as a transfusion product using a novel animal model. *PLoS One* 11:e0166657. doi: 10.1371/journal.pone.0166657

Simpson, C. F., and Kling, J. M. (1967). The mechanism of denucleation in circulating erythroblasts. *J. Cell Biol.* 35, 237–245. doi: 10.1083/jcb.35.1.237

Soni, S., Bala, S., Gwynn, B., Sahr, K. E., Peters, L. L., and Hanspal, M. (2006). Absence of erythroblast macrophage protein (Emp) leads to failure of erythroblast nuclear extrusion. *J. Biol. Chem.* 281, 20181–20189. doi: 10.1074/jbc.M603226200

Swartz, K. L., Wood, S. N., Murthy, T., Ramirez, O., Qin, G., and Pillai, M. M. (2017). E2F-2 promotes nuclear condensation and enucleation of terminally differentiated erythroblasts. *Mol. Cell. Biol.* 37:e00274-16. doi: 10.1128/MCB.00274-16

Syeda, R., Xu, J., Dubin, A. E., Coste, B., Mathur, J., and Huynh, T. (2015). Chemical activation of the mechanotransduction channel Piezo1. *eLife* 4:e07369. doi: 10.7554/eLife.07369

Tchernia, G., Mohandas, N., and Shohet, S. B. (1981). Deficiency of skeletal membrane protein band 4.1 in homozygous hereditary elliptocytosis. Implications for erythrocyte membrane stability. *J. Clin. Invest.* 68, 454–460. doi: 10.1172/JCI110275

Toda, S., Segawa, K., and Nagata, S. (2014). MerTK-mediated engulfment of pyrenocytes by central macrophages in erythroblastic islands. *Blood* 123, 3963–3971. doi: 10.1182/blood-2014-01-547976

Trakarnsanga, K., Griffiths, R. E., Wilson, M. C., Blair, A., Satchwell, T. J., and Meinders, M. (2017). An immortalized adult human erythroid line facilitates sustainable and scalable generation of functional red cells. *Nat. Commun.* 8:14750. doi: 10.1038/ncomms14750

Trakarnsanga, K., Wilson, M. C., Heesom, K. J., Andrienko, T. N., Srisawat, C., and Frayne, J. (2018). Secretory factors from OP9 stromal cells delay differentiation and increase the expansion potential of adult erythroid cells in vitro. *Sci. Rep.* 8:1983. doi: 10.1038/s41598-018-20491-1

Udani, M., Zen, Q., Cottman, M., Leonard, N., Jefferson, S., and Daymont, C. (1998). Basal cell adhesion molecule/lutheran protein. The receptor critical for sickle cell adhesion to laminin. *J. Clin. Invest.* 101, 2550–2558. doi: 10.1172/JCI1204

Ullrich, O., Reinsch, S., Urbe, S., Zerial, M., and Parton, R. G. (1996). Rab11 regulates recycling through the pericentriolar recycling endosome. *J. Cell Biol.* 135, 913–924. doi: 10.1083/jcb.135.4.913

Ulyanova, T., Phelps, S. R., and Papayannopoulou, T. (2016). The macrophage contribution to stress erythropoiesis: when less is enough. *Blood* 128, 1756–1765. doi: 10.1182/blood-2016-05-714527

van den Akker, E., Satchwell, T. J., Pellegrin, S., Daniels, G., and Toye, A. M. (2010a). The majority of the *in vitro* erythroid expansion potential resides in CD_{34}^- cells, outweighing the contribution of CD_{34}^+ cells and significantly increasing the erythroblast yield from peripheral blood samples. *Haematologica* 95, 1594–1598. doi: 10.3324/haematol.2009.019828

van den Akker, E., Satchwell, T. J., Pellegrin, S., Flatt, J. F., Maigre, M., and Daniels, G. (2010b). Investigating the key membrane protein changes during *in vitro* erythropoiesis of protein 4.2 (−) cells (mutations Chartres 1 and 2). *Haematologica* 95, 1278–1286. doi: 10.3324/haematol.2009.021063

van den Akker, E., Satchwell, T. J., Williamson, R. C., and Toye, A. M. (2010c). Band 3 multiprotein complexes in the red cell membrane; of mice and men. *Blood Cells Mol. Dis.* 45, 1–8. doi: 10.1016/j.bcmd.2010.02.019

Vidal, M., Sainte-Marie, J., Philippot, J. R., and Bienvenue, A. (1989). Asymmetric distribution of phospholipids in the membrane of vesicles released during in vitro maturation of guinea pig reticulocytes: evidence precluding a role for "aminophospholipid translocase". *J. Cell. Physiol.* 140, 455–462. doi: 10.1002/jcp.1041400308

Wang, J., Ramirez, T., Ji, P., Jayapal, S. R., Lodish, H. F., and Murata-Hori, M. (2012). Mammalian erythroblast enucleation requires PI3K-dependent cell polarization. *J. Cell Sci.* 125(Pt 2), 340–349. doi: 10.1242/jcs.088286

Wang, J., Wagner-Britz, L., Bogdanova, A., Ruppenthal, S., Wiesen, K., and Kaiser, E. (2013). Morphologically homogeneous red blood cells present a heterogeneous response to hormonal stimulation. *PLoS One* 8:e67697. doi: 10.1371/journal.pone.0067697

Waugh, R. E., Mantalaris, A., Bauserman, R. G., Hwang, W. C., and Wu, J. H. (2001). Membrane instability in late-stage erythropoiesis. *Blood* 97, 1869–1875. doi: 10.1182/blood.V97.6.1869

Waugh, R. E., McKenney, J. B., Bauserman, R. G., Brooks, D. M., Valeri, C. R., and Snyder, L. M. (1997). Surface area and volume changes during maturation of reticulocytes in the circulation of the baboon. *J. Lab. Clin. Med.* 129, 527–535. doi: 10.1016/S0022-2143(97)90007-X

Wickrema, A., Koury, S. T., Dai, C. H., and Krantz, S. B. (1994). Changes in cytoskeletal proteins and their mRNAs during maturation of human erythroid progenitor cells. *J. Cell. Physiol.* 160, 417–426. doi: 10.1002/jcp.1041600304

Wiley, J. S., and Shaller, C. C. (1977). Selective loss of calcium permeability on maturation of reticulocytes. *J. Clin. Invest.* 59, 1113–1119. doi: 10.1172/JCI108735

Wollmann, M., Gerzson, B. M., Schwert, V., Figuera, R. W., and de Oliveira Ritzel, G. (2014). Not available. *Rev. Bras. Hematol. Hemoter.* 36, 25–28. doi: 10.5581/1516-8484.20140009

Yamamoto-Tanaka, M., Makino, T., Motoyama, A., Miyai, M., Tsuboi, R., and Hibino, T. (2014). Multiple pathways are involved in DNA degradation during keratinocyte terminal differentiation. *Cell Death Dis.* 5:e1181. doi: 10.1038/cddis.2014.145

Yang, L., Andrews, D. A., and Low, P. S. (2000). Lysophosphatidic acid opens a Ca^{++} channel in human erythrocytes. *Blood* 95, 2420–2425.

Yokoyama, T., Etoh, T., Kitagawa, H., Tsukahara, S., and Kannan, Y. (2003). Migration of erythroblastic islands toward the sinusoid as erythroid maturation proceeds in rat bone marrow. *J. Vet. Med. Sci.* 65, 449–452. doi: 10.1292/jvms.65.449

Yoshida, H., Kawane, K., Koike, M., Mori, Y., Uchiyama, Y., and Nagata, S. (2005). Phosphatidylserine-dependent engulfment by macrophages of nuclei from erythroid precursor cells. *Nature* 437, 754–758. doi: 10.1038/nature03964

Yuditskaya, S., Suffredini, A. F., and Kato, G. J. (2010). The proteome of sickle cell disease: insights from exploratory proteomic profiling. *Expert Rev. Proteomics* 7, 833–848. doi: 10.1586/epr.10.88

Zarychanski, R., Schulz, V. P., Houston, B. L., Maksimova, Y., Houston, D. S., and Smith, B. (2012). Mutations in the mechanotransduction protein PIEZO1 are associated with hereditary xerocytosis. *Blood* 120, 1908–1915. doi: 10.1182/blood-2012-04-422253

Zermati, Y., Fichelson, S., Valensi, F., Freyssinier, J. M., Rouyer-Fessard, P., and Cramer, E. (2000). Transforming growth factor inhibits erythropoiesis by blocking proliferation and accelerating differentiation of erythroid progenitors. *Exp. Hematol.* 28, 885–894. doi: 10.1016/S0301-472X(00)00488-4

17

Squeezing for Life – Properties of Red Blood Cell Deformability

*Rick Huisjes[1], Anna Bogdanova[2], Wouter W. van Solinge[1], Raymond M. Schiffelers[1], Lars Kaestner[3,4] and Richard van Wijk[1]**

[1] Department of Clinical Chemistry and Haematology, University Medical Center Utrecht, Utrecht University, Utrecht, Netherlands, [2] Red Blood Cell Research Group, Institute of Veterinary Physiology, Vetsuisse Faculty and the Zurich Center for Integrative Human Physiology (ZIHP), University of Zurich, Zürich, Switzerland, [3] Theoretical Medicine and Biosciences, Saarland University, Saarbrücken, Germany, [4] Experimental Physics, Saarland University, Saarbrücken, Germany

***Correspondence:**
Richard van Wijk
r.vanwijk@umcutrecht.nl

Deformability is an essential feature of blood cells (RBCs) that enables them to travel through even the smallest capillaries of the human body. Deformability is a function of (i) structural elements of cytoskeletal proteins, (ii) processes controlling intracellular ion and water handling and (iii) membrane surface-to-volume ratio. All these factors may be altered in various forms of hereditary hemolytic anemia, such as sickle cell disease, thalassemia, hereditary spherocytosis and hereditary xerocytosis. Although mutations are known as the primary causes of these congenital anemias, little is known about the resulting secondary processes that affect RBC deformability (such as secondary changes in RBC hydration, membrane protein phosphorylation, and RBC vesiculation). These secondary processes could, however, play an important role in the premature removal of the aberrant RBCs by the spleen. Altered RBC deformability could contribute to disease pathophysiology in various disorders of the RBC. Here we review the current knowledge on RBC deformability in different forms of hereditary hemolytic anemia and describe secondary mechanisms involved in RBC deformability.

Keywords: deformability, vesiculation, sickle cell anemia, thalassemia, hereditary spherocytosis, enzymopathies, hydration, hemolysis

INTRODUCTION

The primary function of RBCs is to enable respiration in tissues by providing oxygen and removing carbon dioxide via gas exchange in the lungs. During a typical 120 days lifespan of a RBC, it circulates through arteries, veins and small capillaries traveling –in total– a distance of 500 km (Lasch et al., 2000). RBC deformability, i.e., the ability of the RBC to change shape is essential for successful passage through these capillaries and splenic sinuses (Danielczok et al., 2017).

Deformability of RBC depends on the (i) structural properties of the "horizontal" cytoskeletal components such as spectrin (Burton and Bruce, 2011; Nans et al., 2011), (ii) vertical interaction of

Abbreviations: 5-FU, 5-fluorouracil; AC, adenyl cyclase; AMPK, AMP-activated protein kinase; ATP, adenosine triphosphate; Ca^{2+}, calcium; cAMP, cyclic adenosine monophosphate; cGMP, cyclic guanosine monophosphate; Cl^-, chloride; DNA, deoxyribonucleic acid; ET-1, endothelin-1; GAPDH, glyceraldehyde 3-phosphate dehydrogenase; HbS, hemoglobin S; HK, hexokinase; HS, hereditary spherocytosis; IL-10, interleukine-10; K^+, potassium; KCC = K^+-Cl^- cotransporter; KCNN4, calcium-activated potassium channel or Gardos channel; MCHC, mean corpuscular hemoglobin concentration; Mg^{2+}, magnesium; Na^+, sodium; PAF, platelet-activating factor; PDE, phosphodiesterase; PK, pyruvate kinase; PKA, protein kinase A; PKCα, protein kinase C alpha; PS, phosphatidylserine; RBCs, red blood cells; RNA, ribonucleic acid.

cytoskeleton and integral transmembrane complexes that is accomplished by ankyrin, 4.1 and 4.2 protein and the cytosolic domain of band 3 protein (also known as the anion exchanger 1 (AE1) or solute carrier family 4 member 1 (SLC4A1)) (Gallagher, 2004a) and (iii) resistance of the cytosolic pool (i.e., intracellular viscosity, RBC hydration state and surface-volume interaction) (Clark et al., 1983).

Deformability is also affected by metabolic processes controlling ATP levels and redox state. These factors control ion handling by pumps and passive transport pathways (Chu et al., 2012; Bogdanova et al., 2016), proteolytic activity of Ca^{2+}-dependent protease calpain (Bogdanova et al., 2013), and mutations and structural integrity of each element of the membrane architecture (Gallagher, 2004b). Failure to sustain deformability results in shortening of RBC life span and, when not compensated by *de novo* RBC production, in hemolytic anemia.

Therefore, reliable estimation of RBC deformability and understanding of the processes in control of it are essential for evaluation of severity of patients' state and choosing of the optimal therapeutic strategy. This particularly relates to the feasibility of splenectomy as an option to improve or worsen condition of patients with anemic state (Iolascon et al., 2017).

In this review, we provide an overview of the current knowledge on the primary and secondary mechanisms involved in regulation of RBC deformability in hereditary hemolytic anemia. We discuss methodologies that are currently used to assess RBC deformability in the clinical and research laboratories. We link different processes, such as ion channel activity, intracellular energy metabolism and phosphorylation of membrane proteins to RBC deformability and illustrate how these processes are affected in various RBC pathologies, such as sickle cell disease, thalassemia, HS and metabolic defects of RBCs. Finally, we describe the influence of shedding of nano-sized membrane vesicles from the RBC, the oxygenation state of hemoglobin and adaptive responses (such as exercise and high-altitude) on RBC deformability. Increased shedding of RBC vesicles, for example, is a feature of various RBC pathologies and vesicles are increasingly being considered to be a novel biomarker of RBC disorders (Pattanapanyasat et al., 2004; Nantakomol et al., 2012; Alaarg et al., 2013). They are considered to be involved in thrombosis and hemostasis (Biro et al., 2003; Livaja Koshiar et al., 2014) and associated with reduced RBC deformability (Waugh et al., 1992; Bosch et al., 1994).

RBC DEFORMABILITY IN HEREDITARY HEMOLYTIC ANEMIA

Anemia is considered to be hemolytic when RBCs are prematurely cleared from the circulation. Hemolytic anemia can be further subdivided into intra- or extravascular hemolytic anemia, and the underlying cause can be either inherited or acquired. Intravascular hemolysis is, as the name suggests, lysis of RBC in the vasculature. The cause can be hereditary, as seen in sickle cell disease (Pauling and Itano, 1949; Kato et al., 2017), but intravascular hemolysis can also be initiated by certain drugs (Cappellini and Fiorelli, 2008), by mechanical stress (for example through shear forces generated by artificial heart valves), by cold-agglutination (Körmöczi et al., 2006) or as a result of exhaustive exercise (Jordan et al., 1998). Intravascular hemolysis causes the release of hemoglobin into the plasma. Free hemoglobin is toxic and can lead to various clinical manifestations, such as hemoglobinuria, renal dysfunction, pulmonary hypertension and platelet activation (Rother et al., 2005).

Extravascular hemolysis is directly related to reduced RBC deformability. RBCs with reduced deformability fail to pass the spleen, which acts as an RBC quality-control organ (Mebius and Kraal, 2005; Deplaine et al., 2010). The red pulp of the spleen contains narrow inter-endothelial slits (MacDonald et al., 1987). Failure to pass through these narrow slits (Mebius and Kraal, 2005) leads to the uptake and breakdown of RBCs by macrophages (Burger et al., 2012). A number of hereditary RBC disorders result in reduced RBC deformability, which, as a consequence, leads to premature removal of RBCs in the spleen. Removal of RBCs by the spleen is, however, not only dependent on reduced deformability, but also occurs after recognition by macrophages. Senescent RBCs can be recognized and phagocytized by macrophages in the spleen upon binding of autologous antibodies to band 3 (Kay et al., 1983; Kay, 1984), exposure of conformational altered CD47 (Burger et al., 2012) or exposure of PS (Boas et al., 1998).

Hereditary forms of hemolytic anemia can affect the RBC membrane (i.e., HS, elliptocytosis, and pyropoikilocytosis) (Gallagher, 2004a; Perrotta et al., 2008; Da Costa et al., 2013), its metabolism (i.e., enzymopathies) (Zanella and Bianchi, 2000; van Wijk and van Solinge, 2005; Koralkova et al., 2014), cell hemoglobin (i.e., sickle cell anemia, unstable hemoglobin variants) (Higgs et al., 2012; Ware et al., 2017), or cellular hydration (i.e., HS, hereditary xerocytosis or Gardos Channelopathy) (Vives Corrons and Besson, 2001; Albuisson et al., 2013; Andolfo et al., 2013, 2015; Beneteau et al., 2014; Faucherre et al., 2014; Glogowska et al., 2015; Fermo et al., 2017a). While the primary genetic causes of these disorders are often well determined, less is known about the factors triggering the actual hemolysis. Striking examples are sickle cell disease, thalassemia, HS and the metabolic disorders of the RBC. All have well-known and well-studied primary genetic and molecular defects. However, little is known about the secondary mechanisms that may decrease RBC deformability and thereby contribute to the premature removal of these affected RBCs.

For example, the homozygous single point mutation in the *HBB* gene, substituting glutamic acid for valine at position 6 leads to sickle cell disease (Ware et al., 2017). Although the discovery that these RBCs tend to sickle at low oxygen tension was already provided by Hahn and Gillespie (1927), Kenney et al. (1961), it took decades to unravel the processes that contribute to sickle cell dehydration (Lew and Bookchin, 2005; Ataga et al., 2008), decreased deformability and increased endothelial cell adhesion (Alapan et al., 2015, 2016). We still do not understand how does a point mutation in hemoglobin beta chain cause these secondary pathological alterations in density and adhesiveness and how all these changes in turn impact the disease symptoms of the patient. Other examples are the enzymopathies, which are

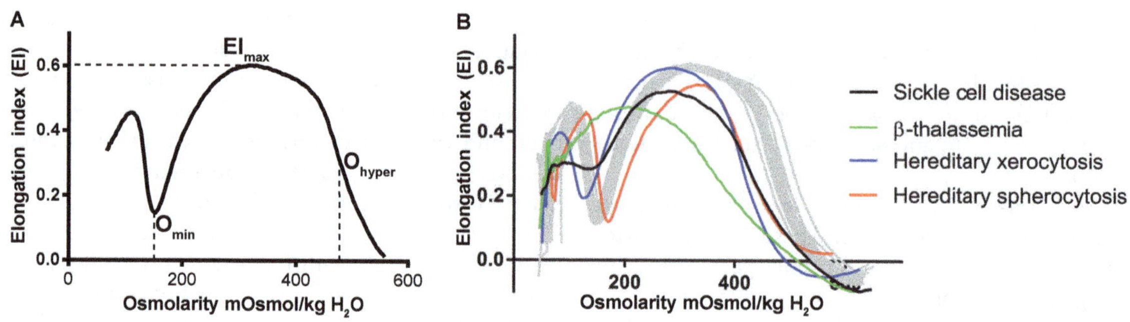

FIGURE 1 | Osmotic gradient ektacytometry as a tool to measure red blood cell (RBC) deformability. The technique is discussed in detail by Clark et al. (1983); Lazarova et al. (2017), and Da Costa et al. (2016). Briefly, during osmotic gradient ektacytometry, the RBC is subjected to an osmotic gradient (range ≈50 mOsmol/kg H_2O – 650 mOsmol/kg H_2O) under constant shear stress, while the elongation index (EI) is measured. The EI corresponds to the deformability at various osmotic conditions. **(A)** the left graph depicts an osmotic gradient ektacytometry curve from a healthy control with various intersection points: the EI_{max} reflects the maximal deformability of the RBC, O_{min} reflects the osmotic fragility and O_{hyper} reflects the (de)hydration state (or intracellular viscosity) of the RBC. **(B)** In the right graph osmotic gradient curves of patients with sickle cell disease (black line), β-thalassemia (green line), hereditary xerocytosis (blue line) and hereditary spherocytosis (red line) and several individual healthy controls (gray lines, $n = 20$) are depicted.

caused by mutations in, for example, PK or HK and lead to a shortage of metabolic energy inside the RBC. Again, although the primary effect on decreased levels of ATP in these diseases is well understood (Zanella et al., 2007), secondary processes such as altered K^+ fluxes (Nathan et al., 1965) and phosphorylation of intracellular proteins (Thali et al., 2010; Wang et al., 2010), need further elucidation.

Moreover, for a substantial number of patients with hereditary hemolytic anemia – the primary causes of disease remain unknown, or were only identified very recently. For these patients, a comprehensive understanding of both primary and secondary defects of the affected RBCs is still lacking. This is illustrated by the recently discovered mutations in patients with hereditary xerocytosis, also known as dehydrated stomatocytosis (Andolfo et al., 2013). In these patients, stomatocytes are typically found in peripheral blood smears. However, the primary molecular cause for the anemia and morphological change of the RBC remained unknown for a long time, let alone that the secondary processes that are involved in the disease process were elucidated. Only recently, it was shown that hereditary xerocytosis was caused by mutations in genes for the mechanosensitive *PIEZO1* channel (Andolfo et al., 2013; Shmukler et al., 2014; Glogowska et al., 2017). Very recently, a mutation in the calcium-activated potassium channel subfamily N member KCNN4 (encoded by the human KCa3.1 gene, and also known as the Gardos channel in RBCs) (Andolfo et al., 2015; Glogowska et al., 2015; Rapetti-Mauss et al., 2015; Fermo et al., 2017a) was shown to cause 'Gardos channelopathy' a disease resembling yet at some points different from hereditary xerocytosis (Fermo et al., 2017a). Only then, the molecular diagnosis of these diseases was established in these patient groups and new insight on RBC deformability and RBC ion homeostasis with respect to ion channel function were obtained. The secondary processes that contribute to RBC clearance in these diseases are now being explored (Fermo et al., 2017a).

TECHNIQUES TO DETERMINE RBC DEFORMABILITY

A currently well-established tool to probe RBC deformability is osmotic gradient ektacytometry, which is routinely used in the diagnosis of patients with hereditary hemolytic anemia. The technique is performed on a Laser-assisted Optical Rotational Cell Analyzer (Lorrca). It assesses RBC deformability, osmotic fragility and cellular hydration status (see **Figure 1**) (Clark et al., 1983; Da Costa et al., 2016; Lazarova et al., 2017; Llaudet-Planas et al., 2017). In osmotic gradient ektacytometry, the maximum RBC deformability is represented by the maximum elongation index (EI_{max}). The O_{min} represents the osmotic value (mOsmol/kg H_2O) where the elongation index (EI) is minimal, corresponding to the 50% lysis point as determined by the classical osmotical fragility test (Clark et al., 1983). The hydration status (or intracellular viscosity) is represented by O_{hyper} (mOsmol/kg H_2O). The value corresponds with the hypertonic osmolarity where the EI is 50% of EI_{max}. The value of these three parameters as well as the shape of the curve is used in the diagnosis of various disorders of the RBC membrane and hydration station (**Figure 1B**).

O_{hyper} correlates with the reciprocal function of the MCHC (Clark et al., 1983). In healthy individuals, during RBC aging increased MCHC is observed and this correlates with decreased RBC deformability (Clark et al., 1983; Bosch et al., 1994). A similar observation has been made for RBCs from patients with sickle cell disease and HS. Also here, a decrease in RBC hydration (i.e., decreased O_{hyper} and increased MCHC) of patient's cells is associated with a decrease in the maximum RBC deformability (EI_{max}) (Clark et al., 1983; Bunn, 1997).

Besides osmotic gradient ektacytometry, there are other methods to measure RBC deformability (Tomaiuolo, 2014). A number of techniques that are also used in diagnostics measures RBC deformability as a function of shear stress, for example the RheoScan-D (Shin et al., 2007), Automated Rheoscope and Cell Analyser (ARCA) (Dobbe et al., 2002) and the deformability measurement module on the Lorrca (Hardeman et al., 1987). The results of RheoScan-D and the deformability measurements (shear-stress module) on the Lorrca were observed to be comparable (Shin et al., 2007). However, RheoScan-D measures RBC deformability under microfluidic conditions after the application of shear stress, while shear-stress on RBCs in the deformability measurements on the Lorrca requires a larger set-up with a rotating cup (Hardeman et al., 1987; Shin et al., 2007). The ARCA measures RBC deformability with a microscope after the application of shear-stress, and therefore has the potential to measure the RBC deformability of subpopulations (Dobbe et al., 2002).

Most direct measurements of single cells include: micropipette (Waugh et al., 1992), atomic force spectroscopy and holographic optical tweezers (HOT) (Steffen et al., 2011; Kaestner et al., 2012). The mechanical probes and the optical approach are complementary since 30 pN is a lower force limit for the mechanical measurements and an upper limit for the HOT in the context of investigating RBCs (Minetti et al., 2013). Currently microfluidic approaches becoming increasingly popular to investigate RBC deformability (Cluitmans et al., 2014; Guo et al., 2014; Picot et al., 2015; Danielczok et al., 2017). While the latter method has the potential to become a routine diagnostic tool, the former single cell methods are mostly dedicated to basic research due to their instrumental complexity.

A further very simple method to measure RBC deformability is the readout of RBC filterability, e.g., by measuring RBC passage through cellulose columns (Oonishi et al., 1997). Unfortunately there is currently no standardized column/readout system on the market that would allow comparison of filterability between diagnostic laboratories. In addition, RBC passage through cellulose columns or filters is highly subjected to changes in cellular volume (such as MCV), which may affect results. A summary of available techniques to measure RBC deformability is depicted in **Table 1**.

DETERMINANTS OF RBC DEFORMABILITY

RBC Hydration

Regulation of RBC Hydration

Red blood cell deformability is highly influenced by RBC volume control and by ion content, both regulated by ion pumps, ion channels, symporters and antiporters (Gallagher, 2013) (see **Figure 2**). When ion channels are open, ions move following their electrochemical gradients, while ion pumps can actively move these ions against the gradient (Gadsby, 2009). Symporters and antiporters may also create secondary ion gradients, but require the pre-existing gradients for at least one type of ions as a driving force to transport the other ion types against the gradient. Symporters transport two (e.g., K^+-Cl^- cotransporter) or more (e.g., Na^+-K^+-$2Cl^-$ cotransporter) ions in the same direction using driving force for one of them, while antiporters (e.g., Na^+/H^+ exchanger or anion exchanger) exchange two ions that move in the opposite direction (Wolfersberger, 1994). These transporters, pumps and channels are crucial in resisting/adapting to local osmotic changes and maintaining RBC volume (Wieth, 1979; Liu et al., 2011; Thomas et al., 2011; Gallagher, 2013; Lew and Tiffert, 2017). RBC volume changes result from differences in osmotic pressure (Sugie et al., 2018), which results in water transport by aquaporins of which AQP1 and AQP3 are found in human RBCs (Yang et al., 2001). Cotransport of water is, however, also possible through the K^+-Cl^- cotransporter (KCC) (Zeuthen and Macaulay, 2012). Volume changes are also associated by in- and efflux of several amino acids and amino-acid derivates, such as taurine (Goldstein and Brill, 1991; Goldstein and Davis, 1994).

As mentioned previously, MCHC is a parameter that reflects the RBC hydration state, and is dependent on the hemoglobin concentration in RBCs, RBC volume, RBC membrane loss and water content. Quick movements of ions and water result in acute changes in MCHC whereas long-term effects on MCHC are often associated with release of hemoglobin-free vesicles. RBC hydration may be quantified using the O_{hyper} value as obtained by osmotic gradient ektacytometry (see **Figure 1** and see section "Techniques to Determine RBC Deformability"). Changes in RBC density detected using cell distribution within Percoll density gradients reflects both membrane loss and the changes in RBC surface-to-volume ratio and alterations in intracellular ion and water content. In-depth morphological analysis could be used as a complementary approach to discriminate between membrane and ion/water loss.

Primary Changes of RBC Hydration

In this section we shall address hereditary hemolytic anemias associated with the changes in the intracellular ion and secondary to the latter changes in water content. One of the players in this type of disorder is a mechano-sensitive PIEZO1 channel, a non-selective cation channel permeable for Ca^{2+} that in turn can activate the calcium activated K^+ channel subfamily N member KCNN4 (or Gardos channel in RBCs) (Kaestner et al., 2018). Thus, hydration state is largely dependent on the shear stress intensity and the hydration state of RBCs from splenectomized and non-splenectomized patients with the same mutation may vary substantially. Furthermore, hydration state is a function of RBC age, young RBCs being more hydrated than the senescent cells (Clark et al., 1983; Lutz et al., 1992).

A RBC disorder characterized by primary hydration changes is hereditary xerocytosis (HX), also known as dehydrated stomatocytosis. HX is a form of hereditary hemolytic anemia, and patients often suffer from iron-overload (Zarychanski et al., 2012). In addition, in many RBC disorders splenectomy relieves symptoms and increases RBC survival, but in HX, splenectomy is contra-indicated as it drastically increases the risks for thrombotic events (Stewart et al., 1996; Jaïs et al., 2003; Iolascon et al., 2017). HX was related to mutations in the mechanosensitive PIEZO1 channel (Zarychanski et al., 2012; Albuisson et al., 2013; Li et al., 2014). PIEZO1 mutations lead to stabilization of the "active" state or destabilization of the "inactive" state of the PIEZO1 protein (Albuisson et al., 2013). These alterations in

TABLE 1 | Overview of techniques to measure RBC deformability.

Method	Principle	Readouts	Advantages	Disadvantages/sources of mistake
Osmotic fragility test (OFT) (Parpart et al., 1947)	The OFT tests RBC lysis at various osmotic conditions. Lysis in OFT depends on critical RBC volume needed for hemoglobin content.	50% lysis point	Relatively easy technique	Requires pre-incubation at 37°C and heparin blood, measurement of population average. pH and temperature of solutions can affect results. Low sensitivity (Bianchi et al., 2012).
Osmotic gradient ektacytometry (Clark et al., 1983; Da Costa et al., 2016; Lazarova et al., 2017)	RBC deformability is constantly measured under constant shear stress while osmotic gradient gradually increases from hypotonic to hypertonic conditions.	Maximum deformability (EI_{max}), RBC hydration (O_{hyper}) and 50% lysis point in OFT (O_{min})	Robust and reproducible, diagnostic technique, enables comparison between laboratories	Measures RBC population average
Shear-stress dependent deformability (Hardeman et al., 1987; Dobbe et al., 2002; Shin et al., 2007)	Measurement of RBC deformability after application of constant or increasing levels stress-stress (i.e., Automated Rheoscope and Cell Analyser (ARCA), RheoScan-D, or deformability on Lorrca).	Elongation index (EI) and maximum deformability EI_{max}	Easy, reproducible and diagnostic techniques Automated Rheoscope and Cell Analyser (ARCA) can measure deformability of subpopulations	RheoScan-D and deformability measurements on Lorrca measures populations average. Automated Rheoscope and Cell Analyser (ARCA) requires a microscope, which leads to number of cells that are out of focus and are rejected from analysis
Atomic force microscopy (AFM) (Yeow et al., 2017)	Scanning technique that uses a tip as a probe to detect morphological changes and changes in deformability. Measures the resistance after application of force.	Elasticity, force, resistance	Single cell technique and AFM can measure RBC deformability at different spots per RBC. Topographic images can be obtained.	Advanced equipment needed and labor extensive, no gold standard
Micropipette (Waugh et al., 1992)	Aspiration of cells or membrane parts.	Surface area, volume, sphericity, elasticity	Single cell technique	Labor intensive
Holographic optical tweezers (HOT) (Steffen et al., 2011; Kaestner et al., 2012)	Usage of highly focused to generate laserbeams to with attractive or repulsive forces.	Depending on set-up; fluidity, elongation, fluorescence microscopy read-out [e.g., Ca^{2+} (fluo-4-AM)]	Low forces can be applied	Advanced equipment needed and labor extensive, no gold standard
Microfluidics (Cluitmans et al., 2014; Guo et al., 2014; Danielczok et al., 2017; Pioot et al., 2015)	RBC suspension is injected in network of microfluidic channels. In these channels RBC are subjected to small pores where RBC deformability is essential.	Depends on microfluidic set-up	Measurement of individual RBCs, RBC deformability measured under relative physiological conditions, various set-ups available	Technique still in development phase, no gold standard available, which hampers comparison between laboratories and reduces interlaboratory reproducibility. RBCs can block microfluidic device
RBC filterability (Oonishi et al., 1997)	RBC needs to pass filter with various pore-sizes. Also various columns are used with different particle and particle sizes (e.g., cellulose, metal beads).	Dependent on set-up: time, lysis, resistance	Relatively easy technique	No standardization available and no standardized commercial technique available. No comparison between laboratories possible. Can be affected by parameters such as MCV.

channel function lead to increased intracellular levels of Ca^{2+} and subsequent KCNN4 (Gardos channel) activation (Cahalan et al., 2015; Danielczok et al., 2017). KCNN4 activation leads to efflux of K^+ and dehydration. The relatively low intracellular levels of K^+ could therefore serve as a biomarker for HX (Zarychanski et al., 2012; Gallagher, 2017). Although PIEZO1 mutations leads to KCNN4 (or Gardos channel) activation, RBCs with mutations in KCNN4 (Gardos channelopathy) exhibit a different pathology (Fermo et al., 2017a). For example, HX caused by mutations in PIEZO1 lead to severe RBC dehydration, which is also shown by a left-shift of O_{hyper} in the osmotic gradient curve (see **Figure 1B** and see section "Techniques to Determine RBC Deformability") while mutations in KCNN4 (or Gardos channel) may cause only slight alterations in the osmotic gradient curve (Fermo et al., 2017b). In addition, RBCs from patients with KCNN4 mutations were found to exhibit increased activity of Na-K-ATPase that is most likely triggered by the increase in the intracellular Na^+ concentrations. The hyperactivated Na, K-pump compensates for the dissipation in Na/K gradients and pumps K^+ back into the cells, but fails to restore normal K^+ content completely (Fermo et al., 2017a). Currently, however, it is difficult to measure intracellular water content or RBC volume

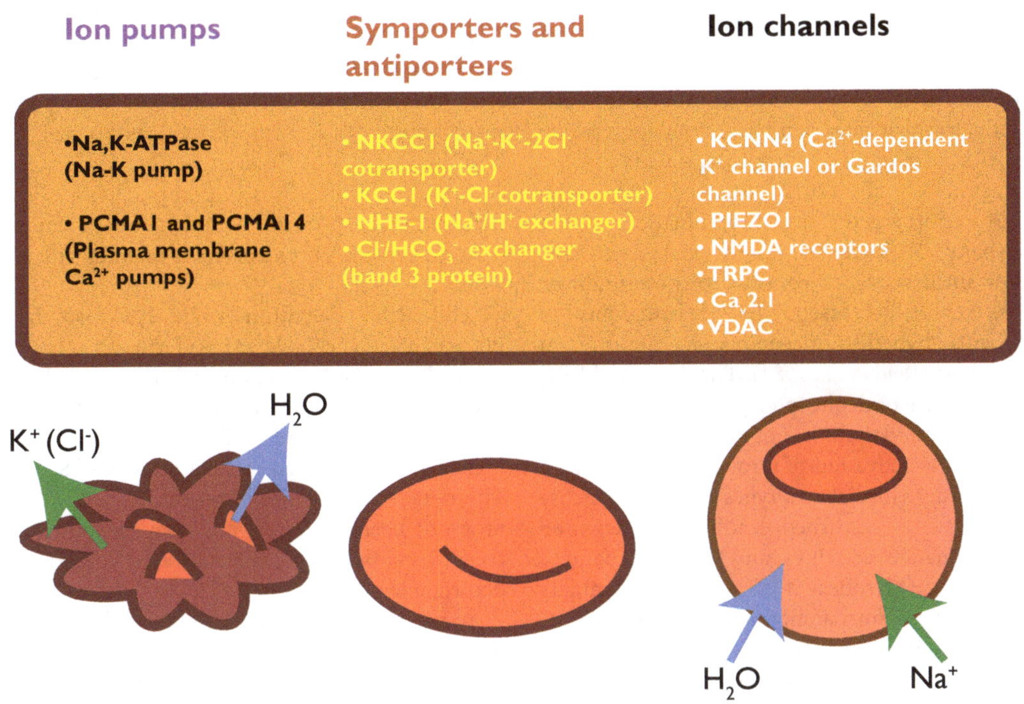

FIGURE 2 | schematic overview of RBC ion pumps (Sachs, 2003; Tiffert et al., 2003), symporters and antiporters (Bernhardt et al., 1988; Wolfersberger, 1994) and ion channels (Bouyer et al., 2012; Kaestner, 2011, 2015).

directly and accurately enough, which makes it challenging to discriminate between water loss and membrane loss.

Cytoskeletal Network

Primary Changes of the Cytoskeletal Network

In addition to the protein defects, described above, that directly disturb the membrane and thereby the ability of the RBC to deform there are also secondary causes affecting membrane (protein) function and, thereby, RBC deformability. Examples of these are membrane protein phosphorylation, RBC density and RBC vesiculation.

The RBC membrane is built from a basic triangular network of α- and β-spectrin molecules connected to band 3, ankyrin and protein 4.1 (Perrotta et al., 2008; Salomao et al., 2008). This network provides the RBC with a certain stability and simultaneously the ability to deform. HS (HS) is characterized by defects in proteins forming the cytoskeletal network or proteins forming ankyrin and junctional complexes. This usually concerns mutations in band 3, protein 4.2, α-spectrin, or ankyrin (Perrotta et al., 2008). These mutations lead to membrane instability, membrane loss through release of hemoglobin-free vesicles, with consequent decreased surface area-to-volume ratio, increase in MCHC and density and formation of spherocytes (Perrotta et al., 2008). Spherocytes show a characteristic loss of RBC deformability, leading to premature removal of these RBCs from the circulation (Perrotta et al., 2008). Hereditary elliptocytosis (HE) is a disorder characterized by disturbances of the horizontal cytoskeletal interactions and are usually caused by mutations in α-spectrin, β-spectrin and protein 4.1R. As the name suggests, the disturbed horizontal interactions lead to the formation of elliptocytes. The majority of HE patients are clinically asymptomatic, but few patients suffer from hemolysis, jaundice and splenomegaly (Da Costa et al., 2013).

Secondary Disturbances of the Cytoskeletal Network

The triangular spectrin network, connected through ankyrin and protein 4.1R to band 3 supports membrane stability and contributes to RBC flexibility and deformability. Tyrosine phosphorylation of in the individual proteins regulates interaction forces between the elements of this network. Tyrosine phosphorylation is regulated by phosphotyrosine kinases and by phosphotyrosine phosphatases. Under normal conditions, protein regulatory tyrosine residues are only phosphorylated to a limited degree (Terra et al., 1998; Zipser et al., 2002). In the RBC membrane, phosphorylation of protein 4.1R, for example, leads to a reduced membrane stability (Muravyov and Tikhomirova, 2013), and phosphorylation of ankyrin regulates its binding to band 3 (Muravyov and Tikhomirova, 2013). The dissociation constant (K_d) between ankyrin and band 3 influences RBC deformability without a loss in elasticity, underlining that cytoskeletal protein phosphorylation has implications on RBC deformability (Anong, 2006).

The effect of phosphorylation of band 3, the most abundant membrane protein, on RBC deformability is not entirely clear. The possible physiological relevance of band 3 protein Tyr phosphorylation state emerges from the fact that it is controlled by hormones such as insulin (Marques et al., 2000) and that it is altered in patients with hemoglobinopathies (Terra et al., 1998). Saldanha et al. (2007) showed that dephosphorylation of band 3 Tyr residues does not affect RBC deformability. It, therefore, appears that phosphorylation of band 3 does not affect RBC deformability directly, but may alter band 3 protein aggregation and its interaction with extracellular matrix components.

Lopes de Almeida et al. (2012) showed that high concentrations of fibrinogen in combination with dephosphorylated band 3, leads to mildly increased RBC deformability at low shear stress. In contrast to these findings, Reid et al. (1984) report decreased RBC deformability in diabetic patients with hyperfibrinogenemia in absence of dephosphorylating agents (Reid et al., 1984). The decreased RBC deformability in the absence of dephosphorylating agents seems to underline that phosphorylation is not involved. However, insulin is implicated in the activation of tyrosine kinases that in turn phosphorylate band 3. In diabetes types I and II, glucose and insulin homeostasis is disturbed leading to increased protein tyrosine phosphatase activities and aberrant band 3 phosphorylation patterns (Marques et al., 2000), potentially leading to reduced RBC deformability and increased RBC turnover. This same principle may also play a role in patients with sepsis, where investigators have shown that tyrosine phosphorylation of band 3 was increased in septic mice and that this increase was accompanied by reduced RBC deformability (Condon et al., 2007).

Band 3 phosphorylation was found to be increased by a rise in intracellular Ca^{2+}-concentrations due to dissociation of phosphotyrosine phosphatase from band 3 (Zipser et al., 2002). Interestingly, sickle cell disease is characterized by an increase in both intracellular Ca^{2+} concentration (Bogdanova et al., 2013) and tyrosine phosphorylation of band 3 (Terra et al., 1998), which potentially could thus influence RBC membrane stability. The importance of band 3 phosphorylation for RBC shape and deformability is highlighted by a number of *in vitro* experiments. For example, morphological changes of RBCs were observed after Tyr-phosphorylation of band 3 mediated by pervanadate (Bordin et al., 1995). In contrast, Ser/Thr-phosphorylation of spectrin, which was selectively induced by okadaic acid did not result in morphological changes (Bordin et al., 1995). Unfortunately, the deformability of RBCs after pervanadate and okadaic treatment was not measured in these studies, but it seems reasonable to assume that RBC deformability is affected since both membrane protein phosphorylation and RBC morphology have been associated with altered RBC deformability (Reid et al., 1984; Chabanel et al., 1987; Hasegawa et al., 1993; Saldanha et al., 2007; Lopes de Almeida et al., 2012).

RBC Hydration Changes Associated With Cytoskeletal Defects

Although reduced RBC deformability in HS mainly results from cytoskeletal disturbances (Perrotta et al., 2008), spherocytes experience dehydration and increased leakage of K^+ (De Franceschi et al., 1997; Gallagher, 2017). To compensate for this increased K^+ leakage, spherocytes are also found to have increased activity of the Na-K pump and the NKCC1 (also known as the Na-K-2Cl cotransporter, coded by gene SLC12A2) (Vives Corrons and Besson, 2001). RBCs of transgenic mice deficient for ankyrin or spectrin show increased activity of the Na-K pump, but normal activities of the NKCC1 and K^+-Cl^- cotransporters (Peters et al., 1999). This contrasts with protein 4.2-deficient mice, where Na-K pump activity is normal, while activities of NKCC1 and K^+-Cl^- cotransporters are increased (Peters et al., 1999). These differences in pump activities between protein 4.2 deficient and spectrin- or ankyrin-deficient mice support the concept that membrane proteins interact with ion channels of the RBC.

The RBC dehydration in HS also involves increased intracellular Ca^{2+} levels (Hertz et al., 2017). Increased intracellular Ca^{2+} correlates with decreased RBC deformability and RBC membrane stiffening (Bogdanova et al., 2013). For example, after *in vitro* ATP-depletion of HS RBCs, Ca^{2+} influx is increased compared to healthy RBCs (Shimoda et al., 1984). The detailed mechanisms beyond this Ca^{2+} influx have up to now not been identified and may include PIEZO1 or NMDA receptors both of which are activated by shear stress in "stiff" less deformable cells.

In protein $4.2^{-/-}$ mice, displaying the HS phenotype, KCNN4 (or known as Gardos channels in RBCs) were noted to be functionally up-regulated, or at least more KCNN4 activity was measured (Peters et al., 1999; De Franceschi et al., 2005). This can be considered as a protective mechanism that leads to an outward flux of K^+ and water from RBCs. This mechanism may compensate for the decreased surface-to-area ratio. Indeed, increased lysis was observed when these RBCs were exposed to KCNN4 (or Gardos-channel) inhibitors (De Franceschi et al., 2005). These findings indicate that KCNN4 is activated in HS in order to facilitate RBC dehydration, which maintains hemoglobin in RBCs at the expense of water. Recent research confirms the finding that RBC dehydration and formation of denser RBCs may protect the RBC in HS from lysis and premature uptake. We observed that mild HS is accompanied with prolonged RBC life-span, relatively mild reductions in RBC deformability and denser RBCs when compared with RBCs from patients with moderate/severe HS (Huisjes et al., 2017a). Most likely, the mild reduction in RBC deformability in patients with mild HS avoids premature splenic uptake and thus may provide the HS RBC time to lose membrane and to become dense.

Red Cell Metabolism

Primary Changes of Red Cell Metabolism

Mature RBCs of healthy individuals lack mitochondria and are therefore entirely dependent on the glycolytic pathway for the production of energy in the form of ATP. In the glycolytic pathway, glucose is converted to lactate by several enzymatic steps (**Figure 3**) (van Wijk and van Solinge, 2005; Koralkova et al., 2014). Key regulatory enzymes in the glycolytic pathway are HK, phosphofructokinase and PK. Hereditary metabolic disorders, or enzymopathies, are disorders impairing cellular energy production and balance, in particular ATP production. ATP is essential in the regulation of RBC deformability, viability, regulatory cascades involving phosphorylation and activity of ion transport involving Na, K-ATPase, and Ca

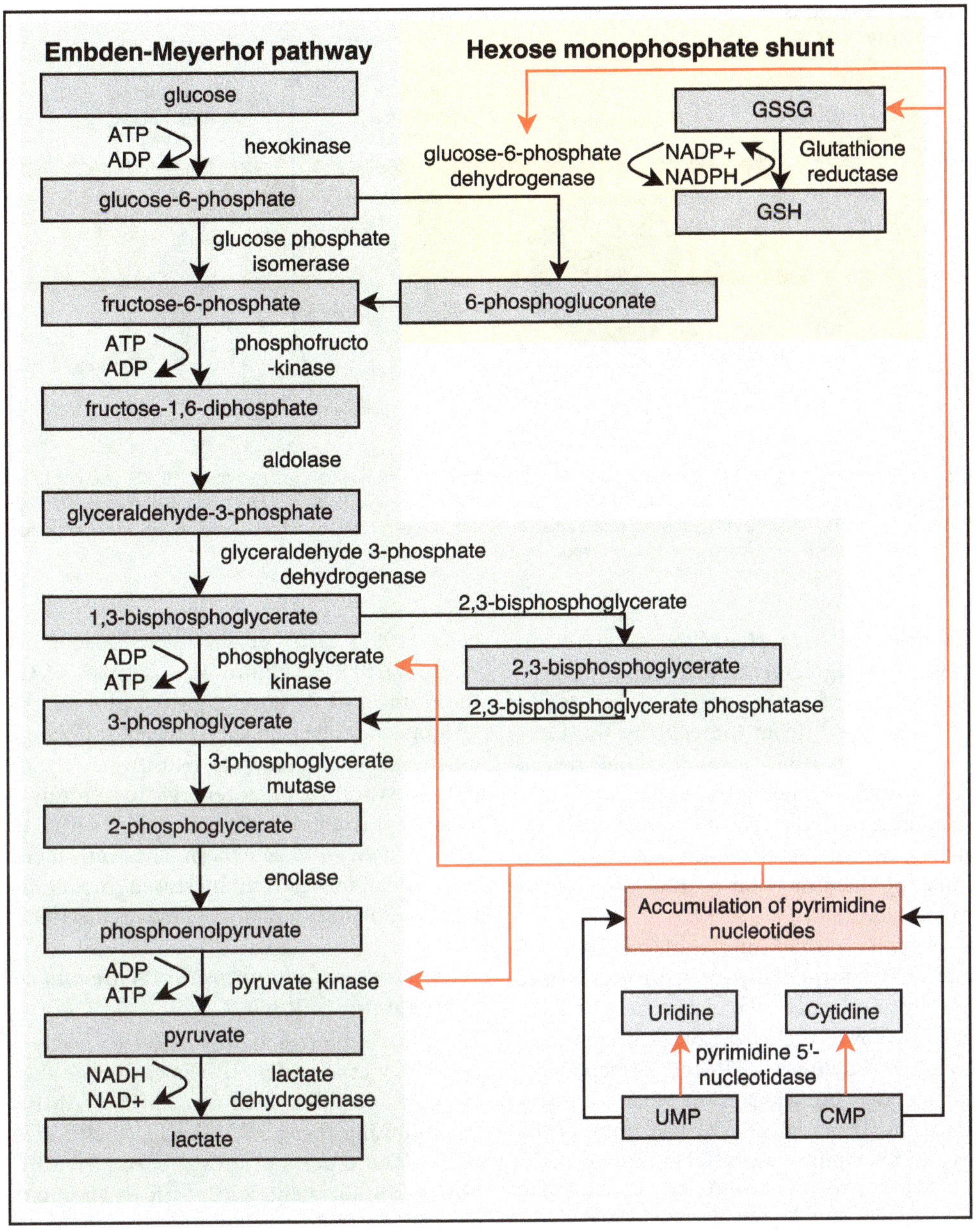

FIGURE 3 | Glycolytic pathway of RBCs is essential for energy metabolism as RBCs lack mitochondria and a nucleus. Enzyme deficiencies can lead to decreased intracellular ATP levels, which possibly reduce RBC deformability. Depicted here are the Embden–Meyerhof pathway, hexose monophosphate shunt and the influence of a pyrimidine 5′-nucleotidase deficiency. Red arrows illustrate negative feedback or reduced production. This illustration is a merged figure adapted from both van Wijk and van Solinge (2005) and Zanella et al. (2006).

ATPase (Weed et al., 1969; Tuvia et al., 1998; Martinov et al., 2000; Fischer et al., 2003; Park et al., 2010; Makhro et al., 2016).

Adenosine triphosphate plays a key role in maintenance of ion gradients and should impact cytoskeletal structure and RBC shape (Tuvia et al., 1998; Park et al., 2010). However, glycolytic enzymopathies usually do not show altered RBC morphology (Koralkova et al., 2014; Huisjes et al., 2017b). For reasons that are not yet well understood, metabolically defective RBCs are prematurely removed by the spleen, causing chronic Hereditary Non-Spherocytic Hemolytic Anemia (HNSHA) (Koralkova et al., 2014).

Several observations point to mechanisms that may be involved in the premature clearance. RBCs from a patient with pyruvate kinase deficiency (PKD) were found to leak K^+ more rapidly and were found to consume ATP at an accelerated rate (Nathan et al., 1965). This most likely contributes to the decreased RBC viability in this disease and could result in reduced RBC deformability (Leblond et al., 1978). A possible explanation for increased clearance of RBCs with metabolic defects is the

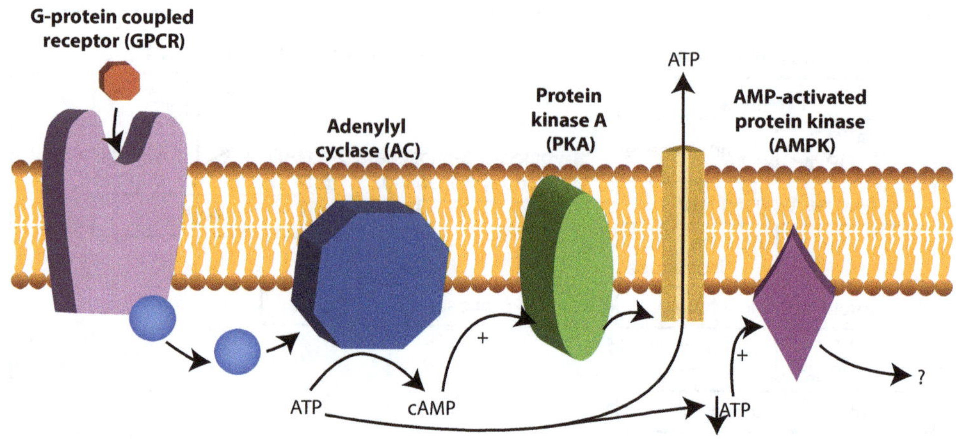

FIGURE 4 | cAMP production by adenylyl cyclase (AC). AC is activated after stimulation by G-protein coupled receptors (GPCR) and converts ATP to cAMP. Examples of GPCRs 2-adrenergic receptor, the lysophosphatidic β in RBCs are the erythrocyte acid (LPA) receptor and the purinergic (P2Y) receptor. cAMP acts as a second messenger in RBCs and among other things stimulate protein kinase A (PKA). Under low ATP concentrations, AMP-activated protein kinase (AMPK) becomes active and can inactivate or activate yet not fully understood processes in RBCs.

imbalance in Ca^{2+} uptake and extrusion (Bogdanova et al., 2013; Hertz et al., 2017). In agreement with the hypothesis that ATP deprivation will cause Ca^{2+} overload due to the inability to actively extrude Ca^{2+} from the cells by the Ca^{2+} pumps, decreased ATP levels in RBCs with metabolic defects were associated with abnormally high intracellular Ca^{2+} and exposure of PS, an important cellular 'eat-me' signal (de Back et al., 2014). Alternatively, defective metabolism may impact the redox state of RBCs making them more susceptible to oxidative stress (Cappellini and Fiorelli, 2008).

Despite the intuitive feeling that intracellular ATP levels should correlate with cellular deformability, evidence for this is so far inconclusive. This may be related to the techniques used. For example, research performed by Karger et al. (2012) did not show any correlation between intracellular ATP and deformability in RBC-concentrates intended for transfusion when assessing deformability by increasing shear stress. On the other hand, studies using viscosity and filterability assays did find correlations between intracellular ATP and deformability and showed that deformability is indeed dependent on intracellular ATP levels (Weed et al., 1969; Fischer et al., 2003). Atomic force microscopy studies also revealed increased membrane stiffness after ATP depletion due to reduced spectrin phosphorylation (Picas et al., 2013). We hypothesize that the different results from these experiments are possibly caused by the fact that ATP is not required for RBCs to elongate after the application of external forces, such as shear stress but ATP might be essential in the process of RBC deformation toward different shapes, as seen in filterability measurements.

Secondary Changes of Metabolism

Cyclic AMP (cAMP) is a second messenger and is derived from ATP. In nucleated human cells, cyclic AMP (cAMP) is synthesized from ATP by adenylate cyclase (AC) upon stimulation by G-protein coupled receptors (GPCR) and there is evidence that this process also occurs in human RBCs (Oonishi et al., 1997; Tuvia et al., 1999; Sprague et al., 2006; Kostova et al., 2015) (see **Figure 4**). Examples of GPCRs on RBCs are the erythrocyte β2-adrenergic receptor (Harrison et al., 2003), the lysophosphatidic acid (LPA) receptor (Wang et al., 2013) and the purinergic (P2Y) receptor (Kostova et al., 2015). The activation of the erythrocyte β2-adrenergic receptor by catecholamines such as epinephrine (or adrenaline) affects RBC deformability (Tuvia et al., 1999). *In vitro* experiments with increased concentration of adrenaline, lead to increased membrane fluctuations and increased RBC filterability (Tuvia et al., 1999).

Intracellular mechanisms that sense and control cellular energy status in RBCs

Phosphodiesterases tightly regulate levels of cAMP in RBCs (Adderley et al., 2011). PDEs catabolize the phosphodiesters in cyclic nucleotides, such as cAMP to AMP or cGMP to GMP. By inhibiting these PDEs, cyclic nucleotides remain intact and active. The reports of cAMP effects on RBC deformability are, however, ambivalent. Recently it was found that sildenafil, which is a PDE inhibitor and well-known for its function in the treatment of erectile dysfunction and pulmonary hypertension, has beneficial effects on RBC deformability in sickle cell disease at low concentrations *in vitro*. Increase in nitric monoxide bioavailability was suggested to improve RBC deformability (Grau et al., 2013; Kuhn et al., 2017). However, increased concentrations of sildenafil impaired sickle RBC filterability (Hagley et al., 2011). Typically, inhibition of cGMP-specific PDE type 5 (PDE-5) by sildenafil reduces the degradation of the second messenger cGMP to GMP and increases smooth muscles relaxation. In RBCs, this PDE-5 inhibition increases not only intracellular levels of cGMP but also preserves intracellular levels of cAMP via the inhibitor activity of cGMP on PDE-3 (see **Figure 5**) (Adderley et al., 2010; Knebel et al., 2013). The effect of increased cAMP levels was also studied using a spleen-like microfiltration system. Increased retention in the microfiltration system, reflecting decreased deformability, was observed after

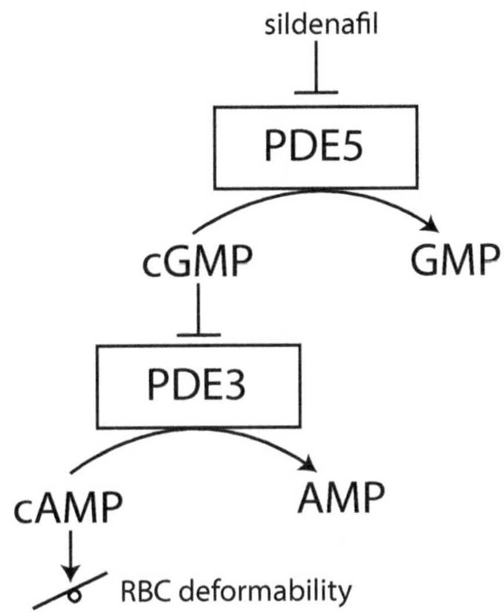

FIGURE 5 | effect of PDE-5 inhibitors, such as sildenafil, on RBC deformability. PDE-5 inhibitors elevate intracellular concentrations of cGMP, thereby indirectly inhibiting PDE3. Inhibition of PDE3 does raise the intracellular concentration of cAMP. Depending on the degree of this intracellular cAMP elevation, RBC deformability can be either increased or decreased.

incubation of RBCs with sildenafil (Ramdani et al., 2015). Moreover, the production of cGMP from GTP is synthesized by guanylate cyclase (Derbyshire and Marletta, 2012). Guanylate cyclase is activated by nitric oxide (NO) and the addition of sodium nitroprusside to RBCs as an artificial nitric oxide donor does prevent Ca^{2+} influx and Ca^{2+}-mediated stiffness of RBCs (Barodka et al., 2014).

In addition, the effect of cAMP on the release of ATP is still under debate. A role for cAMP in the release of ATP to its extracellular environment via PKA was proposed (Sprague et al., 2007; Adderley et al., 2011; Knebel et al., 2013) (see **Figure 4**). Others, however, have attributed the release of ATP solely to hemolysis of the RBC (Sikora et al., 2014) or to release via transporters such as Pannexin 1 (Locovei et al., 2006) or PIEZO1 (Cinar et al., 2015).

Recently AMPK was also found to be present in RBCs (Thali et al., 2010). The exact function of AMPK in RBCs is unknown, however, in other cells, AMPK is essential to balance ATP consumption and ATP production. In muscles and fat AMPK regulates glucose uptake (Mihaylova and Shaw, 2011). Likely, AMPK also regulates these processes in RBCs, as RBCs from $AMPK^{-/-}$ mice were less viable after *in vitro* glucose depletion (Föller et al., 2009). Interestingly, these $AMPK^{-/-}$ mice had increased reticulocytes count, decreased RBC deformability, increased osmotic fragility, increased spleen size and decreased RBC lifespan (Foretz et al., 2010; Wang et al., 2010). This indicates a significant contribution of AMPK in maintaining RBC function and viability. AMPK is an energy-sensing enzyme, which is activated by low AMP: ATP ratios and inhibited by high AMP: ATP ratios (Wang et al., 2003). Under low ATP concentrations, AMP and ADP can bind to AMPK and change its conformation, thereby preventing the protein from activation by phosphorylation (Mihaylova and Shaw, 2011). Chemical agents that increase intracellular levels of cAMP are forskolin and isobutyl-methyl-xanthine (IBMX). Forskolin activates AC and thus leads to increased formation cAMP from ATP, while IBMX inhibits PDEs and maintains cAMP levels. Both forskolin and IBMX lead to AMPK inhibition, which reveals a molecular interaction between cAMP and AMPK activity (Hurley et al., 2006). This interaction could play a role in altered deformability in patients suffering from glycolytic enzymopathies. The low RBC ATP concentrations in these patients would lead to low levels of cAMP and increased intracellular levels of non-phosphorylated (inactive) AMPK.

Phosphorylation of AMPK may also be involved in G6PD-deficiency. G6PD deficiency is the most common RBC enzyme deficiency with over 400 million affected people (Cappellini and Fiorelli, 2008). Deficiency of this enzyme is associated with decreased ability of the RBC to withstand oxidative stress (Cappellini and Fiorelli, 2008; Mangat et al., 2014; Tang et al., 2015). Exposure of normal and G6PD-deficient RBCs to the oxidant diamide leads to a decrease in RBC deformability of the G6PD-deficient RBCs due to the inability of the RBC to maintain the intracellular glutathione-pool (Tang et al., 2015). Depletion of glutathione also leads to activation of AMPK by phosphorylation in G6PD-deficient RBCs. The activation of AMPK in G6PD-deficient RBCs after exposure to oxidative stress is most likely a consequence of ATP-consuming compensation mechanisms after excessive glutathione loss (Tang et al., 2015).

Protein kinase C alpha (PKCα) possibly also regulates RBC deformability. PKCα is involved in the phosphorylation of proteins in the RBC, such as adducin, protein 4.1R and protein 4.9 (George et al., 2010). Moreover, PKCα is involved in stimulation of glucose uptake by phosphorylation of the glucose transporter and participates in the activity of calcium channels (Kanno et al., 1995; George et al., 2010; Wagner-Britz et al., 2013). Consequently, phosphorylation and dephosphorylation of these proteins can be altered upon depletion of glucose. Glucose depletion was found to activate PKCα and this is accompanied by an increase in intracellular Ca^{2+} and, consequently, exposure of the membrane phospholipid PS (Klarl et al., 2006). The phosphorylation of adducin and protein 4.1R by PKCα could change RBC behavior and could influence RBC deformability (George et al., 2010) in a way similar to what is seen, for example, after phosphorylation of band 3 (Saldanha et al., 2007). Interestingly, homology analysis between murine, rat and human showed a conserved region in both liver- and RBC-specific PK for a PKCα binding site (Kanno et al., 1995). PKCα regulates RBC membrane stability and this conserved region for PK indicates a possible role for PK in this process (Kanno et al., 1995). In addition, PK converts phosphoenolpyruvate (PEP) to pyruvate (**Figure 3**) and previously it has been recognized that phosphorylation of PK by cAMP-dependent protein kinases leads to a reduced affinity of PEP for PK, which leads to a reduced production of ATP (Marie et al., 1980). The decreased cAMP and ATP production in metabolic disorders of the RBC, such as PK-deficiency, could subsequently result in disturbed RBC deformability (Leblond et al., 1978).

Role of purines and pyrimidines in RBC deformability

It has been suggested that pools of ATP are intracellular enclosed by the membrane proteins ankyrin, β-spectrin, band 3, and GAPDH, serving as substrates for both the Na^+, K^+-, and Ca^{2+} -pumps (Chu et al., 2012). This indicates an interplay between membrane proteins, energy stores and ion channel function of the RBC. Interestingly, the chemotherapeutic agent 5-FU was shown to induce changes in RBC rigidity, morphology and ion balance, most likely by altering ATP levels in the RBC (Spasojević et al., 2005). 5-FU is a pyrimidine antagonist (Longley et al., 2003) and since purine and pyrimidines play key roles in cellular metabolism and energy homeostasis. 5-FU could, therefore, influence RBC deformability. The activating and feedback mechanisms of purines and pyrimidines on glycolytic enzymes have previously been described by Seider and Kim (1979) and Tomoda et al. (1982). For example, in bovine RBCs incubated with glucose, adenosine stimulated ATP production compared to incubation with glucose alone. Most likely, adenine (i.e., the nucleobase of adenosine) stimulates HK activity (Seider and Kim, 1979). The effect of pyrimidines in RBCs has also been studied in two patients with a pyrimidine 5′-nucleotidase (P5N) deficiency, which lack this enzyme involved in clearance of pyrimidines from the RBC. P5N deficiency increases intracellular concentrations of pyrimidine nucleotides, which eventually leads to hemolytic anemia (Vives L Corrons, 2000). P5N-deficient patients were also found to have increased levels of reduced glutathione (Tomoda et al., 1982). At the same time, pyrimidine 5′-nucleotides (such as cytidine mono-, di-, and triphosphate (CMP, CDP, CTP) or uridine mono-, di-, and triphosphate (UMP, UDP, UTP)) decreased the activity of glucose-6-phosphate dehydrogenase (G6PD, **Figure 3**). As mentioned earlier G6PD activity is crucial in the anti-oxidative defense of RBCs. Indeed, RBCs from P5N-deficient patients were found to be more susceptible to oxidative stress, as reflected by increased formation of Heinz bodies (Tomoda et al., 1982), even despite increased reduced glutathione concentrations. Besides their role as a morphological marker of oxidative stress, Heinz bodies can lead to a decreased deformability by themselves (Hasegawa et al., 1993).

Hemoglobin

Primary Changes of Hemoglobin

Hemoglobin is the main component of the RBC and responsible for the delivery and removal of oxygen and carbon dioxide to and from the tissues, respectively. Intracellular hemoglobin concentrations and its state (polymerization, crystallization, degradation, and oxidation) also defines cytosolic viscosity making up 19.9–22.3 mmol/L in cells of healthy humans. Hemoglobin is composed of two α- and β-hemoglobin molecules together composing a heterotetramer. Disorders of hemoglobin can be subdivided into hemoglobinopathies (e.g., sickle cell anemia) and thalassemias (α- and β-thalassemia) (Galanello and Origa, 2010; Harteveld and Higgs, 2010; Higgs et al., 2012; Ware et al., 2017).

Sickle cell anemia is caused by a single point mutation in the *HBB* gene at position 6 substituting glutamic acid to valine (HbS). This substitution causes formation of HbS polymers of deoxygenated hemoglobin. This transition is usually rapidly reversed upon reoxygenation, but induces progressive damage of membrane driving dehydration to the extreme to the state when HbS polymers do not dissociate as its concentration exceeds it solubility threshold. Destabilization of the membrane and decrease in deformability leads to intravascular hemolysis and to vaso-occlusive events (Ware et al., 2017). Sickle RBCs are poorly deformable (Alapan et al., 2015, 2016) and this is, in part, due to changes in hydration status of the RBC.

In α- and β-thalassemia, α- and β-hemoglobin chains are affected, respectively, which leads to an imbalance in the synthesis of globin chains and to an inability to form sufficient quantities of hemoglobin heterotetramers. The imbalanced synthesis in thalassemia leads to the formation of hemoglobin precipitates, so-called Heinz bodies. RBCs in α-thalassemia show increased hydration (Bunyaratvej et al., 1994; Chui et al., 2003), whereas the hydration of RBCs in β-thalassemia is either decreased or increased (Bunyaratvej et al., 1994; Brugnara and Mohandas, 2013). Both Heinz bodies and the altered hydration state of the RBC are known to impair RBC deformability (Clark et al., 1983; Losco et al., 2001).

Oxygenation of Hemoglobin

The main function of RBCs is to transport oxygen to the tissues in the human body. The oxygenation state of hemoglobin is known to influence various processes of the RBC (Gibson et al., 2000; Stefanovic et al., 2013). Several ion transporters are oxygen sensitive, such as K^+-Cl^- cotransporter (KCC1) and the NKCC1 (Na-K-2Cl cotransporter) (Bogdanova et al., 2009). The function of band 3 seems, however, unaltered upon deoxygenation and oxygenation (Gibson et al., 2000). On the other hand, hemoglobin binds the cytosolic domain of band 3 and this binding is regulated by pH (Eisinger et al., 1982; Chétrite and Cassoly, 1985). Deoxygenation reduces the binding of ankyrin to band 3 and dissociation leads to more freely diffusible band 3 (Stefanovic et al., 2013). In addition, the binding between ankyrin and band 3 is also regulated by 2,3-disphosphoglycerate (2,3-DPG) (Moriyama et al., 1993). 2,3-DPG promotes the dissociation of oxygen from hemoglobin and promotes the release of oxygen from the RBC to the tissues (van Wijk and van Solinge, 2005). In the oxygenated state 2,3-DPG is not bound to hemoglobin and leads to less deformable and more fragile RBCs, while in the deoxygenated state 2,3-DPG is bound to hemoglobin and leads to an increase in RBC deformability and less fragile RBCs (Moriyama et al., 1993). The exact role of the reduced binding between ankyrin and band 3 after deoxygenation and binding of 2,3-DPG to hemoglobin is currently unknown, although it is hypothesized that a mild membrane weakening is beneficial in deoxygenated capillaries to facilitate smooth traveling of the RBC (Stefanovic et al., 2013).

RBC Hydration Changes Associated With Hemoglobin Defects

RBC dehydration in sickle cell anemia

The RBC dehydration in sickle cell anemia is caused by facilitated K^+ loss through hyperactivated KCNN4 (also known as the

Gardos Channel in RBCs) and K^+-Cl^- cotransporter that is not compensated by uptake of equal amounts of Na^+ (Clark et al., 1982; Izumo et al., 1987). Regardless of the ion transport pathway involved, RBC dehydration raises the HbS concentration, thereby affecting the equilibrium of HbS-polymerization and depolymerization in favor of the polymerized version (Eaton and Hofrichter, 1990; Brugnara, 1993). Na/K/ATPase was found to be more active in RBCs from sickle cell disease patients and can contribute to RBC dehydration (Izumo et al., 1987). Dehydration of RBCs in sickle cell disease contributes significantly to the decreased deformability since dehydration promotes the probability of polymerization of HbS by 20–40-fold (Eaton and Hofrichter, 1990) and result in prolonged polymerization of hemoglobin and thus prolonged sickling of RBCs (Brugnara, 1993). Sickled RBCs are far less deformable.

Two mechanisms involved in abnormally high K^+ loss are presented in **Figure 6**. The first mechanism of K^+ loss involves the ubiquitously expressed K-Cl co-transporter (KCC), of which the isoforms KCC1, KCC3, and KCC4 are expressed in human RBCs (Crable et al., 2005).

KCC1, is most often studied in RBCs and referred to as KCC. KCC in RBCs are known to be regulated by intracellular pH, Mg^{2+} concentrations as well as volume and oxygenation states of hemoglobin (Adragna et al., 2004; Khan et al., 2004). Under physiological conditions, KCC activation restores cell volume after swelling, but KCC activation may also respond to the changes in the RBC redox state (Adragna et al., 2004). In healthy RBCs, KCC is oxygen sensitive but only activated at high oxygen tension (pO_2). At low oxygen tension, KCC becomes sensitive to other stimuli (Gibson et al., 1998, 2001; Muzyamba et al., 2006). In sickle cell disease, in contrast, KCC is also activated at low oxygen tension, most likely due to increased phosphorylation of KCC in sickle RBCs (Muzyamba et al., 2006). In addition, KCC activity is intrinsically higher, even in older sickle RBCs (Bize et al., 2003).

The loss of deformability caused by the formation of HbS-polymers at low oxygen tensions (Odièvre et al., 2011) is enhanced by the KCC activation and leads to additional cell shrinkage. The clinical relevance of KCC activity is emphasized by observations in individuals with mild sickle cell disease. In these patients, an increased K-Cl cotransport activity is associated with increased likelihood of hospitalization, because of acute vaso-occlusive problems caused by less deformable dehydrated RBCs (Rees et al., 2015).

One more trigger of K^+ leak from RBCs is the increase in the intracellular Ca^{2+} levels and the activation of Ca^{2+}-sensitive K^+ channels (KCNN4 or known as the Gardos channel in RBCs) (Gallagher, 2017). These channels driving K^+ loss and dehydration are hyperactivated in RBCs of sickle cell disease patients secondary to the high intracellular Ca^{2+} levels (Bookchin and Lew, 1980; Bogdanova et al., 2013) (see **Figure 6**). KCNN4 is expressed in various cell types (Gallagher, 2013) and are inhibited by imidazole antimycotics, such as clotrimazole (McNaughton-Smith et al., 2008). In sickle cell disease, KCNN4 (or known as the Gardos channel in RBCs) is activated by two pathways. Firstly, KCNN4 can be activated by a signaling cascade initially triggered by several cytokines, such as PAF, interleukin-10 (IL-10) and endothelin 1 (ET-1) (Rivera, 2002) also involving activation of PKCα (Rivera et al., 1999; Wagner-Britz et al., 2013). In addition, PAF and ET-1 concentrations are increased in plasma from patients with sickle cell disease and are assumed to contribute to the adhesion of sickle RBCs to endothelium that is responsible for the vaso-occlusive events (Rivera, 2002). Also, these cytokines generate denser RBCs through RBC dehydration after an oxygenation/deoxygenation cycle (Rivera, 2002). Secondly, sickle cell disease patients have increased expression of the NMDA-receptor on their RBC membranes, causing pathological influx of Ca^{2+} after stimulation with receptor agonists (such as glycine and homocysteic acid) (Hänggi et al., 2014) which could contribute to dehydration mediated by KCNN4. Currently, a clinical trial using memantine as a NMDA-receptor antagonist is being tested in sickle cell disease patients (Bogdanova et al., 2017). In addition, the KCNN4 (or Gardos channel) blocker senicapoc (ICA-17043) has recently been tested in sickle cell disease. Senicapoc increased hemoglobin concentrations and hematocrit, and improved RBC hydration. Despite these encouraging findings, this study has been terminated prematurely because senicapoc did not meet its primary efficacy endpoint, defined as a decrease in painful crises (Ataga et al., 2011). From the clinical results obtained with senicapoc it can be hypothesized that the RBC dehydration and changes in RBC hydration after treatment with senicapoc are not causally related to the vaso-occlusive events which are often observed in sickle cell anemia.

Another pathway that increases intracellular Ca^{2+} levels in sickle cell disease is the mechanosensitive PIEZO1 channel (also described at section "Primary Changes of RBC Hydration"). PIEZO1 channels are widely expressed in vertebrates across various cell types and in RBC these channels are responsible for regulation of volume homeostasis upon mechanical signals (Zarychanski et al., 2012; Ge et al., 2015). Sickle RBCs show increased permeability for Ca^{2+} and Mg^{2+} upon deoxygenation. This increased permeability results in an increased deoxygenation-induced cation conductance in sickle cell disease, which can be entirely blocked by GsMTx4 (Ma et al., 2012; Cahalan et al., 2015). The gating modifier GsMTx4 blocks the mechanically sensitive part of PIEZO1 that supports a closed state of this ion channel (Bae et al., 2011), preventing Ca^{2+} influx (Jacques-Fricke et al., 2006).

RBC hydration changes in thalassemia

Three increasingly severe phenotypes can be distinguished in β-thalassemia, i.e., β-thalassemia minor, intermedia and major (Higgs et al., 2012). Intracellular concentrations of Na^+ in RBCs from patients with β-thalassemia minor and β-thalassemia major are comparable with those in RBCs from healthy adults, but K^+ levels are slightly increased (Cividalli et al., 1971). Upon *in vitro* incubation at 37°C, RBCs from patients with β-thalassemia major show increased leakage of K^+ and elevation of intracellular Na^+ levels when compared with healthy RBCs. In RBCs from β-thalassemia minor patients, leakage of K^+ and intracellular Na^+ levels are comparable to the healthy RBCs after *in vitro* incubation at 37°C (Cividalli et al., 1971).

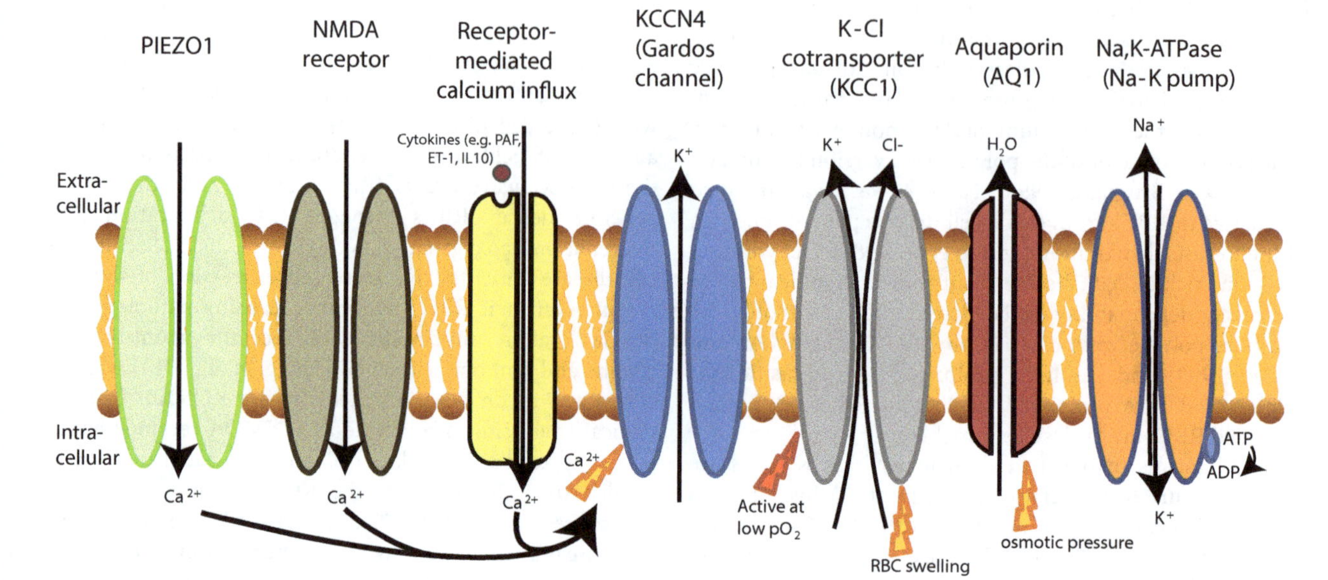

FIGURE 6 | RBC dehydration in sickle cell disease. The Na-K pump (Na, K-ATPase) is more active in sickle RBCs, leading to dehydration as extrusion of 3 Na^+ ions leads to the influx of 2 K^+ ions. Dehydration of sickle cell is initiated by PIEZO1 activation, likely because PIEZO1 is stretch-activation after deoxygenation (Ma et al., 2012). Dehydration in sickle cell disease is also initiated by the upregulation of the NMDA receptor. Both the NMDA receptor and PIEZO1 activation result in Ca^{2+} influx that leads to KCNN4 activation (KCCN4 in RBCs is better known as the Gardos channel). Gardos channel activation in sickle cell disease is also achieved by signaling cascades which respond to increased levels of cytokines. This leads to K^+ and water efflux by aquaporins (AQ1). In sickle cell disease, the K-Cl cotransporter is also activated at low oxygen tensions, causing efflux of K^+ and subsequently loss of water by aquaporins (AQ1), while under normal conditions KCC is only active at normal pO_2. Although water can be cotransported through KCC1 (Zeuthen and Macaulay, 2012), water efflux in RBCs mainly driven by aquaporins (AQ1).

Leakage of K^+ from RBCs in thalassemia is possibly linked to the precipitation of excess α- or β-globin chains inside the RBCs, which is a characteristic feature of this disease. The precipitated globin chains in RBCs can lead to oxidative stress and can affect transport of Na^+ and K^+ in thalassemia RBCs (Olivieri et al., 1994). In both β-thalassemia and α-thalassemia, RBCs show increased efflux of K^+ (Olivieri et al., 1994). Moreover, the amount of hemoglobin aggregates in RBCs is correlated with K^+ efflux (Nathan and Gunn, 1966). The presence of these aggregates reduces RBC deformability (Lubin and Desforges, 1972; Hasegawa et al., 1993) thereby revealing correlation between K^+ fluxes, Heinz body formation, and reduced RBC deformability. The precipitation of globin chains and leakage of K^+ from RBCs in thalassemia is also linked, or may even be augmented, by overload of Ca^{2+} (Shalev et al., 1984; Bookchin et al., 1988).

Another important factor in K^+ loss from RBCs in β-thalassemia involves the K^+-Cl^- cotransporter, which can be affected by oxidative stress (Olivieri et al., 1994). This K^+ loss by the K^+-Cl^- cotransporter is inhibited by increased intracellular concentrations of Mg^{2+} (De Franceschi et al., 1998; Adragna et al., 2004). In a trial with β-thalassemia intermedia patients, dietary Mg^{2+} supplementation did lead to increased intracellular concentrations of Mg^{2+} and to a reduction in the activities for the K^+-Cl^- cotransporter and Na-K pump (Na/K/ATPase). However, Mg^{2+} did not influence the activities of NKCC1 (also known as the Na-K-Cl cotransporter). Although dietary Mg^{2+} supplementation in β-thalassemia patients does not influence the hemoglobin concentration in blood, it does lead to a significant decrease in the absolute reticulocyte number. This is possibly due to improved RBC survival time (De Franceschi et al., 1998).

Little research has been performed on KCNN4 (or also known as the Gardos channel in RBCs) in thalassemia. An exception is the work on a mouse model with a homozygous deletion in the β-globin chain (de Franceschi et al., 1996). These mice were treated with clotrimazole, an antifungal imidazole derivate with KCNN4 blocking properties. During treatment with clotrimazole, hemoglobin concentrations in blood remained constant. In addition, it caused a decrease in MCHC whereas hematocrit and intracellular K^+ levels increased indicating that hydration state of the RBC was restored. Combination of clotrimazole with erythropoietin administration did increase hemoglobin levels in these mice to a higher extent than erythropoietin alone, possibly by promoting proliferation and differentiation during erythropoiesis (de Franceschi et al., 1996).

RBC Vesiculation

Intracellular levels of Ca^{2+} tightly regulate RBC vesiculation and elevated levels of intracellular Ca^{2+} are known to induce PS exposure and RBC vesiculation (Bevers et al., 1992; Nguyen et al., 2011; Fens et al., 2012; Alaarg et al., 2013) (**Figure 7**).

The RBC-vesiculation is a physiological process and leads to reduced RBC deformability. During its 120-day life span, RBC lose membrane surface and hemoglobin content through vesiculation (Werre et al., 2004; Ciana et al., 2017) a process in particular prominent in the youngest RBCs (Greenwalt and

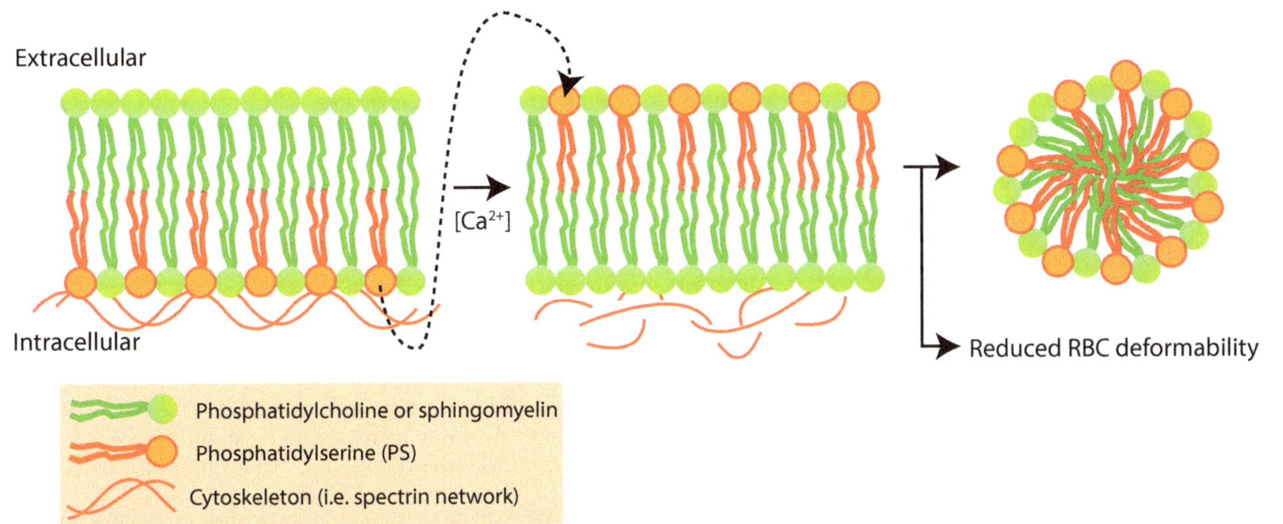

FIGURE 7 | Red blood cell vesiculation is driven by increased concentrations of intracellular Ca^{2+}. Phosphatidylserine (PS) is normally presented in the inner-leaflet of the RBC. Elevated intracellular Ca^{2+} levels activate scramblase and inhibit flippase, leading to phosphatidylserine (PS) externalization and redistribution of membrane and cytoskeletal proteins. PS externalization and protein redistribution leads to vesicle formation and loss of RBC deformability (Alaarg et al., 2013).

Dumaswala, 1988). As membrane is shed, this leads to a decreased surface-to-volume ratio in the RBC. During this RBC aging, hemoglobin-free vesicles are shed which leads to RBC dehydration and older RBCs with increased MCHC (Bosch et al., 1994; Bosman, 2013). Altogether, this leads to a reduction in membrane elasticity and RBC deformability (Linderkamp et al., 1993; Bosch et al., 1994). This implies that there is an important role for vesiculation in RBC deformability.

While RBC-vesiculation is considered a physiological process, RBC vesiculation is increased in various forms of hereditary hemolytic anemia, such as HS and sickle cell disease (Perrotta et al., 2008; Alaarg et al., 2013). In HS, differences in deformability between spectrin/ankyrin-deficient and band 3-deficient RBCs were observed after splenectomy. While splenectomy prevented premature removal of young RBCs from the circulation in both groups, the loss of deformability during RBC-aging was delayed after splenectomy in spectrin/ankyrin-deficient RBCs. This contrasts with band 3-deficient RBCs, where splenectomy did not lead to a delay in the deformability decrease during RBC-aging. This could be explained by the fact that spectrin/ankyrin-deficient RBCs are more prone to shed band 3-containing vesicles. Clustered band 3 is known to induce binding of autologous IgG, which facilitates removal of RBC by macrophages (Kay et al., 1983; Kay, 1984; Willekens et al., 2008). Shedding of band 3-containing vesicles from spectrin/ankyrin-deficient RBCs, therefore, would avoid IgG-opsonisation and clearance of the RBC (Reliene et al., 2002).

Red blood cell vesiculation is suggested as a mechanism to protect the cell from removal from the circulation. By vesiculation, the RBC can shed "eat-me" signals such as PS and specific band 3 cleavage products that react with senescent antigens (Willekens et al., 2008). By shedding these "eat-me" signals, the RBC may escape clearance until the reduction in RBC deformability causes trapping in the spleen. In addition, the lipid bilayer of the RBC is a complex system with various microdomains. These microdomains of the RBC, or so called 'lipid rafts' are specific membrane parts with high concentrations of cholesterol, sphingomyelin and gangliosides (Pike, 2003). These specific lipid rafts have a high abundance of the membrane proteins stomatin, flotillin-1, flottilin-2 (Salzer and Prohaska, 2001) and band 3 (Cai et al., 2012). RBC vesicles shed during storage are enriched in the lipid raft marker stomatin (Salzer et al., 2008) and indicates that specific lipid domains are shed during RBC vesiculation (Leonard et al., 2017).

The relationship between vesiculation and deformability is nicely illustrated by an experiment where chlorpromazine is added to RBCs to stabilize the RBC membrane. During overnight incubation with chlorpromazine at 37°C in a glucose-free buffer, vesiculation is inhibited and RBC deformability is maintained. Without chlorpromazine strong vesiculation of RBCs under these conditions occur as PS is exposed on the RBC surface. The activity of chlorpromazine may be explained by the amphiphilic properties of the molecule directly affecting the RBC membrane (Bütikofer et al., 1989).

High-throughput screening with chemical compound libraries also revealed that RBC-vesiculation can be driven by drugs and chemical compounds. For example, vesiculation of RBCs is driven by certain kinase pathways, including Jak-STAT and protein kinase B. Increased RBC vesiculation is also observed after addition of paclitaxel to blood, probably through its formulation excipient containing Cremophor. Not only RBC vesiculation is influenced by the vehicle Cremophor, but the compound also increases whole blood viscosity and transforms RBC to stomatocytes (Vader et al., 2013).

Adaptive Responses

Exercise leads to increased heart rate as a response to provide tissues with sufficient amount of oxygen. Exercise is accompanied with several stress factors that may affect RBC deformability, such as shear stress, hyperthermia, and glucose consumption (Carlson and Mawdsley, 1986; Szygula, 1990; Smith, 1995; Mairbäurl, 2013). These stress factors can lead to mechanical rupture, stimulated erythropoiesis and can decrease the average RBC age in athletes (Mairbäurl, 2013).

In a study with 24 trained cyclists, RBC deformability was decreased directly after exercise (Oostenbrug et al., 1997). The biology beyond the decrease in RBC deformability is unknown, although increased blood flow may be involved. The change in deformability after exercise can be the results of cytoskeletal changes, such as membrane loss. In addition, decreased levels of haptoglobin and increased levels of bilirubin were observed after marathon races (Jordan et al., 1998; Simpson et al., 2006). On the other hand, RBC deformability seems to be generally increased in well-trained athletes (Mairbäurl, 2013). A study comparing RBC membrane fluidity with the RBC membrane composition in controls and runners observed increased RBC membrane fluidity in endurance runners and sprinters. Although the intake of nutrients was comparable between the running groups and the control group, endurance running was accompanied with reduced concentrations of saturated fatty acids in RBC membranes (Kamada et al., 1993). These results indicate that the RBC can adapt upon exposure to exercise and that these adapted RBCs facilitate exercise and proper delivery of oxygen to the tissues. Interestingly, Smith et al. (1999) observed a higher maximal RBC deformability in elite cyclists when compared with sedentary healthy controls. Also, RBC populations with lower RBC densities were observed in the elite cyclists, which could indicate increased RBC turnover (Smith et al., 1999). A possible explanation for the increased RBC deformability in elite cyclist could be that extreme exercise leads to membrane loss and early RBC uptake, which is likely to be compensated with relatively young and good deformable RBCs. Whether increased RBC deformability would lead to better sports performances is unknown.

Autologous erythropoietin production is stimulated upon exposure to high altitudes. Acute exposure to high altitude, however, does not affect RBC deformability and RBC rheology (Reinhart et al., 1991). The effects of chronic exposure to high altitude seems largely unexplored. RBC deformability related processes were investigated in RBC concentrates obtained from Tibetans living at high altitude and from Tibetans at living at lowland. RBC viscosity was increased, and RBCs were more osmotic fragile in Tibetians living at low altitude when compared to RBC concentrates obtained from their lowland residents (Zhong et al., 2015). The increased viscosity can, however, be affected by increased hemoglobin levels and the decreased osmotic fragility can be affected by the decreased MCV values in Tibetans living at high altitude. The effects of exercise under hypoxia on RBC properties were investigated by Mao et al. (2011). Exercise under hypoxic conditions was found to decrease KCNN4 (or Gardos-channel) modulated deformability and KCNN4 modulated volume and down-regulated the senescence markers CD47 and CD147 (Mao et al., 2011). These results indicate RBC dysfunction after exercise under hypoxia. The dysfunction of RBCs under hypoxic conditions in combination with the erythropoietin-driven increase in RBC production leads to RBCs with relative low densities (Samaja et al., 1993), possibly caused by both increased RBC turnover and increased RBC production.

TABLE 2 | Summary of primary and secondary changes that lead to reduced RBC deformability in hereditary hemolytic anemia.

Anemia group	Disorder	Affected protein	Secondary changes	Deformability
Hemoglobinopathies	Sickle cell anemia	β globin	High intracellular free Ca^{2+} dehydration oxidation, hemolysis, NO scavenging, KCNN4 (Gardos channel) activation, different KCC activity	↓
	Thalassemia	Deficiency in α or β globin chain	High intracellular free Ca^{2+}	↓
Metabolic disorders	Pyruvate kinase deficiency (PKD)	PK	Changes in phosphorylate, low ATP, low cAMP, AMPK activation, intracellular free Ca^{2+} overload	↓, but dependent on technique
	Hexokinase (HK) deficiency	HK		↓, but dependent on technique
	Glucose-6-phosphate-dehydrogenase	G6PD	AMPK activation when in hemolytic crisis	Not affected, but ↓ when in crisis
Structural disorders	Hereditary Spherocytosis	Band 3, ankyrin, SPTA1, SPTB, RhAG, protein 4.1, protein 4.2	Increased MCHC, RBC vesiculation, low intracellular K^+	↓
	Hereditary elliptocytosis	SPTA1, SPTB or protein 4.1	Formation of elliptocytes	↓
Channelopathies	Hereditary xerocytosis	PIEZO1	Low K^+, RBC dehydration	Slightly decreased, mainly dehydrated Splenectomy contra-indicated
	Gardos channelopathy	Gardos channel	Low intracellular K^+, RBC dehydration, increased Ca^{2+}	Slightly decreased, mainly dehydrated

Reduced RBC deformability is noted in the table with ↓.

SUMMARY

Deformability is an important parameter that regulates RBC rheology, its longevity, and efficacy of O_2 transport. Altered deformability is a characteristic feature of multiple forms of hereditary hemolytic anemias and is likely related to the severity of the disease. Factors regulating deformability at the cellular level are dehydration, membrane protein phosphorylation, cytoskeletal integrity, metabolism and the integrity of hemoglobin. Interaction of these factors makes RBCs more or less deformable. Measuring RBC deformability in research and diagnostic laboratories can be challenging as there are many techniques available with all their specific advantages and disadvantages.

Measuring RBC deformability is important from both a diagnostic and research point of view. RBC deformability (i) could provide information about the patient's disease and clinical severity, and (ii) could be a target for pharmacological intervention or predict the toxicity of drugs for patients with hemolytic anemias.

Reduced RBC deformability leads to an inability of the RBC to pass the splenic circulation and leads to premature removal of RBCs from the blood. Altered RBC deformability can be attributed to primary and secondary changes of RBC deformability. Primary changes of RBC deformability are directly related to the disease, such as the membrane weakening in HS or the formation of poorly deformable sickle cells in sickle cell disease. Secondary changes of RBC deformability, such as altered ion fluxes, aberrant membrane protein phosphorylation or RBC vesiculation, are not directly related to the cause of disease. Thus, both primary and secondary causes of RBC deformability can contribute to premature uptake of RBCs in the spleen. In this review and in **Table 2**, we have summarized the current knowledge on primary and secondary mechanisms of RBC deformability in sickle cell anemia, thalassemia, HS, hereditary xerocytosis, and a number of metabolic disorders of the RBC. We have addressed and discussed the effects of ion regulation, ion channels and RBC (de)hydration on RBC deformability. In addition, we discuss the role and current knowledge of the adaptive responses on RBC deformability, intracellular energy-sensing molecules, membrane protein phosphorylation, hemoglobin deoxygenation and RBC vesiculation on RBC deformability. Knowledge about these processes in the RBC will lead to better understanding of the secondary processes involved in premature removal, and could lead to the discovery of new targets for pharmacological treatment. Furthermore, we postulate that a number of currently undiagnosed, patients with hereditary hemolytic anemia may have (genetic) defects in the here discussed secondary pathways or secondary processes that regulate RBC deformability. This review helps to understand the molecular mechanisms that maintain RBC deformability in healthy and diseased individuals, and enumerates the molecular mechanisms that are altered in RBC disorders leading to hereditary hemolytic anemia.

AUTHOR CONTRIBUTIONS

RvW, RS, and WvS encouraged RH to investigate the properties of RBC deformability. RH and RvW wrote the manuscript with support from RS, AB, LK, and WvS.

REFERENCES

Adderley, S. P., Sprague, R. S., Stephenson, A. H., and Hanson, M. S. (2010). Regulation of cAMP by phosphodiesterases in erythrocytes. *Pharmacol. Rep.* 62, 475–482. doi: 10.1016/s1734-1140(10)70303-0

Adderley, S. P., Thuet, K. M., Sridharan, M., Bowles, E. A., Stephenson, A. H., Ellsworth, M. L., et al. (2011). Identification of cytosolic phosphodiesterases in the erythrocyte: a possible role for PDE5. *Med. Sci. Monit.* 17, CR241–CR247. doi: 10.12659/msm.881763

Adragna, N. C., Di Fulvio, M., and Lauf, P. K. (2004). Regulation of K-Cl cotransport: from function to genes. *J. Membr. Biol.* 201, 109–137. doi: 10.1007/s00232-004-0695-6

Alaarg, A., Schiffelers, R. M., van Solinge, W. W., and van Wijk, R. (2013). Red blood cell vesiculation in hereditary hemolytic anemia. *Front. Physiol.* 4:365. doi: 10.3389/fphys.2013.00365

Alapan, Y., Little, J. A., and Gurkan, U. A. (2015). Heterogeneous red blood cell adhesion and deformability in sickle cell disease. *Sci. Rep.* 4:7173. doi: 10.1038/srep07173

Alapan, Y., Matsuyama, Y., Little, J. A., and Gurkan, U. A. (2016). Dynamic deformability of sickle red blood cells in microphysiological flow. *Technology* 4, 71–79. doi: 10.1142/S2339547816400045

Albuisson, J., Murthy, S. E., Bandell, M., Coste, B., Louis-Dit-Picard, H., Mathur, J., et al. (2013). Dehydrated hereditary stomatocytosis linked to gain-of-function mutations in mechanically activated PIEZO1 ion channels. *Nat. Commun.* 4:1884. doi: 10.1038/ncomms2899

Andolfo, I., Alper, S. L., De Franceschi, L., Auriemma, C., Russo, R., De Falco, L., et al. (2013). Multiple clinical forms of dehydrated hereditary stomatocytosis arise from mutations in *PIEZO1*. *Blood* 121, S1–S12. doi: 10.1182/blood-2013-02-482489

Andolfo, I., Russo, R., Manna, F., Shmukler, B. E., Gambale, A., Vitiello, G., et al. (2015). Novel Gardos channel mutations linked to dehydrated hereditary stomatocytosis (xerocytosis). *Am. J. Hematol.* 90, 921–926. doi: 10.1002/ajh.24117

Anong, W. A. (2006). Rate of rupture and reattachment of the band 3-ankyrin bridge on the human erythrocyte membrane. *J. Biol. Chem.* 281, 22360–22366. doi: 10.1074/jbc.M513839200

Ataga, K. I., Reid, M., Ballas, S. K., Yasin, Z., Bigelow, C., James, L. S., et al. (2011). Improvements in haemolysis and indicators of erythrocyte survival do not correlate with acute vaso-occlusive crises in patients with sickle cell disease: a phase III randomized, placebo-controlled, double-blind study of the Gardos channel blocker senicapo. *Br. J. Haematol.* 153, 92–104. doi: 10.1111/j.1365-2141.2010.08520.x

Ataga, K. I., Smith, W. R., De Castro, L. M., Swerdlow, P., Saunthararajah, Y., Castro, O., et al. (2008). Efficacy and safety of the Gardos channel blocker, senicapoc (ICA-17043), in patients with sickle cell anemia. *Blood* 111, 3991–3997. doi: 10.1182/blood-2007-08-110098

Bae, C., Sachs, F., and Gottlieb, P. A. (2011). The mechanosensitive ion channel Piezo1 is inhibited by the peptide GsMTx4. *Biochemistry* 50, 6295–6300. doi: 10.1021/bi200770q

Barodka, V., Mohanty, J. G., Mustafa, A. K., Santhanam, L., Nyhan, A., Bhunia, A. K., et al. (2014). Nitroprusside inhibits calcium-induced impairment of red blood cell deformability. *Transfusion* 54, 434–444. doi: 10.1111/trf.12291

Beneteau, C., Thierry, G., Blesson, S., Le Vaillant, C., Picard, V., Béné, M. C., et al. (2014). Recurrent mutation in the *PIEZO1* gene in two families of hereditary xerocytosis with fetal hydrops. *Clin. Genet.* 85, 293–295. doi: 10.1111/cge.12147

Bernhardt, I., Hall, A. C., and Ellory, J. C. (1988). Transport pathways for monovalent cations through erythrocyte membranes. *Stud. Biophys* 126, 5–21.

Bevers, E. M., Wiedmer, T., Comfurius, P., Shattil, S. J., Weiss, H. J., Zwaal, R. F., et al. (1992). Defective Ca^{2+}-induced microvesiculation and deficient expression of procoagulant activity in erythrocytes from a patient with a bleeding disorder: a study of the red blood cells of Scott syndrome. *Blood* 79, 380–388.

Bianchi, P., Fermo, E., Vercellati, C., Marcello, A. P., Porretti, L., Cortelezzi, A., et al. (2012). Diagnostic power of laboratory tests for hereditary spherocytosis: a comparison study in 150 patients grouped according to molecular and clinical characteristics. *Haematologica* 97, 516–523. doi: 10.3324/haematol.2011.052845

Biro, E., Sturk-Maquelin, K. N., Vogel, G. M. T., Meuleman, D. G., Smit, M. J., Hack, C. E., et al. (2003). Human cell-derived microparticles promote thrombus formation in vivo in a tissue factor-dependent manner. *J. Thromb. Haemost.* 1, 2561–2568. doi: 10.1046/j.1538-7836.2003.00456.x

Bize, I., Taher, S., and Brugnara, C. (2003). Regulation of K-Cl cotransport during reticulocyte maturation and erythrocyte aging in normal and sickle erythrocytes. *Am. J. Physiol. Cell Physiol.* 285, C31–C38. doi: 10.1152/ajpcell.00447.2002

Boas, F. E., Forman, L., and Beutler, E. (1998). Phosphatidylserine exposure and red cell viability in red cell aging and in hemolytic anemia. *Proc. Natl. Acad. Sci. U.S.A.* 95, 3077–3081. doi: 10.1073/pnas.95.6.3077

Bogdanova, A., Berenbrink, M., and Nikinmaa, M. (2009). Oxygen-dependent ion transport in erythrocytes. *Acta Physiol.* 195, 305–319. doi: 10.1111/j.1748-1716.2008.01934.x

Bogdanova, A., Makhro, A., Seiler, E., Max Gass, A., Hegemann, I., and Muller, R. (2017). "N-methyl D-glutamate receptor as a pharmacological target for treatment of sickle cell disease: effect of memantine on red cells of patients on a pilot clinical trail MemSID," in *Proceedings of the 21th Meeting of the Red Cell Society*, Heidelberg.

Bogdanova, A., Makhro, A., Wang, J., Lipp, P., and Kaestner, L. (2013). Calcium in red blood cells-a perilous balance. *Int. J. Mol. Sci.* 14, 9848–9872. doi: 10.3390/ijms14059848

Bogdanova, A., Petrushanko, I. Y., Hernansanz-Agustín, P., and Martínez-Ruiz, A. (2016). "Oxygen Sensing" by Na,K-ATPase: these miraculous thiols. *Front. Physiol.* 7:314. doi: 10.3389/fphys.2016.00314

Bookchin, R. M., and Lew, V. L. (1980). Progressive inhibition of the Ca pump and Ca:Ca exchange in sickle red cells. *Nature* 284, 561–563. doi: 10.1038/284561a0

Bookchin, R. M., Ortiz, O. E., Shalev, O., Tsurel, S., Rachmilewitz, E. A., Hockaday, A., et al. (1988). Calcium transport and ultrastructure of red cells in beta-thalassemia intermedia. *Blood* 72, 1602–1607.

Bordin, L., Clari, G., Moro, I., Dalla Vecchia, F., and Moret, V. (1995). Functional link between phosphorylation state of membrane proteins and morphological changes of human erythrocytes. *Biochem. Biophys. Res. Commun.* 213, 249–257. doi: 10.1006/bbrc.1995.2123

Bosch, F. H., Werre, J. M., Schipper, L., Roerdinkholder-Stoelwinder, B., Huls, T., Willekens, F. L., et al. (1994). Determinants of red blood cell deformability in relation to cell age. *Eur. J. Haematol.* 52, 35–41. doi: 10.1111/j.1600-0609.1994.tb01282.x

Bosman, G. J. (2013). Survival of red blood cells after transfusion: processes and consequences. *Front. Physiol.* 4:376. doi: 10.3389/fphys.2013.00376

Bouyer, G., Thomas, S., and Ege, S. (2012). *Patch-Clamp Analysis of Membrane Transport in Erythrocytes, Patch Clamp Technique.* Available at: https://www.intechopen.com/books/patch-clamp-technique/patch-clamp-analysis-of-membrane-transport-in-erythrocytes

Brugnara, C. (1993). Membrane transport of Na and K and cell dehydration in sickle erythrocytes. *Experientia* 49, 100–109. doi: 10.1007/bf01989413

Brugnara, C., and Mohandas, N. (2013). Red cell indices in classification and treatment of anemias: from M.M. Wintrobes's original 1934 classification to the third millennium. *Curr. Opin. Hematol.* 20, 222–230. doi: 10.1097/MOH.0b013e32835f5933

Bunn, H. F. (1997). Pathogenesis and treatment of sickle cell disease. *N. Engl. J. Med.* 337, 762–769. doi: 10.1056/NEJM199709113371107

Bunyaratvej, A., Fucharoen, S., Greenbaum, A., and Mohandas, N. (1994). Hydration of red cells in alpha and beta thalassemias differs. A useful approach to distinguish between these red cell phenotypes. *Am. J. Clin. Pathol.* 102, 217–222. doi: 10.1093/ajcp/102.2.217

Burger, P., Hilarius-Stokman, P., de Korte, D., van den Berg, T. K., and van Bruggen, R. (2012). CD47 functions as a molecular switch for erythrocyte phagocytosis. *Blood* 119, 5512–5521. doi: 10.1182/blood-2011-10-386805

Burton, N. M., and Bruce, L. J. (2011). Modelling the structure of the red cell membrane. *Biochem. Cell Biol.* 89, 200–215. doi: 10.1139/o10-154

Bütikofer, P., Lin, Z. W., Kuypers, F. A., Scott, M. D., Xu, C. M., Wagner, G. M., et al. (1989). Chlorpromazine inhibits vesiculation, alters phosphoinositide turnover and changes deformability of ATP-depleted RBCs. *Blood* 73, 1699–1704. doi: 10.1128/EC.00038-15

Cahalan, S. M., Lukacs, V., Ranade, S. S., Chien, S., Bandell, M., and Patapoutian, A. (2015). Piezo1 links mechanical forces to red blood cell volume. *eLife* 4:e07370. doi: 10.7554/eLife.07370

Cai, M., Zhao, W., Shang, X., Jiang, J., Ji, H., Tang, Z., et al. (2012). Direct evidence of lipid rafts by in situ atomic force microscopy. *Small* 8, 1243–1250. doi: 10.1002/smll.201102183

Cappellini, M. D., and Fiorelli, G. (2008). Glucose-6-phosphate dehydrogenase deficiency. *Lancet* 371, 64–74. doi: 10.1016/S0140-6736(08)60073-2

Carlson, D. L., and Mawdsley, R. H. (1986). Sports anemia: a review of the literature. *Am. J. Sports Med.* 14, 109–112. doi: 10.1177/036354658601400202

Chabanel, A., Reinhart, W., and Chien, S. (1987). Increased resistance to membrane deformation of shape-transformed human red blood cells. *Blood* 69, 739–743.

Chétrite, G., and Cassoly, R. (1985). Affinity of hemoglobin for the cytoplasmic fragment of human erythrocyte membrane band 3. Equilibrium measurements at physiological pH using matrix-bound proteins: the effects of ionic strength, deoxygenation and of 2,3-diphosphoglycerate. *J. Mol. Biol.* 185, 639–644. doi: 10.1016/0022-2836(85)90076-2

Chu, H., Puchulu-Campanella, E., Galan, J. A., Tao, W. A., Low, P. S., and Hoffman, J. F. (2012). Identification of cytoskeletal elements enclosing the ATP pools that fuel human red blood cell membrane cation pumps. *Proc. Natl. Acad. Sci. U.S.A.* 109, 12794–12799. doi: 10.1073/pnas.1209014109

Chui, D. H., Fucharoen, S., and Chan, V. (2003). Hemoglobin H disease: not necessarily a benign disorder. *Blood* 101, 791–800. doi: 10.1182/blood-2002-07-1975

Ciana, A., Achilli, C., Gaur, A., and Minetti, G. (2017). Membrane remodelling and vesicle formation during ageing of human red blood cells. *Cell. Physiol. Biochem.* 42, 1127–1138. doi: 10.1159/000478768

Cinar, E., Zhou, S., DeCourcey, J., Wang, Y., Waugh, R. E., and Wan, J. (2015). Piezo1 regulates mechanotransductive release of ATP from human RBCs. *Proc. Natl. Acad. Sci. U.S.A.* 112, 11783–11788. doi: 10.1073/pnas.1507309112

Cividalli, G., Locker, H., and Russell, A. (1971). Increased permeability of erythrocyte membrane in thalassemia. *Blood* 37, 716–724.

Clark, M. R., Mohandas, N., and Shohet, S. B. (1982). Hydration of sickle cells using the sodium ionophore Monensin. A model for therapy. *J. Clin. Invest.* 70, 1074–1080. doi: 10.1172/jci110695

Clark, M. R., Mohandas, N., and Shohet, S. B. (1983). Osmotic gradient ektacytometry: comprehensive characterization of red cell volume and surface maintenance. *Blood* 61, 899–910.

Cluitmans, J. C. A., Chokkalingam, V., Janssen, A. M., Brock, R., Huck, W. T. S., and Bosman, G. J. C. G. M. (2014). Alterations in red blood cell deformability during storage: a microfluidic approach. *Biomed Res. Int.* 2014:764268. doi: 10.1155/2014/764268

Condon, M. R., Feketova, E., Machiedo, G. W., Deitch, E. A., and Spolarics, Z. (2007). Augmented erythrocyte band-3 phosphorylation in septic mice. *Biochim. Biophys. Acta* 1772, 580–586. doi: 10.1016/j.bbadis.2007.02.004

Crable, S. C., Hammond, S. M., Papes, R., Rettig, R. K., Zhou, G.-P., Gallagher, P. G., et al. (2005). Multiple isoforms of the KC1 cotransporter are expressed in sickle and normal erythroid cells. *Exp. Hematol.* 33, 624–631. doi: 10.1016/j.exphem.2005.02.006

Da Costa, L., Galimand, J., Fenneteau, O., and Mohandas, N. (2013). Hereditary spherocytosis, elliptocytosis, and other red cell membrane disorders. *Blood Rev.* 27, 167–178. doi: 10.1016/j.blre.2013.04.003

Da Costa, L., Suner, L., Galimand, J., Bonnel, A., Pascreau, T., Couque, N., et al. (2016). Diagnostic tool for red blood cell membrane disorders: assessment of a new generation ektacytometer. *Blood Cells Mol. Dis.* 56, 9–22. doi: 10.1016/j.bcmd.2015.09.001

Danielczok, J. G., Terriac, E., Hertz, L., Petkova-Kirova, P., Lautenschläger, F., Laschke, M. W., et al. (2017). Red blood cell passage of small capillaries is associated with transient Ca^{2+}-mediated adaptations. *Front. Physiol.* 8:979. doi: 10.3389/fphys.2017.00979

de Back, D. Z., Kostova, E. B., van Kraaij, M., van den Berg, T. K., and van Bruggen, R. (2014). Of macrophages and red blood cells; a complex love story. *Front. Physiol.* 5:9. doi: 10.3389/fphys.2014.00009

De Franceschi, L., Cappellini, M. D., Graziadei, G., Manzato, F., Olivieri, O., Corrocher, R., et al. (1998). The effect of dietary magnesium supplementation on the cellular abnormalities of erythrocytes in patients with beta thalassemia intermedia. *Haematologica* 83, 118–125.

De Franceschi, L., Olivieri, O., Miraglia del Giudice, E., Perrotta, S., Sabato, V., Corrocher, R., et al. (1997). Membrane cation and anion transport activities in erythrocytes of hereditary spherocytosis: effects of different membrane protein defects. *Am. J. Hematol.* 55, 121–128. doi: 10.1002/(SICI)1096-8652(199707)55:3<121::AID-AJH1>3.0.CO;2-U

De Franceschi, L., Rivera, A., Fleming, M. D., Honczarenko, M., Peters, L. L., Gascard, P., et al. (2005). Evidence for a protective role of the Gardos channel against hemolysis in murine spherocytosis. *Blood* 106, 1454–1459. doi: 10.1182/blood-2005-01-0368

de Franceschi, L., Rouyer-Fessard, P., Alper, S. L., Jouault, H., Brugnara, C., and Beuzard, Y. (1996). Combination therapy of erythropoietin, hydroxyurea, and clotrimazole in a beta thalassemic mouse: a model for human therapy. *Blood* 87, 1188–1195.

Deplaine, G., Safeukui, I., Jeddi, F., Lacoste, F., Brousse, V., Perrot, S., et al. (2010). The sensing of poorly deformable red blood cells by the human spleen can be mimicked in vitro. *Blood* 117, e88–e95. doi: 10.1182/blood-2010-10-312801

Derbyshire, E. R., and Marletta, M. A. (2012). Structure and regulation of soluble guanylate cyclase. *Annu. Rev. Biochem.* 81, 533–559. doi: 10.1146/annurev-biochem-050410-100030

Dobbe, J. G., Streekstra, G. J., Hardeman, M. R., Ince, C., and Grimbergen, C. A. (2002). Measurement of the distribution of red blood cell deformability using an automated rheoscope. *Cytometry* 50, 313–325. doi: 10.1002/cyto.10171

Eaton, W. A., and Hofrichter, J. (1990). Sickle cell hemoglobin polymerization. *Adv. Protein Chem.* 40, 63–279. doi: 10.1016/S0065-3233(08)60287-9

Eisinger, J., Flores, J., and Salhany, J. M. (1982). Association of cytosol hemoglobin with the membrane in intact erythrocytes. *Proc. Natl. Acad. Sci. U.S.A.* 79, 408–412. doi: 10.1073/pnas.79.2.408

Faucherre, A., Kissa, K., Nargeot, J., Mangoni, M. E., and Jopling, C. (2014). Piezo1 plays a role in erythrocyte volume homeostasis. *Haematologica* 99, 70–75. doi: 10.3324/haematol.2013.086090

Fens, M. H., van Wijk, R., Andringa, G., van Rooijen, K. L., Dijstelbloem, H. M., Rasmussen, J. T., et al. (2012). A role for activated endothelial cells in red blood cell clearance: implications for vasopathology. *Haematologica* 97, 500–508. doi: 10.3324/haematol.2011.048694

Fermo, E., Bogdanova, A., Petkova-Kirova, P., Zaninoni, A., Marcello, A. P., Makhro, A., et al. (2017a). "Gardos Channelopathy": a variant of hereditary Stomatocytosis with complex molecular regulation. *Sci. Rep.* 7:1744. doi: 10.1038/s41598-017-01591-w

Fermo, E., Vercellati, C., Marcello, A. P., Zaninoni, A., van Wijk, R., Mirra, N., et al. (2017b). Hereditary xerocytosis due to mutations in *PIEZO1* gene associated with heterozygous pyruvate kinase deficiency and beta-thalassemia trait in two unrelated families. *Case Rep. Hematol.* 2017:2769570. doi: 10.1155/2017/2769570

Fischer, D. J., Torrence, N. J., Sprung, R. J., and Spence, D. M. (2003). Determination of erythrocyte deformability and its correlation to cellular ATP release using microbore tubing with diameters that approximate resistance vessels *in vivo*. *Analyst* 128, 1163–1168. doi: 10.1039/b308225n

Föller, M., Sopjani, M., Koka, S., Gu, S., Mahmud, H., Wang, K., et al. (2009). Regulation of erythrocyte survival by AMP-activated protein kinase. *FASEB J.* 23, 1072–1080. doi: 10.1096/fj.08-121772

Foretz, M., Guihard, S., Leclerc, J., Fauveau, V., Couty, J.-P., Andris, F., et al. (2010). Maintenance of red blood cell integrity by AMP-activated protein kinase alpha1 catalytic subunit. *FEBS Lett.* 584, 3667–3671. doi: 10.1016/j.febslet.2010.07.041

Gadsby, D. C. (2009). Ion channels versus ion pumps: the principal difference, in principle. *Nat. Rev. Mol. Cell Biol.* 10, 344–352. doi: 10.1038/nrm2668

Galanello, R., and Origa, R. (2010). Beta-thalassemia. *Orphanet J. Rare Dis.* 5, 11. doi: 10.1186/1750-1172-5-11

Gallagher, P. G. (2004a). Hereditary elliptocytosis: spectrin and protein 4.1R. *Semin. Hematol.* 41, 142–164. doi: 10.1053/j.seminhematol.2004.01.003

Gallagher, P. G. (2004b). Update on the clinical spectrum and genetics of red blood cell membrane disorders. *Curr. Hematol. Rep.* 3, 85–91.

Gallagher, P. G. (2013). Disorders of red cell volume regulation. *Curr. Opin. Hematol.* 20, 201–207. doi: 10.1097/MOH.0b013e32835f6870

Gallagher, P. G. (2017). Disorders of erythrocyte hydration. *Blood* 130, 2699–2708. doi: 10.1182/blood-2017-04-590810

Ge, J., Li, W., Zhao, Q., Li, N., Chen, M., Zhi, P., et al. (2015). Architecture of the mammalian mechanosensitive Piezo1 channel. *Nature* 527, 64–69. doi: 10.1038/nature15247

George, A., Pushkaran, S., Li, L., An, X., Zheng, Y., Mohandas, N., et al. (2010). Altered phosphorylation of cytoskeleton proteins in sickle red blood cells: the role of protein kinase C. Rac GTPases, and reactive oxygen species. *Blood Cells Mol. Dis.* 45, 41–45. doi: 10.1016/j.bcmd.2010.02.006

Gibson, J. S., Cossins, A. R., and Ellory, J. C. (2000). Oxygen-sensitive membrane transporters in vertebrate red cells. *J. Exp. Biol.* 203, 1395–1407.

Gibson, J. S., Khan, A., Speake, P. F., and Ellory, J. C. (2001). O_2 dependence of K^+ transport in sickle cells: the effect of different cell populations and the substituted benzaldehyde 12C79. *FASEB J.* 15, 823–832. doi: 10.1096/fj.00-0177com

Gibson, J. S., Speake, P. F., and Ellory, J. C. (1998). Differential oxygen sensitivity of the K+-Cl- cotransporter in normal and sickle human red blood cells. *J. Physiol.* 511(Pt 1), 225–234. doi: 10.1111/j.1469-7793.1998.225bi.x

Glogowska, E., Lezon-Geyda, K., Maksimova, Y., Schulz, V. P., and Gallagher, P. G. (2015). Mutations in the Gardos channel (KCNN4) are associated with hereditary xerocytosis. *Blood* 126, 1281–1284. doi: 10.1182/blood-2015-07-657957

Glogowska, E., Schneider, E. R., Maksimova, Y., Schulz, V. P., Lezon-Geyda, K., Wu, J., et al. (2017). Novel mechanisms of PIEZO1 dysfunction in hereditary xerocytosis. *Blood* 130, 1845–1856. doi: 10.1182/blood-2017-05-786004

Goldstein, L., and Brill, S. R. (1991). Volume-activated taurine efflux from skate erythrocytes: possible band 3 involvement. *Am. J. Physiol.* 260, R1014–R1020. doi: 10.1152/ajpregu.1991.260.5.R1014

Goldstein, L., and Davis, E. M. (1994). Taurine, betaine, and inositol share a volume-sensitive transporter in skate erythrocyte cell membrane. *Am. J. Physiol.* 267, R426–R431. doi: 10.1152/ajpregu.1994.267.2.R426

Grau, M., Pauly, S., Ali, J., Walpurgis, K., Thevis, M., Bloch, W., et al. (2013). RBC-NOS-dependent S-nitrosylation of cytoskeletal proteins improves RBC deformability. *PLoS One* 8:e56759. doi: 10.1371/journal.pone.0056759

Greenwalt, T. J., and Dumaswala, U. J. (1988). Effect of red cell age on vesiculation in vitro. *Br. J. Haematol.* 68, 465–467. doi: 10.1111/j.1365-2141.1988.tb04237.x

Guo, Q., Duffy, S. P., Matthews, K., Santoso, A. T., Scott, M. D., and Ma, H. (2014). Microfluidic analysis of red blood cell deformability. *J. Biomech.* 47, 1767–1776. doi: 10.1016/j.jbiomech.2014.03.038

Hagley, A. C., Younger-Coleman, N. O., Richards, A. A., Nwokocha, C. R., and Pepple, D. J. (2011). The effect of sildenafil on the elasticity of erythrocytes in homozygous sickle cell disease. *Indian J. Med. Sci.* 65, 243–249. doi: 10.4103/0019-5359.107024

Hahn, E. V., and Gillespie, E. B. (1927). Sickle cell anemia. *Arch. Intern. Med.* 39, 233–254. doi: 10.1001/archinte.1927.00130020072006

Hänggi, P., Makhro, A., Gassmann, M., Schmugge, M., Goede, J. S., Speer, O., et al. (2014). Red blood cells of sickle cell disease patients exhibit abnormally high abundance of N-methyl D-aspartate receptors mediating excessive calcium uptake. *Br. J. Haematol.* 167, 252–264. doi: 10.1111/bjh.13028

Hardeman, M. R., Goedhart, P., and Breederveld, D. (1987). Laser diffraction ellipsometry of erythrocytes under controlled shear stress using a rotational viscosimeter. *Clin. Chim. Acta* 165, 227–234. doi: 10.1016/0009-8981(87)90166-5

Harrison, T., Samuel, B. U., Akompong, T., Hamm, H., Mohandas, N., Lomasney, J. W., et al. (2003). Erythrocyte G protein-coupled receptor signaling in malarial infection. *Science* 301, 1734–1736. doi: 10.1126/science.1089324

Harteveld, C. L., and Higgs, D. R. (2010). Alpha-thalassaemia. *Orphanet J. Rare Dis.* 5:13. doi: 10.1186/1750-1172-5-13

Hasegawa, S., Rodgers, G. P., Shio, H., Schechter, A. N., and Uyesaka, N. (1993). Impaired deformability of Heinz body-forming red cells. *Biorheology* 30, 275–286. doi: 10.3233/BIR-1993-303-412

Hertz, L., Huisjes, R., Llaudet-Planas, E., Petkova-Kirova, P., Makhro, A., Danielczok, J. G., et al. (2017). Is increased intracellular calcium in red blood cells a common component in the molecular mechanism causing anemia? *Front. Physiol.* 8:673. doi: 10.3389/FPHYS.2017.00673

Higgs, D. R., Engel, J. D., and Stamatoyannopoulos, G. (2012). Thalassaemia. *Lancet* 379, 373–383. doi: 10.1016/S0140-6736(11)60283-3

Huisjes, R., Petkova-Kirova, P., Makhro, A., Llaudet-Planas, E., Hertz, L., Verhagen, L., et al. (2017a). "In-depth characterization of the red blood cell in hereditary spherocytosis," in *Proceedings of the 21th Meeting of the Red Cell Society*, Heidelberg.

Huisjes, R., van Solinge, W. W., Levin, M. D., van Wijk, R., and Riedl, J. A. (2017b). Digital microscopy as a screening tool for the diagnosis of hereditary hemolytic anemia. *Int. J. Lab. Hematol.* 40, 159–168. doi: 10.1111/ijlh.12758

Hurley, R. L., Barré, L. K., Wood, S. D., Anderson, K. A., Kemp, B. E., Means, A. R., et al. (2006). Regulation of AMP-activated protein kinase by multisite phosphorylation in response to agents that elevate cellular cAMP. *J. Biol. Chem.* 281, 36662–36672. doi: 10.1074/jbc.M606676200

Iolascon, A., Andolfo, I., Barcellini, W., Corcione, F., Garçon, L., De Franceschi, L., et al. (2017). Recommendations regarding splenectomy in hereditary hemolytic anemias. *Haematologica* 102, 1304–1313. doi: 10.3324/haematol.2016.161166

Izumo, H., Lear, S., Williams, M., Rosa, R., and Epstein, F. H. (1987). Sodium-potassium pump, ion fluxes, and cellular dehydration in sickle cell anemia. *J. Clin. Invest.* 79, 1621–1628. doi: 10.1172/JCI112998

Jacques-Fricke, B. T., Seow, Y., Gottlieb, P. A., Sachs, F., and Gomez, T. M. (2006). Ca^{2+} influx through mechanosensitive channels inhibits neurite outgrowth in opposition to other influx pathways and release from intracellular stores. *J. Neurosci.* 26, 5656–5664. doi: 10.1523/JNEUROSCI.0675-06.2006

Jaïs, X., Till, S. J., Cynober, T., Ioos, V., Garcia, G., Tchernia, G., et al. (2003). An extreme consequence of splenectomy in dehydrated hereditary stomatocytosis: gradual thrombo-embolic pulmonary hypertension and lung-heart transplantation. *Hemoglobin* 27, 139–147. doi: 10.1081/HEM-120023377

Jordan, J., Kiernan, W., Merker, H., Wenzel, M., and Beneke, R. (1998). Red cell membrane skeletal changes in marathon runners. *Int. J. Sports Med.* 19, 16–19. doi: 10.1055/s-2007-971873

Kaestner, L. (2011) Cation Channels in Erythrocytes - Historical and Future Perspective. *Open Biol. J.* 4, 27–34.

Kaestner, L. (2015). Channelizing the red blood cell: molecular biology competes with patch-clamp. *Front. Mol. Biosci.* 2:46. doi: 10.3389/fmolb.2015.00046

Kaestner, L., Steffen, P., Nguyen, D. B., Wang, J., Wagner-Britz, L., Jung, A., et al. (2012). Lysophosphatidic acid induced red blood cell aggregation in vitro. *Bioelectrochemistry* 87, 89–95. doi: 10.1016/j.bioelechem.2011.08.004

Kaestner, L., Wang, X., Hertz, L., and Bernhardt, I. (2018). Voltage-activated ion channels in non-excitable cells — a viewpoint regarding their physiological justification. *Front Physiol.* 9:450. doi: 10.3389/fphys.2018.00450

Kamada, T., Tokuda, S., Aozaki, S., and Otsuji, S. (1993). Higher levels of erythrocyte membrane fluidity in sprinters and long-distance runners. *J. Appl. Physiol.* 74, 354–358. doi: 10.1152/jappl.1993.74.1.354

Kanno, H., Morimoto, M., Fujii, H., Tsujimura, T., Asai, H., Noguchi, T., et al. (1995). Primary structure of murine red blood cell-type pyruvate kinase (PK) and molecular characterization of PK deficiency identified in the CBA strain. *Blood* 86, 3205–3210.

Karger, R., Lukow, C., and Kretschmer, V. (2012). Deformability of red blood cells and correlation with ATP content during storage as leukocyte-depleted whole blood. *Transfus. Med. Hemother.* 39, 277–282. doi: 10.1159/000339809

Kato, G. J., Steinberg, M. H., and Gladwin, M. T. (2017). Intravascular hemolysis and the pathophysiology of sickle cell disease. *J. Clin. Invest.* 127, 750–760. doi: 10.1172/JCI89741

Kay, M. M. (1984). Localization of senescent cell antigen on band 3. *Proc. Natl. Acad. Sci. U.S.A.* 81, 5753–5757. doi: 10.1073/pnas.81.18.5753

Kay, M. M., Goodman, S. R., Sorensen, K., Whitfield, C. F., Wong, P., Zaki, L., et al. (1983). Senescent cell antigen is immunologically related to band 3. *Proc. Natl. Acad. Sci. U.S.A.* 80, 1631–1635. doi: 10.1073/pnas.80.6.1631

Kenney, H. W., Smoot, R. T., Trader, J. D., Dowe, C. R., Allain, C. C., and Campbell, T. M. (1961). The sickle cell disease: current status and preliminary research observations. *J. Natl. Med. Assoc.* 53, 137–143.

Khan, A. I., Drew, C., Ball, S. E., Ball, V., Ellory, J. C., and Gibson, J. S. (2004). Oxygen dependence of K^+-Cl^- cotransport in human red cell ghosts and sickle cells. *Bioelectrochemistry* 62, 141–146. doi: 10.1016/j.bioelechem.2003.07.005

Klarl, B. A., Lang, P. A., Kempe, D. S., Niemoeller, O. M., Akel, A., Sobiesiak, M., et al. (2006). Protein kinase C mediates erythrocyte "programmed cell death" following glucose depletion. *Am. J. Physiol. Cell Physiol.* 290, C244–C253. doi: 10.1152/ajpcell.00283.2005

Knebel, S. M., Elrick, M. M., Bowles, E. A., Zdanovec, A. K., Stephenson, A. H., Ellsworth, M. L., et al. (2013). Synergistic effects of prostacyclin analogs and phosphodiesterase inhibitors on cyclic adenosine 3′,5′ monophosphate accumulation and adenosine 3′5′ triphosphate release from human erythrocytes. *Exp. Biol. Med.* 238, 1069–1074. doi: 10.1177/1535370213498981

Koralkova, P., van Solinge, W. W., and van Wijk, R. (2014). Rare hereditary red blood cell enzymopathies associated with hemolytic anemia - pathophysiology, clinical aspects, and laboratory diagnosis. *Int. J. Lab. Hematol.* 36, 388–397. doi: 10.1111/ijlh.12223

Körmöczi, G. F., Säemann, M. D., Buchta, C., Peck-Radosavljevic, M., Mayr, W. R., Schwartz, D. W. M., et al. (2006). Influence of clinical factors on the haemolysis marker haptoglobin. *Eur. J. Clin. Invest.* 36, 202–209. doi: 10.1111/j.1365-2362.2006.01617.x

Kostova, E. B., Beuger, B. M., Klei, T. R. L., Halonen, P., Lieftink, C., Beijersbergen, R., et al. (2015). Identification of signalling cascades involved in red blood cell shrinkage and vesiculation. *Biosci. Rep.* 35:e00187. doi: 10.1042/BSR20150019

Kuhn, V., Diederich, L., Keller, T. C. S., Kramer, C. M., Lückstädt, W., Panknin, C., et al. (2017). Red blood cell function and dysfunction: redox regulation, nitric oxide metabolism, anemia. . *Antioxid. Redox Signal.* 26, 718–742. doi: 10.1089/ars.2016.6954

Lasch, J., Küllertz, G., and Opalka, J. R. (2000). Separation of erythrocytes into age-related fractions by density or size? Counterflow centrifugation. *Clin. Chem. Lab. Med.* 38, 629–632. doi: 10.1515/CCLM.2000.092

Lazarova, E., Gulbis, B., Oirschot, B., and van Wijk, R. (2017). Next-generation osmotic gradient ektacytometry for the diagnosis of hereditary spherocytosis: interlaboratory method validation and experience. *Clin. Chem. Lab. Med.* 55, 394–402. doi: 10.1515/cclm-2016-0290

Leblond, P. F., Coulombe, L., and Lyonnais, J. (1978). Erythrocyte populations in pyruvate kinase deficiency anaemia following splenectomy. II. Cell deformability. *Br. J. Haematol.* 39, 63–70. doi: 10.1111/j.1365-2141.1978.tb07128.x

Leonard, C., Conrard, L., Guthmann, M., Pollet, H., Carquin, M., Vermylen, C., et al. (2017). Contribution of plasma membrane lipid domains to red blood cell (re)shaping. *Sci. Rep.* 7:4264. doi: 10.1038/s41598-017-04388-z

Lew, V. L., and Bookchin, R. M. (2005). Ion transport pathology in the mechanism of sickle cell dehydration. *Physiol. Rev.* 85, 179–200. doi: 10.1152/physrev.00052.2003

Lew, V. L., and Tiffert, T. (2017). On the mechanism of human red blood cell longevity: roles of calcium, the sodium pump, PIEZO1 and Gardos channels. *Front. Physiol.* 8:977. doi: 10.3389/FPHYS.2017.00977

Li, J., Hou, B., Tumova, S., Muraki, K., Bruns, A., Ludlow, M. J., et al. (2014). Piezo1 integration of vascular architecture with physiological force. *Nature* 515, 279–282. doi: 10.1038/nature13701

Linderkamp, O., Friederichs, E., Boehler, T., and Ludwig, A. (1993). Age dependency of red blood cell deformability and density: studies in transient erythroblastopenia of childhood. *Br. J. Haematol.* 83, 125–129. doi: 10.1111/j.1365-2141.1993.tb04642.x

Liu, L., Lei, T., Bankir, L., Zhao, D., Gai, X., Zhao, X., et al. (2011). Erythrocyte permeability to urea and water: comparative study in rodents, ruminants, carnivores, humans, and birds. *J. Comp. Physiol. B* 181, 65–72. doi: 10.1007/s00360-010-0515-5

Livaja Koshiar, R., Somajo, S., Norström, E., Dahlbäck, B., and McMahon, C. (2014). Erythrocyte-derived microparticles supporting activated protein C-mediated regulation of blood coagulation. *PLoS One* 9:e104200. doi: 10.1371/journal.pone.0104200

Llaudet-Planas, E., Vives-Corrons, J. L., Rizzuto, V., Gómez-Ramírez, P., Sevilla Navarro, J., Coll Sibina, M. T., et al. (2017). Osmotic gradient ektacytometry:

a valuable screening test for hereditary spherocytosis and other red blood cell membrane disorders. *Int. J. Lab. Hematol.* 40, 94–102. doi: 10.1111/ijlh.12746

Locovei, S., Bao, L., and Dahl, G. (2006). Pannexin 1 in erythrocytes: function without a gap. *Proc. Natl. Acad. Sci. U.S.A.* 103, 7655–7659. doi: 10.1073/pnas.0601037103

Longley, D. B., Harkin, D. P., and Johnston, P. G. (2003). 5-fluorouracil: mechanisms of action and clinical strategies. *Nat. Rev. Cancer* 3, 330–338. doi: 10.1038/nrc1074

Lopes de Almeida, J. P., Freitas-Santos, T., and Saldanha, C. (2012). Erythrocyte deformability dependence on band 3 protein in an in-vitro model of hyperfibrinogenemia. *Clin. Hemorheol. Microcirc.* 50, 213–219. doi: 10.3233/CH-2010-1433

Losco, P., Nash, G., Stone, P., and Ventre, J. (2001). Comparison of the effects of radiographic contrast media on dehydration and filterability of red blood cells from donors homozygous for hemoglobin A or hemoglobin S. *Am. J. Hematol.* 68, 149–158. doi: 10.1002/ajh.1171

Lubin, A., and Desforges, J. F. (1972). Effect of Heinz bodies on red cell deformability. *Blood* 39, 658–665.

Lutz, H. U., Stammler, P., Fasler, S., Ingold, M., and Fehr, J. (1992). Density separation of human red blood cells on self forming Percoll gradients: correlation with cell age. *Biochim. Biophys. Acta* 1116, 1–10. doi: 10.1016/0304-4165(92)90120-J

Ma, Y.-L., Rees, D. C., Gibson, J. S., and Ellory, J. C. (2012). The conductance of red blood cells from sickle cell patients: ion selectivity and inhibitors. *J. Physiol.* 590, 2095–2105. doi: 10.1113/jphysiol.2012.229609

MacDonald, I. C., Ragan, D. M., Schmidt, E. E., and Groom, A. C. (1987). Kinetics of red blood cell passage through interendothelial slits into venous sinuses in rat spleen, analyzed by in vivo microscopy. *Microvasc. Res.* 33, 118–134. doi: 10.1016/0026-2862(87)90011-2

Mairbäurl, H. (2013). Red blood cells in sports: effects of exercise and training on oxygen supply by red blood cells. *Front. Physiol.* 4:332. doi: 10.3389/fphys.2013.00332

Makhro, A., Huisjes, R., Verhagen, L. P., Mañú-Pereira, M., Llaudet-Planas, E., Petkova-Kirova, P., et al. (2016). Red cell properties after different modes of blood transportation. *Front. Physiol.* 7:288. doi: 10.3389/fphys.2016.00288

Mangat, C., Inoue, S., Saah, E., and Sharman, M. (2014). Acute haemolytic anaemia and myolysis due to G6PD deficiency. *BMJ Case Rep.* 2014:bcr2014203631. doi: 10.1136/bcr-2014-203631

Mao, T.-Y., Fu, L.-L., and Wang, J.-S. (2011). Hypoxic exercise training causes erythrocyte senescence and rheological dysfunction by depressed Gardos channel activity. *J. Appl. Physiol.* 111, 382–391. doi: 10.1152/japplphysiol.00096.2011

Marie, J., Buc, H., Simon, M. P., and Kahn, A. (1980). Phosphorylation of human erythrocyte pyruvate kinase by soluble cyclic-AMP-dependent protein kinases. Comparison with human liver L-type enzyme. *Eur. J. Biochem.* 108, 251–260. doi: 10.1111/j.1432-1033.1980.tb04718.x

Marques, F., Crespo, M. E., Silva, Z. I., and Bicho, M. (2000). Insulin and high glucose modulation of phosphatase and reductase enzymes in the human erythrocytes: a comparative analysis in normal and diabetic states. *Diabetes Res. Clin. Pract.* 47, 191–198. doi: 10.1016/S0168-8227(99)00128-X

Martinov, M. V., Plotnikov, A. G., Vitvitsky, V. M., and Ataullakhanov, F. I. (2000). Deficiencies of glycolytic enzymes as a possible cause of hemolytic anemia. *Biochim. Biophys. Acta* 1474, 75–87. doi: 10.1016/S0304-4165(99)00218-4

McNaughton-Smith, G. A., Burns, J. F., Stocker, J. W., Rigdon, G. C., Creech, C., Arrington, S., et al. (2008). Novel inhibitors of the Gardos channel for the treatment of sickle cell disease. *J. Med. Chem.* 51, 976–982. doi: 10.1021/jm070663s

Mebius, R. E., and Kraal, G. (2005). Structure and function of the spleen. *Nat. Rev. Immunol.* 5, 606–616. doi: 10.1038/nri1669

Mihaylova, M. M., and Shaw, R. J. (2011). The AMPK signalling pathway coordinates cell growth, autophagy and metabolism. *Nat. Cell Biol.* 13, 1016–1023. doi: 10.1038/ncb2329

Minetti, G., Egée, S., Mörsdorf, D., Steffen, P., Makhro, A., Achilli, C., et al. (2013). Red cell investigations: art and artefacts. *Blood Rev.* 27, 91–101. doi: 10.1016/j.blre.2013.02.002

Moriyama, R., Lombardo, C. R., Workman, R. F., and Low, P. S. (1993). Regulation of linkages between the erythrocyte membrane and its skeleton by 2,3-diphosphoglycerate. *J. Biol. Chem.* 268, 10990–10996.

Muravyov, A. V., and Tikhomirova, I. A. (2013). Role molecular signaling pathways in changes of red blood cell deformability. *Clin. Hemorheol. Microcirc.* 53, 45–59. doi: 10.3233/CH-2012-1575

Muzyamba, M. C., Campbell, E. H., and Gibson, J. S. (2006). Effect of intracellular magnesium and oxygen tension on K^+-Cl^- cotransport in normal and sickle human red cells. *Cell. Physiol. Biochem.* 17, 121–128. doi: 10.1159/000092073

Nans, A., Mohandas, N., and Stokes, D. L. (2011). Native ultrastructure of the red cell cytoskeleton by cryo-electron tomography. *Biophys. J.* 101, 2341–2350. doi: 10.1016/j.bpj.2011.09.050

Nantakomol, D., Palasuwan, A., Chaowanathikhom, M., Soogarun, S., and Imwong, M. (2012). Red cell and platelet-derived microparticles are increased in G6PD-deficient subjects. *Eur. J. Haematol.* 89, 423–429. doi: 10.1111/ejh.12010

Nathan, D. G., and Gunn, R. B. (1966). Thalassemia: the consequences of unbalanced hemoglobin synthesis. *Am. J. Med.* 41, 815–830. doi: 10.1016/0002-9343(66)90039-8

Nathan, D. G., Oski, F. A., Sidel, V. W., and Diamond, L. K. (1965). Extreme hemolysis and red-cell distortion in erythrocyte pyruvate kinase deficiency. *N. Engl. J. Med.* 272, 118–123. doi: 10.1056/NEJM196501212720302

Nguyen, D. B., Wagner-Britz, L., Maia, S., Steffen, P., Wagner, C., Kaestner, L., et al. (2011). Regulation of phosphatidylserine exposure in red blood cells. *Cell. Physiol. Biochem.* 28, 847–856. doi: 10.1159/000335798

Odièvre, M.-H., Verger, E., Silva-Pinto, A. C., and Elion, J. (2011). Pathophysiological insights in sickle cell disease. *Indian J. Med. Res.* 134, 532–537.

Olivieri, O., De Franceschi, L., Capellini, M. D., Girelli, D., Corrocher, R., and Brugnara, C. (1994). Oxidative damage and erythrocyte membrane transport abnormalities in thalassemias. *Blood* 84, 315–320.

Oonishi, T., Sakashita, K., and Uyesaka, N. (1997). Regulation of red blood cell filterability by Ca^{2+} influx and cAMP-mediated signaling pathways. *Am. J. Physiol.* 273, C1828–C1834. doi: 10.1152/ajpcell.1997.273.6.C1828

Oostenbrug, G. S., Mensink, R. P., Hardeman, M. R., De Vries, T., Brouns, F., and Hornstra, G. (1997). Exercise performance, red blood cell deformability, and lipid peroxidation: effects of fish oil and vitamin E. *J. Appl. Physiol.* 83, 746–752. doi: 10.1152/jappl.1997.83.3.746

Park, Y., Best, C. A., Auth, T., Gov, N. S., Safran, S. A., Popescu, G., et al. (2010). Metabolic remodeling of the human red blood cell membrane. *Proc. Natl. Acad. Sci. U.S.A.* 107, 1289–1294. doi: 10.1073/pnas.0910785107

Parpart, A. K., Lorenz, P. B., Parpart, E. R., Gregg, J. R., and Chase, A. M. (1947). The osmotic resistance (fragility) of human red cells. *J. Clin. Invest.* 26, 636–640. doi: 10.1172/JCI101847

Pattanapanyasat, K., Noulsri, E., Fucharoen, S., Lerdwana, S., Lamchiagdhase, P., Siritanaratkul, N., et al. (2004). Flow cytometric quantitation of red blood cell vesicles in thalassemia. *Cytometry B Clin. Cytom.* 57, 23–31. doi: 10.1002/cyto.b.10064

Pauling, L., and Itano, H. A. (1949). Sickle cell anemia a molecular disease. *Science* 110, 543–548. doi: 10.1126/science.110.2865.543

Perrotta, S., Gallagher, P. G., and Mohandas, N. (2008). Hereditary spherocytosis. *Lancet* 372, 1411–1426. doi: 10.1016/S0140-6736(08)61588-3

Peters, L. L., Jindel, H. K., Gwynn, B., Korsgren, C., John, K. M., Lux, S. E., et al. (1999). Mild spherocytosis and altered red cell ion transport in protein 4. 2-null mice. *J. Clin. Invest.* 103, 1527–1537. doi: 10.1172/JCI5766

Picas, L., Rico, F., Deforet, M., and Scheuring, S. (2013). Structural and mechanical heterogeneity of the erythrocyte membrane reveals hallmarks of membrane stability. *ACS Nano* 7, 1054–1063. doi: 10.1021/nn303824j

Picot, J., Ndour, P. A., Lefevre, S. D., El Nemer, W., Tawfik, H., Galimand, J., et al. (2015). A biomimetic microfluidic chip to study the circulation and mechanical retention of red blood cells in the spleen. *Am. J. Hematol.* 90, 339–345. doi: 10.1002/ajh.23941

Pike, L. J. (2003). Lipid rafts. *J. Lipid Res.* 44, 655–667. doi: 10.1194/jlr.R200021-JLR200

Ramdani, G., Naissant, B., Thompson, E., Breil, F., Lorthiois, A., Dupuy, F., et al. (2015). cAMP-signalling regulates gametocyte-infected erythrocyte deformability required for malaria parasite transmission. *PLoS Pathog.* 11:e1004815. doi: 10.1371/journal.ppat.1004815

Rapetti-Mauss, R., Lacoste, C., Picard, V. V., Guitton, C., Lombard, E., Loosveld, M., et al. (2015). A mutation in the Gardos channel is associated with hereditary xerocytosis. *Blood* 126, 1273–1280. doi: 10.1182/blood-2015-04-642496

Rees, D. C., Thein, S. L., Osei, A., Drasar, E., Tewari, S., Hannemann, A., et al. (2015). The clinical significance of K-Cl cotransport activity in red cells of patients with HbSC disease. *Haematologica* 100, 595–600. doi: 10.3324/haematol.2014.120402

Reid, H. L., Obi, G. O., and Oli, J. M. (1984). Reduced erythrocyte deformability and hyperfibrinogenemia in Nigerian diabetics with hemoglobin genotype HbAA. *Acta Diabetol. Lat.* 21, 105–114. doi: 10.1007/BF02591099

Reinhart, W. H., Kayser, B., Singh, A., Waber, U., Oelz, O., and Bärtsch, P. (1991). Blood rheology in acute mountain sickness and high-altitude pulmonary edema. *J. Appl. Physiol.* 71, 934–938. doi: 10.1152/jappl.1991.71.3.934

Reliene, R., Mariani, M., Zanella, A., Reinhart, W. H., Ribeiro, M. L., del Giudice, E. M., et al. (2002). Splenectomy prolongs in vivo survival of erythrocytes differently in spectrin/ankyrin- and band 3-deficient hereditary spherocytosis. *Blood* 100, 2208–2215.

Rivera, A. (2002). Modulation of Gardos channel activity by cytokines in sickle erythrocytes. *Blood* 99, 357–363. doi: 10.1182/blood.V99.1.357

Rivera, A., Rotter, M. A., and Brugnara, C. (1999). Endothelins activate Ca^{2+}-gated K^+ channels via endothelin B receptors in CD-1 mouse erythrocytes. *Am. J. Physiol.* 277, C746–C754. doi: 10.1152/ajpcell.1999.277.4.C746

Rother, R. P., Bell, L., Hillmen, P., and Gladwin, M. T. (2005). The clinical sequelae of intravascular hemolysis and extracellular plasma hemoglobin: a novel mechanism of human disease. *JAMA* 293, 1653–1662. doi: 10.1001/jama.293.13.1653

Sachs, J. R. (2003). "Na^+/K^+ Pump," in *Red Cell Membrane Transport in Health and Disease*, eds I. Bernhardt, and J. C. Ellory (Berlin: Springer), 111–137. doi: 10.1007/978-3-662-05181-8_5

Saldanha, C., Silva, A. S., Gonçalves, S., and Martins-Silva, J. (2007). Modulation of erythrocyte hemorheological properties by band 3 phosphorylation and dephosphorylation. *Clin. Hemorheol. Microcirc.* 36, 183–194.

Salomao, M., Zhang, X., Yang, Y., Lee, S., Hartwig, J. H., Chasis, J. A., et al. (2008). Protein 4.1R-dependent multiprotein complex: New insights into the structural organization of the red blood cell membrane. *Proc. Natl. Acad. Sci. U.S.A.* 105, 8026–8031. doi: 10.1073/pnas.0803225105

Salzer, U., and Prohaska, R. (2001). Stomatin, flotillin-1, and flotillin-2 are major integral proteins of erythrocyte lipid rafts. *Blood* 97, 1141–1143. doi: 10.1182/blood.v97.4.1141

Salzer, U., Zhu, R., Luten, M., Isobe, H., Pastushenko, V., Perkmann, T., et al. (2008). Vesicles generated during storage of red cells are rich in the lipid raft marker stomatin. *Transfusion* 48, 451–462. doi: 10.1111/j.1537-2995.2007.01549.x

Samaja, M., Brenna, L., Allibardi, S., and Cerretelli, P. (1993). Human red blood cell aging at 5,050-m altitude: a role during adaptation to hypoxia. *J. Appl. Physiol.* 75, 1696–1701. doi: 10.1152/jappl.1993.75.4.1696

Seider, M. J., and Kim, H. D. (1979). Cow red blood cells. I. Effect of purines, pyrimidines, and nucleosides in bovine red cell glycolysis. *Am. J. Physiol.* 236, C255–C261.

Shalev, O., Mogilner, S., Shinar, E., Rachmilewitz, E. A., and Schrier, S. L. (1984). Impaired erythrocyte calcium homeostasis in beta-thalassemia. *Blood* 64, 564–566.

Shimoda, M., Miyashima, K., and Yawata, Y. (1984). Increased calcium uptake in the red cells of unsplenectomized patients with hereditary spherocytosis: significant contribution of reticulocytosis. *Clin. Chim. Acta* 142, 183–192. doi: 10.1016/0009-8981(84)90378-4

Shin, S., Hou, J. X., Suh, J. S., and Singh, M. (2007). Validation and application of a microfluidic ektacytometer (RheoScan-D) in measuring erythrocyte deformability. *Clin. Hemorheol. Microcirc.* 37, 319–328.

Shmukler, B. E., Vandorpe, D. H., Rivera, A., Auerbach, M., Brugnara, C., and Alper, S. L. (2014). Dehydrated stomatocytic anemia due to the heterozygous mutation R2456H in the mechanosensitive cation channel PIEZO1: a case report. *Blood Cells Mol. Dis.* 52, 53–54. doi: 10.1016/j.bcmd.2013.07.015

Sikora, J., Orlov, S. N., Furuya, K., and Grygorczyk, R. (2014). Hemolysis is a primary ATP-release mechanism in human erythrocytes. *Blood* 124, 2150–2157. doi: 10.1182/blood-2014-05-572024

Simpson, R. J., Florida-James, G. D., Whyte, G. P., Middleton, N., Shave, R., George, K., et al. (2006). The effects of marathon running on expression of the complement regulatory proteins CD55 (DAF) and CD59 (MACIF) on red blood cells. *Eur. J. Appl. Physiol.* 99, 201–204. doi: 10.1007/s00421-006-0326-2

Smith, J. A. (1995). Exercise, training and red blood cell turnover. *Sports Med.* 19, 9–31. doi: 10.2165/00007256-199519010-00002

Smith, J. A., Martin, D. T., Telford, R. D., Ballas, S. K., and John, A. (1999). Greater erythrocyte deformability in world-class endurance athletes Greater erythrocyte deformability in world-class endurance athletes. *Am. J. Physiol.* 276, H2188–H2193.

Spasojević, I., Maksimović, V., Zakrzewska, J., and Bacić, G. (2005). Effects of 5-fluorouracil on erythrocytes in relation to its cardiotoxicity: membrane structure and functioning. *J. Chem. Inf. Model.* 45, 1680–1685. doi: 10.1021/ci0501746

Sprague, R. S., Stephenson, A. H., Bowles, E. A., Stumpf, M. S., and Lonigro, A. J. (2006). Reduced expression of Gi in erythrocytes of humans with type 2 diabetes is associated with impairment of both cAMP generation and ATP release. *Diabetes* 55, 3588–3593. doi: 10.2337/db06-0555

Sprague, R. S., Stephenson, A. H., and Ellsworth, M. L. (2007). Red not dead: signaling in and from erythrocytes. *Trends Endocrinol. Metab.* 18, 350–355. doi: 10.1016/j.tem.2007.08.008

Stefanovic, M., Puchulu-Campanella, E., Kodippili, G., and Low, P. S. (2013). Oxygen regulates the band 3-ankyrin bridge in the human erythrocyte membrane. *Biochem. J.* 449, 143–150. doi: 10.1042/BJ20120869

Steffen, P., Jung, A., Nguyen, D. B., Müller, T., Bernhardt, I., Kaestner, L., et al. (2011). Stimulation of human red blood cells leads to Ca^{2+}-mediated intercellular adhesion. *Cell Calcium* 50, 54–61. doi: 10.1016/j.ceca.2011.05.002

Stewart, G. W., Amess, J. A., Eber, S. W., Kingswood, C., Lane, P. A., Smith, B. D., et al. (1996). Thrombo-embolic disease after splenectomy for hereditary stomatocytosis. *Br. J. Haematol.* 93, 303–310. doi: 10.1046/j.1365-2141.1996.4881033.x

Sugie, J., Intaglietta, M., and Sung, L. A. (2018). Water transport and homeostasis as a major function of erythrocytes. *Am. J. Physiol. Circ. Physiol.* 314, H1098–H1107. doi: 10.1152/ajpheart.00263.2017

Szygula, Z. (1990). Erythrocytic system under the influence of physical exercise and training. *Sports Med.* 10, 181–197. doi: 10.2165/00007256-199010030-00004

Tang, H.-Y., Ho, H.-Y., Wu, P.-R., Chen, S.-H., Kuypers, F. A., Cheng, M.-L., et al. (2015). Inability to maintain GSH pool in G6PD-deficient red cells causes futile AMPK activation and irreversible metabolic disturbance. *Antioxid. Redox Signal.* 22, 744–759. doi: 10.1089/ars.2014.6142

Terra, H. T., Saad, M. J., Carvalho, C. R., Vicentin, D. L., Costa, F. F., and Saad, S. T. (1998). Increased tyrosine phosphorylation of band 3 in hemoglobinopathies. *Am. J. Hematol.* 58, 224–230. doi: 10.1002/(SICI)1096-8652(199807)58:3<224::AID-AJH11>3.0.CO;2-9

Thali, R. F., Tuerk, R. D., Scholz, R., Yoho-Auchli, Y., Brunisholz, R. A., and Neumann, D. (2010). Novel candidate substrates of AMP-activated protein kinase identified in red blood cell lysates. *Biochem. Biophys. Res. Commun.* 398, 296–301. doi: 10.1016/j.bbrc.2010.06.084

Thomas, S. L. Y., Bouyer, G., Cueff, A., Egée, S., Glogowska, E., and Ollivaux, C. (2011). Ion channels in human red blood cell membrane: actors or relics? *Blood Cells Mol. Dis.* 46, 261–265. doi: 10.1016/j.bcmd.2011.02.007

Tiffert, T., Bookchin, R. M., and Lew, V. L. (2003). "Calcium homeostasis in normal and abnormal human red cells," in *Red Cell Membrane Transport in Health and Disease*, eds I. Bernhardt, and J. C. Ellory (Berlin: Springer), 373–405. doi: 10.1007/978-3-662-05181-8_15

Tomaiuolo, G. (2014). Biomechanical properties of red blood cells in health and disease towards microfluidics. *Biomicrofluidics* 8:051501. doi: 10.1063/1.4895755

Tomoda, A., Noble, N. A., Lachant, N. A., and Tanaka, K. R. (1982). Hemolytic anemia in hereditary pyrimidine 5′-nucleotidase deficiency: nucleotide inhibition of G6PD and the pentose phosphate shunt. *Blood* 60, 1212–1218.

Tuvia, S., Levin, S., Bitler, A., and Korenstein, R. (1998). Mechanical fluctuations of the membrane-skeleton are dependent on F-actin ATPase in human erythrocytes. *J. Cell Biol.* 141, 1551–1561. doi: 10.1083/jcb.141.7.1551

Tuvia, S., Moses, A., Gulayev, N., Levin, S., and Korenstein, R. (1999). Beta-adrenergic agonists regulate cell membrane fluctuations of human erythrocytes. *J. Physiol.* 516(Pt 3), 781–792. doi: 10.1111/j.1469-7793.1999.0781u.x

Vader, P., Fens, M. H., Sachini, N., van Oirschot, B. A., Andringa, G., Egberts, A. C., et al. (2013). Taxol(®)-induced phosphatidylserine exposure and microvesicle formation in red blood cells is mediated by its vehicle Cremophor(®) EL. *Nanomedicine* 8, 1127–1135. doi: 10.2217/nnm.12.163

van Wijk, R., and van Solinge, W. W. (2005). The energy-less red blood cell is lost: erythrocyte enzyme abnormalities of glycolysis. *Blood* 106, 4034–4042. doi: 10.1182/blood-2005-04-1622

Vives Corrons, J. L., and Besson, I. (2001). Red cell membrane Na+ transport systems in hereditary spherocytosis: relevance to understanding the increased Na+ permeability. *Ann. Hematol.* 80, 535–539. doi: 10.1007/s002770100342

Vives L Corrons, J. L. (2000). Chronic non-spherocytic haemolytic anaemia due to congenital pyrimidine 5' nucleotidase deficiency: 25 years later. *Best Pract. Res. Clin. Haematol.* 13, 103–118. doi: 10.1053/beha.1999.0060

Wagner-Britz, L., Wang, J., Kaestner, L., and Bernhardt, I. (2013). Protein kinase Ca and P-Type Ca^{2+} Channel $Ca_V2.1$ in red blood cell calcium signalling. *Cell. Physiol. Biochem.* 31, 883–891. doi: 10.1159/000350106

Wang, J., Wagner-Britz, L., Bogdanova, A., Ruppenthal, S., Wiesen, K., Kaiser, E., et al. (2013). Morphologically homogeneous red blood cells present a heterogeneous response to hormonal stimulation. *PLoS One* 8:e67697. doi: 10.1371/journal.pone.0067697

Wang, S., Dale, G. L., Song, P., Viollet, B., and Zou, M.-H. (2010). AMPKalpha1 deletion shortens erythrocyte life span in mice: role of oxidative stress. *J. Biol. Chem.* 285, 19976–19985. doi: 10.1074/jbc.M110.102467

Wang, W., Yang, X., López de Silanes, I., Carling, D., and Gorospe, M. (2003). Increased AMP:ATP ratio and AMP-activated protein kinase activity during cellular senescence linked to reduced HuR function. *J. Biol. Chem.* 278, 27016–27023. doi: 10.1074/jbc.M300318200

Ware, R. E., de Montalembert, M., Tshilolo, L., and Abboud, M. R. (2017). Sickle cell disease. *Lancet* 390, 311–323. doi: 10.1016/S0140-6736(17)30193-9

Waugh, R. E., Narla, M., Jackson, C. W., Mueller, T. J., Suzuki, T., and Dale, G. L. (1992). Rheologic properties of senescent erythrocytes: loss of surface area and volume with red blood cell age. *Blood* 79, 1351–1358.

Weed, R. I., LaCelle, P. L., and Merrill, E. W. (1969). Metabolic dependence of red cell deformability. *J. Clin. Invest.* 48, 795–809. doi: 10.1172/JCI106038

Werre, J. M., Willekens, F. L., Bosch, F. H., de Haans, L. D., van der Vegt, S. G., van den Bos, A. G., et al. (2004). The red cell revisited–matters of life and death. *Cell. Mol. Biol.* 50, 139–145.

Wieth, J. O. (1979). Bicarbonate exchange through the human red cell membrane determined with [14C] bicarbonate. *J. Physiol.* 294, 521–539. doi: 10.1113/jphysiol.1979.sp012944

Willekens, F. L., Werre, J. M., Groenen-Döpp, Y. A., Roerdinkholder-Stoelwinder, B., de Pauw, B., and Bosman, G. J. (2008). Erythrocyte vesiculation: a self-protective mechanism? *Br. J. Haematol.* 141, 549–556. doi: 10.1111/j.1365-2141.2008.07055.x

Wolfersberger, M. G. (1994). Uniporters, symporters and antiporters. *J. Exp. Biol.* 196, 5–6.

Yang, B., Ma, T., and Verkman, A. S. (2001). Erythrocyte water permeability and renal function in double knock out mice lacking aquaporin-1 and aquaporin-3. *J. Biol. Chem.* 276, 624–628. doi: 10.1074/jbc.M008664200

Yeow, N., Tabor, R. F., and Garnier, G. (2017). Atomic force microscopy: from red blood cells to immunohaematology. *Adv. Colloid Interface Sci.* 249, 149–162. doi: 10.1016/j.cis.2017.05.011

Zanella, A., and Bianchi, P. (2000). Red cell pyruvate kinase deficiency: from genetics to clinical manifestations. *Best Pract. Res. Clin. Haematol.* 13, 57–81. doi: 10.1053/beha.1999.0057

Zanella, A., Bianchi, P., Fermo, E., and Valentini, G. (2006). Hereditary pyrimidine 5 '-nucleotidase deficiency: from genetics to clinical manifestations. *Br. J. Haematol.* 133, 113–123. doi: 10.1111/j.1365-2141.2006.05992.x

Zanella, A., Fermo, E., Bianchi, P., Chiarelli, L. R., and Valentini, G. (2007). Pyruvate kinase deficiency: the genotype-phenotype association. *Blood Rev.* 21, 217–231. doi: 10.1016/j.blre.2007.01.001

Zarychanski, R., Schulz, V. P., Houston, B. L., Maksimova, Y., Houston, D. S., Smith, B., et al. (2012). Mutations in the mechanotransduction protein PIEZO1 are associated with hereditary xerocytosis. *Blood* 120, 1908–1915. doi: 10.1182/blood-2012-04-422253

Zeuthen, T., and Macaulay, N. (2012). Transport of water against its concentration gradient: fact or fiction? *WIREs Membr. Transp. Signal.* 1, 373–381. doi: 10.1002/wmts.54

Zhong, R., Liu, H., Wang, H., Li, X., He, Z., Gangla, M., et al. (2015). Adaption to high altitude: an evaluation of the storage quality of suspended red blood cells prepared from the whole blood of Tibetan plateau migrants. *PLoS One* 10:e0144201. doi: 10.1371/journal.pone.0144201

Zipser, Y., Piade, A., Barbul, A., Korenstein, R., and Kosower, N. S. (2002). Ca^{2+} promotes erythrocyte band 3 tyrosine phosphorylation via dissociation of phosphotyrosine phosphatase from band 3. *Biochem. J.* 368, 137–144. doi: 10.1042/BJ20020359

18

Transcriptomic Analysis of Young and Old Erythrocytes of Fish

Miriam Götting and Mikko J. Nikinmaa*

Laboratory of Animal Physiology, Department of Biology, University of Turku, Turku, Finland

***Correspondence:**
Miriam Götting
miriam.gotting@utu.fi

Understanding gene expression changes over the lifespan of cells is of fundamental interest and gives important insights into processes related to maturation and aging. This study was undertaken to understand the global transcriptome changes associated with aging in fish erythrocytes. Fish erythrocytes retain their nuclei throughout their lifetime and they are transcriptionally and translationally active. However, they lose important functions during their lifespan in the circulation. We separated rainbow trout (*Oncorhynchus mykiss*) erythrocytes into young and old fractions using fixed angle-centrifugation and analyzed transcriptome changes using RNA sequencing (RNA-seq) technology and quantitative real-time PCR. We found 930 differentially expressed between young and old erythrocyte fractions; 889 of these showed higher transcript levels in young, while only 34 protein-coding genes had higher transcript levels in old erythrocytes. In particular genes involved in ion binding, signal transduction, membrane transport, and those encoding various enzyme classes are affected in old erythrocytes. The transcripts with higher levels in old erythrocytes were associated with seven different GO terms within biological processes and nine within molecular functions and cellular components, respectively. Our study furthermore found several highly abundant transcripts as well as a number of differentially expressed genes (DEGs) for which the protein products are currently not known revealing the gaps of knowledge in most non-mammalian vertebrates. Our data provide the first insight into changes involved in aging on the transcriptional level and thus opens new perspectives for the study of maturation processes in fish erythrocytes.

Keywords: red blood cells, aging, transcriptome, fish, lifespan, RNA-seq

INTRODUCTION

As in all vertebrates apart from mammals, the erythrocytes in fish are nucleated (Nikinmaa, 1990). Throughout their lifespan, which is between 80 and 500 days (Avery et al., 1992), they appear to be capable of aerobic metabolism, although the respiratory rate decreases with age (Phillips et al., 2000). They are also capable of transcription and translation throughout their lifespan, although, again, the capability decreases with age. The RNA content was significantly lowered by 90% in old erythrocyte fractions while DNA and protein content were unaffected by age (Lund et al., 2000). Young erythrocytes respond much more readily to external stimulation by, e.g., adrenergic drugs than old erythrocytes (Lecklin et al., 2000), and their proportion, which can make up to 50% of the circulating erythrocyte population, increases as a result of temperature stress (Lewis et al., 2012) and changes seasonally (Härdig and Hoglund, 1984). In fish that have recently suffered anemia, the proportion of young RBCs is larger compared to unstressed fish (Lane, 1979).

Associated with the decreased capability to respond to external stimulation, several properties of the erythrocytes are different in young and old erythrocytes. For example, the shape changes from circular to elliptical during maturation (Tavares-Dias, 2006), the membrane of young erythrocytes is more fluid (Lecklin et al., 2000), and old erythrocytes have fewer organelles such as mitochondria (Moyes et al., 2002) and free ribosomes (Phillips et al., 2000).

However, despite these differences in the function and properties of young and old erythrocytes, and although there is a clear difference between the transcriptome of control (11°C) and heat-shocked (1 h at 25°C) erythrocytes (Lewis et al., 2010), quantitative changes in transcription between young and old fish erythrocytes have not been studied earlier. Here we have collected blood from rainbow trout in spring (May) when the proportion of young erythrocytes in the circulation increases with rising ambient water temperature (Härdig and Hoglund, 1984; Alvarez et al., 1994; Houston et al., 1996; Lecklin et al., 2000). We have divided the erythrocytes in young and old cohorts on the basis of the old erythrocytes having higher density than young ones (Lane et al., 1982; Tiano et al., 2000). Since old erythrocytes have higher mean cellular hemoglobin concentration (MCHC) than young ones (Lane et al., 1982), the success of age separation was checked by evaluating MCHC. Thereafter RNA sequencing was carried out and differences in transcriptomes in the young and old cohort evaluated.

MATERIALS AND METHODS

Animals and Blood Sampling Procedure

Rainbow trout (*Oncorhynchus mykiss*, $N = 5$, weight 548.0 ± 70.1 g) were obtained from a commercial hatchery (Finnish Institute for Fisheries and Environment, Parainen, Finland) in May 2016. All procedures were approved by the Finnish Animal Experiment Board (ESAVI/3705/04.10.07/2015). Since the water in the fish tanks of the hatchery is pumped from a nearby bay of the Finnish Archipelago, the water temperature in the tanks follows natural rhythms and is on the rise at this time of the year (K. Malmberg, personal communication). At the date of sampling the water temperature was 14°C.

Fish were netted from the tanks, quickly killed by a blow on the head and blood was sampled by caudal puncture into heparinized syringes, transferred into sterile falcon tubes, and stored on ice. Blood samples were washed three times by repeated re-suspension in rainbow trout saline (128 mM NaCl, 3 mM KCl, 1.5 mM $CaCl_2$, 1.5 mM $MgCl_2$, 20 mM Tris-HCl, pH 7.6 (Nikinmaa and Jensen, 1992) and centrifugation at 800 × g and 10°C for 3 min to remove buffy coat and white blood cells and stored on ice. The erythrocytes were re-suspended in fresh saline at a hematocrit (Hct) of 18–20% and then stored well-aerated over night at 14°C in cell culture flasks (75 cm^2) with open caps to allow equilibration. Fish were weighed and their length was measured.

Erythrocyte Age Class Separation by Density Centrifugation

Density centrifugation of erythrocyte samples followed essentially the procedure described previously (Murphy, 1973; Speckner et al., 1989; Koldkjaer et al., 2004) with minor modifications. A subsample (referred to as "original blood sample") was taken and immediately frozen at −80°C. The rest of the erythrocyte sample was once more washed in saline and then adjusted to a hematocrit of ~80% and transferred into polypropylene tubes (length 47 mm, diameter 4 mm, volume 0.5 ml). Tubes were centrifuged in a fixed-angle rotor (45°) at 16,000 × g and 10°C for 30 min. The tubes were cut into three equally sized parts: the top part, containing the youngest and least dense erythrocyte class fraction, the middle part which was discarded, and the lower part, containing the oldest and most dense erythrocytes. Erythrocyte fractions (50 µl) were transferred into new tubes, diluted with 100 µl rainbow trout saline and frozen at −80°C.

The success of age separation was evaluated by determining the mean cellular hemoglobin concentration (MCHC) of both fractions using conventional methods (centrifugation for haematocrit and cyanmethaemoglobin method for hemoglobin concentration; Speckner et al., 1989; Lund et al., 2000). The MCHC of the putatively old erythrocytes was significantly higher than that of the putatively young erythrocytes ($p = 0.015$) indicating that the age separation was successful.

RNA-Seq of Young and Old Erythrocyte Fractions

Erythrocyte samples of different age were then homogenized in TissueLyser (Qiagen, Austin, USA) with two stainless steel beads for 2 × 60 s at 30 Hz and RNA was isolated using NucleoZol (Macherey-Nagel) according to the manufacturer's instructions. RNA was quantified using a NanoDrop 2000 (Thermo Scientific, Bonn, Germany) and quality was checked with a Fragment Analyzer™. Only samples with $OD_{260/280}$ and $OD_{260/230} > 1.8$ and RIN values higher than 8.7 (range 8.7–9.8) were used in the analyses.

Sequencing libraries were prepared using the Illumina TruSeq Stranded mRNA Sample Preparation Kit and sequenced in two lanes on a HiSeq 3000 instrument at the Finnish Functional Genomics Centre (Turku, Finland) and single-end sequencing chemistry with 50 bp read length.

Bioinformatic Analysis

Base calling on the reads was done using the Bcl2fastq2 software (version 1.8.4). The quality control of raw sequencing reads was performed with FastQC (www.bioinformatics.babraham.ac.uk/projects/fastqc/), and adapters and low quality bases were trimmed by Trimmomatic (Bolger et al., 2014). The read alignment was performed against the reference genome using TopHat v2.1.0 (Kim et al., 2013). We used the Atlantic Salmon genome [ICSASG v2 genome; provided by the International Cooperation to Sequence the Atlantic SalmonGenome (ICSASG; Lien et al., 2016)] as a reference genome because of the status of the higher coverage of the assembly compared to that of the rainbow trout. The number of uniquely aligned reads was between 2.6 and 6.8 M per sample.

The sample correlation values (Spearman's metrics) were between 0.895 and 0.932 (mean 0.910 for young age class, 0.927 for old age class) for all samples.

The gene-wise read counts were normalized using the TMM normalization method of the edgeR R/Bioconductor package before further statistical testing using the Limma R/Bioconductor package. Differentially expressed genes (DEGs) were selected based on a fold change >2 and an FDR (false-discovery-rate) <0.01. Sample pairing (young and old erythrocyte age classes of one individual) was taken into account when building the linear model for statistical testing.

The association between reads and known genes and the number of reads associated with each gene was assessed using the subreads package v1.5.1 (Liao et al., 2014). Differential expression between age classes was analyzed using MA-plots as implemented in DEGseq R package (Wang et al., 2010).

The BLAST2GO software (Götz et al., 2008) was used to predict Gene Ontology (GO) terms for all statistically significant DE genes (FDR < 0.01) and the most abundant genes. Gos are organized hierarchically in terms of biological processes, cellular components and molecular functions. All pseudogenes (labeled with NA) and all tRNAs were removed from the list of DEGs, and the remaining list was subsequently searched against the non-redundant NCBI protein database (NR database) using the BLASTx algorithm (Altschul et al., 1990) with an *E*-value threshold of 10^{-5}, and a maximum of 20 "hit" sequences per query was retained. GO annotations were simplified to a smaller set of high-level GO terms using GO slims as implemented in BLAST2GO.

Differential Expression of Selected Genes Using Quantitative Real-Time PCR (qPCR)

qPCR was used to analyze the expression of selected genes on preparations of young and old erythrocytes relative to the original erythrocyte sample (taken before the fractionation procedure) of five individuals. We selected eight genes which on the basis of earlier research have important functions in fish erythrocytes and designed specific primers (**Table S1**) using the Primer3 software (Koressaar and Remm, 2007; Untergasser et al., 2012) and checked for secondary structures using Beacon Designer Software™ and UNAFold tool (https://eu.idtdna.com/UNAFold). qPCR primers were blasted against the rainbow trout database (NCBI) to ensure specificity.

RNA for qPCR was digested using DNase I (Promega) and 500 ng were reverse transcribed using the RevertAid First Strand Synthesis Kit (Thermo Scientific, Bonn, Germany) using random hexamer primers according to the manufacturer's instructions. cDNA products were amplified in triplicates using the KAPA SYBR® Fast qPCR kit (KapaBiosystems) on a QuantStudio 12K Flex Real-Time PCR System (Thermo Fisher Scientific). Each 10 μL reaction mixture contained 2 μl cDNA template (1:10 or 1:20 dilution) and 0.5 μM of each primer. A two-step cycling protocol was applied: 10 min at 95°C followed by 40 cycles of 15 s at 95°C and 30 s at 60°C and 30 s at 72°C. In a final step, specificity of primers and amplification was evaluated using dissociation curves with a temperature range from 60 to 95°C. All primer pairs generated a single peak in the dissociation curve and PCR efficiency estimated for each primer pair was within the range of 92–105%. Each qPCR plate contained non-template controls to detect potential contamination in reaction mixes. Data were analyzed with the QuantStudio software. Reaction efficiency for each gene was calculated using a standard curve generated from a 1:2 serial dilution of the pooled samples. Standard curve reactions were performed in duplicate. Calculations of relative expression levels with the $2^{-\Delta\Delta CT}$ method (Livak and Schmittgen, 2001) were done in Microsoft Office Excel and the expression of target genes was normalized against *β-actin* (*act*) expression levels. Stability of *β-actin* expression between young, old and original blood sample was assessed using a one-way repeated measures ANOVA ($p = 0.106$) in Real Statistics Resource Pack software (Release 4.3; www.realstatistics.com; Copyright 2013–2015; Zaiontz, 2015). Data are shown relative to the respective mixed blood samples and log2 transformed. All data are expressed as means ± *SD*. Significant differences were assessed first between raw Ct-values of the young, old and originalsamples, and second between the raw Ct-values of the young and old erythrocyte samples using a one-way repeated measures ANOVA after equal variances (Brown–Forsythe) and normality (Shapiro–Wilk test) of data were tested using the Real Statistics Resource Pack software (Release 4.3; www.realstatistics.com; Copyright 2013–2015) in Excel 2010 (Zaiontz, 2015). In cases where tests for equal variances and normality failed we used a non-parametric test (Friedman's test). *Post-hoc* analyses were done with the Holm-Sidak test. Significance was accepted at the $P < 0.05$ level.

RESULTS

Sequencing Statistics

In this study, an average number of 12,197,337 reads (mean young erythrocytes: 11,692,319; mean old erythrocytes 12,702,356) were generated. From the 8,273,888 mapped reads (mean young erythrocytes: 8,192,383; mean old erythrocytes 8,355,393), 54% (young erythrocytes: 49%; mean old erythrocytes 59%) could be uniquely mapped to the reference genome. Only uniquely mapped reads (average 4,469,945; mean young erythrocytes 3,956,287; mean old erythrocytes 4,983,602) were used for the downstream analysis, resulting in 51,226 unigenes.

Most Abundant Genes in Erythrocytes

The 15 most abundant genes (those among the top 10 abundant genes in any sample) account for 9.81–29.35% of all reads (mean young erythrocytes = 23.01 ± 5.76%; mean old erythrocytes = 12.39 ± 1.58%; **Table 1**). Naturally, various hemoglobin subunit transcripts are among them; *hbα* transcripts accounted for 3.46% and *hbß* for 4.56% of all reads. The products of two abundant transcripts in the list are currently not known.

For 13 gene IDs GO terms were found by blast search against the NR database. Seven transcripts were associated

TABLE 1 | Read percentages for the 15 most abundant genes in the erythrocyte samples.

Genbank ID	Gene product	Mean	*SD*	Min	Max
XR_001327939.1	Uncharacterized LOC106601081, transcript variant X4	3.31	1.72	1.66	5.94
XM_014204292.1	Hemoglobin subunit alpha-like	2.39	1.22	1.00	4.44
XM_014186643.1	Hemoglobin subunit beta-like	1.83	0.82	0.55	3.33
NM_001140225.1	EBV-induced G-protein coupled receptor 2	1.67	0.78	0.51	3.29
NA	NA (pseudogene)	1.95	1.06	0.95	3.67
XM_014146046.1	N-terminal EF-hand calcium-binding protein 1-like	1.18	0.17	0.96	1.50
XM_014204291.1	Hemoglobin subunit beta-like	1.54	0.59	0.85	2.75
XM_014192983.1	Hemoglobin subunit alpha-like	1.07	0.39	0.54	1.62
XM_014203987.1	Hemoglobin subunit beta-1-like	0.86	0.48	0.29	1.66
XM_014201444.1	TBC1 domain family member 15-like	0.31	0.10	0.16	0.45
XM_014204289.1	Hemoglobin subunit beta-1-like	0.51	0.28	0.19	0.99
XM_014168090.1	Stathmin-3-like	0.19	0.23	0.04	0.79
XM_014212639.1	Serine protease 27-like	0.20	0.16	0.07	0.58
NM_001279018.1	Hemoglobin subunit beta-1	0.33	0.17	0.18	0.76
XM_014152620.1	Ribosomal RNA small subunit methyltransferase NEP1-like, transcript variant X1	0.34	0.11	0.18	0.50

with the various GO terms related to hemoglobin function (GO:0005833 hemoglobin complex; GO:0005344 oxygen transporter activity; GO:0005506 iron ion binding; GO:0020037 heme binding; GO:0015671 oxygen transport; GO:0019825 oxygen binding). The EBV-induced G-protein coupled receptor 2 (NM_001140225) was assigned to GO terms GO:0016021 (integral component of membrane), GO:0007186 (G-protein coupled receptor signaling pathway), and GO:0002250 (adaptive immune response). The N-terminal EF-hand calcium-binding protein (XM_014146046) was only associated with GO term GO:0005509 (calcium ion binding), while for the transcript of the TBC1 domain family member 15 (XM_014201444) the GO terms GO:0090630 (activation of GTPase activity), GO:0006886 (intracellular protein transport), and GO:0031338 (regulation of vesicle fusion). Stathmin-3 (XM_014168090) was associated with neuron projection development (GO:0031175), cytoplasmic microtubule organization (GO:0031122), regulation of microtubule polymerization or depolymerization (GO:0031110), regulation of GTPase activity (GO:0043087), negative regulation of Rac protein signal transduction (GO:0035021), and microtubule depolymerization (GO:0007019). Serine protease 27 (XM_014212639) is assigned to proteolysis (GO:0006508), and ribosomal RNA small subunit methyltransferase NEP1 (XM_014152620) with methylation (GO:0032259).

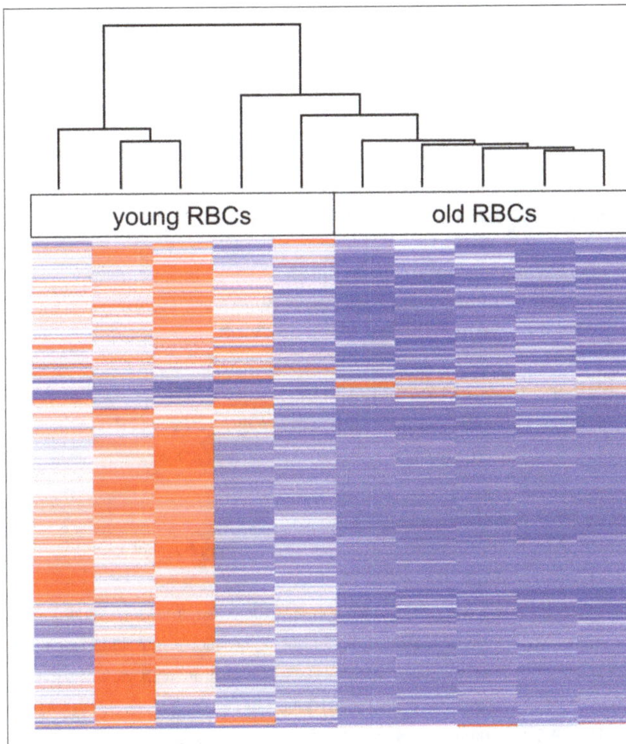

FIGURE 1 | Heat map of age-related changes in gene expression of erythrocytes (RBCs) with hierarchical clustering (complete linkage method with Euclidean distance measure) of all biological replicates. Red indicates highest expression and blue indicates lowest expression.

Aging Results in Lower Transcript Levels

The DEGs between young and old RBCs were identified by selecting a threshold of > two-fold change in expression level (FDR < 0.01). There was a large shift in transcript abundance between young and old erythrocyte samples (**Figure 1**). The total number of DEGs was 930; 889 (95.6%) of which show higher transcript levels in young erythrocytes (**Figure 1**; **Table S2**), while only 41 (4.4%) have higher transcript levels in old erythrocytes (**Figure 1**; **Table 2**). Positive $\log_2$-fold changes of transcripts in old erythrocytes did not exceed 2.05 (**Table 2**). The three genes with the highest $\log_2$-fold changes were the transmembrane protein 215 (XM_014194795), the cancer susceptibility candidate 1, transcript variant X2 (XM_014153053), and the corin, serine peptidase (XM_014206310). Negative $\log_2$-fold changes of five genes with unknown products were up to −6.5 in old erythrocytes (**Table S2**).

TABLE 2 | List of genes with significantly higher transcript levels in old vs. young erythrocyte fractions.

Genbank ID	Gene product	Log2 fold change	*p*-value FDR adjusted	Mean RPKM young fractions	Mean RPKM old fractions
XM_014133936.1	Adaptor protein, phosphotyrosine interaction, PH domain and leucine zipper containing 1, transcript variant X1	1.816	2.52E-08	0.399	1.462
XM_014189649.1	Retinal degeneration 3-like, transcript variant X1	1.418	1.79E-101	81.412	215.543
XM_014210752.1	Protein RD3-like	1.439	1.20E-22	4.092	10.991
XM_014127483.1	Huntingtin-interacting protein 1-related protein-like	1.66	4.04E-08	0.347	1.065
NA	tRNA-Thr	2.061	4.11E-05	0.055	0.982
NM_001141783.1	60S ribosomal protein L4-A	1.52	2.69E-06	0.397	1.068
XM_014194795.1	Transmembrane protein 215	2.048	1.37E-04	0	0.377
XM_014141736.1	Uncharacterized LOC106569954	1.912	1.22E-04	0.066	0.265
XM_014171620.1	Uncharacterized LOC106585433, transcript variant X2	1.896	1.22E-04	0.122	0.549
XM_014153053.1	Cancer susceptibility candidate 1, transcript variant X2	1.927	2.47E-04	0	0.556
NA	tRNA-Thr	1.357	2.91E-06	0.71	1.906
XM_014167525.1	Gap junction delta-2 protein-like	1.32	4.64E-07	4.176	12.823
XM_014206310.1	Corin, serine peptidase	1.92	3.49E-04	0	1.307
XR_001320426.1	Uncharacterized LOC106568984	1.16	1.15E-17	3.978	9.113
XM_014135536.1	SUZ domain-containing protein 1-like	1.651	1.93E-04	0.421	1.377
XM_014200511.1	Protein argonaute-3-like, transcript variant X1	1.165	3.42E-11	1.805	4.151
XM_014181495.1	E3 ubiquitin-protein ligase RNF6-like, transcript variant X2	1.183	1.23E-09	1.051	2.421
XM_014173518.1	Frizzled-5-like	1.502	1.73E-04	0.244	0.716
NM_001195818.1	Sterol regulatory element binding transcription factor 1	1.038	1.49E-23	14.103	28.79
XM_014199009.1	Protein RD3-like	1.476	2.27E-04	0.2	0.55
XM_014191191.1	Autophagy-related protein 9A-like, transcript variant X1	1.148	6.44E-08	2.63	5.709
XM_014212078.1	Transcription factor COE3-like, transcript variant X2	1.173	7.30E-07	1.187	2.613
XM_014212670.1	Alpha-N-acetylgalactosaminide alpha-2,6-sialyltransferase 2-like, transcript variant X1	1.365	1.88E-04	0.122	0.337
XM_014208326.1	Fructose-2,6-bisphosphatase TIGAR B-like	1.146	1.16E-06	1.731	3.853
XM_014194237.1	Mitochondrial import inner membrane translocase subunit tim16-like, transcript variant X2	1.028	6.54E-11	7.329	15.124
XM_014153345.1	G1/S-specific cyclin-D2-like	1.003	1.87E-15	29.248	66.339
XM_014197815.1	Kinesin-like protein KIF3B	1.315	3.18E-04	0.554	1.399
XM_014125557.1	Laminin subunit beta-4-like, transcript variant X2	1.041	2.90E-07	2.665	6.388
XM_014135839.1	Transmembrane protein 9-like, transcript variant X2	1.045	4.37E-07	1.397	2.819
NA	NA	1.265	2.25E-04	0.822	2.033
XR_001322670.1	Uncharacterized LOC106579519	1.236	3.66E-04	0.237	0.606
XM_014205641.1	Transmembrane protein 181, transcript variant X1	1.061	3.58E-05	4.582	9.641
XM_014176665.1	Uncharacterized LOC106588004	1.095	7.95E-05	1.626	3.606
XM_014126943.1	E3 ubiquitin-protein ligase NEDD4-like, transcript variant X4	1.02	1.12E-05	0.677	1.462
XM_014171405.1	Myosin regulatory light chain 2, ventricular/cardiac muscle isoform-like	1.006	1.11E-05	0.76	1.484
XM_014177327.1	Retinoic acid receptor RXR-beta-A, transcript variant X15	1.108	2.23E-04	0.67	1.45
XR_001319380.1	Uncharacterized LOC106563995	1.147	3.61E-04	1.049	2.501
XM_014171986.1	Anthrax toxin receptor 1-like, transcript variant X2	1.027	5.61E-05	1.187	2.49
XM_014140667.1	Peroxiredoxin, transcript variant X1	1.094	3.05E-04	0.748	1.619
NA	tRNA-Met	1.023	3.57E-04	1.903	4.085
XM_014147553.1	leucine rich repeat containing 23, transcript variant X2	1.007	2.77E-04	1.777	3.506

Functional Classification of DEGs

The gene annotation tool BLAST2GO (Götz et al., 2008), was used to annotate identified DEGs. The input list for the transcripts with higher levels in young erythrocytes contained 742 IDs (**Table S2**) and for 478 IDs GO annotation terms were found (**Figures 2A–C**). Eleven terms belonged to the biological process group (**Figure 2A**), 6 GO terms to the cellular component group (**Figure 2C**) and 5 GO terms to the molecular function group (**Figure 2B**). The largest three subcategories in the biological group were cellular processes (209 IDs), metabolic processes (151 IDs) and single-organism processes (138 IDs). In the molecular function category 140 IDs were associated with

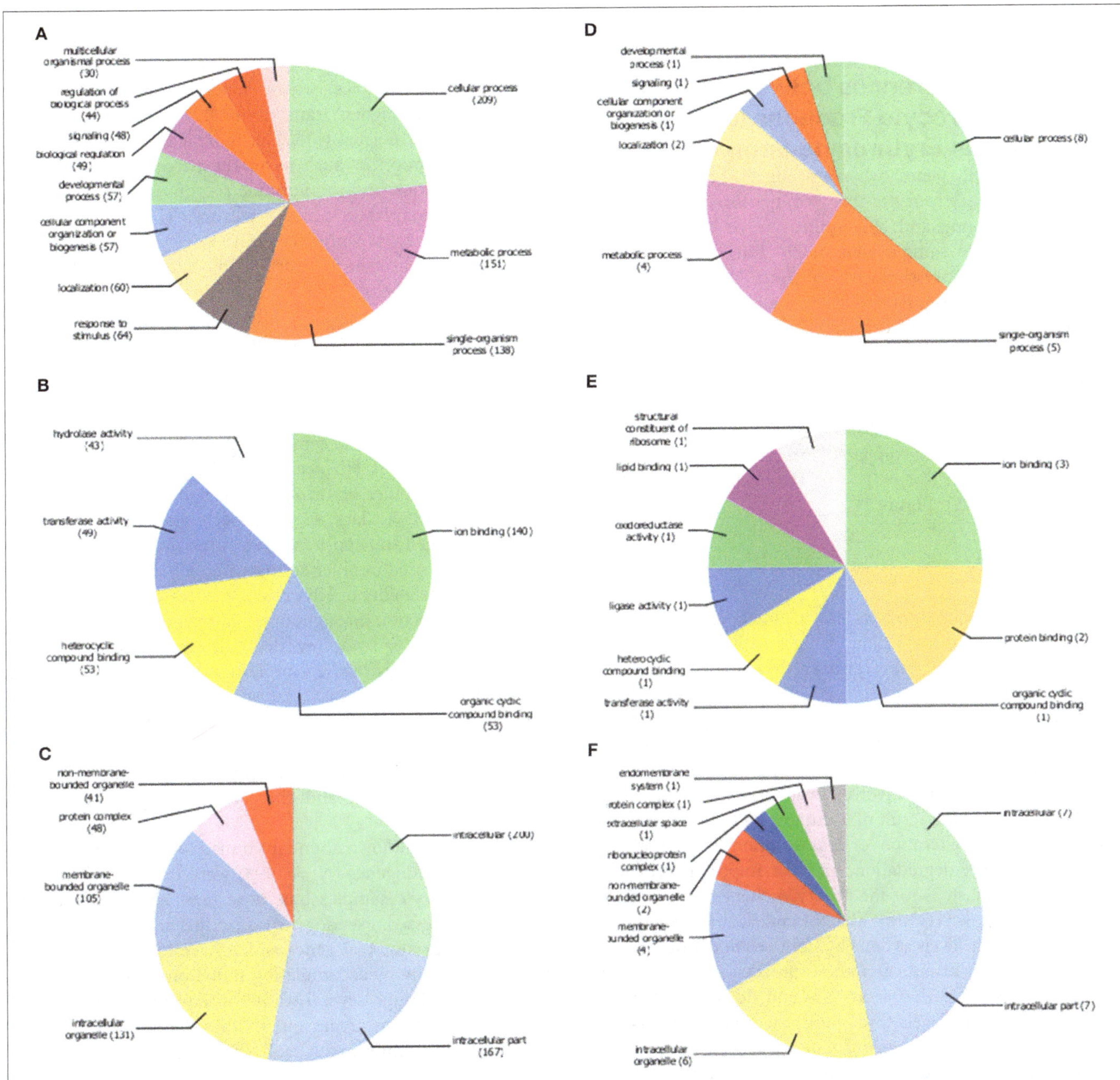

FIGURE 2 | Gene ontology (GO) terms associated with young **(A–C)** and old **(D–F)** erythrocyte age classes. Pie charts were generated at level 2 for biological process **(A,D)**, and level 3 for molecular function **(B,E)** and cellular component **(C,F)** by Blast2GO using 742 transcripts with higher levels in young erythrocytes (**Table S2**; pie charts **A–C**) and 34 transcripts with higher levels in old erythrocytes (**Table 2**; pie charts **D–F**) as input.

ion binding, and in cellular component category, 4 enriched GO terms were found: intracellular (200 IDs), intracellular part (167 IDs), membrane-bounded organelle (105 IDs) and intracellular organelle (191 IDs) were enriched terms in the cellular component.

The input list of the transcripts with higher levels in old erythrocytes contained 34 IDs (**Table 2**), for 18 IDs a total of 25 Gene ontology (GO) annotation terms were identified where 7 were within biological process (**Figure 2D**), and 9 each in cellular component (**Figure 2F**) and molecular function (**Figure 2E**). For 16 IDs no GO terms could be found. GO terms were enriched for cellular process (8 IDs), single-organism process (5 IDs) and metabolic process (4 IDs) in the biological process category. In the metabolic function category, no enriched GO terms were found and with each of the GO terms 1–3 IDs were associated. Intracellular components (7 IDs), membrane-bounded organelle

(4 IDs) and intracellular organelle (6 IDs) were enriched terms in the cellular component.

Expression Differences between Young and Old Erythrocyte Fractions in Relation to the Original Erythrocyte Sample

We selected eight genes whose products have important functions in fish erythrocytes for a comparison of expression levels between young and old erythrocyte fractions with the original erythrocyte sample with qPCR. Raw data were first normalized to the expression levels of *β-actin*, and then related to the values of the original erythrocyte sample and finally $\log_2$ transformed. The levels of expression of the genes are shown in **Figure 3**. The statistical analyses between young, old and original erythrocyte samples revealed four genes with significant differences: *gbx* ($p = 0.0408$), β_{3b}-*ar* ($p = 0.0111$), *gapdh* ($p = 0.0150$), and *hsp70* ($p = 0.007$). When only young and old erythrocyte fractions were compared, three of the genes remained significantly different: β_{3b}-*ar* ($p = 0.0159$), *gapdh* ($p = 0.0253$), and *hsp70* ($p = 0.0351$; **Figure 3**).

DISCUSSION

In fish, circulating erythrocytes are a population of different age classes, and their proportion changes with season and as a result of environmental stress (Härdig and Hoglund, 1984; Lewis et al., 2012). Maturation of fish erythrocytes in the circulation is associated with marked changes in many aspects of their physiology. We analyzed these changes on the transcriptomic level in young and old erythrocytes in order to get insights into the yet unknown pathways involved in aging. Changes in cellular transcript levels are the result of a number of tightly controlled processes, such as alteration of transcription rate, transcript stability, or mRNA degradation, and the importance of each of these regulatory steps for the observed changes in transcript levels is not yet known (Götting and Nikinmaa, 2017). Measuring cellular steady-state levels as done by RNA-seq does not take into account alterations in either of these processes (Hayles et al., 2010). Thus, we avoid the terms "up- and downregulated" for changes in transcript levels throughout the manuscript, as it is not known if any of the steps is regulated or just changes.

Our results revealed that aging in fish erythrocytes is accompanied by a decrease in transcript levels of a number of genes. It was shown earlier that the rate of transcription and the cellular RNA content decreases during maturation of nucleated non-mammalian erythrocytes (Grasso et al., 1977; Wiersma and Cox, 1985; Lund et al., 2000). High transcriptional and translational activity is required in young, immature erythrocyte because they gradually undergo changes in cell shape, membrane rigidity and other properties until maturation (e.g., Lecklin et al., 2000; Tavares-Dias, 2006). In contrast, in old, mature erythrocytes the need for gene transcription and protein synthesis is much lower and the necessary machinery, such as ribosomes is very low (Lane et al., 1982; Phillips et al., 2000). A total of 51,226 unigenes could be identified in the present study but we found only 930 (1.8%) DEGs. Most of the DEGs (95.6%) had significantly decreased levels in old erythrocytes and the overall gene expression is much more variable between young erythrocyte samples than between old erythrocyte samples, which appear more homogeneous (**Figure 1**). The higher transcriptional variability in young erythrocytes is associated with their more active roles in various physiological processes such as in the perception of external stimuli, adaptation and the immune response compared to the terminally differentiated, mature erythrocyte (Lecklin et al., 2000; Koldkjaer et al., 2004; Morera et al., 2011).

The most abundant transcripts in terms of number and expression level belonged to hemoglobin (Hb). Fish exhibit a remarkable multiplicity of Hbs with different functional properties, such as differences in O_2-affinity and sensitivity to allosteric regulators, which provide an important molecular strategy for adapting to a changing environment (Weber, 1990). During aging some hemoglobin subunit transcripts decrease significantly, while others remain at the same level. It has been reported earlier that Hb accumulates in erythrocytes during maturation and older erythrocytes are tightly packed with Hb (Bastos et al., 1977; Clark, 1988). Older erythrocytes thus serve merely as oxygen transporters. Even if the overall *hb* transcript levels are decreased in older erythrocytes, a long transcript half-life and a high stability of Hb protein ensures adequate synthesis for required function throughout the lifespan in the circulation.

Surprisingly, our study revealed that for two of the 15 most abundant transcripts in the samples the products and thus the function is not known. A blast search revealed a total of 7 transcript variants for the locus LOC106601081, and a blastx search using the unknown protein product of transcript variant 1 (XM_014192985) as query, found no hits. Further studies are required to identify and characterize the function of this transcript.

The second unknown abundant transcript is a pseudogene. A number of pseudogenes ($N = 1993$) were found to be present in the erythrocyte samples but more than half of them were only little expressed. Pseudogene transcripts are very often non-functional copies of real genes which have lost some or all of their functionality by accumulating mutations that disable, e.g., translation. Although several studies discussed the existence of pseuogenes in various organisms, another source of pseudogenes is the read alignment step during RNA-seq data analysis (Tonner et al., 2012).

Other abundant transcripts have functions in the intracellular protein transport and GTPase activation (TBC1 domain family member 15), calcium ion binding (N-terminal EF-hand calcium-binding protein) or the cytoplasmic microtubule organization (Stathmin-3). Furthermore, highly abundant transcripts of the serine protease 27, responsible for proteolysis, and of the ribosomal RNA small subunit methyltransferase NEP1, involved in methylation, were found. Among the genes with abundant levels only the transcripts of genes encoding EBV-induced G-protein coupled receptor 2 are significantly reduced by 88% in old erythrocytes, suggesting an impairment of the G-protein coupled receptor signaling pathway and a massively reduced adaptive immune response in old erythrocytes. An earlier study revealed already that nucleated erythrocytes play an active role in

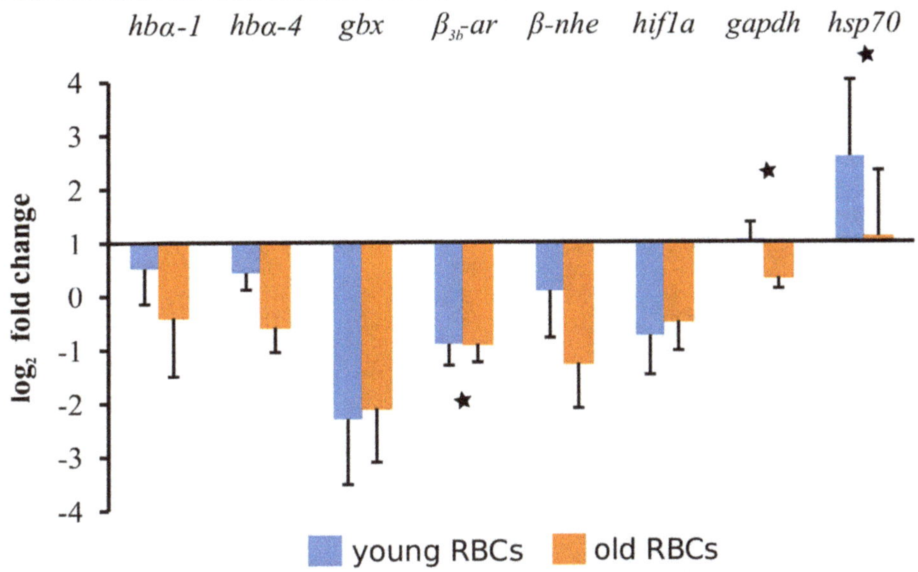

FIGURE 3 | Comparative gene expression levels between young and old erythrocytes (RBCs). Expression of eight target genes was normalized to *β-actin* as a reference gene and then related to the expression of the respective gene in the original erythrocyte sample taken before the fractionation procedure. Gene abbreviations are *hbα-1*, *hemoglobin α-1*; *hbα-4*, *hemoglobin α-4*; *gbx*, *globin x1*; β_{3b}*-ar*, β_{3b}*-adrenergic receptor*; *β-nhe*, *β-Na*$^+$*/H*$^+$*-exchanger*; *hif1a*, *hypoxia inducible factor 1a*; *gapdh*, *glyceraldehyde-3-phosphate dehydrogenase*; *hsp70*, *inducible heat shock protein 70 kDa*. Statistically significant differences between means of young and old erythrocyte fractions is shown by $^*p < 0.05$.

the immune response (Morera et al., 2011), but according to our results this is probably mostly restricted to young erythrocytes.

Age-dependent decreases in transcript levels of proteins involved in many molecular pathways were found in the present study (**Figure 4**). In particular genes whose products have functions in ion binding and DNA-binding or in signaling and membrane transport have significantly reduced transcript levels in old erythrocytes. Several enzyme classes (e.g., kinases, oxidoreductases, peptidases) seem to be affected as well. Earlier studies found that mRNA levels of carbonic anhydrase and Cl^-/HCO_3-exchanger (AE1) decrease with age (Lund et al., 2000), and also enzyme activity levels of carbonic anhydrase, citrate synthase, cytochrome oxidase and lactate dehydrogenase in rainbow trout RBCs (Lund et al., 2000; Phillips et al., 2000) are lower.

Only a small proportion of the DEGs ($N = 41$; 4.4%) showed higher levels in old erythrocytes. Among them, 34 are protein-coding and only for three the products are currently not known, although their $\log_2$-fold changes are comparably high. Two of the three genes with the highest $\log_2$-fold changes are integral components of the membrane. Currently little is known about the transmembrane protein 215 (XM_014194795) and its function. It is conserved among vertebrate species and is expressed in mouse bipolar cells (Park et al., 2017). An attractive speculation is, because of the increase of its transcription in old cells, that it is involved in the age-dependent removal of cells from circulation. For the corin, serine peptidase (XM_014206310; **Table 1**) the blastx search against the NR database revealed a hit of the atrial natriuretic peptide-converting enzyme of *Oreochromis niloticus,* which is involved in proteolysis and serine-type endopeptidase activity. For the cancer susceptibility candidate 1, transcript variant X2 (XM_014153053) no blastx hits and thus no annotations were found. For almost half of the DEGs with higher levels in old erythrocytes ($N = 16$; 47%) no GO terms could be retrieved from the databases revealing the gaps in knowledge for non-mammalian non-model organisms.

Using quantitative real-time PCR we analyzed the changes of eight genes, which have important functions in fish erythrocytes, in young and old fractions and compared them to the original erythrocyte sample. Four transcripts (β_{3b}*-ar*, *gapdh*, *gbx*, and *hsp70*) had significantly different levels between the young, old and the original sample. When only young and old fractions were compared, three transcripts were found to be significantly different (β_{3b}*-ar*, *gapdh*, and *hsp70*; **Figure 3**), which are not among the DEGs in the RNA-seq results (**Table S2**). This is due to the different statistical cutoffs applied for the RNA-seq data (FDR adjusted *p*-value, see Materials and Methods section) vs. a significance level of $p < 0.05$ used in the qPCR. When using the not-adjusted *T*-test *p*-value for the RNA-seq data, β_{3b}*-ar* and *gapdh* also have significant different levels in young and old fractions ($p = 0.02$ and $p = 0.03$, respectively), while *hsp70* remained non-significant ($p = 0.05$). The other transcripts (*hbα-1*, *hbα-4*, *hif1a*, and *β-nhe*) studied showed the same results as the RNA-seq data and were not different between age class fractions.

The higher β_{3b}*-ar* transcript levels in young fractions and the decrease with age is in accordance with earlier reported results and explains why the response of older, mature erythrocytes to external stimuli such as catecholamines is impaired (Cossins and Richardson, 1985; Lecklin et al., 2000). β_{3b}*-ar* transcript

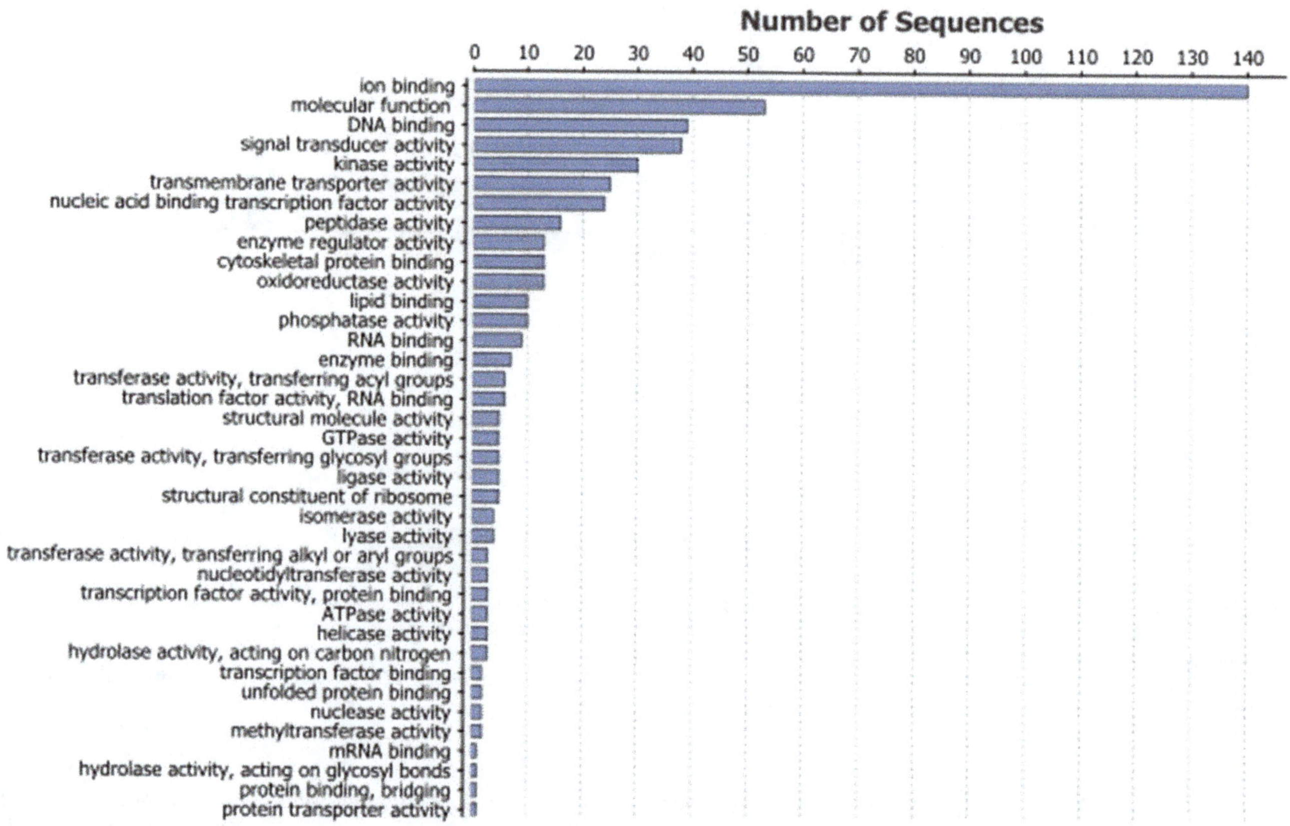

FIGURE 4 | Most frequent GO terms associated with the 742 DEGs with lower transcript levels in old erythrocytes.

levels in rainbow trout vary with season, showing high levels in summer (May to October) and low levels in winter (December to May) (Koldkjaer et al., 2004). Although β_{3b}-*ar* mRNA was not compared between young and old erythrocyte fractions by Koldkjaer et al. (2004), the observed increase in mRNA can be mainly attributed to the increased proportion of young erythrocytes in the in spring.

Older erythrocytes have a lower ability to produce stress proteins during the recovery period after heat shock (Lund et al., 2000). We found significantly higher transcript levels for the heat shock protein 70 kDa in young erythrocytes in both qPCR and RNA-seq data, but transcript levels of HSF-1 and Hsc71 were unaffected by cell age. This is in contrast to earlier study reporting lower transcript levels for the heat shock cognate 71 kDa (Hsc71) and the heat shock factor (HSF) in old erythrocytes compared to younger ones (Lund et al., 2000).

CONCLUSION

The mechanisms and characteristics which finally promote the removal of erythrocytes from the circulation and their destruction are still not known in fish. We found only a small proportion of DEGs between young and old fractions suggesting that even rather subtle changes in gene expression can have significant impact on a wide variety of molecular functions and the cell fate. The diversity of transcripts found in both erythrocyte age classes implies that the physiological roles of nucleated erythrocytes go far beyond the already known functions in oxygen transport and immune response. Hence, our data provide a rich resource for future investigations on the regulation of aging in fish and in particular fish erythrocytes and help to uncover additional physiological functions.

DATA DEPOSITION

The RNA-seq data have been deposited at the NCBI Gene Expression Omnibus (GEO) with the accession number GSE106570.

AUTHOR CONTRIBUTIONS

MG and MN: conceived the study and wrote the paper; MG: performed the experiments and analyzed the data.

ACKNOWLEDGMENTS

We thank Kurt Malmberg (Ammattiopisto Livia/Yrkesinstitut Livia) for providing the rainbow trout. Additionally, we thank V. Vainio and J. Ruohomäki for help with lab work. We acknowledge the Finnish Functional Genomics Centre and the Bioinformatics Unit at the Turku Centre for Biotechnology and Biocenter Finland for their help in plate run services, RNA sequencing and in data analysis. The Units are supported by University of Turku, Åbo Akademi University, and Biocenter Finland. We would like to thank the two reviewers for their valuable comments on an earlier version of the article.

REFERENCES

Altschul, S. F., Gish, W., Miller, W., Myers, E. W., and Lipman, D. J. (1990). Basic local alignment search tool. *J. Mol. Biol.* 215, 403–410. doi: 10.1016/S0022-2836(05)80360-2

Alvarez, F., Flaño, E., Villena, A. J., Zapata, A., and Razquin, B. E. (1994). Seasonal intrathymic erythropoietic activity in trout. *Dev. Comp. Immunol.* 18, 409–420.

Avery, E. H., Lee, B. L., Freedland, R. A., and Cornelius, C. E. (1992). Bile pigments in gallbladder and freshly-secreted hepatic duct bile from fed and fasted rainbow trout, *Oncorhynchus mykiss. Comp. Biochem. Physiol. Comp. Physiol.* 101, 857–861.

Bastos, R. N., Volloch, Z., and Aviv, H. (1977). Messenger RNA population analysis during erythroid differentiation: a kinetical approach. *J. Mol. Biol.* 110, 191–203.

Bolger, A. M., Lohse, M., and Usadel, B. (2014). Trimmomatic: a flexible trimmer for Illumina sequence data. *Bioinformatics* 30, 2114–2120. doi: 10.1093/bioinformatics/btu170

Clark, M. R. (1988). Senescence of red blood cells: progress and problems. *Physiol. Rev.* 68, 503–554.

Cossins, A. R., and Richardson, P. A. (1985). Adrenalin-induced Na+/H+ exchange in' trout erythrocytes and its effects upon oxygen-carrying capacity. *J. Exp. Biol.* 118, 229–246.

Götting, M., and Nikinmaa, M. (2017). *In vitro* study on the regulation of cellular mRNA levels by changes in transcription rate and transcript stability in fish red blood cells. *Comp. Biochem. Physiol. Part B Biochem. Mol. Biol.* 213, 35–44. doi: 10.1016/j.cbpb.2017.07.006

Götz, S., García-Gómez, J. M., Terol, J., Williams, T. D., Nagaraj, S. H., Nueda, M. J., et al. (2008). High-throughput functional annotation and data mining with the Blast2GO suite. *Nucleic Acids Res.* 36, 3420–3435. doi: 10.1093/nar/gkn176

Grasso, J. A., Chromey, N. C., and Moxey, C. F. (1977). Biochemical characterization of RNA and protein synthesis in erythrocyte development. *J. Cell Biol.* 73, 206–222.

Härdig, J., and Hoglund, L. B. (1984). Seasonal variation in blood components of reared Baltic salmon, *Salmo salar* L. *J. Fish Biol.* 24, 565–579. doi: 10.1111/j.1095-8649.1984.tb04827.x

Hayles, B., Yellaboina, S., and Wang, D. (2010). Comparing transcription rate and mRNA abundance as parameters for biochemical pathway and network analysis. *PLoS ONE* 5:e9908. doi: 10.1371/journal.pone.0009908

Houston, A. H., Dobric, N., and Kahurananga, R. (1996). The nature of hematological response in fish. *Fish Physiol. Biochem.* 15, 339–347. doi: 10.1007/BF02112361

Kim, D., Pertea, G., Trapnell, C., Pimentel, H., Kelley, R., and Salzberg, S. L. (2013). TopHat2: accurate alignment of transcriptomes in the presence of insertions, deletions and gene fusions. *Genome Biol.* 14:R36. doi: 10.1186/gb-2013-14-4-r36

Koldkjaer, P., Pottinger, T. G., Perry, S. F., and Cossins, A. R. (2004). Seasonality of the red blood cell stress response in rainbow trout (*Oncorhynchus mykiss*). *J. Exp. Biol.* 207, 357–367. doi: 10.1242/jeb.00747

Koressaar, T., and Remm, M. (2007). Enhancements and modifications of primer design program Primer3. *Bioinformatics* 23, 1289–1291. doi: 10.1093/bioinformatics/btm091

Lane, H. C. (1979). Some haematological responses of normal and splenectomized rainbow trout Salmo gairdneri to a 12% blood loss. *J. Fish Biol.* 14, 159–164. doi: 10.1111/j.1095-8649.1979.tb03505.x

Lane, H. C., Weaver, J. W., Benson, J. A., and Nichols, H. A. (1982). Some age related changes of adult rainbow trout, Salmo gairdneri Rich., peripheral erythrocytes separated by velocity sedimentation at unit gravity. *J. Fish Biol.* 21, 1–14. doi: 10.1111/j.1095-8649.1982.tb02818.x

Lecklin, T., Tuominen, A., and Nikinmaa, M. (2000). The adrenergic volume changes of immature and mature rainbow trout (*Oncorhynchus mykiss*) erythrocytes. *J. Exp. Biol.* 203, 3025–3031.

Lewis, J. M., Hori, T. S., Rise, M. L., Walsh, P. J., and Currie, S. (2010). Transcriptome responses to heat stress in the nucleated red blood cells of the rainbow trout (*Oncorhynchus mykiss*). *Physiol. Genomics* 42, 361–373. doi: 10.1152/physiolgenomics.00067.2010

Lewis, J. M., Klein, G., Walsh, P. J., and Currie, S. (2012). Rainbow trout (*Oncorhynchus mykiss*) shift the age composition of circulating red blood cells towards a younger cohort when exposed to thermal stress. *J. Comp. Physiol. B. Biochem. Syst. Environ. Physiol.* 182, 663–671. doi: 10.1007/s00360-012-0650-2

Liao, Y., Smyth, G. K., and Shi, W. (2014). featureCounts: an efficient general purpose program for assigning sequence reads to genomic features. *Bioinformatics* 30, 923–930. doi: 10.1093/bioinformatics/btt656

Lien, S., Koop, B. F., Sandve, S. R., Miller, J. R., Kent, M. P., Nome, T., et al. (2016). The Atlantic salmon genome provides insights into rediploidization. *Nature* 533, 200–205. doi: 10.1038/nature17164

Livak, K. J., and Schmittgen, T. D. (2001). Analysis of relative gene expression data using real-time quantitative PCR and the $2^{-\Delta\Delta C}$T Method. *Methods* 25, 402–408. doi: 10.1006/meth.2001.1262

Lund, S. G., Phillips, M. C., Moyes, C. D., and Tufts, B. L. (2000). The effects of cell ageing on protein synthesis in rainbow trout (*Oncorhynchus mykiss*) red blood cells. *J. Exp. Biol.* 203, 2219–2228.

Morera, D., Roher, N., Ribas, L., Balasch, J. C., Doñate, C., Callol, A., et al. (2011). RNA-seq reveals an integrated immune response in nucleated erythrocytes. *PLoS ONE* 6:e26998. doi: 10.1371/journal.pone.0026998

Moyes, C. D., Sharma, M. L., Lyons, C., Leary, S. C., Leon, M., Petrie, A., et al. (2002). Origins and consequences of mitochondrial decline in nucleated erythrocytes. *Biochim. Biophys. Acta. Mol. Cell Res.* 1591, 11–20. doi: 10.1016/S0167-4889(02)00224-0

Murphy, J. R. (1973). Influence of temperature and method of centrifugation on the separation of erythrocytes. *J. Lab. Clin. Med.* 82, 334–41.

Nikinmaa, M. (1990). *Vertebrate Red Blood Cells : Adaptations of Function to Respiratory Requirements.* Berlin; New York, NY: Springer-Verlag.

Nikinmaa, M., and Jensen, F. (1992). Inhibition of adrenergic proton extrusion in rainbow trout red cells by nitrite-induced methaemoglobinaemia. *J. Comp. Physiol. B. Biochem. Syst. Environ. Physiol.* 162, 424–429. doi: 10.1007/BF00258964

Park, K. U., Randazzo, G., Jones, K. L., Brzezinski, J. A. IV. (2017). Gsg1, Trnp1, and Tmem215 Mark Subpopulations of Bipolar Interneurons in the Mouse Retina. *Invest. Ophthalmol. Vis. Sci.* 58, 1137–1150. doi: 10.1167/iovs.16-19767

Phillips, M. C., Moyes, C. D., and Tufts, B. L. (2000). The effects of cell ageing on metabolism in rainbow trout (*Oncorhynchus mykiss*) red blood cells. *J. Exp. Biol.* 203, 1039–1045.

Speckner, W., Schindler, J. F., and Albers, C. (1989). Age-dependent changes in volume and haemoglobin content of erythrocytes in the carp (*Cyprinus carpio* L.). *J. Exp. Biol.* 141, 133–149.

Tavares-Dias, M. (2006). A morphological and cytochemical study of erythrocytes, thrombocytes and leukocytes in four freshwater teleosts. *J. Fish Biol.* 68, 1822–1833. doi: 10.1111/j.1095-8649.2006.01089.x

Tiano, L., Ballarini, P., Santoni, G., Wozniak, M., and Falcioni, G. (2000). Morphological and functional changes of mitochondria from density separated trout erythrocytes. *Biochim. Biophys. Acta* 1457, 118–128. doi: 10.1016/S0005-2728(00)00071-2

Tonner, P., Srinivasasainagendra, V., Zhang, S., and Zhi, D. (2012). Detecting transcription of ribosomal protein pseudogenes in diverse human tissues from RNA-seq data. *BMC Genomics* 13:412. doi: 10.1186/1471-2164-13-412

Untergasser, A., Cutcutache, I., Koressaar, T., Ye, J., Faircloth, B. C., Remm, M., et al. (2012). Primer3–new capabilities and interfaces. *Nucleic Acids Res.* 40:e115. doi: 10.1093/nar/gks596

Wang, L., Feng, Z., Wang, X., Wang, X., and Zhang, X. (2010). DEGseq: an R package for identifying differentially expressed genes from RNA-seq data. *Bioinformatics* 26, 136–138. doi: 10.1093/bioinformatics/btp612

Weber, R. (1990). "Functional significance and structural basis of multiple hemoglobins with special reference to ectothermic vertebrates," in *Animal Nutrition and Transport Processes Comparative and Environmental Aspects. Comp. Physiol. 6. Transport, Respiration and Excretion*, eds. J. Truchot and B. Lahlou (Basel: Karger) 58–75.

Wiersma, P. A., and Cox, G. S. (1985). Synthesis of messenger-like RNA in avian erythrocyte nuclei. *Arch. Biochem. Biophys.* 242, 90–103.

Zaiontz, C. (2015). *Real Statistics Using Excel.* Available online at: www.realstatistics.com

19

The Action of Red Cell Calcium Ions on Human Erythrophagocytosis *in Vitro*

Pedro J. Romero* and Concepción Hernández-Chinea

Laboratory of Membrane Physiology, Faculty of Sciences, Institute of Experimental Biology, Central University of Venezuela, Caracas, Venezuela

***Correspondence:**
Pedro J. Romero
romepe@yahoo.com

In the present work we have studied *in vitro* the effect of increasing red cell Ca^{2+} ions on human erythrophagocytosis by peripheral monocyte-derived autologous macrophages. In addition, the relative contribution to phagocytosis of phosphatidylserine exposure, autologous IgG binding, complement deposition and Gárdos channel activity was also investigated. Monocytes were obtained after ficoll-hypaque fractionation and induced to transform by adherence to glass coverslips, for 24 h at 37°C in a RPMI medium, containing 10% fetal calf serum. Red blood cells (RBC) were loaded with Ca^{2+} using 10 μM A23187 and 1 mM Ca-EGTA buffers, in the absence of Mg^{2+}. Ca^{2+}-loaded cells were transferred to above coverslips and incubated for 2 h at 37°C under various experimental conditions, after which phagocytosis was assessed by light microscopy. Confirming earlier findings, phagocytosis depended on internal Ca^{2+}. Accordingly; it was linearly raised from about 2–15% by increasing the free Ca^{2+} content of the loading solution from 0.5 to 20 μM, respectively. Such a linear increase was virtually doubled by the presence of 40% autologous serum. At 7 μM Ca^{2+}, the phagocytosis degree attained with serum was practically equal to that obtained with either 2 mg/ml affinity-purified IgG or 40% IgG-depleted serum. However, phagocytosis was reduced to levels found with Ca^{2+} alone when IgG-depleted serum was inactivated by heat, implying an involvement of complement. On the other hand, phagocytosis in the absence of serum was markedly reduced by preincubating macrophages with phosphatidylserine-containing liposomes. In contrast, a similar incubation in the presence of serum affected it partially whereas employing liposomes made only of phosphatidylcholine essentially had no effect. Significantly, the Gárdos channel inhibitors clotrimazole (2 μM) and TRAM-34 (100 nM) fully blocked serum-dependent phagocytosis. These findings show that a raised internal Ca^{2+} promotes erythrophagocytosis by independently triggering phosphatidylserine externalization, complement deposition and IgG binding. Serum appeared to stimulate phagocytosis in a way dependent on Gárdos activity. It seems likely that Ca^{2+} promoted IgG-binding to erythrocytes via Gárdos channel activation. This can be an important signal for clearance of senescent human erythrocytes under physiological conditions.

Keywords: erythrophagocytosis, internal calcium, autologous serum, red blood cells, Gárdos channel

INTRODUCTION

The normal human red blood cell (RBC) ages in the blood stream while circulating ceaselessly for a finite lifespan of nearly 120 days (Berlin and Berk, 1975). Aging appears as a continuous process of multifactorial origin, becoming abruptly interrupted by splenic retention of the senescent RBC. The sequestered cell is immediately recognized and phagocytosed by resident macrophages (Rifkind, 1966; Mebius and Kraal, 2005). Although many different hypotheses have accumulated over the years, the mechanisms responsible for trapping, recognition and destruction of aged cells are not completely elucidated (Clark, 1988; Bratosin et al., 1998; Antonelou et al., 2010; Lutz and Bogdanova, 2013). Suggested age-related changes involved in these mechanisms include dehydration with augmented cell density, decreased size, vesiculation, increased oxidative stress, band 3 clustering, band 3 phosphorylation, increased membrane IgG content and loss of membrane phospholipid asymmetry (Low et al., 1985; Lutz et al., 1987; Ciana et al., 2004; Willekens et al., 2008; Franco et al., 2013; Lutz and Bogdanova, 2013).

One of the current hypotheses that has great consensus is based upon IgG attachment to the RBC membrane and its recognition for macrophage clearance via Fc receptor interaction (Arese et al., 2005; Bosman et al., 2005; Lutz and Bogdanova, 2013). It is well-known that IgG accumulates on the outer membrane surface as the RBC ages (Lutz and Stringaro-Wipf, 1983). A small fraction of IgG binds significantly to α-galactosyl residues of presumably membrane glycolipids in aged RBCs (Galili et al., 1984). Another fraction is bound to a neo-antigenic region located on band 3 protein, which becomes progressively expressed during cell aging. This region corresponds to a distinct interdimeric band 3 epitope exposing binding sites for low-affinity autologous IgG, which is formed upon oligomerization and clustering of band 3 aggregates during RBC senescence (Lutz et al., 1984; Kannan et al., 1991; Lutz, 2012). Additionally, it has been shown that bivalent IgG binding to interdimeric band 3 potentiates the opsonizing IgG action on RBCs by recruiting C3b, a critical complement component, thus compensating for its low-affinity binding characteristic (Lutz, 2012).

The proportion of natural IgG antibodies bound to band 3 was found about a half of that associated to α-galactosyl residues, whereas the rest constituting about 70% of the total showed an unknown specificity (Sorette et al., 1991).

Another proposed hypothesis that originally had a great impact for involving a classical apoptosis hallmark, relates to the asymmetrical distribution of membrane phospholipids, a "sine qua non" characteristic of normal living cells. Of particular importance in this context is phosphatidylserine (PS), which accumulates in the inner membrane leaflet by action of an aminophospholipid translocase (APLT), a P_4-type ATPase (Bitbol et al., 1987; Morrot et al., 1990). Externalization of PS is a widely accepted signal for macrophage recognition and phagocytosis of apoptotic and effete cells (Schroit et al., 1985; McEvoy et al., 1986; Fadok et al., 1992; Kiefer and Snyder, 2000; Segawa and Nagata, 2015). The specific recognition of surface exposed PS occurs by direct interactions with membrane macrophage receptors such as stabilin-2 (Park et al., 2008) or Tim-1/Tim-4 (Kobayashi et al., 2007) and indirect ones, via serum proteins that act as bridging opsonins such as lactadherin (Hanayama et al., 2002), thrombospondin-1, growth arrest-specific 6 (Gas-6) and protein S to $\alpha_v\beta_{3/5}$ integrins and TAM tyrosine kinase receptors on macrophages (de Back et al., 2014; Segawa and Nagata, 2015).

In addition to the already mentioned exposure of natural antibodies-binding neoantigenic regions and surface PS, another unique signal for RBC removal has been proposed. This involves CD47, a transmembrane RBC glycoprotein that interacts with signal regulatory protein α (SIRP α) on macrophages blocking erythrophagocytosis (Oldenborg et al., 2000). However, in "artificially aged" RBCs (oxidatively treated) phagocytosis was stimulated by $F(ab)_2$ anti-CD47, which prevented binding of oxidized CD47 to SIRPα. A similar effect seemed to be elicited by thrombospondin-1(TSP1), a known CD47 natural physiological ligand. It was therefore proposed that CD47 could act like a switch promoting or inhibiting phagocytosis, depending on whether TSP1 becomes bound or not (Oldenborg et al., 2000; Burger et al., 2012). It has been suggested that TSP1 binding to CD47 may be responsible for *in vivo* clearance of senescent RBCs.

An interesting hypothesis has been raised recently; drawing attention on the likely possibility that removal tagging signals on circulating RBCs may pass undetected because of their rapid dismissal. It was shown that the aging RBC decreases its membrane content of spectrin and flotillin-2, a lipid raft marker (Ciana et al., 2017). It was also found that vesicles induced by Ca^{2+}-A23187 treatment were depleted of flotillin-2. It was proposed by above authors, that vesicles would contain a balanced lipid-bilayer/cytoskeletal protein ratio so that their release should occur without affecting the biconcave-disk shape of the cell. The hypothesis has been put forward that the continuous removal of vesicles by resident macrophages and the "pitting" splenic action during RBC aging, would reduce the cell size down to a minimum with a consequent increased rigidity (Ciana et al., 2017). This would lead to sequestration at the narrow splenic slits, recognition of accumulated tagging signals and finally clearance by phagocytosis.

On the other hand, earlier works stressed the importance of an elevated internal free Ca^{2+} as possible triggering signal for the events leading to clearance of senescent RBCs (Romero, 1978; Romero and Romero, 1999a; Bosman et al., 2005; Bogdanova et al., 2013). This idea finds support first, on the raised internal Ca^{2+} occurring during RBC aging as result of a steadily increased entry into cells having a progressive pumping deficiency (Romero and Romero, 1997, 1999b; Lew et al., 2007). Secondly, such a Ca^{2+} rise appears as common denominator of most of above mentioned age-related changes (Elgsaeter et al., 1976; Allan and Michell, 1977; Turrini et al., 1991; Kiefer and Snyder, 2000; Lang K. S. et al., 2003; Bogdanova et al., 2013).

Contrary to what would be expected from an abrupt clearance process, tagging signals steadily accumulate during the RBC lifespan. It is generally assumed that they trigger cell removal after reaching a threshold, as suggested for IgG binding where a few hundred molecules seem required (Bosman et al., 2005). In contrast with this view, previous work proposed a key role for the Gárdos channel (also known as KCNN4, KCa3.1,

IKCa1) in the earlier events of senescent RBC clearance (Romero and Romero, 1999a). Accordingly, the channel would act as a molecular transducer between a monotonic signal (steadily rise in free internal Ca) and an "all-or-none" change (abrupt, self-generated Ca^{2+} increase, caused by membrane hyperpolarization due to channel opening) required for both a time-dependent sequestration and recognition of the aged cell. Essential to this view is the existent factual relationship between an increased Ca^{2+} content, activity of the Gárdos channel and cellular dehydration, referred to recently as the central paradigm of erythrocyte volume homeostasis (Martinac and Cox, 2017). Hence, a circulation-dependent raised cell Ca^{2+} above threshold levels (*caused by pressure or shear stress*) promotes erythrocyte dehydration by activating the Gárdos channel.

The purpose of the present study is to address the role that a raised free internal Ca^{2+} might possibly have on the clearance of aged cells, by studying *in vitro* its action on human erythrophagocytosis by peripheral monocyte-derived autologous macrophages under various experimental conditions. A complex action of Ca^{2+} was revealed, presumably involving phosphatidylserine externalization, IgG binding, complement activation and Gárdos channel activity.

MATERIALS AND METHODS

All reagents of the best quality available were purchased mainly from Sigma-Aldrich Corp., St Louis, USA. Protein A-sepharose CL-4B was obtained from GE Healthcare, Uppsala, Sweden. Fetal calf serum (FCS) was from GIBCO BRL, New York, USA. The pH of all solutions was adjusted at room temperature (RT) to ± 0.02 units. Fresh human blood (mainly 0+) was used, obtained from healthy subjects of both sexes, equally represented and mostly with ages between 35 and 55 years old.

Isolation of Peripheral Blood Monocytes

Blood (10 ml) was collected by venipuncture in the presence of citrate (3.8%) and mixed with equal vol of phosphate-buffered saline (PBS) (310 mOsm/kg H_2O, 150 mM NaCl + 20 mM (Na/K) phosphate buffer, pH 7.4), supplemented with 2 mM EDTA-Na_2 and 10 mM glucose. The diluted blood was deposited on top of a ficoll-hypaque (FH) layer (density = 1.0775 g/ml) at a vol ratio blood/FH of 1:0.5 and spun down at 900 g for 30 min at RT. The cells banding at the serum-FH interphase were removed carefully and washed by resuspension in PBS medium supplemented as above and centrifuging at a sequentially decreasing low force (300, 200 and twice at 100 g). The fraction obtained consisted mainly of mononuclear cells (MNC) (>90%).

MNCs were resuspended in RPMI 1640-medium containing 0.03% glutamine and supplemented with 10% (vol/vol) heat-inactivated FCS plus antibiotics (100 U/ml penicillin G and 100 μg/ml streptomycin sulfate). Cells were enumerated in a Neubauer chamber and adjusted to a density of 3 × 10^6 cells/ml with supplemented-RPMI medium (MNC suspension). Viable cells were routinely determined by trypan blue exclusion (Freshney, 1987). Viability always exceeded 98%.

To promote cell adherence and induce macrophage transformation, aliquots of the above MNC suspension (70 μl) were seeded on glass coverslips, deposited inside 6-holes culture dishes and placed in an air-CO_2 incubator. After 1 h at 37°C under a 5% CO_2-humidified air atmosphere, 2 ml of warm RPMI medium supplemented as above were added to each well and incubation further continued for up to 24 h.

Loading Erythrocytes with Ca^{2+}

Erythrocytes from above FH fractionation (approx. 200 μl from the bottom of RBCs pellet) were separated and stored overnight in PBS plus 10 mM glucose and antibiotics. They were then washed once with PBS and thrice with a choline medium, containing (mM): choline Cl, 109; KCl, 5; Tris-HCl, 20 (pH 7.4). RBCs were loaded with Ca^{2+} by incubating in choline medium (1% hematocrit) for 30 min at 37°C under moderate shaking, in the presence of 10 μM A23187 for uniform Ca^{2+} permeabilization (Dagher and Lew, 1988) and 1 mM Ca-EGTA buffers, set at different Ca/EGTA ratios to obtain 0–20 μM ionized Ca (Fabiato and Fabiato, 1979). After loading, the ionophore was removed by washing once with 100 vols of choline medium containing 2 mg bovine serum albumin (BSA)/ml and twice with a similar medium but having 0.5 mg BSA/ml. RBCs were further washed twice with PBS to remove the remnant BSA and finally suspended in RPMI. Erythrocytes were enumerated in a Neubauer chamber and diluted with RPMI to about 50 times the number of monocytes/coverslip.

Since Mg^{2+} is also transported by A23187 (Reed and Lardy, 1972), this ion was omitted from the Ca^{2+}-loading media in order to inactivate the Ca^{2+} pump. As a reference control, in some experiments Mg^{2+} was added to the loading medium at 0.15 mM, a concentration set at equilibrium with a −12 mV membrane potential (Flatman and Lew, 1980). Thereby, no net Mg^{2+} movements were expected during RBCs loading.

Obtention of Autologous Serum (AS)

A parallel blood sample (10 ml) was collected without anticoagulant and allowed to clot at 37°C for 2 h. Thereafter, it was centrifuged at 3,000 g for 20 min at RT and kept at 4°C for 1 h before serum withdrawal. The AS was stored at −20°C until use on the following day.

Affinity Purification of IgG

Sepharose-coupled protein A was treated as recommended by the manufacturers and further used as described next. Briefly, it was washed several times with 50 mM Tris-HCl buffer (pH 7.0) by centrifuging 3 min at 500 g. One ml of this slurry sediment was packed at 15,000 g for 15 min. The supernatant was replaced by 500 μl of AS, the suspension mixed and left shaking for 15 min at RT. After packing as just described, the supernatant consisting of IgG-depleted serum was recovered, supplemented with antibiotics and preserved at −20°C until use. The total protein content of supernatants was usually 27–30 mg/ml.

The remaining sediment was washed five times with 50 mM Tris-HCl buffer (pH 7.0) and packed at 15,000 g as described before. To elute bound IgG, it was added 500 μl of 0.1 M citric acid (pH 3.0); the suspension mixed and left shaking for 15 min at RT. After which, the mixture was packed as above, the supernatant containing eluted IgG was recovered and neutralized to pH 7.0-7.5 by adding appropriate amounts of 1M Tris-HCl solution (pH 9.0). The IgG solution obtained was supplemented with (mM): NaCl, 150; $CaCl_2$, 2; $MgCl_2$, 1; plus antibiotics, and finally stored at −20°C until use. This solution generally contained 8–9 mg protein/ml. The efficiency of the process was checked by SDS-PAGE, using 10% polyacrylamide gels in the presence of 1% (vol/vol) 2-mercaptoethanol (Laemmli, 1970). Protein concentration was estimated using the Lowry method (Lowry et al., 1951). Equal amounts (20 μg) of protein were loaded per track for electrophoretic assays.

Preparation of Liposomes

Small unilamellar liposomes were prepared by sonication essentially as described by Fadok et al. (1992). The lipids, PS (L-α-phosphatidyl-L-serine) and L-α-dimyristoyl phosphatidylcholine (PC) were dissolved in chloroform at a molar ratio PS/PC of 3:7 and roto-evaporated at 50–60°C under reduced pressure. The dry material was resuspended in minimal medium of composition to be described later and vigorously shaken. The mixture was subsequently sonicated for two 10 min-cycles at 1°C, in a Braun-Sonic 2000 sonicator (Fisher Scientific Products, Pittsburgh PA). The clear liposomal suspension (2 mM total lipid) was stored at −20°C until use. Liposomes containing only PC were used as control.

Erythrophagocytosis Assays

After adherence, coverslips were washed five times with warm RPMI medium to remove non-adherent cells. The RBCs (loaded or not with Ca^{2+}) were suspended in RPMI medium supplemented or not with 40% (vol/vol) AS or other additions. This suspension was deposited on macrophages-attached coverslips and incubated for 2 h at 37°C in a 5% CO_2 humidified-air incubator. Thereafter, non-adherent RBCs were removed from coverslips by washing thrice with PBS and the attached cells were fixed with 2.5% glutaraldehyde in 0.15 M (Na/K) phosphate buffer (pH 7) for 15 min at RT. Subsequently, they were Wright-stained using conventional methods and observed under a light microscope (Nikon Eclipse E400).

In some experiments, macrophages were preincubated with PC- or mixed (PS + PC)-liposomes (200 μM total lipid content), for 30 min at 37°C in RPMI medium, in a 5% CO_2 humidified-air incubator. After washing five times with warm RPMI medium, macrophages were challenged with 7 μM Ca^{2+}-loaded RBCs and phagocytosis then assayed in a similar medium in the presence and absence of 40% AS, as described above.

Erythrophagocytosis was quantified (in percent) by scoring the number of macrophages having not only ingested but also attached RBCs, the latter considered an early step of the phagocytic process (Elliott and Ravichandran, 2010). At least 10^3 macrophages counts were accumulated for each condition to minimize counting error, except for experiments with liposomes where 300 cells were scored.

In some assays, the RMPI medium employed for phagocytosis was replaced by a minimal medium containing (mM): NaCl, 140; KCl, 5; $CaCl_2$, 2; $MgCl_2$, 1; Hepes (pH 7.5), 10; glucose, 10; penicillin G, 100 U/ml and streptomycin, 100 μg/ml, leading to no significantly different results (not shown).

Statistical Analysis

Data were analyzed using GraphPad Prism Version 5.01 software for Windows. Statistical analysis was performed by unpaired two-tailed *t*-test when 2 groups were compared or 1-way ANOVA with Bonferroni post-tests when comparing more than 2 groups. Statistical significance of the data was defined as follows: $P > 0.05$ (n.s), $P \leq 0.05$ (*), $P \leq 0.01$ (**), $P \leq 0.001$ (***). Each experiment presented corresponded to a different donor.

ETHICS

The present study was approved by the Bioethics Committee of the Faculty of Sciences, Central University of Venezuela. Investigations were carried out in accordance with the principles of the 2013 Declaration of Helsinki. Written informed consent was obtained from all blood donors participating in this study.

RESULTS

Effects of Ca^{2+} and AS on Erythrophagocytosis

Early work showed the requirement of both internal Ca^{2+} and presence of AS for phagocytosis of human RBCs by leukocytes *in vitro* (Romero and Romero, 1999a). This study, however, employed ghosts from the two cell types involved, a condition that may have obscured in part the conclusions drawn. With the interest of confirming these observations under more physiological conditions, intact RBCs were loaded with Ca^{2+} by means of the ionophore A23187 and exposed to monocyte-derived autologous macrophages. In addition, to assess a possible effect of Mg^{2+}, phagocytosis was studied on cells treated or not with this ion during loading.

As reported in **Table 1**, with RBCs loaded in the virtual absence of both Ca^{2+} and Mg^{2+}, the phagocytosis degree was about 2%, and tended to become reduced to a half when 0.15 mM Mg^{2+} was also added with the ionophore. Phagocytosis of these cells was significantly stimulated 2.5-fold by adding 40% AS to the assay medium whereas it remained unaltered if Mg^{2+} was present during loading.

In contrast, after loading with 20 μM Ca^{2+} and no Mg^{2+}, phagocytosis increased high significantly by nearly 900% and became additionally stimulated 2-fold by adding serum (**Table 1**). On the other hand, with 100 μM Ca^{2+} and Mg^{2+} present during loading, phagocytosis was only enhanced by about 400% and serum almost trebled this effect. The extent of phagocytosis attained without AS in these cells was not significantly different from that of cells loaded in the nominal absence of divalent cations, thus suggesting they contain almost a comparable very-low ionized Ca concentration.

These results show first, that free internal Ca^{2+} is required for phagocytosis and that serum enhances its effect, thus confirming previous findings. Secondly, cells loaded in the nominal absence of both Ca^{2+} and $Mg^{2+}$are more prone to become phagocytosed with serum present. This increased propensity to phagocytosis is

TABLE 1 | The effect on phagocytosis of Mg omission during erythrocyte loading.

Additions to loading medium			Addition to assay medium	*P*
Ca^{2+} (µM)	0 Mg	0.15 Mg (mM)	AS (40%)	
0	1.70 ± 0.85^{a} (6)	0.76 ± 0.23^{e} (3)	−	(a-b)*
				(a-e)$^{n.s}$
				(a-g)$^{n.s}$
	4.30 ± 2.65^{b} (6)	0.98 ± 0.23^{f} (3)	+	(e-f)$^{n.s}$
				(b-f)*
				(b-d)***
20	14.6 ± 4.82^{c} (5)	-	−	(c-a)***
				(c-d)*
	27.0 ± 4.94^{d} (4)	-	+	(d-a)***
100	-	2.70 ± 0.30^{g} (3)	−	(g-h)*
				(g-e)***
	-	9.0 ± 2.54^{h} (3)	+	(h-f)**
				(h-b)*

RBCs were loaded with and without Ca in choline medium, in the absence and presence of Mg. When Ca was present, it was added at 20 and 100 µM free concentrations in solutions lacking or not Mg, respectively. Loaded cells were then assayed for phagocytosis in RPMI medium to which autologous serum (AS) was added or not. The phagocytosis degree (in percent) is presented as mean value ± SD of mean from the number of experiments shown in parenthesis. The probability (P) derived from statistical comparison of the data indicated with letters is also given. The degree of significance rises with increasing number of asterisks and (n.s) denotes not significant. See the text for further details.

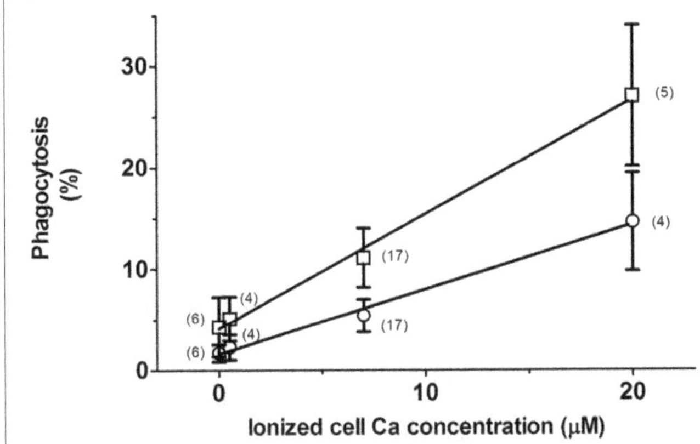

FIGURE 1 | Stimulation of erythrophagocytosis by internal Ca and autologous serum. RBCs were loaded with 0, 0.5, 7, and 20 µM ionic Ca concentrations in a choline medium without Mg. The extent of phagocytosis (in percent) after incubation without (circles) or with 40% AS (squares) is given as mean values of the number of experiments shown within parenthesis. Vertical bars represent ± 1SD of mean. Collected results from different experiments are given. The curves drawn correspond to linear regression lines, whose determination coefficients (r^2) are 0.997 and 0.994 for data from cells incubated with and without serum, respectively.

also attained by omitting Mg^{2+} during Ca^{2+} loading. Thirdly, phagocytosis is markedly diminished when loading with high ionic Ca^{2+} in the presence of Mg^{2+}.

Subsequent experiments were performed only on cells loaded with Ca^{2+} in the absence of Mg^{2+}.

Dependence of Phagocytosis on Intracellular Ca^{2+}

With the interest of determining the dependence of phagocytosis on internal Ca^{2+}, RBCs were loaded with 0, 0.5, 7, and 20 µM ionized Ca^{2+} concentrations. The process was then assayed in RPMI medium, to which 40% AS was added or not.

The extent of phagocytosis followed a strict linear relationship (correlation coefficient $r^2 = 0.994$) with the free Ca^{2+} content of cells (**Figure 1**). Accordingly, it was increased from about 2 to nearly 15% by raising Ca^{2+} from 0 to 20 µM, respectively. Addition of serum further stimulated phagocytosis by almost 100%, while keeping the relationship linear ($r^2 = 0.997$). These results clearly indicate that phagocytosis depends monotonically on the ionic cell Ca^{2+} content, whether in absence or presence of serum.

Effects of Preliminary Incubation of Macrophages with Liposomes

The results presented above undoubtedly show that phagocytosis is stimulated by a rise in the free Ca^{2+} content of erythrocytes. This ion is a well-known modulator of PS externalization in human RBCs (Bitbol et al., 1987; Williamson et al., 1992), which in turn constitutes an important signal for macrophage recognition and erythrocyte removal (Schroit et al., 1985). To investigate if the Ca^{2+} action is related to PS exposure, macrophages were preincubated with PS-containing liposomes in RPMI medium. As control, macrophages were similarly exposed to PC liposomes. After washing, macrophages were challenged with 7 µM Ca^{2+}-loaded RBCs, in the presence and absence of 40% AS.

As was expected, after exposing macrophages to PC-containing liposomes, the extent of phagocytosis was not much different to that obtained with untreated ones. Thus, the mean phagocytosis value from two separate experiments was 7.5 and 11.9%, without and with serum, respectively (compare with data of **Figure 1**). In marked contrast, after pretreating macrophages with PS-containing liposomes, the corresponding phagocytosis only amounted to 2.4 and 6.4%, respectively. These results demonstrate that phagocytosis of Ca^{2+}-loaded RBCs is selectively affected by previous exposure of macrophages to a PS carrier, being almost fully blocked in the absence of AS whilst partially affected in its presence.

Influence on Phagocytosis of Serum IgG Removal and Autologous IgG Supply

To study whether stimulation of phagocytosis by AS depends essentially on the IgG content, the latter was selectively removed from serum by adsorption to protein A. This procedure appeared satisfactorily accomplished when monitored by SDS-PAGE analyses, producing two fractions: one corresponding to IgG-depleted serum and the other consisting of purified IgG. These were tested on RBCs loaded with 7 µM free Ca^{2+}.

As was expected, phagocytosis increased high significantly from nearly 6 to about 12% after adding either 40% AS or 2 mg/ml purified IgG (**Figure 2**). To our surprise, it was similarly stimulated by IgG-depleted AS. This effect, however, was completely abolished by heating depleted serum for 30 min at 55°C. Thus, phagocytosis reached about 5% under this condition, a value not statistically different from that obtained without serum (**Figure 2**).

Microscopic observations showed that RBCs having different degrees of shrinking were phagocytosed following above treatments. Cell shapes varied from echinocytes to smooth spheres in spite that they were homogenously loaded with Ca^{2+}. No preferential shape to be phagocytosed was evident. **Figure 3** illustrates some aspects of this process under the various conditions studied.

The above results demonstrate that the stimulatory action of AS can be replaced with equal potency by affinity-purified autologous IgG. The findings also show that enhancement of Ca^{2+}-dependent phagocytosis by IgG-depleted serum seems related to complement activity.

Action of Gárdos Channel Blockers

Early work has proposed an involvement of the Gárdos channel in the physiological dismissal of senescent RBCs (Romero and Romero, 1999a). Therefore, it was of interest to assess the effect on phagocytosis of some inhibitors of this channel. When incorporated, they were present throughout the whole experimental procedure, at concentrations at least 10 times higher than their corresponding IC_{50}. Two selective blockers were chosen. The potent inhibitor clotrimazole (CLT) was the first to be tested on RBCs loaded with 0.5 and 7 μM ionized Ca. Phagocytosis was assayed with and without 40% AS, in the presence and absence of 2 μM CLT.

As expected, adding AS to 7 μM Ca^{2+}-loaded cells brought about a highly significant stimulation of phagocytosis to nearly 10% (**Figure 4**). Remarkably, this action was fully blocked by CLT. Thus, the extent of phagocytosis obtained with serum plus CLT was about 4%, a value not statistically different from that of control cells without serum. These results were reproduced employing RBCs loaded with 0.5 μM Ca^{2+}, but a lower phagocytosis degree was attained (**Figure 4**).

Almost identical findings were obtained by replacing CLT with TRAM-34, a highly selective channel blocker. Accordingly, in three separate experiments on cells loaded with 7 μM Ca^{2+}, phagocytosis (in percent ± 1 SD of mean) was significantly increased from 5.6 ± 1.35 to 10.1 ± 2.08 ($P < 0.05$) when 40% AS was added. In contrast, in the presence of 100 nM TRAM, the extent of phagocytosis without and with serum did not differ

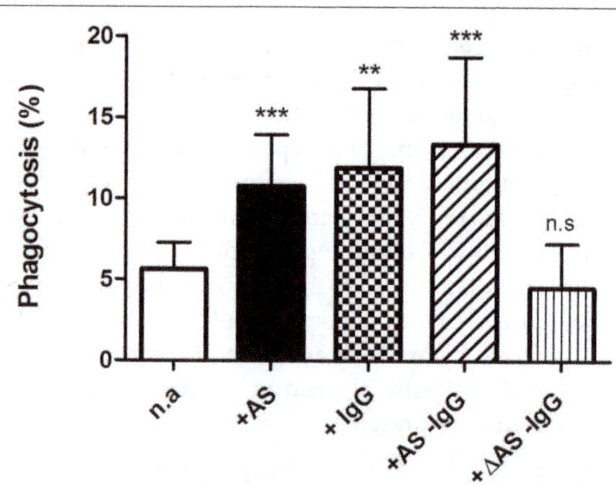

FIGURE 2 | Parallel enhancement of erythrophagocytosis by IgG and serum IgG depletion. Phagocytosis of 7 μM Ca-loaded cells was assessed (in percent) after 2 h incubation in RPMI medium, with no addition (n.a) or after adding 40% autologous serum (+AS), 2 mg/ml purified IgG (+IgG), 40% IgG-depleted serum (+AS −IgG), or 40% IgG-depleted serum inactivated by heat (+ΔAS −IgG). Results from ten experiments are shown as mean value ± 1SD of mean, except for purified IgG and heat inactivation conditions where only four experiments are included. Vertical bars indicate the SD. Asterisks number denotes statistical significance and n.s stands for not significant. See the text for further details.

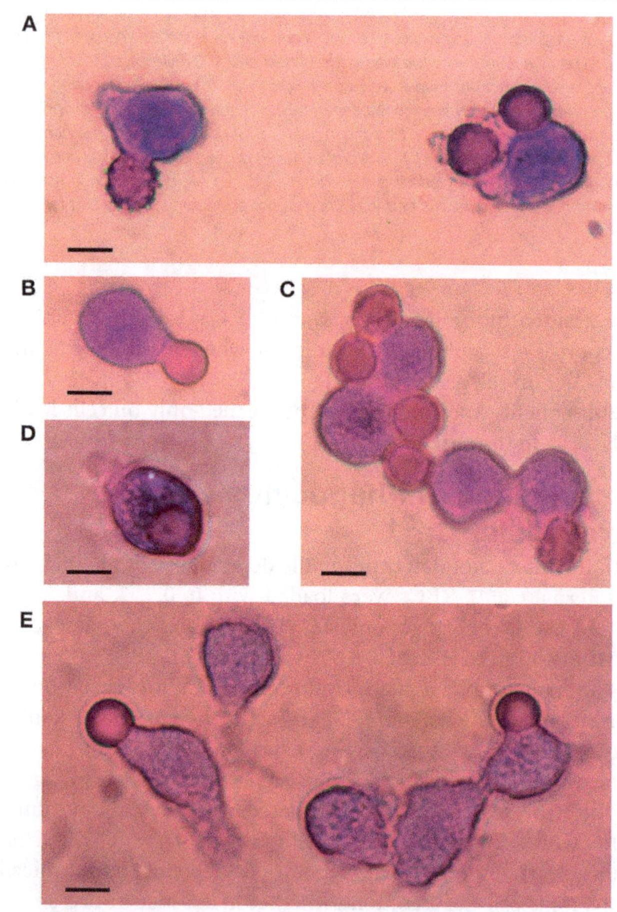

FIGURE 3 | Phagocytosis of Ca^{2+}-loaded RBCs. Illustrative images of Wright-stained cells are shown in this composite figure. Ca^{2+}-loaded RBCs (7 μM) were incubated for 2 h in RPMI medium, in the absence **(A)** and presence of AS **(B)**, affinity-purified IgG **(C)**, IgG-depleted serum **(D)** and inactivated IgG-depleted serum **(E)**. Notice late stages of echinocytes: crenated and smooth spheres, undergoing phagocytosis. Bars represent 10 μm.

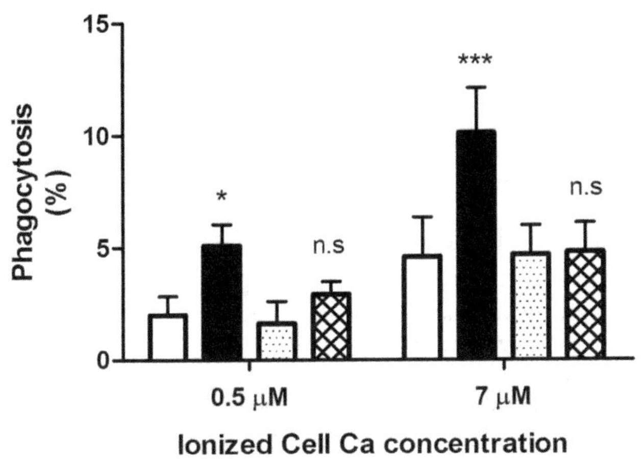

FIGURE 4 | Blocking by clotrimazole of serum-dependent erythrophagocytosis. RBCs were loaded with 0.5 and 7 μM ionic Ca concentrations in a choline medium, with and without 2 μM clotrimazole. Phagocytosis of loaded cells was determined (in percent) following incubation in RPMI medium without (white and dotted columns) and with 40% AS (black and cross-hatched columns), in the presence (dotted and cross-hatched columns) and absence (white and black columns) of clotrimazole. Cells were treated with the azole throughout the whole experiment. Results from five experiments are shown as mean value ± 1SD of mean. Vertical bars indicate the SD. Asterisks number denotes statistical significance and n.s stands for not significant. See the text for further details.

statistically from each other ($P > 0.05$), amounting to 4.4 ± 1.53 and 2.7 ± 2.15, respectively.

The above results clearly demonstrate that Gárdos channel blockers inhibit selectively the stimulatory activity of AS on phagocytosis, strongly indicating an involvement of this channel.

DISCUSSION

A common finding with normal human RBCs is the increase of internal Ca^{2+} that occurs during cell aging (Shiga et al., 1985; Aiken et al., 1992; Romero et al., 1997; Lew et al., 2007), thus suggesting a cause-effect interrelation. Modification of internal Ca^{2+} by ionophore loading was employed here as a model for studying some aspects of RBC aging leading to phagocytic clearance. Accordingly, cells were loaded by incubating with EGTA-buffered low-μM free Ca^{2+} concentrations instead of mM levels (i.e., 1–2 mM), that most likely would promote eryptosis (Lang K. S. et al., 2003; Lang et al., 2005; Romero, 2011). These cells were subsequently challenged with activated macrophages under various conditions, to gain insight into the mechanisms through which Ca^{2+} might promote erythrophagocytosis.

Effect on Phagocytosis of Mg^{2+} Omission and Influence of Ca^{2+}

In order to establish a reliable relation between phagocytosis and free internal Ca^{2+}, loading with this ion was accomplished by using the divalent cation selective ionophore A23187 in Mg^{2+}-free choline medium, which would simultaneously deplete RBCs of Mg^{2+}. It should be stressed that by lacking ATP-Mg, the true Ca^{2+} pump substrate, Mg^{2+}-depleted cells are incapable of extruding Ca^{2+} (Schatzmann and Vincenzi, 1969). Therefore, internal Ca^{2+} is kept constant during phagocytosis. We did not attempt to measure intracellular Ca^{2+} in these cells. However, the ionized concentration should equal that present in the loading medium, if no major changes of internal pH take place.

On the other hand, the lack of Mg^{2+} during loading with A23187 in Na-containing media causes RBC membrane disturbances leading to increased mechanical fragility and enhanced permeability (Romero, 1974). The final outcome is hemolysis since the ionophore also catalyzes rapid Na transport in the complete absence of divalent cations (Flatman and Lew, 1977). These effects are markedly reduced or blunted by replacing Na by choline or adding low Mg^{2+} or Ca^{2+} concentrations to the loading medium (Flatman and Lew, 1977).

The present study showed that RBCs exposed to ionophore in the virtual absence of both Ca^{2+} and Mg^{2+}, were phagocytosed to an equal low-extent than cells whose free internal Mg^{2+} was kept at normal levels by adding Mg^{2+} during loading, thus suggesting a comparable cell behavior. However, such a basal phagocytosis was increased significantly on AS addition whilst it was not affected if Mg^{2+} was present during loading. This observation indicates that some membrane alterations may have taken place in (Ca^{2+} + Mg^{2+})-depleted cells, despite they apparently maintained normal integrity and permeability after ionophore removal. Since these changes appeared evident on serum addition, it seems likely that new antigenic epitopes or binding sites became accessible on these cells.

Confirming and extending previous findings (Romero and Romero, 1999a), basal phagocytosis was stimulated significantly by rising ionized Ca in Mg^{2+}-depleted RBCs. Of note, erythrocytes loaded with 100 μM Ca^{2+} in the presence of Mg^{2+} were less prone to phagocytosis than those cells loaded with five times less free Ca^{2+} but in the absence of Mg^{2+}. Such dissimilarities in phagocytic extents can be attributed indeed to active Ca^{2+} extrusion. In spite of a rapid ATP breakdown occurring by Ca^{2+} pump activity during loading, Mg^{2+}-containing cells would restore their ATP content through glycolysis as substrates become available during cell handling and phagocytosis. Under such conditions, however, the amount of free Ca^{2+} remaining in cells is unknown.

The extent of phagocytosis attained after loading Mg^{2+}-depleted cells with 0.5 μM free Ca^{2+}, was not much at variance with that reported for young human RBCs employing a roughly comparable phagocytosis model (Luján-Brajovich et al., 2009). This may lend some support for validating the use of above cells in our present study.

The results shown here disclose Ca^{2+} as first messenger of a chain of events leading to phagocytosis. Accordingly, its action appears multiple, promoting activation of various processes such as PS externalization, IgG binding, complement deposition and Gárdos channel activity, which shall be discussed separately.

Dependence of Phagocytosis on Ca^{2+}-Associated PS Exposure

Our results have clearly shown that phagocytosis of Mg^{2+}-depleted, Ca^{2+}-loaded cells was blocked after preincubating macrophages with liposomes that contained a mixture of PS plus PC. No such an effect was found when they were made of PC as the only phospholipid. Remarkably, phagocytosis was almost fully inhibited in the absence of AS whilst partially affected in its presence. These results suggest that two distinct processes are involved: one that occurs with no serum present and which is selectively blocked by PS. The other seems unrelated to PS and expressed in presence of serum, as referred to later. These findings are in agreement with the stereospecific inhibition of apoptotic-lymphocyte phagocytosis by liposomes containing the L-serine form of PS (Fadok et al., 1992). They strongly indicate that PS externalization mediates phagocytosis of Mg^{2+}-depleted cells loaded with Ca^{2+}.

Since APLT is inactive in above cells due to both Ca^{2+} presence and lack of ATP-Mg, the true enzyme substrate (Morrot et al., 1990), stimulation by Ca^{2+} of phospholipid scramblase (TMEM16F) readily leads to PS exposure (Williamson et al., 1992; Bratton et al., 1997; Williamson, 2015). This appears the main mechanism for PS externalization on Mg^{2+}-depleted RBCs. Contribution of other known mechanisms seems unlikely for the following considerations. First, it is recognized that Gárdos channel activity promotes PS exposure on human RBCs (Lang P. A. et al., 2003; Wesseling et al., 2016). However, a similar action on Ca^{2+}-loaded, Mg^{2+}-depleted cells is highly improbable since phagocytosis was unaltered by adding Gárdos channel inhibitors in the absence of AS, as shall be discussed later. Additionally, such findings also discard the possibility of a shrinkage-related PS externalization, as reported for RBCs under hyperosmotic shock (Lang et al., 2004). Secondly, it is known that protein kinase Cα activity is involved in PS exposure on human RBCs (de Jong et al., 2002). Nonetheless, recent work showed that selective enzyme inhibitors (chelerytine, calphostin) hardly affect the PS externalization induced by A23187 plus Ca^{2+} in above cells (Wesseling et al., 2016), thereby indicating that protein kinase Cα is not responsible for PS scrambling in Ca^{2+}-loaded, Mg^{2+}-depleted RBCs.

Significantly, due to the intrinsic characteristic of being Mg^{2+}-depleted cells, their phagocytosis dependence on PS exposure disclosed by our aging model, roughly resembles that of eryptosis, a process evoked at much higher Ca^{2+} levels (Lang et al., 2005). Unlike with the latter, however, the extent of PS externalization does not increase during the normal RBC lifespan (Boas et al., 1998; Lutz, 2004; Willekens et al., 2008; Ghashghaeinia et al., 2012; Franco et al., 2013), thus demonstrating that it is not tagging signal for clearance of senescent RBCs. Nonetheless, it is still an open question as to whether PS becomes exposed on those cells already sequestered, that become inaccessible to analyses. Such an answer obviously cannot be tested experimentally for ethical reasons. Perhaps, the cell model used here may help in approaching this problem.

On the other hand, erythrocyte vesicles bearing PS and IgG are shed from the membrane during the normal RBC lifespan, in a way presumably associated to PS externalization (Willekens et al., 2008). Microvesicles are also produced when RBCs are exposed to the combined action of A23187 plus Ca^{2+} (Allan and Michell, 1977). We have observed no vesicles in our preparation that may have interfered with the phagocytosis assay as PS-containing liposomes did. Most probably, this was due to their dismissal by the low centrifugal force employed for cell wash following ionophore loading.

Action on Phagocytosis of Serum IgG Removal and Autologous IgG supply

Very early work has shown the need of AS for promoting erythrophagocytosis by leukocytes *in vitro* (Greendyke et al., 1963). It is also widely known the general requirement of erythrocyte opsonization for phagocytosis by professional macrophages (de Back et al., 2014). In accordance with this assertion and confirming previous work (Romero and Romero, 1999a), phagocytosis of Ca^{2+}-loaded RBCs was further enhanced by addition of 40% AS. This effect, like that attained without serum, exhibited a linear relationship with increasing ionized Ca, thus revealing a monotonic nature of activation. At all Ca^{2+} concentrations tested the magnitude of stimulation by AS doubled that obtained in its absence. We did not explore other serum concentrations, not knowing if that presently employed was the optimal.

Notably, the extent of phagocytosis reached with either 2 mg/ml purified IgG or 40% IgG-depleted serum, was practically identical to that attained with AS. The former IgG concentration is roughly equivalent to that of IgG present in 40% AS (about 3 mg/ml). These findings demonstrate on the one hand, that serum can be replaced by IgG stimulating phagocytosis with equal potency, thereby suggesting that its action can be accounted for by its IgG content. On the other hand, they also show that phagocytosis can be equally enhanced with similar potency by serum in a non-IgG dependent way. The latter action was suppressed by preheating IgG-depleted serum under conditions well established to inactivate the complement system (Soltis et al., 1979); strongly suggesting that complement activity is involved in such stimulation. In addition, the findings indicate that IgG is not needed for complement-stimulated phagocytosis of Mg^{2+}-depleted Ca^{2+}-loaded RBCs. This action was not studied further. Other normal serum factors that may be required for erythrophagocytosis could also be affected by heating.

Taking into consideration all preceding findings it becomes evident that at least, Ca^{2+} promotes phagocytosis of Mg^{2+}-depleted RBCs via three apparently independent processes. The first is elicited in the absence of serum, and is mediated through PS exposure. The second is related to AS stimulation and presumably is mediated mostly by IgG, and the third one, corresponds to that associated with complement activation. The latter two processes seem to exert a sort of additive action on the former.

Erythrophagocytosis Inhibition by Gárdos Channel Blockers

The main finding of the present work was the action on phagocytosis of two Gárdos channel inhibitors. First, the azole containing compound CLT that at 2 μM, completely inhibited serum-dependent phagocytosis of cells loaded with 0.5 and 7 μM free Ca^{2+}. This compound is a well-known potent channel inhibitor (IC_{50} = 50 nM in normal RBCs) (Alvarez et al., 1992). Though selective, however, it is a non-specific inhibitor since its interactions with a wide number of unrelated targets possessing dissimilar CLT affinities have been reported (Thomas et al., 1999; Klokouzas et al., 2001; Zhang et al., 2002).

The second blocker used, TRAM-34, is a triphenylmethane compound possessing a pyrazole moiety instead of an azole one, for which neither inhibits cytochrome P450-dependent enzymes nor exhibit the toxic CLT side effects. TRAM-34 is a highly-selective Gárdos channel inhibitor, having an IC_{50} = 20 nM (Wulff et al., 2000). This compound at 100 nM fully inhibited the AS-dependent phagocytosis of 7 μM Ca^{2+}-loaded RBCs, thus confirming above findings with CLT.

The inhibitory effect of CLT and TRAM-34 just described clearly demonstrates a specific participation of the Gárdos channel in erythrophagocytosis. As these compounds fully blocked phagocytosis only in the presence of AS, the results disclose a peculiar involvement of this channel.

Possible Involvement of the Gárdos Channel in Erythrophagocytosis

It is widely recognized that band 3 aggregations occurs in RBCs exposed to oxidative stress, with resultant IgG binding and complement deposition (Low et al., 1985; Lutz et al., 1987; Turrini et al., 1991; Lutz, 2012). Based on these findings, some consensus has been reached for the proposal that oxidative stress, acting via band 3 peroxidation of cytosolic domain and concomitant binding of met-hemoglobin and hemichromes, may be the physiological trigger for such aggregation (Low et al., 1985; Arese et al., 2005; Lutz, 2012; Lutz and Bogdanova, 2013; Mohanty et al., 2014). In addition to these effects, oxidative stress or defects of antioxidative defense also enhance RBC Ca^{2+} entry (Lang K. S. et al., 2003), thus involving this ion in the above process.

It is quite feasible that Ca^{2+} can promote band 3 aggregation in Mg^{2+}-depleted cells, as demonstrated by its action on the distribution of intramembrane particles in human RBC ghosts (Elgsaeter et al., 1976), believed to consist of band 3 macromolecular complexes (Verkleij and Ververgaert, 1978). Interaction of Ca^{2+} with cytoskeletal proteins is known to loosen the cytoskeleton network, weakening its anchorage to integral membrane proteins (Bogdanova et al., 2013). Consequently, a larger number of band 3 dimers are freed to move within the lipid bilayer plane, becoming capable of forming multimers and higher aggregates.

It is conceivable that upon Gárdos channel activation, the consequent membrane deformation and presumably hydrophobic mismatch imposed by dehydration, acting in concert with the loosening of band 3 cytoskeletal anchorage, may drive clustering of band 3 aggregates. The latter would lead to an increased IgG binding and presumably complement deposition, thus signaling macrophages for recognition and phagocytosis (Turrini et al., 1991; Lutz, 2004; Arese et al., 2005). This may explain the selective inhibition of AS-dependent phagocytosis by Gárdos channel inhibitors reported in the present study, and place the findings into a physiological context.

It is quite remarkable that a wide variety of hemolytic anemia, including sickle cell disease, thalassemia, Gárdos channelopathy, and both hereditary spherocytosis and xerocytosis, are associated to RBC Ca^{2+} overloading (Bookchin et al., 1988; Lew et al., 2002; Fermo et al., 2017; Hertz et al., 2017). The fate of such pathological cells, like that of senescent cells is to become phagocytosed by macrophages. Thus, it is not surprising a convergence of tagging signals in these cells for macrophage clearance. Aging and eryptosis may share the same final mechanisms for RBC dismissal (Romero, 2011). Along the same idea, recent work have put forward the hypothesis that an increased internal Ca^{2+} is the common component in the mechanism causing an accelerated RBCs clearance in some hemolytic anemia (Hertz et al., 2017).

In conclusion, the results presented in this work indicate that a rise in free internal Ca^{2+} is fundamental for promoting phagocytosis by autologous macrophages *in vitro*.

AUTHOR CONTRIBUTIONS

PR and CH-C contribute equally in designing, performing and analyzing the experimental data.

ACKNOWLEDGMENTS

The authors wish to express their gratitude to the volunteers that participated as subjects in the present study.

REFERENCES

Aiken, N., Satterlee, J. D., and Galey, W. R. (1992). Measurement of intracellular Ca^{2+} in young and old human erythrocytes using ^{19}F-NMR spectroscopy. *Biochim. Biophys. Acta* 1136, 155–160. doi: 10.1016/0167-4889(92)90251-6

Allan, D., and Michell, R. H. (1977). Calcium ion-dependent diacylglycerol accumulation in erythrocytes is associated with microvesiculation but not with efflux of potassium ions. *Biochem. J.* 166, 495–499. doi: 10.1042/bj1660495

Alvarez, J., Montero, M., and Garcia-Sancho, J. (1992). High affinity inhibition of Ca^{2+}-dependent K^+ channels by cytochrome P-450 inhibitors. *J. Biol. Chem.* 267, 11789–11793.

Antonelou, M. H., Kriebardis, A. G., and Papassideri, I. S. (2010). Aging and death signalling in mature red cells: from basic science to transfusion practice. *Blood Transfus.* 8(Suppl. 3), s39–s47. doi: 10.2450/2010.007S

Arese, P., Turrini, F., and Schwarzer, E. (2005). Band 3/complement-mediated recognition and removal of normally senescent and pathological human erythrocytes. *Cell. Physiol. Biochem.* 16, 133–146. doi: 10.1159/000089839

Berlin, N. I., and Berk, P. D. (1975). "The biological life of the red cell," in *The Red Blood Cell*, ed D. M. Surgenor (New York; San Francisco; London: Academic Press), 957–1019.

Bitbol, M., Fellmann, P., Zachowski, A., and Devaux, P. F. (1987). Ion regulation of phosphatidylserine and phosphatidylethanolamine outside-inside translocation in human erythrocytes. *Biochim. Biophys. Acta* 904, 268–282. doi: 10.1016/0005-2736(87)90376-2

Boas, F. E., Forman, L., and Beutler, E. (1998). Phosphatidylserine exposure and red cell viability in red cell aging and in hemolytic anemia. *Proc. Natl. Acad. Sci. U.S.A.* 95, 3077–3081. doi: 10.1073/pnas.95.6.3077

Bogdanova, A., Makhro, A., Wang, J., Lipp, P., and Kaestner, L. (2013). Calcium in red blood cells - a perilous balance. *Int. J. Mol. Sci.* 14, 9848–9872. doi: 10.3390/ijms14059848

Bookchin, R. M., Ortiz, O. E., Shalev, O., Tsurei, S., Rachmilewitz, E. A., Hockaday, A., et al. (1988). Calcium transport and ultrastructure of red cells in betathalassemia intermedia. *Blood* 72, 1602–1607.

Bosman, G. J., Willekens, F. L., and Were, J. M. (2005). Erythrocyte aging: a more than superficial resemblance to apoptosis? *Cell. Physiol. Biochem.* 16, 1–8. doi: 10.1159/000087725

Bratosin, D., Mazurier, J., Tissier, J. P., Estaquier, J., Huart, J. J., Ameisen, J. C., et al. (1998). Cellular and molecular mechanisms of senescent erythrocyte phagocytosis by macrophages. A review. *Biochimie* 80, 173–185. doi: 10.1016/S0300-9084(98)80024-2

Bratton, D. L., Fadok, V. A., Richter, D. A., Kailey, J. M., Guthrie, L. A., and Henson, P. M. (1997). Appearance of phosphatidylserine on apoptotic cells requires calcium-mediated nonspecific flip-flop and is enhanced by loss of the aminophospholipid translocase. *J. Biol. Chem.* 272, 26159–26165. doi: 10.1074/jbc.272.42.26159

Burger, P., Hilarius-Stokman, P., de Korte, D., van den Berg, T. K., and van Bruggen, R. (2012). CD47 functions as a molecular switch for erythrocyte phagocytosis. *Blood* 119, 5512–5521. doi: 10.1182/blood-2011-10-386805

Ciana, A., Achilli, C., Gaur, A., and Minetti, G. (2017). Membrane remodelling and vesicle formation during ageing of human red blood cells. *Cell. Physiol. Biochem.* 42:1127–1138. doi: 10.1159/000478768

Ciana, A., Minetti, G., and Balduini, C. (2004). Phosphotyrosine phosphatases acting on band 3 in human erythrocytes of different age: PTP1B processing during cell ageing. *Bioelectrochemistry* 62, 169–173. doi: 10.1016/j.bioelechem.2003.07.004

Clark, M. R. (1988). Senescence of red blood cells, progress and problems. *Physiol. Rev.* 68, 503–555.

Dagher, G., and Lew, V. L. (1988). Maximal calcium extrusion capacity and stoichiometry of the human red cell calcium pump. *J. Physiol.* 407, 569–586. doi: 10.1113/jphysiol.1988.sp017432

de Back, D. Z., Kostova, E. B., van Kraaij, M., van den Bergand, T. K., and van Bruggen, R. (2014). Of macrophages and red blood cells; a complex love story. *Front. Physiol.* 5:9. doi: 10.3389/fphys.2014.00009

de Jong, K., Rettig, M. P., Low, P. S., and Kuypers, F. A. (2002). Protein kinase C activation induces phosphatidylserine exposure on red blood cells. *Biochemistry* 41, 12562–12567. doi: 10.1021/bi025882o

Elgsaeter, A., Shotton, D. M., and Branton, D. (1976). Intramembrane particle aggregation in erythrocyte ghosts. II. The influence of spectrin aggregation. *Biochim. Biophys. Acta* 426, 101–122. doi: 10.1016/0005-2736(76)90433-8

Elliott, M. R., and Ravichandran, K. S. (2010). Clearance of apoptotic cells: implications in health and disease. *J. Cell Biol.* 189, 1059–1070. doi: 10.1083/jcb.201004096

Fabiato, A., and Fabiato, F. (1979). Calculator programs for computing the composition of the solutions containing multiple metals and ligands used for experiments in skinned muscle cells. *J. Physiol. (Paris)* 75, 463–505.

Fadok, V. A., Voelker, D. R., Campbell, P. A., Cohen, J. J., Bratton, D. L., and Henson, P. M. (1992). Exposure of phosphatidylserine on the surface of apoptotic lymphocytes triggers specific recognition and removal by macrophages. *J. Immunol.* 148, 2207–2216.

Fermo, E., Bogdanova, A., Petkova-Kirova, P., Zaninoni, A., Marcello, A. P., Makhro, A., et al. (2017). 'Gardos Channelopathy': a variant of hereditary stomatocytosis with complex molecular regulation. *Sci. Rep.* 7:1744. doi: 10.1038/s41598-017-01591-w

Flatman, P. W., and Lew, V. L. (1977). Does ionophore A23187 mediate Na transport in the absence of divalent cations? *Nature* 270, 444–445. doi: 10.1038/270444a0

Flatman, P. W., and Lew, V. L. (1980). Magnesium buffering in intact human red blood cells measured using the ionophore A23187. *Nature (Lond.)* 305, 13–30. doi: 10.1113/jphysiol.1980.sp013346

Franco, R. S., Puchulu-Campanella, M. E., Barber, L. A., Palascak, M. B., Joiner, C. H., Low, P. S., et al. (2013). Changes in the properties of normal human red blood cells during *in vivo* aging. *Am. J. Hematol.* 88, 44–51. doi: 10.1002/ajh.23344

Freshney, R. (1987). *Culture of Animal Cells: A Manual of Basic Technique*. New York, NY: Alan R. Liss Inc.

Galili, U., Rachmilewitz, E. A., Peleg, A., and Flechner, I. (1984). A unique natural human IgG antibody with anti-α-galactosyl specificity. *J. Exp. Med.* 160, 1519–1531. doi: 10.1084/jem.160.5.1519

Ghashghaeinia, M., Cluitmans, J. C., Akel, A., Dreischer, P.,Toulany, M., Koberle, M., et al. (2012). The impact of erythrocyte age on eryptosis. *Br. J. Haematol.* 157, 606–614. doi: 10.1111/j.1365-2141.2012.09100.x

Greendyke, R. M., Brierty, R. E., Swisher, S. M., Trabold, N., and Ryser, R. (1963). *In vitro* studies on erythrophagocytosis. *Blood* 22, 295–312.

Hanayama, R., Tanaka, M., Miwa, K., Shinohara, A., Iwamatsu, A., and Nagata, S. (2002). Identification of a factor that links apoptotic cells to phagocytes. *Nature* 417, 182–187. doi: 10.1038/417182a

Hertz, L., Huisjes, R., Llaudet-Planas, E., Petkova-Kirova, P., Makhro, A., Danielczok, J. G., et al. (2017). Is increased intracellular calcium in red blood cells a common component in the molecular mechanism causing anemia? *Front. Physiol.* 8:673. doi: 10.3389/fphys.2017.00673

Kannan, R., Yuan, J., and Low, P. S. (1991). Isolation and partial characterization of antibody and globin-enriched complexes from membranes of dense human erythrocytes. *Biochem. J.* 278, 57–62. doi: 10.1042/bj2780057

Kiefer, C. R., and Snyder, L. M. (2000). Oxidation and erythrocyte senescence. *Curr. Opin. Hematol.* 7, 113–116. doi: 10.1097/00062752-200003000-00007

Klokouzas, A., Barrand, M. A., and Hladky, S. B. (2001). Effects of clotrimazole on transport mediated by multidrug resistance associated protein 1 (MRP1) in human erythrocytes and tumour cells. *Eur. J. Biochem.* 268, 6569–6577. doi: 10.1046/j.0014-2956.2001.02611.x

Kobayashi, N., Karisola, P., Pena-Cruz, V., Dorfman, D. M., Jinushi, M., Umetsu, S. E., et al. (2007).TIM-1and TIM-4 glycoproteins bind phosphatidylserine and mediate uptake of apoptotic cells. *Immunity* 27, 927–940. doi: 10.1016/j.immuni.2007.11.011

Laemmli, U. K. (1970). Cleavage of structural proteins during the assembly of the head of bacteriophage T4. *Nature (Lond.)* 227, 680–685. doi: 10.1038/227680a0

Lang, K. S., Duranton, C., Poehlmann, H., Myssina, S., C, Bauer, C., Lang, F., et al. (2003). Cation channels trigger apoptotic death of erythrocytes. *Cell Death Differ.* 10, 249–256. doi: 10.1038/sj.cdd.4401144

Lang, K. S., Lang, P. A., Bauer, C., Duranton, C., Wieder, T., Huber, S. M., et al. (2005). Mechanisms of suicidal erythrocyte death. *Cell Physiol. Biochem.* 15, 195–202. doi: 10.1159/000086406

Lang, K. S., Myssina, S., Brand, V., Sandu, C., Lang, P. A., Berchtold, S., et al. (2004). Involvement of ceramide in hyperosmotic shock-induced death of erythrocytes. *Cell Death Differ.* 11, 231–243. doi: 10.1038/sj.cdd.4401311

Lang, P. A., Kaiser, S., Myssina, S., Wieder, T., Lang, F., and Huber, S. M. (2003). Role of Ca^{2+}-activated K^+ channels in human erythrocyte apoptosis. *Am. J. Physiol. Cell Physiol.* 285, C1553–C1560. doi: 10.1152/ajpcell.00186.2003

Lew, V. L., Daw, N., Etzion, Z., Tiffert, T., Muoma, A., Vanagas, L., et al. M. (2007). Effects of age-dependent membrane transport changes on the homeostasis of senescent human red blood cells. *Blood* 110, 1334–1342. doi: 10.1182/blood-2006-11-057232

Lew, V. L., Etzion, Z., and Bookchin, R. M. (2002). Dehydration response of sickle cells to sickling-induced Ca. *Blood* 99, 2578–2585. doi: 10.1182/blood.V99.7.2578

Low, P. S., Waugh, S. M., Zinke, K., and Drenckhahn, D. (1985). The role of hemoglobin denaturation and Band 3 clustering in red blood cell aging. *Science* 227, 531–533. doi: 10.1126/science.2578228

Lowry, O. H., Rosebrough, N. J., Farr, A. L., and Randall, R. J. (1951). Protein measurements with the Folin phenol reagent. *J. Biol. Chem.* 193, 265–275.

Luján-Brajovich, M., Rucci, A., Acosta, I. L., Cotorruelo, C., García-Borrás, S., Racca, L., et al. (2009). Effects of aging on antioxidant response and phagocytosis in senescent erythrocytes. *Immunol. Invest.* 38, 551–559. doi: 10.1080/08820130902888383

Lutz, H. A., Bussolino, F., Flepp, R., Fasler, S., Stammler, P., Kazatchkine, M. D., et al. (1987). Naturally occurring anti-band-3 antibodies and complement together mediate phagocytosis of oxidatively stressed human erythrocytes. *Proc. Natl. Acad. Sci. U.S.A.* 84, 7368–7372. doi: 10.1073/pnas.84.21.7368

Lutz, H. U. (2004). Innate immune and non-immune mediators of erythrocyte clearance. *Cell. Mol. Biol.* 50, 107–116.

Lutz, H. U. (2012). Naturally occurring anti-Band 3 antibodies in clearance of senescent and oxidatively stressed human red blood cells. *Transfus. Med. Hemother.* 39, 321–327. doi: 10.1159/000342171

Lutz, H. U., and Bogdanova, A. (2013). Mechanisms tagging senescent red blood cells for clearance in healthy humans. *Front. Physiol.* 4:387. doi: 10.3389/fphys.2013.00387

Lutz, H. U., Flepp, R., and Stringaro-Wipf, G. (1984). Naturally occurring autoantibodies to exoplasmic and cryptic regions of band 3 protein, the major integral membrane protein of human red blood cells. *J. Immunol.* 133, 2610–2618.

Lutz, H. U., and Stringaro-Wipf, G. (1983). Senescent red cell-bound IgG is attached to band 3 protein. *Biomed. Biochim. Acta* 42, 117–121.

Martinac, B., and Cox, C. D. (2017). "Mechanosensory transduction: focus on ion channels," in *Reference Module in Life Sciences: Comprehensive Biophysics,* ed H.-X. Zhou (Oxford, UK: Elsevier Inc), 1–47.

McEvoy, L., Williamson, P., and Schlegel, R. A. (1986). Membrane phospholipid asymmetry as a determinant of erythrocyte recognition by macrophages. *Proc. Natl. Acad. Sci. U.S.A.* 83, 3311–3315. doi: 10.1073/pnas.83.10.3311

Mebius, R. E., and Kraal, G. (2005). Structure and function of the spleen. *Nature Immunol.* 5, 606–616. doi: 10.1038/nri1669

Mohanty, J. G., Nagababu, E., and Rifkind, J. M. (2014). Red blood cell oxidative stress impairs oxygen delivery and induces red blood cell aging. *Front. Physiol.* 5:84. doi: 10.3389/fphys.2014.00084

Morrot, G., Zachowski, A., and Devaux, P. F. (1990). Partial purification and characterization of the human erythrocyte Mg^{2+}-ATPase. A candidate aminophospholipid translocase. *FEBS Lett.* 266, 29–32. doi: 10.1016/0014-5793(90)81498-D

Oldenborg, P. A., Zheleznyak, A., Fang, Y. F., Lagenaur, C. F., Gresham, H. D., and Lindberg, F. P. (2000). Role of CD47 as a marker of self on red blood cells. *Science* 288, 2051–2054. doi: 10.1126/science.288.5473.2051

Park, S. Y., Jung, M. Y., Kim, H. J., Lee, S. J., Kim, S. Y., Lee, B. H., et al. (2008). Rapid cell corpse clearance by stabilin-2, a membrane phosphatidylserine receptor. *Cell Death Differ.* 15, 192–201. doi: 10.1038/sj.cdd.4402242

Reed, P. W., and Lardy, H. A. (1972). A23187: a divalent cation ionophore. *J. Biol. Chem.* 247, 6970–6977.

Rifkind, R. A. (1966). Destruction of injured red cells *in vivo. Am. J. Med.* 41, 711–723. doi: 10.1016/0002-9343(66)90032-5

Romero, P. J. (1974). The role of membrane-bound magnesium in the permeability of ghosts to K^+. *Biochim. Biophys. Acta* 339, 116–125. doi: 10.1016/0005-2736(74)90337-X

Romero, P. J. (1978). Is the Ca^{2+}-sensitive K^+ channel under metabolic control in human red cells? *Biochim. Biophys. Acta* 507, 178–181. doi: 10.1016/0005-2736(78)90385-1

Romero, P. J. (2011). "Calcium and cell ageing: the human red cell as a model," in *Advances in Medicine and Biology*, ed L. V. Bernhart (New York, NY: Nova Science Publisher Inc.), 24, 1–133.

Romero, P. J., and Romero, E. A. (1997). Differences in Ca^{2+} pumping activity between sub-populations of human red cells. *Cell Calcium* 21, 353–358. doi: 10.1016/S0143-4160(97)90028-2

Romero, P. J., and Romero, E. A. (1999a). The role of calcium metabolism in human red blood cell ageing: a proposal. *Blood Cells Mol. Dis.* 25, 9–19. doi: 10.1006/bcmd.1999.0222

Romero, P. J., and Romero, E. A. (1999b). The effect of cell ageing on Ca^{2+} influx into human red cells. *Cell Calcium* 26, 131–137. doi: 10.1054/ceca.1999.0063

Romero, P. J., Romero, E. A., and Winkler, B, M. D. (1997). Ionic calcium content of light and dense human red cells separated by Percoll density gradients. *Biochim. Biophys. Acta* 1323, 23–28. doi: 10.1016/S0005-2736(96)00141-1

Schatzmann, H. J., and Vincenzi, F. F. (1969). Calcium movements across the membrane of human red cells. *J. Physiol.* 201, 369–395. doi: 10.1113/jphysiol.1969.sp008761

Schroit, A. J., Madsen, J. W., and Tanaka, Y. (1985). *In vivo* recognition and clearance of red blood cells containing phosphatidylserine in their plasma membranes. *J. Biol. Chem.* 260, 5131–5138.

Segawa, K., and Nagata, S. (2015). An apoptotic 'Eat Me' signal: phosphatidylserine exposure. *Trends in Cell Biology* 25, 639–650. doi: 10.1016/j.tcb.2015.08.003

Shiga, T., Sekiya, M., Maeda, N., Kon, K., and Okazawa, M. (1985). Cell age-dependent changes in deformability and calcium accumulation of human erythrocytes. *Biochim. Biophys. Acta* 814, 289–299. doi: 10.1016/0005-2736(85)90447-X

Soltis, R. D., Hasz, D., Morris, M. J., and Wilson, I. D. (1979). The effect of heat inactivation of serum on aggregation of immunoglobulins. *Immunology* 36, 37–45.

Sorette, M. P., Galili, U., and Clark, M. R. (1991). Comparison of serum anti-band 3 and anti-gal antibody binding to density-separated human red blood cells. *Blood* 77, 628–636.

Thomas, G. P., Karmazyn, M., , Zygmunt, A. C., Antzelevitch, C., and Narayanan, N. (1999). The antifungal antibiotic clotrimazole potently inhibits L-type calcium current in guinea-pig ventricular myocytes. *Br. J. Pharmacol.* 126, 1531–1533. doi: 10.1038/sj.bjp.0702475

Turrini, F., Arese, P., Yuan, J., and Low, P. S. (1991). Clustering of integral membrane proteins of the human erythrocyte membrane stimulates autologous IgG binding, complement deposition, and phagocytosis. *J. Biol. Chem.* 266, 23611–23617.

Verkleij, A. J., and Ververgaert, P. H. (1978). Freeze-fracture morphology of biological membranes. *Biochim. Biophys. Acta* 515, 303–327. doi: 10.1016/0304-4157(78)90017-5

Wesseling, M. C., Wagner-Britz, L., Nguyen, D. B., Asanidze, S., Mutua, J., Mohamed, N., et al. (2016). Novel insights in the regulation of phosphatidylserine exposure in human red blood cells. *Cell. Physiol. Biochem.* 39, 1941–1954. doi: 10.1159/000447891

Willekens, F. L. A., Werre, J. M., Groenen-Döpp, Y. A. M., Roerdinkholder-Stoelwinder, B., de Pauw, B., and Bosman, G. J. (2008). Erythrocyte vesiculation: a self-protective mechanism? *Br. J. Haematol.* 141, 549–556. doi: 10.1111/j.1365-2141.2008.07055.x

Williamson, P. (2015). Phospholipid scramblases. *Lipid Insights* 8, 41–44. doi: 10.4137/LPI.S31785

Williamson, P., Kulick, A., Zachowski, A., Schlegel, R. A., and Devaux, P. F. (1992). Ca^{2+} induces transbilayer redistribution of all major phospholipids in human erythrocytes. *Biochemistry* 31, 6355–6360. doi: 10.1021/bi00142a027

Wulff, H., Miller, M. J., Hänsel, W., Grissmer, S., Cahalan, M. D., and Chandy, K. G. (2000). Design of a potent and selective inhibitor of the intermediate-conductance Ca^{2+}-activated K^+ channel, IKCa1: a potential immunosuppressant. *Proc. Natl. Acad. Sci. U.S.A.* 97, 8151–8156. doi: 10.1073/pnas.97.14.8151

Zhang, W., Ramamoorthy, Y., Kilicarslan, T., Nolte, H., Tyndale, R. F., and Sellers, E. M. (2002). Inhibition of cytochromes P450 by antifungal imidazole derivatives. *Drug Metab. Dispos.* 30, 314–318. doi: 10.1124/dmd.30.3.314

20

Continuous Change in Membrane and Membrane-Skeleton Organization During Development from Proerythroblast to Senescent Red Blood Cell

Giampaolo Minetti[1], Cesare Achilli[1], Cesare Perotti[2] and Annarita Ciana[1]*

[1] *Laboratori di Biochimica, Dipartimento di Biologia e Biotecnologie, Università degli Studi di Pavia, Pavia, Italy,* [2] *Servizio Immunoematologia e Medicina Trasfusionale, Fondazione IRCCS Policlinico San Matteo, Pavia, Italy*

Correspondence:
Giampaolo Minetti
minetti@unipv.it

Within the context of erythropoiesis and the possibility of producing artificial red blood cells (RBCs) *in vitro*, a most critical step is the final differentiation of enucleated erythroblasts, or reticulocytes, to a fully mature biconcave discocyte, the RBC. Reviewed here is the current knowledge about this fundamental maturational process. By combining literature data with our own experimental evidence we propose that the early phase in the maturation of reticulocytes to RBCs is driven by a membrane raft-based mechanism for the sorting of disposable membrane proteins, mostly the no longer needed transferrin receptor (TfR), to the multivesicular endosome (MVE) as cargo of intraluminal vesicles that are subsequently exocytosed as exosomes, consistently with the seminal and original observation of Johnstone and collaborators of more than 30 years ago (Pan BT, Johnstone RM. Cell. 1983;33:967-978). According to a strikingly selective sorting process, the TfR becomes cargo destined to exocytosis while other molecules, including the most abundant RBC transmembrane protein, band 3, are completely retained in the cell membrane. It is also proposed that while this process could be operating in the early maturational steps in the bone marrow, additional mechanism(s) must be at play for the final removal of the excess reticulocyte membrane that is observed to occur in the circulation. This processing will most likely require the intervention of the spleen, whose function is also necessary for the continuous remodeling of the RBC membrane all along this cell's circulatory life.

Keywords: artificial red blood cells, reticulocyte maturation, red blood cell ageing, multivesicular endosome, membrane rafts, fluid phase endocytosis, autophagy, spleen

> "In fact, it may almost be true to say that the red cell continuously changes until its senescent properties are recognized and it is eliminated from the circulation."
>
> (Ahn and Johnstone, 1991)

INTRODUCTION

Recapitulation of erythroid differentiation and amplification *in vitro* is an actively investigated topic for the potentially revolutionary impact on regeneration and transfusion medicine, for all the conditions where reintegration of functional blood volume is required. Significant advancements in the field have made it possible to expand and differentiate *in vitro* erythroid precursors to the stage of enucleation, starting from progenitor cells of various origin: embryonic stem cells (Lu et al., 2008; Ma et al., 2008); adult circulating CD34$^+$ cells (Migliaccio et al., 2002; Neildez-Nguyen et al., 2002; Giarratana et al., 2011; Griffiths et al., 2012b); CD34$^-$ mononuclear cells (MNC) (van den Akker et al., 2010; Tirelli et al., 2011); umbilical cord blood (Neildez-Nguyen et al., 2002; Leberbauer et al., 2005; Miharada et al., 2006; Baek et al., 2008; Kupzig et al., 2017) or even immortalized cell lines (Hiroyama et al., 2008; Trakarnsanga et al., 2017).

Paramount for the possibility of developing a simplified *in vitro* culture of RBCs was the discovery that the last stage in erythroblast development, the expulsion of the nucleus, is an intrinsic property of the erythroblast that does not require an erythroblastic island to occur. In fact, the central macrophage in the island appears to be actively involved, at this stage, only in the phagocytosis of the extruded nucleus (Koury et al., 1988; Qiu et al., 1995; Ji et al., 2010). Although it is possible that significant scale-up will require co-culture with bone marrow stromal cells (Giarratana et al., 2005; Mountford et al., 2010; Rousseau et al., 2014), to date differentiation to the reticulocyte (retic) stage can be obtained in liquid cultures using only soluble factors and it is reasonable that in a relatively short time the target concentration of 5×10^7 cells/ml could be reached (Rousseau et al., 2014). Yet, full development of the retic to a mature biconcave RBC under artificial conditions appears to still be a major challenge (Giarratana et al., 2005, 2011; Koury et al., 2005; Miharada et al., 2006). A number of reviews are available on the erythroblastic island and erythroid differentiation (Mountford et al., 2010; An and Mohandas, 2011; Anstee et al., 2012; Griffiths et al., 2012a; de Back et al., 2014; Satchwell et al., 2015a; Mankelow et al., 2016; Moras et al., 2017). The present article reviews the literature on retic maturation, one of the unsolved problems of erythropoiesis (Chasis et al., 1989; Koury et al., 1989; Blanc and Vidal, 2010; Ney, 2011), seen as a continuum of differential remodeling of the lipid bilayer and of the membrane-skeleton that leads to the mature circulating RBC first and then to the senescent RBC, and focusing on aspects of membrane topology and selectivity of protein sorting.

SORTING OF PROTEINS DURING ENUCLEATION

In early seminal work, synthesis of RBC membrane proteins was described to occur asynchronously in avian and murine RBCs (Lazarides and Moon, 1984; Hanspal and Palek, 1987; Hanspal et al., 1992). In murine erythroblasts, band 3 synthesis, through a complex dynamics of trafficking from internal membranes to the plasma membrane of dimeric and tetrameric forms of the protein (Hanspal et al., 1998), was completed while the translation of spectrins was still in progress. More recent studies of human erythropoiesis have revealed that band 3 is synthesized early (Gautier et al., 2016) and assembled into multiprotein complexes, especially with protein 4.2, in the intracellular compartment (Satchwell et al., 2011). In a study (Chen et al., 2009) carried out with murine erythroblasts infected with the anemia-inducing strain of Friend erythroleukemia virus (FVA cells) (Koury et al., 1984), many RBC proteins were followed throughout maturation from proerythroblast to retic. Three patterns of protein turnover were observed for integral proteins. The levels of some proteins, including band 3 and glycophorin A (GPA), increased toward the late orthochromatic stage, those of others (CD44, Lu, ICAM-4, and β1 integrin) decreased throughout differentiation, and still others, among which the transferrin receptor (TfR or CD71), remained stable. Of the membrane-skeletal proteins all were shown to increase steadily except for actin, which decreased from proerythroblast to retic (Chen et al., 2009). Similar results were obtained with human erythroblasts (Hu et al., 2013). Comparative transcriptome and expression analysis of human and murine erythroid differentiation (An et al., 2014; Satchwell et al., 2015a; Gautier et al., 2016) is beginning to shed more light on this developmental program and its interspecies differences, which are responsible for generating the heterogeneous phenotypes seen in RBCs of different mammals (Ahn and Johnstone, 1991). Moreover, additional useful information would come from analysis of retic transcriptome, evaluated at different stages of retic maturation (Goh et al., 2007; Malleret et al., 2013).

Whatever the set of membrane proteins with which developing erythroblasts arrive at the orthochromatic stage, this composition will undergo a major redistribution with the enucleation event. This concept was already clear in early seminal studies carried out mostly in mice. Concerning transmembrane proteins, in enucleating mouse erythroblasts isolated from bone marrow, band 3 was shown to partition at a higher concentration in the membrane surrounding the nucleus, than in the membrane of the incipient retic. On the other hand, GPA, the second most abundant integral protein of the RBC membrane, was found to be equally distributed between these two domains of the membrane at enucleation (**Figure 1A**; Geiduschek and Singer, 1979). In erythroblasts isolated from rat bone marrow a similar partition pattern was described (Skutelsky and Farquhar, 1976).

More recently, GPA was found to partition almost exclusively to the retic during enucleation of FVA cells, possibly because of transiently increased connectivity, of unknown origin, of GPA to the spectrin skeleton (Lee et al., 2004). It should be observed that the cell model adopted may influence the results obtained. Many studies were carried out with FVA cells that may not exactly represent physiological erythroid differentiation. Nevertheless, this scenario was largely confirmed in a recent proteomic study of protein distribution during human erythroblast enucleation, although e.g., the restriction of band 3 to the retic membrane seemed to be less defined than what seen in the murine model (Bell et al., 2013).

Concerning membrane-skeletal proteins, they all partition to the retic by a remarkably selective sorting process whose mechanism remains unknown (Geiduschek and Singer, 1979; Zweig et al., 1981; Wickrema et al., 1994; Bell et al., 2013).

SORTING OF PROTEINS DURING RETIC-TO-RBC MATURATION

A major remodeling of the reticulocyte in the maturation to RBC entails the loss of approximately 20% plasma membrane and the continued removal of residual intracellular components.

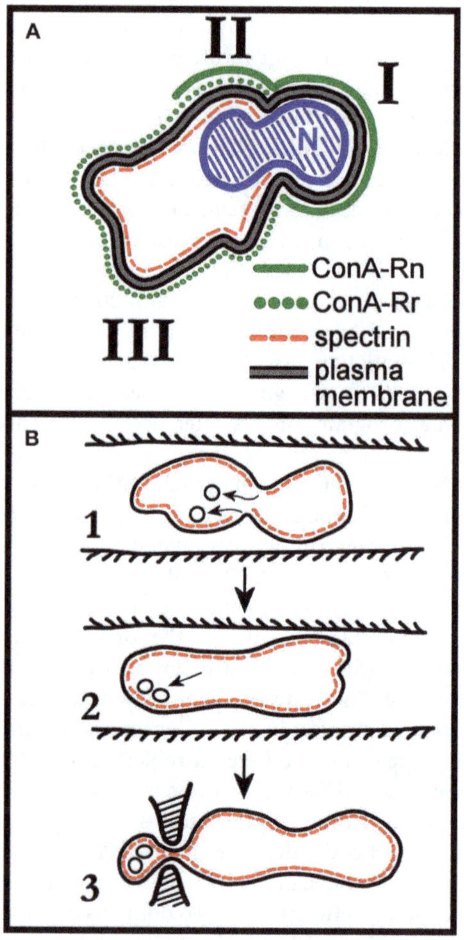

FIGURE 1 | (A) Schematic distribution of membrane proteins in the enucleating mouse erythroblast. Roman numerals I, II, and III correspond to the domains identified by the authors of the work (Geiduschek and Singer, 1979). Domain III corresponds to the incipient reticulocyte. The nucleus (N), not completely extruded, shows the characteristic constriction which separates domain I from domain II. As discussed in the text of the cited work, two classes of ConA receptors (ConA is a lectin that binds to band3, so ConA receptors are band 3 molecules) are assumed to be present in the erythroblast membrane, with ConA-Rn (but not ConA-Rr) present in domain I; both ConA-Rn and ConA-Rr in the membrane of domain II; and ConA-Rr (but not ConA-Rn) in domain III. Most strikingly, spectrin is confined to domains II and III. Re-drawn from Geiduschek and Singer (1979). **(B)** Rudimentary early depiction of a model for the remodeling of the cell membrane during retic maturation to RBC *in vivo*. Panel 1 depicts the invaginations of spectrin-free domains of the retic membrane occurring in the circulation, and their subsequent endocytosis. In panel 2, the endocytosed vesicles are pictured as associating with the membrane either to fuse with it or to be exocytosed. In panel 3, the exocytosis of vesicles in a larger, spectrin-containing body is pictured as occurring by mediation of the spleen. Re-drawn from Zweig et al. (1981).

Concerning membrane-skeletal proteins, they are thought to be largely retained in the maturing RBC through retic-to-RBC transition (Tokuyasu et al., 1979; Pan and Johnstone, 1983). A recent study on stress murine retics documents this in detail (Liu J. et al., 2010). Here all the main membrane-skeletal proteins (α-spectrin, β-spectrin, ankyrin R, protein 4.1R, membrane-associated actin, protein 4.2, p55, tropomodulin, protein 4.9) were found to be unchanged between retics and RBCs. Other cytoskeletal components declined (myosin, tropomyosin, adducin) and some of them were completely lost (tubulin, cytosolic actin). Concerning transmembrane proteins, a decline of Na^+/K^+ATPase, NHE1, GPA, CD47, Duffy, and Kell was observed, together with the complete loss of CD71 and of ICAM4. Interestingly and surprisingly, the following proteins were found to be increased in the membrane of the mature RBC: band 3, GPC, Rh, RhAG, XK, and GPA (for GPA, only the subset of molecules that act as receptor for the TER-119 antibody; Kina et al., 2000). This phenomenon was not commented further in the cited paper (Liu J. et al., 2010) (for a plausible explanation see below). A more recent proteomic analysis of human retics obtained by *in vitro* expansion and differentiation in *in vitro* culture of cord blood-derived $CD34^+$ cells, largely confirmed a similar pattern of protein partitioning between cultured retics and the autologous mature RBCs recovered from cord blood (Wilson et al., 2016).

MODELS OF RETICULOCYTE MATURATION

The loss of retic's excess membrane was originally proposed to occur through the mechanism depicted in **Figure 1B**, for which hints were already available since the 1960's (Kent et al., 1966; Holroyde and Gardner, 1970). Here the excess surface area first invaginates as endocytic spectrin-free vesicles, which are then hypothetically removed as the content of a larger spectrin-containing vesicle, possibly with the active intervention of the spleen. Later, Johnstone et al. (Pan and Johnstone, 1983; Johnstone, 2005) and Stahl and co-workers (Harding et al., 1984, 2013) almost at the same time discovered that in maturing retics a special endosomal compartment is formed, named multivesicular endosome or body (MVE, MVB), which contains intraluminal vesicles (ILVs) carrying the TfR and other selected transmembrane proteins, but lacking band 3 and GPA. Fusion of the MVE with the plasma membrane and exocytosis of the ILVs is the process though which maturing retics dispose of no longer needed membrane proteins. Although the discovery by Johnstone and co-workers was seminal for subsequent understanding of endocytic processes and vesicular trafficking and may explain the loss of most of the TfR, it does not account entirely for the loss of membrane surface area from retic to mature RBC (see below).

According to the current view of the vesicular trafficking around the complex endosomal compartment, several endocytic processes exist in eukaryotic cells, clathrin-dependent and -independent, for the purpose of captating extracellular components and for the internal needs of the cell of turning over plasma membrane constituents. Thus, the endocytic vesicles produced by clathrin-mediated endocytosis, caveolar endocytosis, flotillin-dependent endocytosis and Arf6-dependent endocytosis all fuse generating a common compartment, the early (sorting) endosome (Otto and Nichols, 2011; Bohdanowicz and Grinstein, 2013; Johannes et al., 2015). From the sorting endosome, a MVE can form that can take two different routes: one is fusion with the lysosome for complete hydrolytic degradation of the ILVs; the other is fusion with the plasma membrane for discharging the ILVs, that can now be defined as exosomes (Cocucci and Meldolesi, 2015), in the extracellular space.

Topologically, the orientation of transmembrane proteins in ILVs and exosomes is the same as in the plasma membrane (right-side-out) and as in ectosomes (intended as vesicles released extracellularly directly from the plasma membrane), whereas it is opposite in endocytic vesicles (inside-out).

There are therefore two steps at which proteins must be sorted along the above-described pathway. The first entails the selection at the plasma membrane for endocytosis. In the specific of retic maturation, endocytosis of TfR from the plasma membrane. The next sorting step occurs on the membrane of the sorting endosome where the TfR must be again selected among other membrane proteins to be inserted in ILVs. This process is mediated by a special molecular machinery based on ESCRT protein complexes (Gruenberg and Stenmark, 2004; Kowal et al., 2014) although an ESCRT-independent, ceramide-based mechanism has also been described (Trajkovic et al., 2008).

Concerning the sorting of plasma membrane proteins, as mentioned in the previous section, an increase in band 3 and GPC was observed in the maturation of mouse retics to RBCs by Western blotting of whole cell proteins, normalizing the quantity of sample by loading the same amount of cholesterol for RBCs and retics (Liu J. et al., 2010). Whereas, a decline of proteins during the retic-to-RBC transition can be easily accepted, their stability or increase in a membrane that is at the same time decreasing in size is less easily understood, especially for a complex multi-pass transmembrane protein like band 3. This is certainly not due to *de novo* synthesis in a cell that is progressively dismantling its internal translational apparatus and consuming the molecular machinery required for vesicular trafficking and where band 3 was synthesizes and already partially assembled in complexes in earlier erythroblastic stages (van den Akker et al., 2011). As the decrease in membrane surface area that occurs in the retic-to-RBC maturation is of the same order of magnitude as the observed "increase" in band 3 and GPC, the latter can only be explained by the increase in concentration that follows a selective loss of cholesterol (and other components different from band 3) by the retic in the process. Previous and independently obtained evidence exists on stable amounts of band 3 in retics and RBCs, despite the large difference in surface area between the two cell types (Foxwell and Tanner, 1981), pointing to a peculiar and as yet unknown mechanism for such selective retention of band 3 in the membrane of maturing retics that must be capable of discriminating between two almost equally abundant transmembrane proteins, band 3 with approximately 1.2×10^6 copies/cell and CD71 with approximately 8×10^5 copies/cell (Van Bockxmeer and Morgan, 1979) and completely get rid of the latter while largely saving the former.

To explain the selective retention in the reticulocyte membrane of such abundant transmembrane proteins as band 3, GPA, RhAG, GPC, CD47, a mechanism based on the formation of stable multiprotein complexes among the above-mentioned species, with the association to components of the membrane-skeleton (Satchwell et al., 2015b, 2016) could be conceived. This mechanism would work by mechanically preventing incorporation of the bulky protein complexes into endovesicles. However, this is difficult to reconcile with the evidence that, for instance, some subpopulations of band 3 molecules or even band 3 complexes (with 4.2 and ankyrin), may still move around unanchored to the skeleton in retics (due to the extra membrane present at this stage, that cannot be supported by a membrane-skeleton of smaller area). Moreover, even in fully mature normal RBCs there is a significant 30% of band 3 molecules which is highly mobile, being not anchored to the skeleton. This population of band 3 molecules should be in principle free to leave the cell if size reduction was driven by a non-specific mechanism, but it is not: band 3 (as well as GPA and GPC) are not found in exosomes derived from ILVs in MVEs, as discovered already by Johnstone and co-workers.

There is actually one particular experimental model in which a peculiarly sharp segregation of different membrane proteins is observed, and that is during the isolation of membrane rafts as detergent resistant membrane (DRM). When DRMs are properly isolated from RBCs, they meet the canonical requirements for membrane rafts of being enriched in cholesterol, sphingolipids and specific classes of proteins like GPI-linked proteins, flotillins and stomatin, to name only the most relevant. In addition, and strikingly, they are completely devoid of band 3 and GPC (Ciana et al., 2005, 2011, 2013, 2014; Crepaldi Domingues et al., 2009; Domingues et al., 2010; Achilli et al., 2011; Minetti et al., 2013).

We infer from literature data and from our own experimental evidence that the step at which band 3, GPC, and GPA (Johnstone, 1992) are selected for being retained in the plasma membrane at the retic-to-RBC transition is in the trafficking of MVEs, and implies a mechanism based on differential partitioning of a given transmembrane protein into the membrane raft phase. To the best of our knowledge this is the first time that a membrane raft-based process for the sorting of membrane proteins during retic maturation is proposed.

At the plasma membrane the TfR is selected as the cargo of clathrin-coated vesicles with the mediation of the adaptin AP-2 (Liu A. P. et al., 2010; Kelly and Owen, 2011). The same route of entry is contemplated in early work of Johnstone (1992). It is accepted notion that clathrin-mediated endocytosis occurs at regions of the membrane that exclude lipid rafts, whereas caveolin-mediated and possibly other forms of endocytosis include micro- nano-domains of typical raft composition (Rajendran and Simons, 2005). In a recent study on mesenchymal stem cells, lipid rafts and TfR were found to co-localize in the MVB membrane, and it was concluded that they were ferried there together in the same clathrin-coated vesicles that were endocytosed from the plasma membrane (Tan et al., 2013). However, because of the accepted notion that rafts do not partition in clathrin-coated vesicles, it is more likely that diverse components of the plasma membrane converge in a single MVB coming from different endocytic routes. Plenty of evidence indeed exists on the presence of membrane raft markers in the exosomes. GPI linked proteins (a typical raft marker) were detected in TfR-containing exosomes already by Johnstone (1992); in exosomes released *in vitro* by rat "stress" retics, and also from retics from human patients, canonical raft markers such as flotillin, stomatin, ganglioside GM1 were found enriched (de Gassart et al., 2003). All this clearly suggests that a pathway must exist, different from the clathrin-coated mediated one, for delivering raft material to the MVB first and then to the exosomes (the scenario described above is depicted in **Figure 2A**). Incidentally, these other raft-dependent endocytic vesicles could be responsible for the disposal of other transmembrane proteins that do not follow the clathrin-dependent pathway. Unfortunately, in the cited studies the membrane of the MVB was never characterized for the presence of band 3, GPA or GPC, so the possibility has never been evaluated that band 3 (plus GPC and GPA) actually reaches the MVB via any of the various endocytic pathways, but then it is excluded from the ILVs because the discriminating step occurs at the level of the budding of ILVs inside the MVB. At this latter step, the selection mechanism could be based on different affinities of a given protein for the raft phase (maybe exploiting the ESCRT-independent route mentioned above; Trajkovic et al., 2008). According to this mechanism, band 3 would not be inserted in exosomes, but will be entirely recycled to the plasma membrane at the time the MVB fuses with it (this alternative scenario is depicted in **Figure 2B**). Experimentally answering this question would be important to understand the selectivity of the whole process. It would also clarify whether the exclusion of band 3, GPC, and GPA from membrane rafts is due to an intrinsic property of these proteins, and what is the role played by the membrane-skeleton in this scenario.

Along this line, a number of other issues still have to be solved concerning the maturation of retics to RBCs. What is the role played by the membrane-skeleton when, after enucleation, in the immature retic the heavy intracellular vesicular traffic must efficiently endocytose and circulate endocytic vesicles to generate the MVEs and then move the latter to the plasma membrane for the final fusion and the release of exosomes? Is this taking place because the membrane-skeleton is still completely or partially unanchored to the bilayer? Or is the spectrin network temporarily detached from the bilayer only locally where endocytic vesicles form? The first scenario is more likely, because portions of the retic membrane must be still floating unattached to the membrane-skeleton, making it more likely to be a site where endocytic formation is not hindered

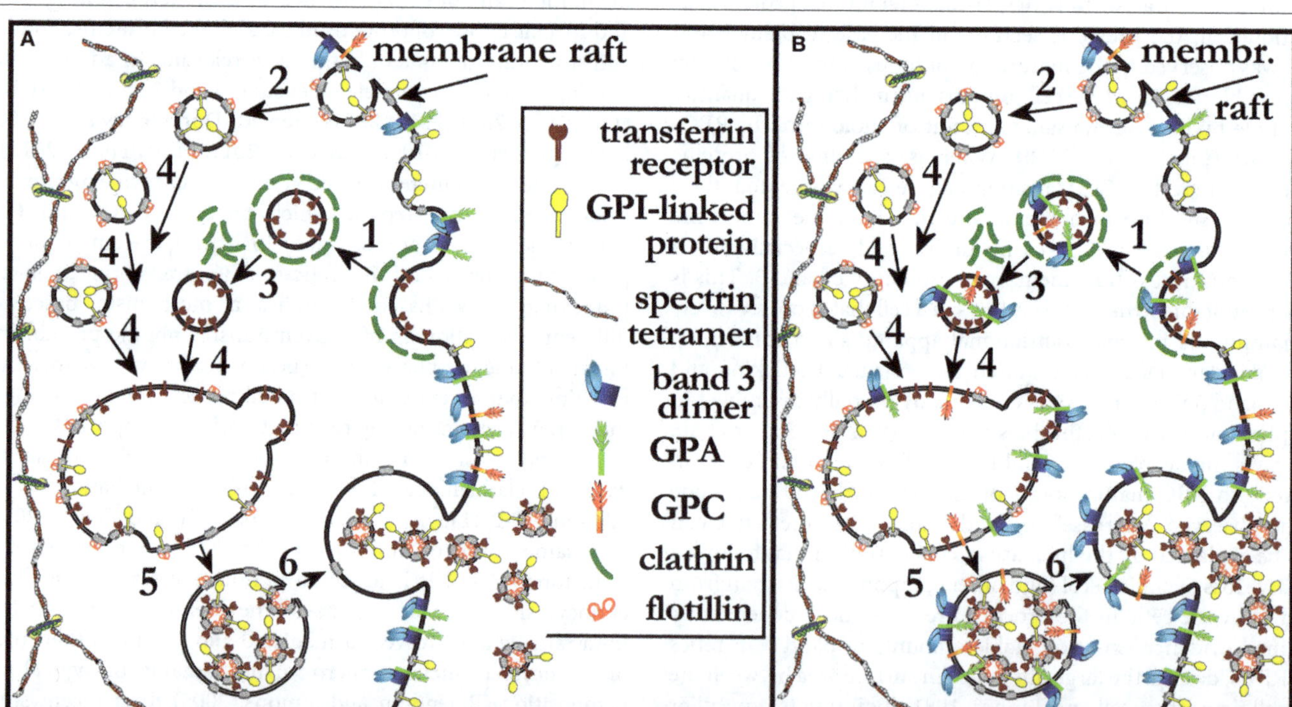

FIGURE 2 | (A) A model extended from that proposed by Johnstone et al. (Johnstone, 2005). Reticulocytes mature through the release of TfR-containing exosomes from MVEs. Clathrin coated vesicles and lipid rafts have been added to the original scenario, to show that TfR is recruited at clathrin-coated pits and endocytosed in clathrin-coated vesicles (1) that do not contain membrane rafts nor band 3, GPC, or GPA. Parallel routes of endocytosis must exist that deliver membrane raft components to the MVB while, again, excluding band 3, GPC and GPA (2). After shedding of the clathrin coat (3) from clathrin-coated vesicles, all vesicles converge and fuse (4) in a single early endosome, which is soon converted into a MVB with the endovesiculation of ILVs that contain both membrane raft components and TfR (5). The membrane of the MVB becomes thus depleted of TfR and membrane raft constituents, including cholesterol and sphingolipids, The MVB eventually fuses with the plasma membrane and releases the ILVs that are now defined as exosomes. The bulky structure of the spectrin skeleton is depicted as separated from the scenario where this vesicular trafficking occurs. In **(B)** a different pathway is proposed whereby band 3, GPC, and GPA can reach the MVB membrane coming from, for instance, clathrin-coated vesicles, but then are not packaged into ILVs and exosomes because of their inability to partition to the raft phase. Band 3, GPC, and GPA are therefore returned to the plasma membrane with the fusion of the MVB with it. See text for additional details.

by a bulky spectrin network. In this respect, there appear to be significant differences in the ontogeny of primitive and definitive erythroblasts, whereby, at least in the mice model, primitive erythroblasts enucleate intravascularly, after having circulated for some time without a fully assembled membrane-skeleton (therefore with a less deformable cell structure). In definitive erythropoiesis, instead, erythroblasts do not enucleate until just before leaving the bone marrow and circulate with a stable membrane-skeleton, and therefore with higher deformability, although with an excess lipid bilayer that must be shed by the circulating retic. In both cases, for stable membrane-skeleton assembly, a switch to the expression of the mature spliceoform of protein 4.1R appears to be fundamental (Huang et al., 2017). However, the timing and modalities for the establishment of a stable membrane-skeleton in erythropoiesis before and after enucleation are still poorly understood.

Another possible trafficking pathway has been recently described adding complexity to the process of retic maturation. Here, endovesiculation (not better characterized as being or not clathrin-dependent) would produce GPA-positive endosomes that would then fuse with a late autophagosome. The latter, in turn, will be "extruded" from the cell by "crossing" the plasma membrane while maintaining its topology. Through this process it would be possible for the retic to eliminate additional membrane area as large vesicles, which are phosphatidylserine-positive because of their inside-out nature. Curiously, the fate of TfR was not followed in these works, so it is not possible to ascertain whether it is also part of the membrane that is lost by this mechanism. Several topological aspects, however, remain poorly defined and render this membrane trafficking route difficult to comprehend (Griffiths et al., 2012a,b; Mankelow et al., 2016).

It is interesting to note that the TfR was very likely recycled, together with transferrin, through several rounds of receptor-mediated-endocytosis for iron captation during differentiation from proerythroblast, whereas, at the retic-to-RBC transition it is instead routed to the MVE for eventual discharge from the cell. It is still a mystery how the cell can perform this switch in the routing of the same type of cargo, the TfR, at different stages of cell differentiation. It is also still unclear what is the relative contribution of the exosome pathway and other, possibly spleen-mediated pathways for the removal of excess TfR and membrane extension at the various stages of retic maturation.

Concluding on the relative enrichment in band 3 in the membrane of the mature RBC with respect to that of the retic (Liu J. et al., 2010), this would result from the selective loss of cholesterol as part of the membrane raft phase that is selectively eliminated with the exosomes. As seen in **Figure 2**, in fact, a profound imbalance in the composition of the lipid bilayer that is returned to the plasma membrane (when the MVB fuses with it) with respect to the membrane that is lost as exosomes, is generated along this membrane trafficking route. This hypothesis predicts, and to the best of our knowledge there are no data in the literature that answer this question, that the lipid composition of the plasma membrane should also change during maturation from retic to RBC, with a decrease in the ratio of (sphingolipids + cholesterol) to glycerophospholipids, and a decrease in membrane-raft associated proteins.

Importantly, the enrichment in band 3 described above as based on raft trafficking and previous evidence obtained on mature RBCs concerning the complete absence of band 3 and GPC from the DRM fraction, corroborates the long debated and never settled hypothesis (Sonnino and Prinetti, 2013) that DRMs are a good representation of membrane rafts (Ciana et al., 2014).

CONCLUSIONS

It is unlikely that apparently autonomous mechanisms like the MVE-based trafficking or others like the ones involving autophagy, are the only processes through which retics eliminate their excess membrane. The reason for this is 2-fold: first, it is unclear for how long these mechanisms could be sustained in a cell that is progressively losing its molecular components, including the ones that organize MVE or autophagosome assembly (Gruenberg and Stenmark, 2004). In fact, at the same time that the plasma membrane is remodeled, additional processes are at play for the disposal of intracellular soluble components, likely through proteolytic processes including the ubiquitin/proteasome-mediated pathway, and residual organelles through autophagy and other routes (Moras et al., 2017). Ubiquitin was originally discovered in stress-retics from rabbit (Ciehanover et al., 1978), the ubiquitination/proteasome pathway is present and active to a very late stage (Liu J. et al., 2010; Neelam et al., 2011; Gautier et al., 2016), caspases and calpain are expressed in RBCs. The MVE-based mechanism was first described to occur in sheep stress retics, and it is probable that under physiological conditions it occurs predominantly in the bone marrow phase of retic maturation (R1). Maybe this could only be observed in circulating retics (R2) if they were the result of accelerated erythropoiesis and precocious egression from the bone marrow as it occurs in response to extensive phlebotomy or phenylhydrazine treatment. In fact, most of the TfR appears to be lost in R1 retics through the MVE pathway (Malleret et al., 2013), yet some is lost by circulating retics. Second, circulating retics require a functioning spleen for full maturation. It is therefore highly probable that under physiological conditions the MVE-based mechanism operates when retics are still in the bone marrow, and only partially, if at all, in R2 retics. Therefore, other as yet unidentified mechanisms should take over the duty of completing retic maturation. It is likely that this would imply the intervention of the spleen because the spleen is essential for the final steps in the topogenesis of a mature RBC membrane, with a biconcave discocyte shape and an optimized ratio of lipid bilayer to underlying membrane-skeleton. The spleen is also needed for the continuous processing of mature RBCs until they are cleared from the circulation (Crosby and Benjamin, 1957; Crosby, 1959; Kent et al., 1966; Holroyde and Gardner, 1970; Shattil and Cooper, 1972; Lux and John, 1977; Groom et al., 1991; Gifford et al., 2003).

The mechanism will also have to be capable of acting with some selectivity because residual TfR molecules will have to be removed from the surface of R2 retics, probably with a pinching action similar to that depicted in **Figure 1B**. Whether this is the actual mechanism and whether it also involves the recognition of membrane micro- nano-domains (membrane rafts) remains to be established.

On a methodological note, in times when the study of circulating micro-particles has become of age (Herring et al., 2013), assessing the origin of such entities is of importance for isolation and characterization. As RBC-derived micro-particles are usually recognized and isolated because they express GPA on their surface, any vesicles released by retics as exosomes would escape detection because exosomes originating from MVE appear not to contain GPA (Johnstone, 1992).

We have recently supported with novel experimental evidence the old notion that maturation and aging of circulating RBCs also require an intervention of the spleen (Ciana et al., 2017a,b; Kaestner and Minetti, 2017). In short, we have observed a disproportionate loss of flotillin-2 with respect to the loss in surface area that occurs during the ageing *in vivo* of normal human RBCs (approximately −17%). If this loss occurred through membrane vesiculation according to known spontaneous processes of ectosome release from RBCs, vesicles obtained *in vitro* from RBCs should contain flotillin-2 enriched with respect to the parent cell plasma membrane. Instead, we have observed the opposite. Moreover, we have observed that spectrin and other membrane-skeletal proteins decline with RBC ageing on a per-cell basis. This should not happen if ageing RBCs lost membrane as spectrin-free vesicles.

It should be noted that such splenic function may not be limited to a mechanical action on the RBC, but may require active recognition and removal of selected portions of the cell. To date, protocols for producing artificial RBCs succeed in the generation of significant amounts of enucleated erythroblasts. Complete maturation to a biconcave disc, however, has not been described to date to occur *in vitro* (Giarratana et al., 2011). It would be interesting to verify whether and to what extent the MVE-based mechanism is at play in artificially produced retics.

An advantage for transfusion medicine would be that, with the infusion of a cohort of synchronized "young" RBCs, the problem of the dramatic loss of up to 25% of stored RBCs in the first 24 h from transfusion should be solved or strongly attenuated. However, the infusion of blood units composed only of retics could pose an excessive burden on the recipient's spleen, which will have to process circulating retics at a much higher rate than the 1% retics per day that occurs under normal conditions. Therefore, full retic-to-RBC conversion may be required for clinical approval of artificial RBCs for transfusion purposes. It remains to be evaluated whether final maturation could be achieved by mimicking a mechanical splenic function or whether a fully biomimetic "artificial spleen" is required for this important maturational step.

AUTHOR CONTRIBUTIONS

GM conceived the review and wrote a first draft, CA contributed to discussing the draft, to drawing the figures and writing the revised manuscript, CP discussed and contributed to writing the revised versions, AC conceived the manuscript and contributed to all revision phases with dicussions and writing of the text and figures.

ACKNOWLEDGMENTS

This work was supported by the EU Commission Horizon 2020 Marie Skłodowska-Curie Actions Innovative Training Networks project RELEVANCE Grant Agreement N. 675115.

REFERENCES

Achilli, C., Ciana, A., Balduini, C., Risso, A., and Minetti, G. (2011). Application of gelatin zymography for evaluating low levels of contaminating neutrophils in red blood cell samples. *Anal. Biochem.* 409, 296–297. doi: 10.1016/j.ab.2010.10.019

Ahn, J., and Johnstone, R. M. (1991). Synthesis of the transferrin receptor in peripheral sheep reticulocytes: evidence for incomplete oligosaccharide processing. *Adv. Exp. Med. Biol.* 307, 3–13. doi: 10.1007/978-1-4684-5985-2_1

An, X., and Mohandas, N. (2011). Erythroblastic islands, terminal erythroid differentiation and reticulocyte maturation. *Int. J. Hematol.* 93, 139–143. doi: 10.1007/s12185-011-0779-x

An, X., Schulz, V. P., Li, J., Wu, K., Liu, J., Xue, F., et al. (2014). Global transcriptome analyses of human and murine terminal erythroid differentiation. *Blood* 123, 3466–3477. doi: 10.1182/blood-2014-01-548305

Anstee, D. J., Gampel, A., and Toye, A. M. (2012). *Ex-vivo* generation of human red cells for transfusion. *Curr. Opin. Hematol.* 19, 163–169. doi: 10.1097/MOH.0b013e328352240a

Baek, E. J., Kim, H. S., Kim, S., Jin, H., Choi, T. Y., and Kim, H. O. (2008). *In vitro* clinical-grade generation of red blood cells from human umbilical cord blood CD34+ cells. *Transfusion* 48, 2235–2245. doi: 10.1111/j.1537-2995.2008.01828.x

Bell, A. J., Satchwell, T. J., Heesom, K. J., Hawley, B. R., Kupzig, S., Hazell, M., et al. (2013). Protein distribution during human erythroblast enucleation *in vitro*. *PLoS ONE* 8:e60300. doi: 10.1371/journal.pone.0060300

Blanc, L., and Vidal, M. (2010). Reticulocyte membrane remodeling: contribution of the exosome pathway. *Curr. Opin. Hematol.* 17, 177–183. doi: 10.1097/MOH.0b013e328337b4e3

Bohdanowicz, M., and Grinstein, S. (2013). Role of phospholipids in endocytosis, phagocytosis, and macropinocytosis. *Physiol. Rev.* 93, 69–106. doi: 10.1152/physrev.00002.2012

Chasis, J. A., Prenant, M., Leung, A., and Mohandas, N. (1989). Membrane assembly and remodeling during reticulocyte maturation. *Blood* 74, 1112–1120.

Chen, K., Liu, J., Heck, S., Chasis, J. A., An, X., and Mohandas, N. (2009). Resolving the distinct stages in erythroid differentiation based on dynamic changes in membrane protein expression during erythropoiesis. *Proc. Natl. Acad. Sci. U.S.A.* 106, 17413–17418. doi: 10.1073/pnas.0909296106

Ciana, A., Achilli, C., Balduini, C., and Minetti, G. (2011). On the association of lipid rafts to the spectrin skeleton in human erythrocytes. *Biochim. Biophys. Acta* 1808, 183–190. doi: 10.1016/j.bbamem.2010.08.019

Ciana, A., Achilli, C., Gaur, A., and Minetti, G. (2017a). Membrane remodelling and vesicle formation during ageing of human red blood cells. *Cell. Physiol. Biochem.* 42, 1127–1138. doi: 10.1159/000478768

Ciana, A., Achilli, C., Hannoush, R. N., Risso, A., Balduini, C., and Minetti, G. (2013). Freely turning over palmitate in erythrocyte membrane proteins is not responsible for the anchoring of lipid rafts to the spectrin skeleton: a study with bio-orthogonal chemical probes. *Biochim. Biophys. Acta* 1828, 924–931. doi: 10.1016/j.bbamem.2012.11.029

Ciana, A., Achilli, C., and Minetti, G. (2014). Membrane rafts of the human red blood cell. *Mol. Membr. Biol.* 31, 47–57. doi: 10.3109/09687688.2014.896485

Ciana, A., Achilli, C., and Minetti, G. (2017b). Spectrin and other membrane-skeletal components in human red blood cells of different age. *Cell. Physiol. Biochem.* 42, 1139–1152. doi: 10.1159/000478769

Ciana, A., Balduini, C., and Minetti, G. (2005). Detergent-resistant membranes in human erythrocytes and their connection to the membrane-skeleton. *J. Biosci.* 30, 317–328. doi: 10.1007/BF02703669

Ciehanover, A., Hod, Y., and Hershko, A. (1978). A heat-stable polypeptide component of an ATP-dependent proteolytic system from reticulocytes. *Biochem. Biophys. Res. Commun.* 81, 1100–1105. doi: 10.1016/0006-291X(78)91249-4

Cocucci, E., and Meldolesi, J. (2015). Ectosomes and exosomes: shedding the confusion between extracellular vesicles. *Trends Cell Biol.* 25, 364–372. doi: 10.1016/j.tcb.2015.01.004

Crepaldi Domingues, C., Ciana, A., Buttafava, A., Balduini, C., de Paula, E., and Minetti, G. (2009). Resistance of human erythrocyte membranes to Triton X-100 and C12E8. *J. Membr. Biol.* 227, 39–48. doi: 10.1007/s00232-008-9142-4

Crosby, W. H. (1959). Normal functions of the spleen relative to red blood cells: a review. *Blood* 14, 399–408.

Crosby, W. H., and Benjamin, N. R. (1957). Siderocytes and the Spleen. *Blood* 12, 165–170.

de Back, D. Z., Kostova, E. B., van Kraaij, M., van den Berg, T. K., and van Bruggen, R. (2014). Of macrophages and red blood cells; a complex love story. *Front. Physiol.* 5:9. doi: 10.3389/fphys.2014.00009

de Gassart, A., Geminard, C., Fevrier, B., Raposo, G., and Vidal, M. (2003). Lipid raft-associated protein sorting in exosomes. *Blood* 102, 4336–4344. doi: 10.1182/blood-2003-03-0871

Domingues, C. C., Ciana, A., Buttafava, A., Casadei, B. R., Balduini, C., de Paula, E., et al. (2010). Effect of cholesterol depletion and temperature on the isolation of detergent-resistant membranes from human erythrocytes. *J. Membr. Biol.* 234, 195–205. doi: 10.1007/s00232-010-9246-5

Foxwell, B. M., and Tanner, M. J. (1981). Synthesis of the erythrocyte anion-transport protein. Immunochemical study of its incorporation into the plasma membrane of erythroid cells. *Biochem. J.* 195, 129–137. doi: 10.1042/bj1950129

Gautier, E. F., Ducamp, S., Leduc, M., Salnot, V., Guillonneau, F., Dussiot, M., et al. (2016). Comprehensive proteomic analysis of human erythropoiesis. *Cell Rep.* 16, 1470–1484. doi: 10.1016/j.celrep.2016.06.085

Geiduschek, J. B., and Singer, S. J. (1979). Molecular changes in the membranes of mouse erythroid cells accompanying differentiation. *Cell* 16, 149–163. doi: 10.1016/0092-8674(79)90196-X

Giarratana, M. C., Kobari, L., Lapillonne, H., Chalmers, D., Kiger, L., Cynober, T., et al. (2005). *Ex vivo* generation of fully mature human red blood cells from hematopoietic stem cells. *Nat. Biotechnol.* 23, 69–74. doi: 10.1038/nbt1047

Giarratana, M. C., Rouard, H., Dumont, A., Kiger, L., Safeukui, I., Le Pennec, P. Y., et al. (2011). Proof of principle for transfusion of *in vitro*-generated red blood cells. *Blood* 118, 5071–5079. doi: 10.1182/blood-2011-06-362038

Gifford, S. C., Frank, M. G., Derganc, J., Gabel, C., Austin, R. H., Yoshida, T., et al. (2003). Parallel microchannel-based measurements of individual erythrocyte areas and volumes. *Biophys. J.* 84, 623–633. doi: 10.1016/S0006-3495(03)74882-6

Goh, S. H., Josleyn, M., Lee, Y. T., Danner, R. L., Gherman, R. B., Cam, M. C., et al. (2007). The human reticulocyte transcriptome. *Physiol. Genomics* 30, 172–178. doi: 10.1152/physiolgenomics.00247.2006

Griffiths, R. E., Kupzig, S., Cogan, N., Mankelow, T. J., Betin, V. M., Trakarnsanga, K., et al. (2012a). The ins and outs of human reticulocyte maturation: autophagy and the endosome/exosome pathway. *Autophagy* 8, 1150–1151. doi: 10.4161/auto.20648

Griffiths, R. E., Kupzig, S., Cogan, N., Mankelow, T. J., Betin, V. M., Trakarnsanga, K., et al. (2012b). Maturing reticulocytes internalize plasma membrane in glycophorin A-containing vesicles that fuse with autophagosomes before exocytosis. *Blood* 119, 6296–6306. doi: 10.1182/blood-2011-09-376475

Groom, A. C., Schmidt, E. E., and MacDonald, I. C. (1991). Microcirculatory pathways and blood flow in spleen: new insights from washout kinetics, corrosion casts, and quantitative intravital videomicroscopy. *Scanning Microsc.* 5, 159–174.

Gruenberg, J., and Stenmark, H. (2004). The biogenesis of multivesicular endosomes. *Nat. Rev. Mol. Cell Biol.* 5, 317–323. doi: 10.1038/nrm1360

Hanspal, M., Golan, D. E., Smockova, Y., Yi, S. J., Cho, M. R., Liu, S. C., et al. (1998). Temporal synthesis of band 3 oligomers during terminal maturation of mouse erythroblasts. Dimers and tetramers exist in the membrane as preformed stable species. *Blood* 92, 329–338.

Hanspal, M., Hanspal, J. S., Kalraiya, R., Liu, S. C., Sahr, K. E., Howard, D., et al. (1992). Asynchronous synthesis of membrane skeletal proteins during terminal maturation of murine erythroblasts. *Blood* 80, 530–539.

Hanspal, M., and Palek, J. (1987). Synthesis and assembly of membrane skeletal proteins in mammalian red cell precursors. *J. Cell Biol.* 105, 1417–1424. doi: 10.1083/jcb.105.3.1417

Harding, C., Heuser, J., and Stahl, P. (1984). Endocytosis and intracellular processing of transferrin and colloidal-gold transferrin in rat reticulocytes: demonstration of a pathway for receptor shedding. *Eur. J. Cell Biol.* 35, 256–263.

Harding, C. V., Heuser, J. E., and Stahl, P. D. (2013). Exosomes: looking back three decades and into the future. *J. Cell Biol.* 200, 367–371. doi: 10.1083/jcb.201212113

Herring, J. M., McMichael, M. A., and Smith, S. A. (2013). Microparticles in health and disease. *J. Vet. Intern. Med.* 27, 1020–1033. doi: 10.1111/jvim.12128

Hiroyama, T., Miharada, K., Sudo, K., Danjo, I., Aoki, N., and Nakamura, Y. (2008). Establishment of mouse embryonic stem cell-derived erythroid progenitor cell lines able to produce functional red blood cells. *PLoS ONE* 3:e1544. doi: 10.1371/journal.pone.0001544

Holroyde, C. P., and Gardner, F. H. (1970). Acquisition of autophagic vacuoles by human erythrocytes. Physiological role of the spleen. *Blood* 36, 566–575.

Hu, J., Liu, J., Xue, F., Halverson, G., Reid, M., Guo, A., et al. (2013). Isolation and functional characterization of human erythroblasts at distinct stages: implications for understanding of normal and disordered erythropoiesis *in vivo*. *Blood* 121, 3246–3253. doi: 10.1182/blood-2013-01-476390

Huang, Y. S., Delgadillo, L. F., Cyr, K. H., Kingsley, P. D., An, X., McGrath, K. E., et al. (2017). Circulating primitive erythroblasts establish a functional, protein 4.1R-dependent cytoskeletal network prior to enucleating. *Sci. Rep.* 7:5164. doi: 10.1038/s41598-017-05498-4

Ji, P., Yeh, V., Ramirez, T., Murata-Hori, M., and Lodish, H. F. (2010). Histone deacetylase 2 is required for chromatin condensation and subsequent enucleation of cultured mouse fetal erythroblasts. *Haematologica* 95, 2013–2021. doi: 10.3324/haematol.2010.029827

Johannes, L., Parton, R. G., Bassereau, P., and Mayor, S. (2015). Building endocytic pits without clathrin. *Nat. Rev. Mol. Cell Biol.* 16, 311–321. doi: 10.1038/nrm3968

Johnstone, R. M. (1992). The jeanne manery-fisher memorial lecture 1991. Maturation of reticulocytes: formation of exosomes as a mechanism for shedding membrane proteins. *Biochem. Cell Biol.* 70, 179–190. doi: 10.1139/o92-028

Johnstone, R. M. (2005). Revisiting the road to the discovery of exosomes. *Blood Cells Mol. Dis.* 34, 214–219. doi: 10.1016/j.bcmd.2005.03.002

Kaestner, L., and Minetti, G. (2017). The potential of erythrocytes as cellular aging models. *Cell Death Differ.* 24, 1475–1477. doi: 10.1038/cdd.2017.100

Kelly, B. T., and Owen, D. J. (2011). Endocytic sorting of transmembrane protein cargo. *Curr. Opin. Cell Biol.* 23, 404–412. doi: 10.1016/j.ceb.2011.03.004

Kent, G., Minick, O. T., Volini, F. I., and Orfei, E. (1966). Autophagic vacuoles in human red cells. *Am. J. Pathol.* 48, 831–857.

Kina, T., Ikuta, K., Takayama, E., Wada, K., Majumdar, A. S., Weissman, I. L., et al. (2000). The monoclonal antibody TER-119 recognizes a molecule associated with glycophorin A and specifically marks the late stages of murine erythroid lineage. *Br. J. Haematol.* 109, 280–287. doi: 10.1046/j.1365-2141.2000.02037.x

Koury, M. J., Koury, S. T., Kopsombut, P., and Bondurant, M. C. (2005). *In vitro* maturation of nascent reticulocytes to erythrocytes. *Blood* 105, 2168–2174. doi: 10.1182/blood-2004-02-0616

Koury, M. J., Sawyer, S. T., and Bondurant, M. C. (1984). Splenic erythroblasts in anemia-inducing Friend disease: a source of cells for studies of erythropoietin-mediated differentiation. *J. Cell. Physiol.* 121, 526–532. doi: 10.1002/jcp.1041210311

Koury, S. T., Koury, M. J., and Bondurant, M. C. (1988). Morphological changes in erythroblasts during erythropoietin-induced terminal differentiation *in vitro*. *Exp. Hematol.* 16, 758–763.

Koury, S. T., Koury, M. J., and Bondurant, M. C. (1989). Cytoskeletal distribution and function during the maturation and enucleation of mammalian erythroblasts. *J. Cell Biol.* 109, 3005–3013. doi: 10.1083/jcb.109.6.3005

Kowal, J., Tkach, M., and Thery, C. (2014). Biogenesis and secretion of exosomes. *Curr. Opin. Cell Biol.* 29, 116–125. doi: 10.1016/j.ceb.2014.05.004

Kupzig, S., Parsons, S. F., Curnow, E., Anstee, D. J., and Blair, A. (2017). Superior survival of *ex vivo* cultured human reticulocytes following transfusion into mice. *Haematologica* 102, 476–483. doi: 10.3324/haematol.2016.154443

Lazarides, E., and Moon, R. T. (1984). Assembly and topogenesis of the spectrin-based membrane skeleton in erythroid development. *Cell* 37, 354–346. doi: 10.1016/0092-8674(84)90364-7

Leberbauer, C., Boulmé, F., Unfried, G., Huber, J., Beug, H., and Müllner, E. W. (2005). Different steroids co-regulate long-term expansion versus terminal differentiation in primary human erythroid progenitors. *Blood* 105, 85–94. doi: 10.1182/blood-2004-03-1002

Lee, J. C., Gimm, J. A., Lo, A. J., Koury, M. J., Krauss, S. W., Mohandas, N., et al. (2004). Mechanism of protein sorting during erythroblast enucleation: role of cytoskeletal connectivity. *Blood* 103, 1912–1919. doi: 10.1182/blood-2003-03-0928

Liu, A. P., Aguet, F., Danuser, G., and Schmid, S. L. (2010). Local clustering of transferrin receptors promotes clathrin-coated pit initiation. *J. Cell Biol.* 191, 1381–1393. doi: 10.1083/jcb.201008117

Liu, J., Guo, X., Mohandas, N., Chasis, J. A., and An, X. (2010). Membrane remodeling during reticulocyte maturation. *Blood* 115, 2021–2027. doi: 10.1182/blood-2009-08-241182

Lu, S. J., Feng, Q., Park, J. S., Vida, L., Lee, B. S., Strausbauch, M., et al. (2008). Biologic properties and enucleation of red blood cells from human embryonic stem cells. *Blood* 112, 4475–4484. doi: 10.1182/blood-2008-05-157198

Lux, S. E., and John, K. M. (1977). Isolation and partial characterization of a high molecular weight red cell membrane protein complex normally removed by the spleen. *Blood* 50, 625–641.

Ma, F., Ebihara, Y., Umeda, K., Sakai, H., Hanada, S., Zhang, H., et al. (2008). Generation of functional erythrocytes from human embryonic stem cell-derived definitive hematopoiesis. *Proc. Natl. Acad. Sci. U.S.A.* 105, 13087–13092. doi: 10.1073/pnas.0802220105

Malleret, B., Xu, F., Mohandas, N., Suwanarusk, R., Chu, C., Leite, J. A., et al. (2013). Significant biochemical, biophysical and metabolic diversity in circulating human cord blood reticulocytes. *PLoS ONE* 8:e76062. doi: 10.1371/journal.pone.0076062

Mankelow, T. J., Griffiths, R. E., Trompeter, S., Flatt, J. F., Cogan, N. M., Massey, E. J., et al. (2016). The ins and outs of reticulocyte maturation revisited: the role of autophagy in sickle cell disease. *Autophagy* 12, 590–591. doi: 10.1080/15548627.2015.1125072

Migliaccio, G., Di Pietro, R., di Giacomo, V., Di Baldassarre, A., Migliaccio, A. R., Maccioni, L., et al. (2002). *In vitro* mass production of human erythroid cells from the blood of normal donors and of thalassemic patients. *Blood Cells Mol. Dis.* 28, 169–180. doi: 10.1006/bcmd.2002.0502

Miharada, K., Hiroyama, T., Sudo, K., Nagasawa, T., and Nakamura, Y. (2006). Efficient enucleation of erythroblasts differentiated *in vitro* from hematopoietic stem and progenitor cells. *Nat. Biotechnol.* 24, 1255–1256. doi: 10.1038/nbt1245

Minetti, G., Egée, S., Mörsdorf, D., Steffen, P., Makhro, A., Achilli, C., et al. (2013). Red cell investigations: art and artefacts. *Blood Rev.* 27, 91–101. doi: 10.1016/j.blre.2013.02.002

Moras, M., Lefevre, S. D., and Ostuni, M. A. (2017). From erythroblasts to mature red blood cells: organelle clearance in mammals. *Front. Physiol.* 8:1076. doi: 10.3389/fphys.2017.01076

Mountford, J., Olivier, E., and Turner, M. (2010). Prospects for the manufacture of red cells for transfusion. *Br. J. Haematol.* 149, 22–34. doi: 10.1111/j.1365-2141.2010.08079.x

Neelam, S., Kakhniashvili, D. G., Wilkens, S., Levene, S. D., and Goodman, S. R. (2011). Functional 20S proteasomes in mature human red blood cells. *Exp. Biol. Med. (Maywood)* 236, 580–591. doi: 10.1258/ebm.2011.010394

Neildez-Nguyen, T. M., Wajcman, H., Marden, M. C., Bensidhoum, M., Moncollin, V., Giarratana, M. C., et al. (2002). Human erythroid cells produced *ex vivo* at large scale differentiate into red blood cells *in vivo*. *Nat. Biotechnol.* 20, 467–472. doi: 10.1038/nbt0502-467

Ney, P. A. (2011). Normal and disordered reticulocyte maturation. *Curr. Opin. Hematol.* 18, 152–157. doi: 10.1097/MOH.0b013e328345213e

Otto, G. P., and Nichols, B. J. (2011). The roles of flotillin microdomains–endocytosis and beyond. *J. Cell Sci.* 124, 3933–3940. doi: 10.1242/jcs.092015

Pan, B. T., and Johnstone, R. M. (1983). Fate of the transferrin receptor during maturation of sheep reticulocytes *in vitro*: selective externalization of the receptor. *Cell* 33, 967–978. doi: 10.1016/0092-8674(83)90040-5

Qiu, L. B., Dickson, H., Hajibagheri, N., and Crocker, P. R. (1995). Extruded erythroblast nuclei are bound and phagocytosed by a novel macrophage receptor. *Blood* 85, 1630–1639.

Rajendran, L., and Simons, K. (2005). Lipid rafts and membrane dynamics. *J. Cell Sci.* 118, 1099–1102. doi: 10.1242/jcs.01681

Rousseau, G. F., Giarratana, M. C., and Douay, L. (2014). Large-scale production of red blood cells from stem cells: what are the technical challenges ahead? *Biotechnol. J.* 9, 28–38. doi: 10.1002/biot.201200368

Satchwell, T. J., Bell, A. J., Hawley, B. R., Pellegrin, S., Mordue, K. E., van Deursen, C. T., et al. (2016). Severe Ankyrin-R deficiency results in impaired surface retention and lysosomal degradation of RhAG in human erythroblasts. *Haematologica* 101, 1018–1027. doi: 10.3324/haematol.2016.146209

Satchwell, T. J., Bell, A. J., Pellegrin, S., Kupzig, S., Ridgwell, K., Daniels, G., et al. (2011). Critical band 3 multiprotein complex interactions establish early during human erythropoiesis. *Blood* 118, 182–191. doi: 10.1182/blood-2010-10-314187

Satchwell, T. J., Bell, A. J., and Toye, A. M. (2015a). The sorting of blood group active proteins during enucleation. *ISBT Sci. Ser.* 10, 163–168. doi: 10.1111/voxs.12127

Satchwell, T. J., Hawley, B. R., Bell, A. J., Ribeiro, M. L., and Toye, A. M. (2015b). The cytoskeletal binding domain of band 3 is required for multiprotein complex formation and retention during erythropoiesis. *Haematologica* 100, 133–142. doi: 10.3324/haematol.2014.114538

Shattil, S. J., and Cooper, R. A. (1972). Maturation of macroreticulocyte membranes *in vivo*. *J. Lab. Clin. Med.* 79, 215–227.

Skutelsky, E., and Farquhar, M. G. (1976). Variations in distribution of con A receptor sites and anionic groups during red blood cell differentiation in the rat. *J. Cell Biol.* 71, 218–231. doi: 10.1083/jcb.71.1.218

Sonnino, S., and Prinetti, A. (2013). Membrane domains and the "lipid raft" concept. *Curr. Med. Chem.* 20, 4–21. doi: 10.2174/0929867311320010003

Tan, S. S., Yin, Y., Lee, T., Lai, R. C., Yeo, R. W., Zhang, B., et al. (2013). Therapeutic MSC exosomes are derived from lipid raft microdomains in the plasma membrane. *J. Extracell. Vesicles* 2:22614. doi: 10.3402/jev.v2i0.22614

Tirelli, V., Ghinassi, B., Migliaccio, A. R., Whitsett, C., Masiello, F., Sanchez, M., et al. (2011). Phenotypic definition of the progenitor cells with erythroid differentiation potential present in human adult blood. *Stem Cells Int.* 201:602483. doi: 10.4061/2011/602483

Tokuyasu, K. T., Schekman, R., and Singer, S. J. (1979). Domains of receptor mobility and endocytosls in the membranes of neonatal human erythrocytes and reticulocyles are deficient in spectrin. *J. Cell Biol.* 80, 481–486. doi: 10.1083/jcb.80.2.481

Trajkovic, K., Hsu, C., Chiantia, S., Rajendran, L., Wenzel, D., Wieland, F., et al. (2008). Ceramide triggers budding of exosome vesicles into multivesicular endosomes. *Science* 319, 1244–1247. doi: 10.1126/science.1153124

Trakarnsanga, K., Griffiths, R. E., Wilson, M. C., Blair, A., Satchwell, T. J., Meinders, M., et al. (2017). An immortalized adult human erythroid line facilitates sustainable and scalable generation of functional red cells. *Nat. Commun.* 8:14750. doi: 10.1038/ncomms14750

Van Bockxmeer, F. M., and Morgan, E. H. (1979). Transferrin receptors during rabbit reticulocyte maturation. *Biochim. Biophys. Acta* 584, 76–83. doi: 10.1016/0304-4165(79)90237-X

van den Akker, E., Satchwell, T. J., Pellegrin, S., Daniels, G., and Toye, A. M. (2010). The majority of the *in vitro* erythroid expansion potential resides in $CD34^-$ cells, outweighing the contribution of $CD34^+$ cells and significantly increasing the erythroblast yield from peripheral blood samples. *Haematologica* 95, 1594–1598. doi: 10.3324/haematol.2009.019828

van den Akker, E., Satchwell, T. J., Pellegrin, S., Flatt, J. F., Maigre, M., Daniels, G., et al. (2011). Investigating the key membrane protein changes during *in vitro* erythropoiesis of protein 4.2 (-) cells (mutations Chartres 1 and 2). *Haematologica* 95, 1278–1286. doi: 10.3324/haematol.2009.021063

Wickrema, A., Koury, S. T., Dai, C. H., and Krantz, S. B. (1994). Changes in cytoskeletal proteins and their mRNAs during maturation of human erythroid progenitor cells. *J. Cell. Physiol.* 160, 417–426. doi: 10.1002/jcp.1041600304

Wilson, M. C., Trakarnsanga, K., Heesom, K. J., Cogan, N., Green, C., Toye, A. M., et al. (2016). Comparison of the proteome of adult and cord erythroid cells, and changes in the proteome following reticulocyte maturation. *Mol. Cell. Proteomics.* 15, 1938–1946. doi: 10.1074/mcp.M115.057315

Zweig, S. E., Tokuyasu, K. T., and Singer, S. J. (1981). Membrane-associated changes during erythropoiesis. On the mechanism of maturation of reticulocytes to erythrocytes. *J. Supramol. Struct. Cell. Biochem.* 17, 163–181. doi: 10.1002/jsscb.380170207

21

Voltage-Activated Ion Channels in Non-Excitable Cells—A Viewpoint Regarding their Physiological Justification

Lars Kaestner[1,2]*, *Xijia Wang*[3], *Laura Hertz*[4] *and Ingolf Bernhardt*[3]

[1] Theoretical Medicine and Biosciences, Saarland University, Homburg, Germany, [2] Experimental Physics, Saarland University, Saarbrücken, Germany, [3] Laboratory of Biophysics, Saarland University, Saarbrücken, Germany, [4] Medical Faculty, Institute for Molecular Cell Biology, Saarland University, Homburg, Germany

Keywords: red blood cells, $Ca_V2.1$, Piezo1, hSK4 (KCNN4), Calcium signaling, Gardos-channelopathy

***Correspondence:**
Lars Kaestner
lars_kaestner@me.com

It is a well-known fact that voltage-activated ion channels are expressed in non-excitable cells (Jagannathan et al., 2002; Piskorowski et al., 2008; Sontheimer, 2008). However, their putative physiological functions and the regulation of their activity in non-excitable cells are controversial topics (Stokes et al., 2004; Badou et al., 2013). This also holds true for red blood cells (RBCs).

In the context of investigating ion transport across the membrane of RBCs, especially in low ionic strength media, the existence of ion transport dependent on the membrane potential was reported for the first time approximately 50 years ago (Donlon and Rothstein, 1969). In an investigation based on comparative physiology, it became evident that the low ionic strength-induced cation permeability in RBCs is not due to electrodiffusion but due to a transport protein-based process (Halperin et al., 1990; Bernhardt et al., 1991). Later, in addition to the $K^+(Na^+)/H^+$ exchanger (Richter et al., 1997; Kummerow et al., 2000), the existence of a voltage-activated non-selective cation channel was functionally demonstrated utilizing the patch-clamp technique (Christophersen and Bennekou, 1991; Kaestner et al., 1999; Rodighiero et al., 2004). At present, the molecular identity of this particular channel remains unknown (Kaestner, 2011; Bouyer et al., 2012), and it has alternatively been proposed to reflect a conductance state of the voltage-dependent anion channel (VDAC) (Bouyer et al., 2011). On the other hand, evidence for the existence of a number of voltage-activated Ca^{2+} channels that are abundant in RBCs has been reported (Pinet et al., 2002; Romero et al., 2006), and the most convincing evidence is for $Ca_V2.1$, based on molecular biology data (Western blot) (Andrews et al., 2002) and, presumably, $Ca_V2.1$-specific pharmacological interactions (ω-agatoxinTK) (Andrews et al., 2002; Wagner-Britz et al., 2013). Nevertheless, so far, we and others have failed to obtain direct functional evidence for the existence of $Ca_V2.1$ or other voltage-activated Ca^{2+} channels in RBCs by patch-clamp techniques.

Although RBCs are undoubtedly non-excitable cells, sudden changes in membrane potential occur, when increased cation permeability is induced. This is the case because the resting membrane potential is determined by Cl^- conductance (Hunter, 1977; Lassen et al., 1978). For example, when the Gardos channel (Gardos, 1958; Hoffman et al., 2003) is activated, the resting membrane potential changes from approximately −10 to −90 mV (Tiffert et al., 2003). The physiological function of the Gardos channel remained elusive for decades, until it was discovered that it is a major component of the suicidal process of RBCs (Kaestner and Bernhardt, 2002; Lang et al., 2003; Bogdanova et al., 2013) triggered by Ca^{2+} entry (Yang et al., 2000; Kaestner et al., 2004), resulting in cell shrinkage (Begenisich et al., 2004; Lew et al., 2005), and phosphatidylserine exposure (Chung et al., 2007; Nguyen et al., 2011). Only very recently was the interplay between the mechanosensitive channel Piezo1 and the Gardos channel established (Faucherre et al., 2013; Cahalan et al., 2015; Danielczok et al., 2017a), showing a Ca^{2+}-mediated response when RBCs pass through constrictions such as small capillaries.

Since patch-clamp protocols for $Ca_V2.1$ in RBCs are lacking, imaging approaches based on the Ca^{2+} fluorophore Fluo-4 are the method of choice (Minetti et al., 2013). The sudden change in membrane potential following Gardos channel activation suggests that there is a link between Gardos channel activity and voltage-activated channels. Such an interplay was already demonstrated in a recent publication showing an 80% reduction in lysophosphatidic acid (LPA)-induced Ca^{2+} entry by the Gardos channel blocker charybdotoxin (Figure 4A in Wesseling et al., 2016). It would be nice to show $Ca_V2.1$ activity in direct response to Gardos channel activation. This is challenging because the activation stimulus for the Gardos channel (an increase in intracellular Ca^{2+}) is the same parameter used to measure $Ca_V2.1$ activity. However, Gardos channel activity is increased in patients carrying a mutation that affects the calmodulin-binding site (R352H) (Rapetti-Mauss et al., 2015; Fermo et al., 2017). This could be used as a model to investigate the putative interplay between the Gardos channel and $Ca_V2.1$. One would expect an increase in $Ca_V2.1$ activity due to increased Gardos channel activity. Consequently, intracellular Ca^{2+} levels should be elevated in the RBCs of these patients, which indeed is the case (Figure 6 in Fermo et al., 2017). The finding that only a subpopulation of cells showed increased Ca^{2+} levels (Fermo et al., 2017) can probably be explained by the highly heterogeneous distribution of the participating channels, which is well-established for the Gardos channel (Grygorczyk et al., 1984; Lew et al., 2005) but is also likely to apply to other channels in RBCs (Kaestner, 2015).

Nevertheless, we are still left with one peculiarity: According to previous investigations, $Ca_V2.1$ activation is induced by depolarization (Catterall, 2011), not by hyperpolarization, which is the outcome of Gardos channel activity. However, hyperpolarization is a requirement to switch $Ca_V2.1$ channels from the inactivated state to the closed state, which is a prerequisite to subsequently transition to the open state (Catterall, 2000) (**Figure 1A**). Closing of the Gardos channels after their initial activation could well provide the necessary conditions for subsequent depolarisation to activate $Ca_V2.1$. Since the hypothetical switching behavior of the Gardos channel would be crucial for the activation of $Ca_V2.1$, we would like to discuss this aspect in more detail. We envision three principle modes by which this switching could occur:

(i) Because channel activity is a stochastic event and because the number of Gardos channels per RBC is rather low (in the single digit numbers; Grygorczyk et al., 1984; Wolff et al., 1988), depolarisation could be the result of stochastic Gardos channel closures. This hypothesis is supported by the rather sparse whole cell patch-clamp recordings of Gardos channel activity in human RBCs (Qadri et al., 2011; Kucherenko et al., 2012, 2013; Fermo et al., 2017). Whole cell current traces do not show a smooth appearance but rather a flickering pattern similar to that observed with single channel recordings, especially at higher (positive and negative) membrane potentials.

(ii) When looking at Gardos channel-induced changes in the membrane potential of cell populations, a gradual Ca^{2+} concentration-dependent effect can be seen (Baunbaek and Bennekou, 2008), i.e., the hyperpolarisation observed in RBC suspensions is a gradual Ca^{2+} concentration-dependent effect. However, the abovementioned study (Baunbaek and Bennekou, 2008) as well as another report (Seear and Lew, 2011) showed that the activation of the Gardos channel at the cellular level is an all-or-none response. This means that the gradual change in membrane potential would be the result of the summation of cells with open or closed Gardos channels. Taking into consideration that the Ca^{2+} pump (Schatzmann, 1973) continuously operates in response to any increase in intracellular Ca^{2+} levels, one would imagine that the state of the Gardos channels is exclusively modulated by variations in intracellular Ca^{2+} concentrations. Hence, the switching behavior of the Gardos channel would be the direct consequence of continuous variations in RBC intracellular Ca^{2+} concentrations.

(iii) Localized interactions between the Gardos channel and $Ca_V2.1$ in RBCs could occur in lipid rafts or nanodomains, as is the case with closely related ion transporters in other cell types, for example, within the fuzzy space or dyadic cleft in myocytes (Lines et al., 2006). Although RBCs do not possess membrane-constricted subspaces, there are indications for functional compartments in the immediate vicinity of the plasma membrane (Chu et al., 2012). Colocalization of ion channels is common in excitable cells (Rasband and Shrager, 2000; Bers, 2002). For RBCs, it is still unknown if the different ion channels colocalize or cluster to allow their interaction in nanodomains. However, in support of this idea is the observation that local activation of mechanosensitive channels (most likely Piezo 1) by patch-clamp micropipettes resulted in local activation (single-channel recordings) of the Gardos channel (Dyrda et al., 2010).

Although the previous three lines of argumentation are to some extent speculative and although we are unable to favor one over the others, we believe it is worthwhile to share our thoughts with both the RBC and Ca_V channel research communities in this opinion article. The concerted activity of channels is essential in numerous physiological mechanisms, such as the generation of action potentials in neurons (Rojas et al., 1970), excitation-contraction coupling in the heart (Bers, 2002), and during the formation of the immunological synapse (Quintana et al., 2006). In RBCs, there is evidence that the Gardos channel is activated in response to the opening of Piezo1 (Dyrda et al., 2010; Danielczok et al., 2017a), but the inverse process may also occur; activation of the Gardos channel may induce Piezo1 activity. Since Gardos channel activation is supposed to be associated with RBC volume changes, this effect is likely to activate the mechanosensitive channel Piezo1.

To imagine what may happen when Piezo1 is activated, we need to consider the membrane potential. Activation of Piezo1, which is a non-selective cation channel, would lead to a disruption of the hyperpolarisation induced by the Gardos channel, thus preventing voltage activation of $Ca_V2.1$. Therefore, if Piezo1 is closed, $Ca_V2.1$ activation would be facilitated, resulting in increased intracellular Ca^{2+} compared to control

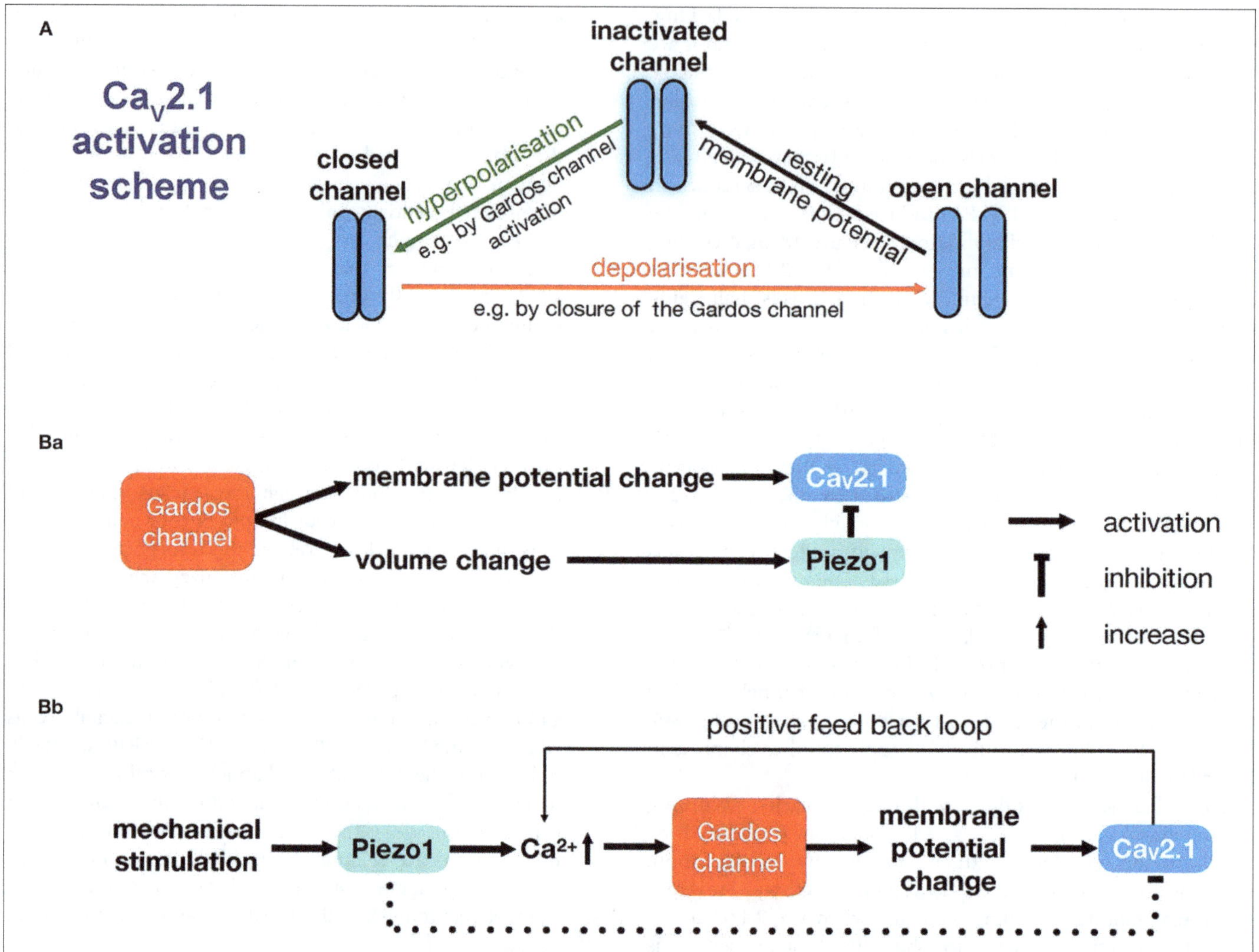

FIGURE 1 | Interplay between $Ca_V2.1$, Piezo1 and the Gardos channel. **(A)** Activation scheme for the $Ca_V2.1$ channel modulated by underlying Gardos channel activity. **(B)** Proposed interactions between $Ca_V2.1$, the Gardos channel and Piezo1. **(Ba)** illustrates a mechanism that is compatible with the measurements presented in Wesseling et al. (2016) and that explains the pathophysiological events seen in Gardos channelopathy (Fermo et al., 2017). **(Bb)** illustrates a sequence of events that is more likely to be relevant to physiological mechanical stimulation conditions in the circulation (Faucherre et al., 2013; Cahalan et al., 2015; Danielczok et al., 2017a). Whether Piezo1 would exert an inhibitory effect in this scenario is an open question, and therefore, this is depicted with a dashed line. For more details, see the main text.

conditions. We propose two scenarios explaining the interplay between the Gardos channel, $Ca_V2.1$ and Piezo1 (**Figure 1B**).

The first scenario takes into account the RBCs of patients carrying the R352H mutation (Rapetti-Mauss et al., 2015; Fermo et al., 2017) or the V282M/E mutation (Andolfo et al., 2015; Glogowska et al., 2015; Rapetti-Mauss et al., 2015). The RBCs of these patients show increased baseline Gardos channel activity, which is schematically sketched in **Figure 1Ba**. This sequence of events can be initiated by the abovementioned mutations or by an increase in intracellular Ca^{2+} independent of mechanical stress, e.g., by NMDA receptor activity (Makhro et al., 2013), TRPC channel openings (Danielczok et al., 2017b), or VDAC activity (Bouyer et al., 2011).

The second scenario envisions an alternative, independent sequence of events. Piezo1 may indirectly modulate $Ca_V2.1$ activity, as outlined in **Figure 1Bb**. If Piezo1 is the source of the increase in intracellular Ca^{2+}, then subsequent Gardos channel activity would induce the opening of $Ca_V2.1$ channels, while Piezo1 channels might still be in an inactivated state. It is likely that Piezo1 channels would remain inactive. After mechanical stimulation, inactivation occurs within 100 ms (Wu et al., 2017), and channel reopening would require a new (repetitive; not lasting) mechanical stimulation (Lewis et al., 2017). Whether the volume change induced by mechanical stress is sufficient for repetitive activation remains unclear, and therefore, the inhibitory effect by Piezo1 is indicated by a dashed line in **Figure 1Bb**. This mechanism (**Figure 1Bb**) might explain the long-lasting Ca^{2+} signal seen after mechanical stimulation and reported in this Research Topic (Danielczok et al., 2017a).

In summary, here, we propose several reasonable mechanisms (**Figure 1**) to explain how voltage-activated (Ca^{2+}) channels could fulfill a physiological function in non-excitable RBCs. We hope to initiate a discussion on this topic and to encourage further investigations beyond the content of this paper.

AUTHOR CONTRIBUTIONS

LK designed the experimental approach. XW and LH performed and analyzed the experiments. IB and LK supervised the experiments. LK wrote the manuscript. LH and IB revised the manuscript.

ACKNOWLEDGMENTS

The research leading to this opinion has received funding from the European Seventh Framework Program under grant agreement number 602121 (CoMMiTMenT) and the European Framework Horizon 2020 under grant agreement number 675115 (RELEVANCE).

REFERENCES

Andolfo, I., Russo, R., Manna, F., Shmukler, B. E., Gambale, A., Vitiello, G., et al. (2015). Novel Gardos channel mutations linked to dehydrated hereditary stomatocytosis (xerocytosis). *Am. J. Hematol.* 90, 921–926. doi: 10.1002/ajh.24117

Andrews, D. A., Yang, L., and Low, P. S. (2002). Phorbol ester stimulates a protein kinase C-mediated agatoxin-TK-sensitive calcium permeability pathway in human red blood cells. *Blood* 100, 3392–3399. doi: 10.1182/blood.V100.9.3392

Badou, A., Jha, M. K., Matza, D., and Flavell, R. A. (2013). Emerging roles of L-type voltage-gated and other calcium channels in T lymphocytes. *Front. Immunol.* 4:243. doi: 10.3389/fimmu.2013.00243

Baunbaek, M., and Bennekou, P. (2008). Evidence for a random entry of Ca2+ into human red cells. *Bioelectrochemistry* 73, 145–150. doi: 10.1016/j.bioelechem.2008.04.006

Begenisich, T., Nakamoto, T., Ovitt, C. E., Nehrke, K., Brugnara, C., Alper, S. L., et al. (2004). Physiological roles of the intermediate conductance, Ca^{2+}-activated potassium channel Kcnn4. *J. Biol. Chem.* 279, 47681–47687. doi: 10.1074/jbc.M409627200

Bernhardt, I., Hall, A. C., and Ellory, J. C. (1991). Effects of low ionic strength media on passive human red cell monovalent cation transport. *J. Physiol.* 434, 489–506.

Bers, D. M. (2002). Cardiac excitation-contraction coupling. *Nature* 415, 198–205. doi: 10.1038/415198a

Bogdanova, A., Makhro, A., Wang, J., Lipp, P., and Kaestner, L. (2013). Calcium in red blood cells-a perilous balance. *Int. J. Mol. Sci.* 14, 9848–9872. doi: 10.3390/ijms14059848

Bouyer, G., Cueff, A., Egée, S., Kmiecik, J., Maksimova, Y., Glogowska, E., et al. (2011). Erythrocyte peripheral type benzodiazepine receptor/voltage-dependent anion channels are upregulated by *Plasmodium falciparum*. *Blood* 118, 2305–2312. doi: 10.1182/blood-2011-01-329300

Bouyer, G., Thomas, S., and Egée, S. (2012). "Patch-clamp analysis of membrane transport in erythrocytes," in *Patch Clamp Technique* (Rijeka: InTech), 171–202.

Cahalan, S. M., Lukacs, V., Ranade, S. S., Chien, S., Bandell, M., and Patapoutian, A. (2015). Piezo1 links mechanical forces to red blood cell volume. *Elife* 4:e07370. doi: 10.7554/eLife.07370

Catterall, W. A. (2000). Structure and regulation of voltage-gated Ca^{2+} channels. *Annu. Rev. Cell Dev. Biol.* 16, 521–555. doi: 10.1146/annurev.cellbio.16.1.521

Catterall, W. A. (2011). Voltage-gated calcium channels. *Cold Spring Harb. Perspect. Biol.* 3:a003947. doi: 10.1101/cshperspect.a003947

Christophersen, P., and Bennekou, P. (1991). Evidence for a voltage-gated, non-selective cation channel in the human red cell membrane. *Biochim. Biophys. Acta* 1065, 103–106.

Chu, H., Puchulu-Campanella, E., Galan, J. A., Tao, W. A., Low, P. S., and Hoffman, J. F. (2012). Identification of cytoskeletal elements enclosing the ATP pools that fuel human red blood cell membrane cation pumps. *Proc. Natl. Acad. Sci. U.S.A.* 109, 12794–12799. doi: 10.1073/pnas.1209014109

Chung, S. M., Bae, O. N., Lim, K. M., Noh, J. Y., Lee, M. Y., Jung, Y. S., et al. (2007). Lysophosphatidic acid induces thrombogenic activity through phosphatidylserine exposure and procoagulant microvesicle generation in human erythrocytes. *Arterioscler. Thromb. Vasc. Biol.* 27, 414–421. doi: 10.1161/01.ATV.0000252898.48084.6a

Danielczok, J. G., Terriac, E., Hertz, L., Petkova-Kirova, P., Lautenschläger, F., Laschke, M. W., et al. (2017a). Red blood cell passage of small capillaries is associated with transient Ca^{2+}-mediated adaptations. *Front. Physiol.* 8:979. doi: 10.3389/fphys.2017.00979

Danielczok, J., Hertz, L., Ruppenthal, S., Kaiser, E., Petkova-Kirova, P., Bogdanova, A., et al. (2017b). Does erythropoietin regulate TRPC channels in red blood cells? *Cell. Physiol. Biochem.* 41, 1219–1228. doi: 10.1159/000464384

Donlon, J. A., and Rothstein, A. (1969). The cation permeability of erythrocytes in low ionic strength media of various tinicities. *J. Membr. Biol.* 1, 37–52.

Dyrda, A., Cytlak, U., Ciuraszkiewicz, A., Lipinska, A., Cueff, A., Bouyer, G., et al. (2010). Local membrane deformations activate Ca^{2+}-dependent K+ and anionic currents in intact human red blood cells. *PLoS ONE* 5:e9447. doi: 10.1371/journal.pone.0009447

Faucherre, A., Kissa, K., Nargeot, J., Mangoni, M. E., and Jopling, C. (2013). Piezo1 plays a role in erythrocyte volume homeostasis. *Haematologica* 99, 70–75. doi: 10.3324/haematol.2013.086090

Fermo, E., Bogdanova, A., Petkova-Kirova, P., Zaninoni, A., Marcello, A. P., Makhro, A., et al. (2017). "Gardos Channelopathy": a variant of hereditary Stomatocytosis with complex molecular regulation. *Sci. Rep.* 7:1744. doi: 10.1038/s41598-017-01591-w

Gardos, G. (1958). The function of calcium in the potassium permeability of human erythrocytes. *Biochim. Biophys. Acta.* 30, 653–654.

Glogowska, E., Lezon-Geyda, K., Maksimova, Y., Schulz, V. P., and Gallagher, P. G. (2015). Mutations in the Gardos channel (KCNN4) are associated with hereditary xerocytosis. *Blood* 126, 1281–1284. doi: 10.1182/blood-2015-07-657957

Grygorczyk, R., Schwarz, W., and Passow, H. (1984). Ca^{2+}-activated K^+ channels in human red cells. Comparison of single-channel currents with ion fluxes. *Biophys. J.* 45, 693–698. doi: 10.1016/S0006-3495(84)84211-3

Halperin, J. A., Brugnara, C., Van Ha, T., and Tosteson, D. C. (1990). Voltage-activated cation permeability in high-potassium but not low-potassium red blood cells. *Am. J. Physiol. Cell Physiol.* 258, 1169–1172.

Hoffman, J. F., Joiner, W., Nehrke, K., Potapova, O., Foye, K., and Wickrema, A. (2003). The hSK4 (KCNN4) isoform is the Ca^{2+}-activated K^+ channel (Gardos channel) in human red blood cells. *Proc. Natl. Acad. Sci. U.S.A.* 100, 7366–7371. doi: 10.1073/pnas.1232342100

Hunter, M. J. (1977). Human erythrocyte anion permeabilities measured under conditions of net charge transfer. *J. Physiol.* 268, 35–49. doi: 10.1111/(ISSN)1469-7793

Jagannathan, S., Publicover, S. J., and Barratt, C. L. (2002). Voltage-operated calcium channels in male germ cells. *Reproduction* 123, 203–215. doi: 10.1530/rep.0.1230203

Kaestner, L. (2011). Cation channels in erythrocytes - historical and future perspective. *Open Biol. J.* 4, 27–34. doi: 10.2174/1874196701104010027

Kaestner, L. (2015). Channelizing the red blood cell: molecular biology competes with patch-clamp. *Front. Mol. Biosci.* 2:46. doi: 10.3389/fmolb.2015.00046

Kaestner, L., and Bernhardt, I. (2002). Ion channels in the human red blood cell membrane: their further investigation and physiological relevance. *Bioelectrochemistry* 55, 71–74. doi: 10.1016/S1567-5394(01)00164-5

Kaestner, L., Bollensdorff, C., and Bernhardt, I. (1999). Non-selective voltage-activated cation channel in the human red blood cell membrane. *Biochim. Biophys. Acta* 1417, 9–15.

Kaestner, L., Tabellion, W., Lipp, P., and Bernhardt, I. (2004). Prostaglandin E2 activates channel-mediated calcium entry in human erythrocytes: an indication for a blood clot formation supporting process. *Thromb. Haemostasis* 92, 1269–1272. doi: 10.1267/THRO04061269

Kucherenko, Y. V., Wagner-Britz, L., Bernhardt, I., and Lang, F. (2013). Effect of chloride channel inhibitors on cytosolic Ca^{2+} levels and Ca^{2+}-activated K^+ (Gardos) channel activity in human red blood cells. *J. Membr. Biol.* 246, 315–326. doi: 10.1007/s00232-013-9532-0

Kucherenko, Y., Zelenak, C., Eberhard, M., Qadri, S. M., and Lang, F. (2012). Effect of casein kinase 1α activator pyrvinium pamoate on erythrocyte ion channels. *Cell. Physiol. Biochem.* 30, 407–417. doi: 10.1159/000339034

Kummerow, D., Hamann, J., Browning, J. A., Wilkins, R., Ellory, J. C., and Bernhardt, I. (2000). Variations of intracellular pH in human erythrocytes via $K^+(Na^+)/H^+$ exchange under low ionic strength conditions. *J. Membr. Biol.* 176, 207–216. doi: 10.1007/s002232001089

Lang, K. S., Duranton, C., Poehlmann, H., Myssina, S., Bauer, C., Lang, F., et al. (2003). Cation channels trigger apoptotic death of erythrocytes. *Cell Death Differ.* 10, 249–256. doi: 10.1038/sj.cdd.4401144

Lassen, U. V., Pape, L., and Vestergaard-Bogind, B. (1978). Chloride conductance of the amphiuma red cell membrane. *J. Membr. Biol.* 39, 27–48.

Lew, V. L., Tiffert, T., Etzion, Z., Perdomo, D., Daw, N., Macdonald, L., et al. (2005). Distribution of dehydration rates generated by maximal Gardos-channel activation in normal and sickle red blood cells. *Blood* 105, 361–367. doi: 10.1182/blood-2004-01-0125

Lewis, A. H., Cui, A. F., McDonald, M. F., and Grandl, J. (2017). Transduction of repetitive mechanical stimuli by Piezo1 and Piezo2 ion channels. *Cell Rep.* 19, 2572–2585. doi: 10.1016/j.celrep.2017.05.079

Lines, G. T., Sande, J. B., Louch, W. E., Mørk, H. K., Grøttum, P., and Sejersted, O. M. (2006). Contribution of the $Na^+/Ca2^+$ exchanger to rapid Ca^{2+} release in cardiomyocytes. *Biophys. J.* 91, 779–792. doi: 10.1529/biophysj.105.072447

Makhro, A., Hänggi, P., Goede, J. S., Wang, J., Brüggemann, A., Gassmann, M., et al. (2013). N-methyl D-aspartate (NMDA) receptors in human erythroid precursor cells and in circulating red blood cells contribute to the intracellular calcium regulation. *Am. J. Physiol. Cell Physiol.* 305, C1123–C1138. doi: 10.1152/ajpcell.000 31.2013

Minetti, G., Egée, S., Mörsdorf, D., Steffen, P., Makhro, A., Achilli, C., et al. (2013). Red cell investigations: art and artefacts. *Blood Rev.* 27, 91–101. doi: 10.1016/j.blre.2013.02.002

Nguyen, D. B., Wagner-Britz, L., Maia, S., Steffen, P., Wagner, C., Kaestner, L., et al. (2011). Regulation of phosphatidylserine exposure in red blood cells. *Cell. Physiol. Biochem.* 28, 847–856. doi: 10.1159/000335798

Pinet, C., Antoine, S., Filoteo, A. G., Penniston, J. T., and Coulombe, A. (2002). Reincorporated plasma membrane Ca^{2+-}ATPase can mediate B-Type Ca^{2+} channels observed in native membrane of human red blood cells. *J. Membr. Biol.* 187, 185–201. doi: 10.1007/s00232-001-0163-5

Piskorowski, R., Haeberle, H., Panditrao, M. V., and Lumpkin, E. A. (2008). Voltage-activated ion channels and Ca(2+)-induced Ca (2+) release shape Ca (2+) signaling in Merkel cells. *Pflugers Arch.* 457, 197–209. doi: 10.1007/s00424-008-0496-3

Qadri, S. M., Kucherenko, Y., and Lang, F. (2011). Beauvericin induced erythrocyte cell membrane scrambling. *Toxicology* 283, 24–31. doi: 10.1016/j.tox.2011.01.023

Quintana, A., Schwarz, E. C., Schwindling, C., Lipp, P., Kaestner, L., and Hoth, M. (2006). Sustained activity of CRAC channels requires translocation of mitochondria to the plasma membrane. *J. Biol. Chem.* 281, 40302–40309. doi: 10.1074/jbc.M607896200

Rapetti-Mauss, R., Lacoste, C., Picard, V., Guitton, C., Lombard, E., Loosveld, M., et al. (2015). A mutation in the Gardos channel is associated with hereditary xerocytosis. *Blood* 126, 1273–1280. doi: 10.1182/blood-2015-04-642496

Rasband, M. N., and Shrager, P. (2000). Ion channel sequestration in central nervous system axons. *J. Physiol.* 525 (Pt 1), 63–73. doi: 10.1111/j.1469-7793.2000.00063.x

Richter, S., Hamann, J., Kummerow, D., and Bernhardt, I. (1997). The monovalent cation "leak" transport in human erythrocytes: an electroneutral exchange process. *Biophys. J.* 73, 733–745.

Rodighiero, S., De Simoni, A., and Formenti, A. (2004). The voltage-dependent nonselective cation current in human red blood cells studied by means of whole-cell and nystatin-perforated patch-clamp techniques. *Biochim. Biophys. Acta* 1660, 164–170. doi: 10.1016/j.bbamem.2003.11.011

Rojas, E., Bezanilla, F., and Taylor, R. E. (1970). Demonstration of sodium and potassium conductance changes during a nerve action potential. *Nature* 225, 747–748.

Romero, P. J., Romero, E. A., Mateu, D., Hernández, C., and Fernández, I. (2006). Voltage-dependent calcium channels in young and old human red cells. *Cell Biochem. Biophys.* 46, 265–276. doi: 10.1385/CBB:46:3:265

Schatzmann, H. J. (1973). Dependence on calcium concentration and stoichiometry of the calcium pump in human red cells. *J. Physiol.* 235, 551–569.

Seear, R. V., and Lew, V. L. (2011). IKCa agonist (NS309)-elicited all-or-none dehydration response of human red blood cells is cell-age dependent. *Cell Calcium* 50, 444–448. doi: 10.1016/j.ceca.2011.07.005

Sontheimer, H. (2008). An unexpected role for ion channels in brain tumor metastasis. *Exp. Biol. Med.* 233, 779–791. doi: 10.3181/0711-MR-308

Stokes, L., Gordon, J., and Grafton, G. (2004). Non-voltage-gated L-type Ca2+ channels in human T cells: pharmacology and molecular characterization of the major alpha pore-forming and auxiliary beta-subunits. *J. Biol. Chem.* 279, 19566–19573. doi: 10.1074/jbc.M401481200

Tiffert, T., Bookchin, R. M., and Lew, V. L. (2003). "Calcium homeostasis in normal and abnormal human red cells," in *Red Cell Membrane Transport in Health and Disease*, eds I. Bernhardt and C. Ellory (Berlin; Heidelberg; New York, NY: Springer Verlag), 373–405.

Wagner-Britz, L., Wang, J., Kaestner, L., and Bernhardt, I. (2013). Protein kinase Cα and P-type Ca channel CaV2.1 in red blood cell calcium signalling. *Cell. Physiol. Biochem.* 31, 883–891. doi: 10.1159/000350106

Wesseling, M. C., Wagner-Britz, L., Nguyen, D. B., Asanidze, S., Mutua, J., Mohamed, N., et al. (2016). Novel insights in the regulation of phosphatidylserine exposure in human red blood cells. *Cell. Physiol. Biochem.* 39, 1941–1954. doi: 10.1159/000447891

Wolff, D., Cecchi, X., Spalvins, A., and Canessa, M. (1988). Charybdotoxin blocks with high affinity the Ca-activated K^+ channel of Hb A and Hb S red cells: individual differences in the number of channels. *J. Membr. Biol.* 106, 243–252.

Wu, J., Young, M., Lewis, A. H., Martfeld, A. N., Kalmeta, B., and Grandl, J. (2017). Inactivation of mechanically activated Piezo1 ion channels is determined by the C-terminal extracellular domain and the inner pore helix. *Cell Rep.* 21, 2357–2366. doi: 10.1016/j.celrep.2017.10.120

Yang, L., Andrews, D. A., and Low, P. S. (2000). Lysophosphatidic acid opens a Ca(++) channel in human erythrocytes. *Blood* 95, 2420–2425. Available online at: http://www.bloodjournal.org/content/95/7/2420/tab-article-info

Permissions

All chapters in this book were first published by Frontiers; hereby published with permission under the Creative Commons Attribution License or equivalent. Every chapter published in this book has been scrutinized by our experts. Their significance has been extensively debated. The topics covered herein carry significant findings which will fuel the growth of the discipline. They may even be implemented as practical applications or may be referred to as a beginning point for another development.

The contributors of this book come from diverse backgrounds, making this book a truly international effort. This book will bring forth new frontiers with its revolutionizing research information and detailed analysis of the nascent developments around the world.

We would like to thank all the contributing authors for lending their expertise to make the book truly unique. They have played a crucial role in the development of this book. Without their invaluable contributions this book wouldn't have been possible. They have made vital efforts to compile up to date information on the varied aspects of this subject to make this book a valuable addition to the collection of many professionals and students.

This book was conceptualized with the vision of imparting up-to-date information and advanced data in this field. To ensure the same, a matchless editorial board was set up. Every individual on the board went through rigorous rounds of assessment to prove their worth. After which they invested a large part of their time researching and compiling the most relevant data for our readers.

The editorial board has been involved in producing this book since its inception. They have spent rigorous hours researching and exploring the diverse topics which have resulted in the successful publishing of this book. They have passed on their knowledge of decades through this book. To expedite this challenging task, the publisher supported the team at every step. A small team of assistant editors was also appointed to further simplify the editing procedure and attain best results for the readers.

Apart from the editorial board, the designing team has also invested a significant amount of their time in understanding the subject and creating the most relevant covers. They scrutinized every image to scout for the most suitable representation of the subject and create an appropriate cover for the book.

The publishing team has been an ardent support to the editorial, designing and production team. Their endless efforts to recruit the best for this project, has resulted in the accomplishment of this book. They are a veteran in the field of academics and their pool of knowledge is as vast as their experience in printing. Their expertise and guidance has proved useful at every step. Their uncompromising quality standards have made this book an exceptional effort. Their encouragement from time to time has been an inspiration for everyone.

The publisher and the editorial board hope that this book will prove to be a valuable piece of knowledge for researchers, students, practitioners and scholars across the globe.

List of Contributors

Virgilio L. Lew and Teresa Tiffert
Physiological Laboratory, Department of Physiology, Development and Neuroscience, University of Cambridge, Cambridge, United Kingdom

Laura Hertz, Polina Petkova-Kirova and Jens G. Danielczok
Research Centre for Molecular Imaging and Screening, Medical School, Saarland University, Homburg, Germany
Institute for Molecular Cell Biology, Saarland University, Homburg, Germany

Esther Llaudet-Planas, Maria del Mar Mañú-Pereira and Joan-Lluis Vives Corrons
Red Blood Cell Defects and Hematopoietic Disorders Unit, Josep Carreras Leukaemia Research Institute, Barcelona, Spain

Asya Makhro and Anna Bogdanova
Red Blood Cell Research Group, Institute of Veterinary Physiology, Vetsuisse Faculty and the Zurich Center for Integrative Human Physiology (ZIHP), University of Zurich, Zurich, Switzerland

Stephane Egee
Centre National de la Recherche Scientifique, UMR 8227 Comparative Erythrocyte's Physiology, Roscoff, France
Université Pierre et Marie Curie, Sorbonne Universités, Roscoff, France
Laboratoire d'Excellence GR-Ex, Roscoff, France

Emmanuel Terriac and Franziska Lautenschläger
Experimental Physics, Saarland University, Saarbrücken, Germany
Leibniz Institute for New Materials, Saarbrücken, Germany

Matthias W. Laschke
Institute for Clinical and Experimental Surgery, Saarland University, Homburg, Germany

Joanna F. Flatt and Lesley J. Bruce
Bristol Institute for Transfusion Sciences, NHS Blood and Transplant, Bristol, United Kingdom

Lena Wiegmann
The Interface Group, Institute of Physiology, University of Zurich, Zurich, Switzerland

Diane A. de Zélicourt
The Interface Group, Institute of Physiology, University of Zurich, Zurich, Switzerland
National Center of Competence in Research, Kidney CH, Zurich, Switzerland

Oliver Speer
Division of Haematology, University Children's Hospital Zurich, Zurich, Switzerland

Alissa Muller
Department of Health Sciences and Technology, ETH Zurich, Zurich, Switzerland

Jeroen S. Goede
Department of Haematology, Kantonsspital Winterthur, Winterthur, Switzerland
Zurich Center for Integrative Human Physiology, University of Zurich, Zurich, Switzerland

Burkhardt Seifert
Department of Biostatistics, Epidemiology, Biostatistics and Prevention Institute, University of Zurich, Zurich, Switzerland

Vartan Kurtcuoglu
The Interface Group, Institute of Physiology, University of Zurich, Zurich, Switzerland
National Center of Competence in Research, Kidney CH, Zurich, Switzerland
Zurich Center for Integrative Human Physiology, University of Zurich, Zurich, Switzerland
Neuroscience Center Zurich, University of Zurich, Zurich, Switzerland

Emily S. Hartman and Julien Papoin
Laboratory of Developmental Erythropoiesis, Center for Autoimmune, Musculoskeletal and Hematopoietic Diseases, The Feinstein Institute for Medical Research, Manhasset, NY, United States

Elena C. Brindley
Laboratory of Developmental Erythropoiesis, Center for Autoimmune, Musculoskeletal and Hematopoietic Diseases, The Feinstein Institute for Medical Research, Manhasset, NY, United States
Donald and Barbara Zucker School of Medicine at Hofstra/Northwell, Hempstead, NY, United States

Steven L. Ciciotte, Yue Zhao and Luanne L. Peters
The Jackson Laboratory, Bar Harbor, ME, United States

Lionel Blanc
Laboratory of Developmental Erythropoiesis, Center for Autoimmune, Musculoskeletal and Hematopoietic Diseases, The Feinstein Institute for Medical Research, Manhasset, NY, United States
Department of Molecular Medicine and Pediatrics, Donald and Barbara Zucker School of Medicine at Hofstra/Northwell, Hempstead, NY, United States

Anna Zaninoni, Elisa Fermo, Cristina Vercellati, Anna P. Marcello, Alberto Zanella, Wilma Barcellini and Paola Bianchi
UOC Oncoematologia, UOS Fisiopatologia delle Anemie, Fondazione IRCCS Ca' Granda Ospedale Maggiore Policlinico, Milan, Italy

Dario Consonni
UO Epidemiologia, Fondazione IRCCS Ca' Granda Ospedale Maggiore Policlinico, Milan, Italy

Agostino Cortelezzi
UOC Oncoematologia, UOS Fisiopatologia delle Anemie, Fondazione IRCCS Ca' Granda Ospedale Maggiore Policlinico, Milan, Italy
Università degli Studi di Milano, Milan, Italy

Tomasz Walski, Natalia Trochanowska-Pauk and Małgorzata Komorowska
Department of Biomedical Engineering, Faculty of Fundamental Problems of Technology, Wrocław University of Science and Technology, Wrocław, Poland
Regional Specialist Hospital in Wrocław, Research and Development Centre, Wrocław, Poland

Anna Drohomirecka
Regional Specialist Hospital in Wrocław, Research and Development Centre, Wrocław, Poland
Institute of Cardiology, Warsaw, Poland

Jolanta Bujok and Albert Czerski
Regional Specialist Hospital in Wrocław, Research and Development Centre, Wrocław, Poland
Department of Animal Physiology and Biostructure, Faculty of Veterinary Medicine, Wrocław University of Environmental and Life Sciences, Wrocław, Poland

Grzegorz Wąż
Regional Specialist Hospital in Wrocław, Research and Development Centre, Wrocław, Poland
Medinet Heart Center Ltd., Wrocław, Poland

Romuald Cichoń
Medinet Heart Center Ltd., Wrocław, Poland

Michał Gorczykowski
Department of Internal Medicine and Clinic of Diseases of Horses, Dogs and Cats, Faculty of Veterinary Medicine, Wrocław University of Environmental and Life Sciences, Wrocław, Poland

Ryszard Grygorczyk
Medicine, Université de Montréal, Montreal, QC, Canada

Sergei N. Orlov
Biology, M. V. Lomonosov Moscow State University, Moscow, Russia

Kat S. Moore and Marieke von Lindern
Department of Hematopoiesis, Sanquin Research, and Landsteiner Laboratory, Amsterdam UMC, Amsterdam, Netherlands

Joames K. F. Leal, Merel J. W. Adjobo-Hermans and Giel J. C. G. M. Bosman
Department of Biochemistry, Radboud University Medical Center, Nijmegen, Netherlands

Heimo Mairbäurl
Medical Clinic VII, Sports Medicine, Translational Lung Research Center, German Center for Lung Research, University Hospital Heidelberg, Heidelberg, Germany

Gregory Barshtein
Faculty of Medicine, Biochemistry Department, Hebrew University of Jerusalem, Jerusalem, Israel

Dan Arbell
Pediatric Surgery, Hadassah-Hebrew University Medical Center, Jerusalem, Israel

Leonid Livshits
Faculty of Medicine, Biochemistry Department, Hebrew University of Jerusalem, Jerusalem, Israel
Institute of Veterinary Physiology, University of Zurich, Zürich, Switzerland

Alexander Gural
Blood Bank, Hadassah-Hebrew University Medical Center, Jerusalem, Israel

Julien Delobel, Aurélie Hübner and Corinne Benay
Laboratoire de Recherche sur les Produits Sanguins, Recherche et Développement Produits, Transfusion Interrégionale CRS, Épalinges, Switzerland

Michel Prudent, Niels Lion and Jean-Daniel Tissot
Laboratoire de Recherche sur les Produits Sanguins, Recherche et Développement Produits, Transfusion Interrégionale CRS, Épalinges, Switzerland
Faculté de Biologie et de Médecine, Université de Lausanne, Lausanne, Switzerland

Martina Moras, Sophie D. Lefevre and Mariano A. Ostuni
UMR-S1134 Integrated Biology of Red Blood Cell, INSERM, Université Paris Diderot, Sorbonne Paris Cité, Institut National de la Transfusion Sanguine, Laboratoire d'Excellence GR-Ex, Paris, France

Elina Ovchynnikova, Francesca Aglialoro, Marieke von Lindern and Emile van den Akker
Department of Hematopoiesis, Sanquin Research, Amsterdam, Netherlands
Landsteiner Laboratory, Academic Medical Center, University of Amsterdam, Amsterdam, Netherlands

Rick Huisjes, Wouter W. van Solinge, Raymond M. Schiffelers and Richard van Wijk
Department of Clinical Chemistry and Haematology, University Medical Center Utrecht, Utrecht University, Utrecht, Netherlands

Anna Bogdanova
Red Blood Cell Research Group, Institute of Veterinary Physiology, Vetsuisse Faculty and the Zurich Center for Integrative Human Physiology (ZIHP), University of Zurich, Zürich, Switzerland

Lars Kaestner
Theoretical Medicine and Biosciences, Saarland University, Saarbrücken, Germany
Experimental Physics, Saarland University, Saarbrücken, Germany
Theoretical Medicine and Biosciences, Saarland University, Homburg, Germany

Miriam Götting and Mikko J. Nikinmaa
Laboratory of Animal Physiology, Department of Biology, University of Turku, Turku, Finland

Pedro J. Romero and Concepción Hernández-Chinea
Laboratory of Membrane Physiology, Faculty of Sciences, Institute of Experimental Biology, Central University of Venezuela, Caracas, Venezuela

Giampaolo Minetti, Cesare Achilli and Annarita Ciana
Laboratori di Biochimica, Dipartimento di Biologia e Biotecnologie, Università degli Studi di Pavia, Pavia, Italy

Cesare Perotti
Servizio Immunoematologia e Medicina Trasfusionale, Fondazione IRCCS Policlinico San Matteo, Pavia, Italy

Xijia Wang and Ingolf Bernhardt
Laboratory of Biophysics, Saarland University, Saarbrücken, Germany

Laura Hertz
Medical Faculty, Institute for Molecular Cell Biology, Saarland University, Homburg, Germany

Index

www.ingramcontent.com/pod-product-compliance
Lightning Source LLC
LaVergne TN
LVHW082156200926
848484LV00008B/2172